Phlébologie
— 92 —
Phlebology

2

British Library Cataloguing in Publication Data
A catalogue record for this book is available from the British Library

ISBN 086196 357 1

Éditions John Libbey Eurotext
6, rue Blanche, 92120 Montrouge, France
Tél. : (1) 47 35 85 52

John Libbey and Company Ltd
13, Smith Yard, summerley Street,
London SW18 4HR, England
Tél. : (1) 947 27 77

John Libbey CIC
Via L. Spallanzani, 11
00161, Rome, Italy
Tél. : (06) 862 289

Phlébologie
—— 92 ——
Phlebology

XIe Congrès Mondial
Union Internationale de Phlébologie
XIth World Congress

30 août-4 septembre, 1992
Montréal August 30-September 4, 1992

Coordinateurs / Editors
P. Raymond-Martimbeau
R. Prescott
M. Zummo

Volume 2

John Libbey EUROTEXT

Union Internationale de Phlébologie

Président d'honneur-fondateur/Honorary President and Founder	R. Tournay †
Comité d'honneur/Honorary Committee :	H.R. Van der Molen
	Gl. Bassi †
	J. Van der Stricht
Président/President :	A. Davy
Vice-Présidents/Vice-Presidents :	U. Brunner
	M. Horakova
	J. Kuiper
	J. Salvador Marques
	S. Umansky
Secrétaire Général/General Secretary :	P. Wallois
Trésorier/Treasurer :	J. Follereau

Comité organisateur du congrès/*Congress Organizing Committee*

Président d'honneur/Honorary Presidents :	G. Cloutier
	J.C. Ménard
Président directeur général/President General Director :	R. Prescott

Comité organisateur/*Organizing Committee*

Président/President :	M. Zummo
Secrétaire Général/General Secretary :	P. Raymond-Martimbeau
Trésorier/Treasurer :	E. Bernier
Membres/Members :	R. Bernard
	C. Choulnard
	L. Grondin
	J.F. Mercier

Comité scientifique/*Scientific Committee*

Président/President :	P. Raymond-Martimbeau
Vice-président/Vice-President :	C. Choulnard
Secrétaire Général/General Secretary :	J. Leclerc
Membres/Members :	J.F. Mercier
	R. Parent
	A. Roussin
	B. Scalabrini
	J. Trudel

Comité de soutien financier/*Fund raising Committee*

Président fondateur/Founding President :	P. Raymond-Martimbeau

Comité consultatif International/*International Advisory Committee*

G. Acsady (Hongrie/Hungaray)
E. Altman Canestri (Argentine/Argentina)
E. Anguero Wagner (Paraguay)
P. Bacci (Italie/Italy)
P. Balas (Grèce/Greece)
M. Bartolo (Italie/Italy)
V. Batchvarova (Bulgarie/Bulgaria)
G. Benovese (Italie/Italy)
J. Bergan (États-Unis/United States)
W. Blättler (Suisse/Switzerland)
M. Bravo (Chili/Chile)
E. Brizzio (Argentine/Argentina)
N. Browse (Royaume Uni/United Kingdom)
U. Brunner (Suisse/Switzerland)
A. Butie (États-Unis/United States)
E. Canestri (Argentine/Argentina)
P. Carinici (Italie/Italy)
P. Choi (Hong Kong)
C. Chouinard (Canada)
D. Christopoulos (Grèce/Greece)
G. Cloutier (Canada)
F. Cockett (Royaume Uni/United Kingdom)
J. Coget (France)
P. Conrad (Australie/Australia)
A. Davy (France)
D. De Anna (Italie/Italy)
W. de Groot (États-Unis/United States)
L. del Aquilla Hoyoz (Pérou/Peru)
A. Diaz (Équateur/Equator)
G. Donadi (Italie/Italy)
I. Donini (Italie/Italy)
J. Dormandy (Royaume Uni/United Kingdom)
J. Dortu (France)
D. Fillipin (Argentine/Argentina)
H. Fisher (Allemagne/Germany)
J. Follerean (France)
A. Fronck (États-Unis/United States)
V. Gasbarro (Italie/Italy)
G. Genovese (Italie/Italy)
M. Gligora (Yougoslavie/Yugoslavia)
M. Goldman (États-Unis/United States)
R. Gregorian (U.R.S.S./U.S.S.R.)
J. Gruffaz (France)
W. Hach (Allemagne/Germany)
M. Hme (États-Unis/Unites States)
J. Hobbs (Royaume Uni/United Kingdom)
M. Hoe (Singapoure/Singapore)
M. Holdi (Allemagne/Germany)
H. Horakova (Tchécoslovaquie/Czechoslovakia)
S. Hwang (Hong Kong)
P. Ignat (Roumanie/Romania)
G. Jantet (Royaume Uni/United Kingdom)
J. Jimenez Cossio (Espagne/Spain)
G. Johnson (États-Unis/United States)
N. Kluken (Allemagne/Germany)
M. Krishnan (Malaisie/Malaysia)
J. Kuiper (Pays-Bas/Netherlands)
G. Lalande (Philippines)
P. Langeron (France)
J. Latrose (Espagne/Spain)
A. Lechter (Colombie/Columbia)
P. Levitcharov (Bulgarie/Bulgaria)
S. Mancini (Italie/Italy)
W. Marley (États-Unis/United States)
F. Mathiesen (Scandinavie/Scandinavia)
J. Natali (France)
D. Negus (Royaume Uni/United Kingdom)
H. Newmann (Pays-Bas/Netherlands)
C. Olivier (France)
?. Olzensky (Pologne/Poland)
P. Ouvry (France)
C. Papendieck (Argentine/Argentina)
H. Partsch (Autriche/Austria)
L. Peirera (Brésil/Brazil)
M. Perrin (France)
J. Picard (France)
R. Prescott (Canada)
P. Raymond-Martimbeau (Canada)
H. Reid Lewis (Jamaïque/Jamaica)
R. Rettori (France)
R. Romero (Mexique/Mexico)
S. Rose (Royaume Uni/United Kingdom)
N. Rosli (Argentine/Argentina)
P. Sainte-Luce (Guadeloupe)
J. Salvador Marques (Portugal)
?. Samaniego (Espagne/Spain)
C. Sanchez (Argentine/Argentina)
M. Santos Gaston (Espagne/Spain)
G. Sapin (France)
V. Savelief (U.R.S.S./U.S.S.R.)
W. Schneider (Allemagne/Germany)
U. Schultz-Ehrenburg (Allemagne/Germany)
A. Scuderi (Brézil/Brazil)
R. Simkin (Argentine/Argentina)
S. Skaguchi (Japon/Japan)
R. Stemmer (France)
P. Thibault (Australie/Australia)
L. Thiery (Belgique/Belgium)
L. Tojino (Philippines)
L. Tretbar (États-Unis/United States)
R. Tullij (Brésil/Brazil)
G. Tuscano (Italie/Italy)
J. Ulloa Dominguez (Colombie/Columbia)
S. Umansky (Espagne/Spain)
H. van der Molen (Pays-Bas/Netherlands)
J. van der Stricht (Belgique/Belgium)
J. Villavicencio (États-Unis/United States)
P. Wallois (France)
T. Wupperman (Allemagne/Germany)
P. Zamboni (Italie/Italy)
F. Zucarelli (France)
M. Zummo (Canada)

SOMMAIRE/*CONTENTS*

Volume 2

XIII. TRAITEMENT MÉDICAL/*MEDICAL TREATMENT*

A. Pharmacologie/*Pharmacology*

c. Complications/*Complications*

C. Traitement compressif/*Compressive treatment*

C. Résultats/*Results*

D. Complications/*Complications*

B. Veines superficielles/*Superficial veins*

XVIII. TRAITEMENT DES MALADIES THROMBO-EMBOLIQUES/ *THROMBO-EMBOLIC DISORDER TREATMENT*

XIII.
TRAITEMENT MÉDICAL
MEDICAL TREATMENT

A. Pharmacologie / *Pharmacology*

Phlébologie 92. Eds P. Raymond-Martimbeau, R. Prescott, M. Zummo.
John Libbey Eurotext, Paris © 1992, pp. 709-711

Antioxidant properties of S 5682

Marcelle Damon, Benoît Cypriani, Christian Le Doucen, Benjamin Limasset*, Marie-Luce Carrié, André Crastes de Paulet*

*INSERM U.58, 60, rue de Navacelles, * Laboratoire de Biochimie A, Institut de Biologie, 34090 Montpellier, France.*

Polymorphonuclear neutrophils participate to the amplification of inflammatory processes through their ability to generate toxic reactive oxygen species which are inactivated by cellular antioxydant systems in physiological conditions (Weiss, 1989). Flavonoids are known to be able to supply to these protector systems. Their inhibitory effect depends on their structure (Robak et al., 1988). The present work was undertaken to study the inhibitory effect of S 5682 (Daflon 500) a purified preparation of disomin (90 %) and hesperidin (10 %) solubilized by clathrate formation with β hydroxycyclodextrin molecules (cyclodextrin) on the release of oxygen species by in vitro phorbol myristate acetate (PMA)-stimulated neutrophils. Enzymatic and chemical technics were used to investigate the mecanism by which it develops its inhibitory effect.

METHODS

Preparation of neutrophil suspension :
Heparinized blood was collected from healthy donors by venipuncture. Neutrophils were separated and purified by centrifugation on discontinuous Percoll gradient. Erythrocyte contamination was ruled out by lysis and neutrophils were collected after centrifugation in phosphate buffer saline (50mM, pH 7.4) containing 1 mM Mg^{++} and 1.5 mM Ca^{++}. The cell viability as shown by trypan blue test, and the purity of neutrophils were > 95 %.

Chemiluminescence (CL) determination :
1) CL was measured according to the method previously described by Allen (Methods on Enzymology, 1986) using a LKB Wallac luminometer (model 1251). Two luminophores were used: luminol which reacts with the whole set of oxygen species and lucigenin which is $O2^{\cdot -}$ specific. After luminophores were added to the cell suspension in the luminometer at 37°C without or with different concentrations of S 5862 or cyclodextrin, a measure was done before stimulation, then PMA was added and CL was measured until maximal (CL peak) value was obtained. The effect of S 5862 was compared to that of 2 enzymes involved in transformation of initial signal (superoxide dismutase (SOD) and catalase) and to NaN_3 which inhibits myeloperoxidase (MPO). Various other flavonoids were also studied. A same work was realized using 2 oxygen species metabolites: hydrogen peroxide (H_2O_2) and OCl^- known to be generated through MPO activity.
2) SOD activity was determined by lucigenin-dependent CL according to the method described by Corbisier et al. (Annal. Biochem., 1987). The effect of S 5862 and cyclodextrin was compared to that of potassium cyanide known to inhibit SOD activity.

Enzymatic and chemical techniques :
1) $O_2^{\cdot -}$ and H_2O_2 formation were performed on cellular sytem (PMA-stimulated cells) and

acellular systems such as xanthin/xanthin oxidase (X/XO) for $O_2{\cdot}^-$ generation, glucose/glucose oxidase (G/GO)for H_2O_2. The $O_2{\cdot}^-$ generation was carried out using superoxide dismutase inhibitable reduction of ferricytochrome c according to McCord et al.(J. Biol. Chem., 1969). H_2O_2 formation was evaluated using extinction of continuous fluorescence of reduced scopoletin according to Boveris et al.(Annal. Biochem.,1977).
2) Oxygen formation through H_2O_2 breakdown was measured on a polarograph using a Clark oxygen electrode. The catalase was tested as comparative compound.
3) UV spectrum analysis : The UV spectrum modifications of S 5682 and cyclodextrin by H_2O_2 were analyzed every 2 min during 28 min in the presence or the abscence of HRP. The modifications promoted by OCl^- were evaluated during 5 min for various concentrations of S 5682

RESULTS

S-5682 had no inhibitory effect on lucigenin-dependent CL which was inhibited by SOD and enhanced by NaN_3 and S-5682. Conversely, a dose-dependent inhibition of luminol-amplified CL by S 5682 was observed with IC50 = 5.10^{-5}M. The same result was obtained with NaN3. SOD and catalase had a lower effect. Cyclodextrin had no effect. These results showed that S 5682 had the same effect as NaN3 which inhibits the MPO-dependent formation of OCl^-. Moreover, whereas diosmetin, quercetin and fisetin inhibited CL with any luminophore, S 5682 as hesperetin enhanced lucigenin-dependent CL. This results was confirmed by spectrophotometric analysis of $O2{\cdot}^-$ formation in cellular and acellular (X/XO) systems . No effect was observed on SOD activity.
Direct contact of H_2O_2 with luminol induced a very sharp response which was inhibited in a dose-dependent manner by S 5682 (IC50 = 5.10^{-6}M). The same dose-dependent inhibition was observed when HRP was added (IC50 = 3.10^{-6}M). The OCl^- CL was inhibited by S 5682 with IC50 = 7. 10^{-5}M. Cyclodextrin had no effect.
S 5682 inhibited the formation of H_2O_2 obtained in cell and cell free (G/GO) systems. IC50 were 1.6 10^{-6}M and 2.10^{-6}M respectively. However, the formation of O_2 was not observed when S 5682 was in direct contact with H_2O_2.
No modification of UV spectrum was obtained when H_2O_2 was added alone to S 5682. Conversely, The UV spectrum was modified when HRP was added with H_2O_2 (decrease of the absorbance at 346 nm, fig.1). Same modifications were observed in the presence of OCl^- (fig.2).

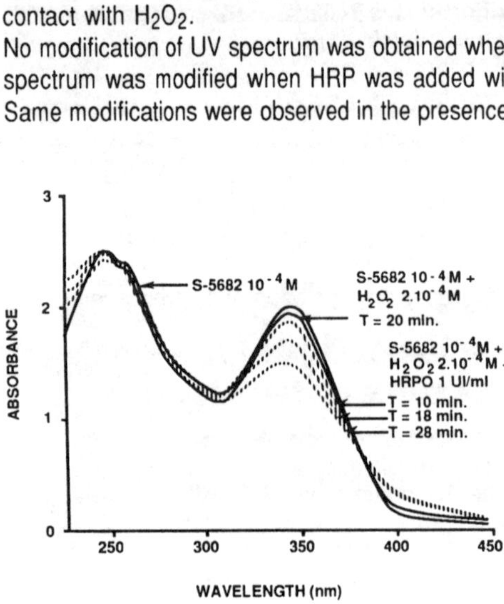

Figure 1

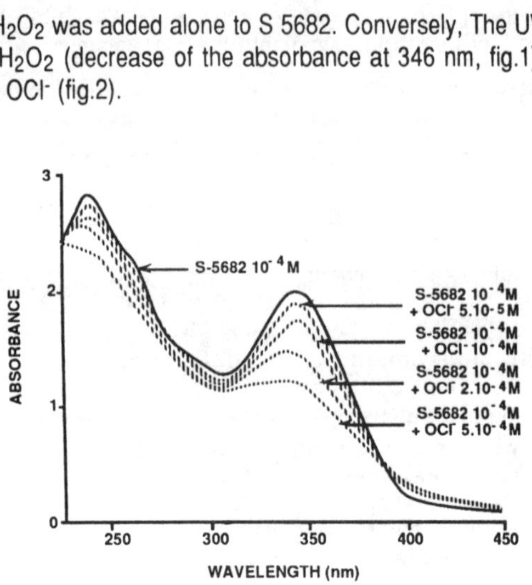

Figure 2

DISCUSSION

Knowing that S 5682 reduced luminol-dependent CL triggered by PMA-stimulated neutrophils, we tried to localize S 5682 targets and to characterize the functional mechanisms of this compound.

S 5682 increased slightly lucigenin-dependent CL but did not decrease acellular $O_2^{.-}$ formation as hesperetin did, whereas quercetin, known to inhibit PKC activity (Gschwendt et al.,Biochem. Biophys. Res. Commun., 1983), rutin, fisetin and diosmetin decreased it (Ferriola et al., Biochem. Pharmacol., 1989). S 5682 did not reduce SOD activity.

On the contrary, S 5682 reduced the release of H_2O_2 in the acellular system and after neutrophil stimulation. This compound was more efficient than catalase and as efficient as NaN3 in inhibiting luminol-dependent CL. But the reaction was dependent on the weak H_2O_2 transformation. Thus in these conditions, H_2O_2 alone did not modify the S 5682 UV spectrum. Conversely, when HRP was added to the reaction mixture, the CL values were higher. S 5682 inhibited the CL induced by H_2O_2 and its UV spectrum was modified, suggesting that S 5682 may be active in the H_2O_2-OCl^--MPO system. The results obtained with OCl^- confirms this hypothesis since CL was decreased and S 5682 UV spectrum was modified by OCl^-. The enhancement of $O_2^{.-}$ formation by S 5682 might be explained by reduced utilization of $O_2^{.-}$ either through inibited MPO as NaN3 effect or through NADPH oxidase stimulation, since OCl^- has a negative feedback effect on this enzyme activity (Edwards et al., J. Clin. Lab. Immunol., 1986).

To conclude, S 5682 affects in a same manner the product coming from H_2O_2 transformation and OCl^-; It migh inhibit MPO activity.

REFERENCES

Allen, R.C. (1986) : Phagocytic leucocyte oxygenation activities and chemiluminescence : a kinetic approach to analysis. Methods in Enzymology 133: 449-507.

Boveris, A., Martino, E., and Stoppani, A.M.(1977) : Evaluation of horseradish peroxidase-scopoletin method for the measurement of hydrogen peroxide formation in biological systems. Annal Biochem. 80: 145-158.

Corbisier, P., Houbio, A., and Remacle J.(1987) : A new technique for highly sensitive detection of superoxide dismutase activity by chemiluminescence. Annal Biochem. 164: 240-247.

Edwards, S.W., and Swan, T.F. (1986) : Regulation of superoxide generation by myeloperoxidase during the respiratory burst of human neutrophils. Biochem. J. 237: 601-604.

Ferriola, P.C., Cody, V., and Middleton E.(1989) : Protein kinase C inhibition by plant flavonoids. Kinetic mechanisms and structure-activity relationships. Biochem. Pharmacol. 38: 1617-1624.

Gschwendt, M., Horn, F., Kittstein, W., and Marks, F.(1983) : Inhibition of the calcium-and phospholipid-dependent protein kinase activity from mouse brain cytosol by quercetin. Biochem. Biophys. Res. Commun. 117: 444-447.

McCord, J.M., and Fridovich, I. (1969) : Superoxide dismutase. An enzymatic function for erythrocuprein (hemocuprein). J. Biol. Chem. 144: 6049-6055.

Robak, J, and Gryglewski, J.R. (1988) : Flavonoids are scavengers of superoxide anions. Biochem. Biophys. Res. Commun. 37: 837-841.

Weiss, S.J. (1989) : Tissue destruction by neutrophils. New Engl. J. Med. 320: 365-376.

Phlébologie 92. Eds P. Raymond-Martimbeau, R. Prescott, M. Zummo.
John Libbey Eurotext, Paris © 1992, pp. 712-714

Effects of S 5682 on the response to exogenous norepinephrine on varicose veins and normal veins with histological alterations

N. Juteau, F. Bakri, G. Narcisse, M. Thiollet*, Y. Tsouderos*, G. Lange**, J.P. Cron***

*U.F.R. de Pharmacie de Tours et I.M.T., B.P. 253, 37702 St-Pierre-des-Corps Cedex, France. * I.R.I.S., B.P. 126, 92200 Neuilly-sur-Seine Cedex, France. ** Cabinet de Phlébologie, 2, quai d'Orléans, 37000 Tours, France. *** Clinique St-Gatien, 37000 Tours, France.*

INTRODUCTION

Several authors (Docherty, 1987 ; Godfraind and Morel, 1988 ; Müller-Schweinitzer, 1988) considere the human saphenous vein as a preparation of a great relevance in human pharmacology. Particularly, it seems of interest to study on this in vitro preparation the effects of a venotropic drug, S 5682*, used in the treatment of venous insufficiency. Nevertheless, the use of human tissues in pharmacology remains complex because numerous parameters have to be taken into account (sexe, age, prior drug therapy...). In order to try and obtain more homogenous populations, investigations were performed with important sample sizes and rings were classified according to their histological characteristics ; data were analysed after this classification. In an attempt to recreate "pathological conditions" the experiments were carried out in metabolic acidosis (pH 6.4).Vanhoutte and Clement (1968), Verbeuren et al. (1978), Rinaldi et al. (1987) reported that metabolic acidosis depressed the contractile activity of vascular smooth muscles. Edvinsson and Sercombe (1976), Dacey and Duling (1982) showed on isolated cerebral vessels, that reducing the extracellular pH decreased the vasoconstrictor response to agonists such as norepinephrine and serotonine. In different isolated arterial preparations in which adrenergic receptors are mainly of the α_1 type, Williamson et al. (1960), Edvinsson et al. (1976), Medgett et al. (1987) showed that the responses to norepinephrine are unaffected by a reduction in pH whereas in arterial preparations with essentially α_2 adrenoceptors, contractile responses to norepinephrine are markedly inhibited under acidotic conditions. In our laboratory, Bakri et al. (unpublished data) showed that acidosis caused significant reduction of the contractile response of both "normal" and "varicose" veins to norepinephrine (NE). The purpose of this work was to study under acidosis conditions, the effect of S 5682 towards norepinephrine on the contractile response of different histological types of human venous rings.

* Daflon 500 mg, Detralex, Capiven, Arvenum 500)

METHODS

Human saphenous veins were obtained from two distinct clinical sources : "Normal veins" from patients undergoing coronary artery bypass graft surgery and "varicose veins" from conservative varicose vein surgery. Veins were stored overnight in Krebs-Henseleit solution at 4°C before use. The composition of this solution was, in mM : NaCl 118.3, KCl 4.7, $MgSO_4$ 1.2, KH_2PO_4 1.2, $NaHCO_3$ 25.0, $CaCl_2$ 1.2, glucose 11.1. The venous segments were cut into rings and suspended for isometric tension recording in 20 ml organ baths filled with Krebs-Henseleit (37°C) continuously aerated with 95 % O_2 - 5 % CO_2 (pH 7.4).

After having achieved a preload of 1.5 to 2 g for "normal veins" and 1 to 1.5 g "varicose veins", the preparations were allowed to equilibrate for 45 min and then, KCl (60 mM) was added in equimolar replacement of NaCl. This constituted a validation test for the venous rings reactivity. After a 40 min equilibration period, the experimental protocol in acidosis was applied.

• Experimental protocol :

Acidosis (pH 6.4) was performed by lowering the HCO_3^- concentration of the Krebs-Henseleit solution at a constant pCO_2. In these conditions, cumulative concentration response curves for NE were established in the presence or the absence of S 5682 (10^{-5} M) added 20 min previously to the organ bath. In each experiment, control and treatment rings were investigated at the same time. Histological studies were performed following the pharmacological experiments and a histological classification of the tested rings was established.

• Drugs used :
Flavonoid S 5682 (Laboratoires Servier - micronised fraction composed of 90 % diosmin and 10 % hesperidin), sodium hydroxyde (PROLABO), arterenol bitartrate (SIGMA). S 5682 was dissolved in a 1N NaOH solution ; further dilutions being made in Krebs solution just before use. The final pH in organ baths was shown not to be modified by the addition of vehicle which did not affect either the baseline tension.

• Data analysis :
Results were expressed as a percentage of maximal response to NE for each curve. The EC_{50} (concentration producing 50 % of the maximum contraction) of NE was determined for each group. Data were compared by a two-way analysis of variance and Newman-Keul's test.

RESULTS AND DISCUSSION

• The histological study of the venous rings revealed that clinically "normal veins" were actually divided into a group including "near-normal" rings and another comprising rings with "prevaricose lesions". Otherwise, clinically "varicose veins" were divided into "near-normal" rings and rings showing "advanced varicose process". The results corresponding to these four histological groups were analysed (Table 1).

• Under acidosis conditions, S 5682 induced a shift of the concentration-response curves for NE towards lower concentrations comparatively to its vehicle, regardless of the clinical origin of the veins (JUTEAU et al., 1992).
This potentiation was significant on clinically "varicose veins" irrespective of their histological grouping (Fig N° 2) and for clinically "normal veins" with histological alterations (Fig. N° 1). To assess the validity of this work, the vehicle group was compared with a control group under acidosis conditions and there was no significant difference between these two groups.

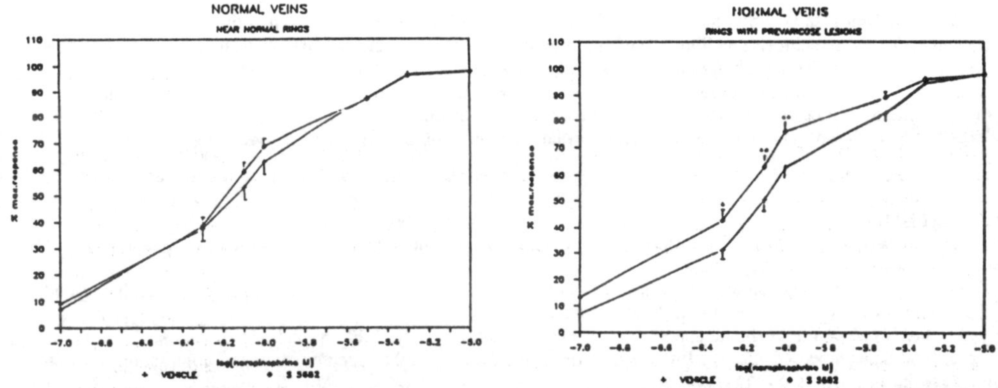

Fig. 1 : Effect of S 5682 (10^{-5} M) on the contractile response to NE under acidosis conditions in clinically "normal" saphenous veins. Mean ± s.e.m. (8 < n < 15)
Newman Keuls ' test S 5682/ vehicle. ▲ $p < 0.025$; ▲▲ $p < 0.01$; ▲▲▲ $p < 0.001$

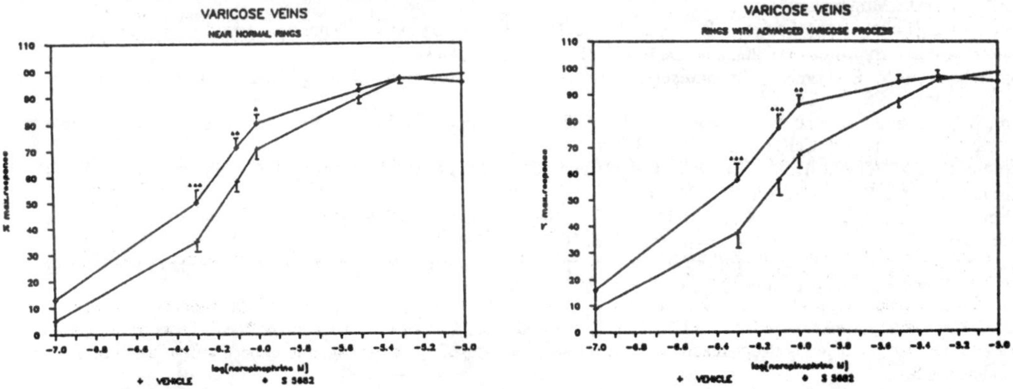

Fig. 2 : Effect of S 5682 (10^{-5} M) on the contractile response to NE under acidosis conditions in clinically "varicose" saphenous veins. Mean ± s.e.m. (10 < n < 14)
Newman Keuls ' test S 5682/ vehicle. ▲ $p < 0.025$; ▲▲ $p < 0.01$; ▲▲▲ $p < 0.001$

Clinical origin :	NORMAL VEIN		VARICOSE VEIN	
Histological grouping	Near-normal rings	Rings with prevaricose lesions	Near normal rings	Rings with advanced varicose process
Vehicle/NE	7.2×10^{-7} M n = 15	8.2×10^{-7} M n = 8	6.5×10^{-7} M n = 11	6.5×10^{-7} M n = 12
S 5682/NE	6.2×10^{-7} M n = 15	4.9×10^{-7} M n = 9	3.9×10^{-7} M n = 13	3.3×10^{-7} M n = 11

EC_{50} of NE, under acidosis conditions (pH 6.4), obtained for each histological group, in presence or absence of S 5682

TABLE 1

To conclude, the present results show that S 5682 (10^{-5} M) makes up for the decreased contractile reactivity of human saphenous vein under severe acidosis conditions. Furthermore the combination of the pharmacological and histological data leads us to conclude that, under these conditions, the potentializing activity of S 5682 towards norepinephrine is increased in proportion with the pathological status of the venous rings. Works are currently in progress, in our laboratory, to precise on one hand the exact mechanisms involved in the reduction of the contractile activity of the human saphenous vein under acidosis conditions and on the other hand, to explain the differential activities of S 5682 in these conditions.

BIBLIOGRAPHIE

Branco, D. and Osswald, W. (1988) : The influence of Ruscus extract on the uptake and metabolism of noradrenaline in the normal and varicose human saphenous vein. Phlebology, 3, 33-39.

Dacey, F. and Duling, B. (1982) : studies of isolated cerebral arteries. In : Heistad, D., Marcus, M. (eds). Cerebral blood flow. Effect of nerves and neurotransmitters. Elsevier, New-York.

Docherty, J.R. (1987) : The use of the human saphenous vein in pharmacology. TIPS. 8, 358-361.

Edvinsson, L. and Sercombe, R. (1976) : Influence of pH and pCO_2 on alpha-receptor mediated contraction in brain vessels. Acta physiol. scand. 97, 325-331.

Godfraind, T. and Morel, N. (1988) : Tissue specificity of dihydropyridine-type calcium antagonists in human isolated tissues. TIPS. 9, 37-39.

Juteau, N., Bakri, F., Rigaudy, P., Pillion, G., Genre, O., Cron, J.P. (1992) : The human saphenous vein in pharmacology : effect of a new flavonoidic fraction on norepinephrine induced contraction. Oral communication in XI World Congress. Montreal. 1992.

Medgett, I.C., Hicks,. P.E., Langer,. S.Z. (1987) : Effect of acidosis on α_1- and α_2- adrenoceptor mediated vasoconstrictor responses in isolated arteries. Eur. J. pharmacol. 135, 443-447.

Müller-Schweinitzer, E. (1988) : Cryopreservation : a useful technique for storing tissues for pharmacological investigations. TIPS. 9, 221-223.

Rinaldi, G.J., Amado Cattaneo, E., Cingolani, H.E. (1987) : Interaction between calcium and hydrogen ions in canine coronary arteries. J. Mol. Cell. Cardiol. 19, 773-784.

Vanhoutte, P. and Clément, D. (1968) : Effect of pH and pCO_2 changes on the reactivity of isolated venous smooth muscle. Arch. int. Physiol. Bioch. 76, 144-146.

Verbeuren, T.J., Janssens, W.J., Vanhoutte, P.M. (1978) : Effects of moderate acidosis on adrenergic neurotransmission in canine saphenous vein. J. pharmacol. Exp. Ther. 206, 105-114.

Williamson, A.W.R. and Moore, F.D. (1960) : Norepinephrine sensitivity of isolated rabbit aorta strips in solutions of varying pH and electrolyte content. Am. J. Physiol. 198, 1157.

Phlébologie 92. Eds P. Raymond-Martimbeau, R. Prescott, M. Zummo.
John Libbey Eurotext, Paris © 1992, pp. 715

The extend of the edema protective effect of horse chestnut seed extract

M. Steiner

University Freiburg i. Br., Dept. of Gynecology and Obstetrics, Hugstetterstr. 55, D-7800 Freiburg i. Br., Germany.

Numerous studies have demonstrated that horse chestnut seed extract (Venostasin retard) is mobilizing existing peripheral venous edemas safely and reliably within one or two weeks. In our own double blind, randomized, cross-over, comperative study va. placebo, we observed 20 female patients between the ages of 20 to 40 years suffering from pregnancy related leg volume measured by waterplethysmography. A five day wash-out phase was followed by two test phases of 14 days. 10 patients have been in the verum beginner as well as in the placebo beginner group. Results: The leg volume was shown to be unchanging under placebo therapy and even increasing following a verum period. Under verum the volume decreased 128.6 rep. 114.0 ml. Assumning that the average leg by may hold about 500.0 ml edema fluid, the reduction of about 120.0 ml means a 25% reduction of edema vlume. Other papers show an approximately reduction fo 38% under therapy by a medical stocking of compression class II. In comparison to that standard, an oral therapy by Venostasin shows a 65%-effect of that being possible und physical therapy.

Phlébologie 92. Eds P. Raymond-Martimbeau, R. Prescott, M. Zummo.
John Libbey Eurotext, Paris © 1992, pp. 716-718

In vitro free radical scavenging and antioxidant activity of hemisynthetic diosmin

S. Bervoas Martin, M. Finet

Innothera, Department of Pharmacology, 10, avenue Paul Vaillant Couturier, 94111 Arcueil Cedex, France.

INTRODUCTION

Free radicals and especially reactive oxygen species modify properties of various biomolecules and can thus promote tissue damage. They have been involved in the pathological processes of a widespread range of diseases, in particular , in degenerative vascular disorders (Negre et al., 1989, Deby et al., 1989). However, no real proof has been yet provided, particularly because of difficulties related to their detection in biological tissues.

The aim of the present work was to quantify the antiradical activity of hemisynthetic diosmin and some of its potential metabolites and to evaluate their mechanism of action, by comparison with references.

Hemisynthetic Diosmin (DIOVENOR®) is a flavone derivative indicated in chronic venous insufficiency. It has been demonstrated that at therapeutic doses, Diosmin modifies noradrenaline metabolism in human saphenous vein (Osswald et al., 1991).

MATERIALS AND METHODS

- Global free radical scavenging activity was studied by a method measuring the radicalar form reduction of 1,1-diphenyl-2-picrylhydrazyl (DPPH), a stable free radical,method modified from Lamaison et al., (1988).
- Superoxide anion scavenging activity was studied by a method using nitroblue tetrazolium (NBT) and a superoxide anion generator, method modified from Yuting et al., (1990).
- Antioxidant activity was investigated using a lipid peroxydation model based on iron induced lipid peroxidation of a linoleic acid emulsion, method modified from Sutherland et al., (1982).

REFERENCES

DPPH MODEL % INHIBITION

	10^{-3} M	10^{-5} M	10^{-7} M
VIT. E	- 96.4 ± 0.3	- 34.8 ± 0.0	- 0.7 ± 0.2
BHT	- 94.5 ± 0.0	- 5.7 ± 0.3	- 1.2 ± 0.0
N - PROPYLGALLATE	- 96.8 ± 0.1	- 79.6 ± 0.2	- 0.9 ± 0.0
PYROGALLOL	- 95.0 ± 0.1	- 53.73± 0.1	- 1.2 ± 0.2

NBT MODEL % INHIBITION

	10^{-3} M	10^{-4} M	10^{-5} M	10^{-6} M
P-BENZOQUINONE	- 99.5 ± 0.1	- 99.0 ± 0.2	- 22.6 ± 0.1	- 8.3 ± 0.0
N-PROPYL GALLATE	NT	- 41.6 ± 0.3	- 24.2 ± 0.7	- 5.3 ± 0.5

LA MODEL % INHIBITION

	10^{-4} M	10^{-5} M	10^{-6} M	10^{-7} M
VIT. E	- 85.7 ± 5.7	- 77.5 ± 1.2	- 50.9 ± 1.8	- 15.7 ±1.2
BHT	- 98.8 ± 3.9	- 95.5 ± 0.7	- 92.2 ± 0.1	- 2.7 ±4.4
N - PROPYLGALLATE	- 94.1 ± 1.1	- 86.5 ± 0.6	- 68.2 ± 0.4	—

DIOSMIN AND POTENTIAL METABOLITES

DPPH MODEL % INHIBITION

	10^{-3} M	10^{-5} M	10^{-7} M
DIOSMIN	- 19.4 ± 0.2	- 0.6 ± 0.3	- 0.6 ± 0.0
DIOSMETIN	- 15.9 ± 0.1	- 0.3 ± 0.0	NA
P-HYDROXYBENZOIC ACID	- 2.0 ± 0.0	- 0.6 ± 0.1	- 0.2 ± 0.0
PROTOCATECHIC ACID	- 91.4 ± 0.6	- 32.0 ± 0.8	- 0.8 ± 0.0
CAFEIC ACID	- 100.4 ± 0.0	- 53.6 ± 0.0	- 1.4 ± 0.0
FERULIC ACID	- 95.2 ± 0.0	- 22.2 ± 0.0	- 0.2 ± 0.0
3-HYDROXYPHENYLPROPIONIC ACID	- 5.1 ± 0.0	- 0.1 ± 0.0	- 0.1 ± 0.0
HOMOPROTOCATECHIC ACID	- 96.6 ± 0.0	- 72.6 ± 0.3	- 1.3 ± 0.0
M-COUMARINIC ACID	- 3.5 ± 0.0	- 0.6 ± 0.0	- 0.6 ± 0.1
ISOFERULIC ACID	- 26.4 ± 0.0	- 2.5 ± 0.0	NA
HIPPURIC ACID	- 2.7 ± 0.5	- 0.5 ± 0.0	NA
ORTHOHYDROXYHIPPURIC ACID	- 2.4 ± 0.3	- 1.1 ± 0.0	NA
BENZOIC ACID	- 2.5 ± 0.0	NA	NA
ALPHA-HYDROXYHIPPURIC ACID	- 4.3 ± 0.3	- 0.9 ± 0.0	0.6 ± 0.1

NBT MODEL % INHIBITION

	10^{-3} M	10^{-4} M	10^{-5} M	10^{-6} M
DIOSMIN	- 59.8 ± 5.9	- 34.5 ± 0.9	- 13.8 ± 1.7	- 2.8 ± 0.0
DIOSMETIN	—	- 16.7 ± 0.1	- 6.0 ± 0.8	- 5.8 ± 0.4
PROTOCATECHIC ACID	- 51.9 ± 2.0	- 20.8 ± 3.0	- 6.2 ± 0.3	- 5.5 ± 0.8
HOMOPROTOCATECHIC ACID	- 72.5 ± 2.8	- 9.6 ± 0.1	NA	NA
CAFEIC ACID	- 91.2 ± 1.1	- 26.0 ± 0.5	- 2.0 ± 1.1	- 0.6 ± 2.7
FERULIC ACID	- 16.9 ± 9.5	- 4.1 ± 1.3	- 2.7 ± 1.1	NA

LA MODEL % INHIBITION

	10^{-4} M	10^{-5} M	10^{-6} M	10^{-7} M
DIOSMIN	- 93.7 ± 0.8	- 71.5 ± 1.3	- 29.5 ± 0.2	NA
DIOSMETIN	- 98.9 ± 1.7	- 62.2 ± 0.8	- 25.7 ± 0.2	NA
PROTOCATECHIC ACID	- 81.7 ± 3.8	- 70.0 ± 0.6	- 5.1 ± 2.5	NA
HOMOPROTOCATECHIC ACID	- 76.5 ± 2.3	- 73.7 ± 2.1	- 13.7 ± 4.2	- 3.5 ± 2.6
CAFEIC ACID	- 81.6 ± 0.4	- 81.5 ± 0.9	- 34.4 ± 1.9	NA
FERULIC ACID	- 84.1 ± 8.8	- 48.1 ± 0.0	- 6.7 ± 3.2	NA

NT = Not tested

NA = No activity

Assays and controls were made in triplicates and percentages of inhibition were calculated (results expressed as mean ± s.e.m.).

RESULTS

In the DPPH model, Diosmin and Diosmetin (its aglycone) showed a very low activity. Among all the potential metabolites of Diosmin tested, only few ones showed an effect similar to that of the references.
In the NBT model, Diosmin and Diosmetin showed noticeable activities. The activity of the other compounds was lower than that observed for the references, except for cafeic acid.
In the linoleic acid model, Diosmin , Diosmetin and the potential metabolites showed an important antioxidant activity. ED50 values calculated for Diosmin and Diosmetin were respectively equal to 5.4 ± 0.8 uM and 7.0 ± 0.5 uM, these values being close to those of Vitamin E and BHT, respectively equal to 1.0 ± 1.5 uM and 5.6 ± 2.2 uM.

DISCUSSION

These results suggest that Diosmin can act either directly as an antioxidant or as a superoxide anion scavenger, or indirectly through phenolic compounds considered as potential metabolites. Even though Diosmin metabolism has not been fully elucidated, previous studies performed in man have allowed to clearly identify homoprotocatechic acid and cafeic alcohol as Diosmin metabolites.
These antiradical properties of Diosmin could explain some of its pharmacological properties and particularly the anti-inflammatory actions, which are observed at high doses.

REFERENCES

Deby C. et al.(1989) : Are antilipoperoxidant and antiradicalar activities in the varicose veins correlated with the antioxidant amount : the case of tocopherol. Phlébologie'89, 677-679

Lamaison J.L. et al.(1988): Activités antiradicalaires in vitro d'huiles essentielles .Plantes Méd. Phytotherap., XXII, 231-234

Negre A. et al.(1989) : Additional antilipoperoxidative properties of ascorbic acid, alphatocopherol and rutin in membrane-like systems and cell cultures. Phlébologie'89, 59-61

Osswald W. et al.(1991): Diosmin theapy alters the in vitro metabolism of noradrenaline by the varicose human saphenous vein. Pharmacological Res., 24:3, 253-256

Sutherland M.N. et al. (1982) : .Arch. Biochem. Biophys.,214,1-11

Yuting C. et al.(1990) : Flavonoids as superoxide scavengers and antioxidants. Free Rad.Biol.Méd.,9, 19-21

Phlébologie 92. Eds P. Raymond-Martimbeau, R. Prescott, M. Zummo.
John Libbey Eurotext, Paris © 1992, pp. 719-721

Hemisynthetic diosmin protects against vascular hyperpermeability induced by 17ß oestradiol in female rat

C. Dacquet, J. Sannier, M. Finet

Innothera, Department of Pharmacology, 10, avenue Paul-Vaillant-Couturier, 94111 Arcueil Cedex, France.

INTRODUCTION

High oestrogen doses lead to an excessive permeability in cutaneous microcirculation (Merlen and Sarteel, 1979). The aim of this work was to study the effects of an hemisynthetic flavone derivative, Diosmin (Diovenor ®), on the modification of local vascular permeability induced by intradermal administration of 17 ß oestradiol on female rat.

MARERIALS AND METHODS

Animals

Female Wistar rats weighing 180-200 g were used in all the experiments. Rats had free access to water and food. They were anesthetized by diethylether.

Drugs

17 ß oestradiol was solubilized in sesame oil before being administrated sub-cutaneously under a volume equal to 0.1 ml.

Diosmin was dissolved in dimethylsulfoxide to have a final concentration of 20 mg/kg in 0.1 ml.

Extravasation measurement

1 ml of 0.5 % Evans blue solution was injected intravenously to the anesthetized rats.Immediately after, 17 ß oestradiol doses (0.1, 1, 2 or 4 mg) were administrated intradermaly in the abdomen skin. One hour later, rats were sacrified. Skin macula corresponding to the injection site was carefully cut. Measurement of the extravasation was carried on whole macula according to Beach and Steinetz method (1961).

Vascular permeability was determined by measuring the optic density expressed by the protein extravasation marked by Evans blue. Results were expressed as µg of Evans blue extracted.

Statistics

All results are expressed as arithmetic mean ± s.e.m. Student's t test was used for differences between the Diosmin treatment and those with its solvent.

RESULTS

High 17 ß oestradiol sub-cutaneous doses (0.1, 1, 2 and 4 mg) increased significantly the local vascular permeability on the female rat. Measured one hour after the administration, the increase of vascular permeability was respectively equal to 15, 17, 22 and 27 % ($n=8-24$, $p<0.05$) compared to control animals.The vascular hyperpermeability seems to be proportional to the administrated doses.

Diosmin (20 mg/kg) administrated in prevention two hours before the measurement reduced significantly (- 20 %, $p<0.05$, $n=16$) the vascular permeability induced by the administration of 17 ß oestradiol (ID 2 mg), whereas its solvent was without effect on the increased local vascular permeability.

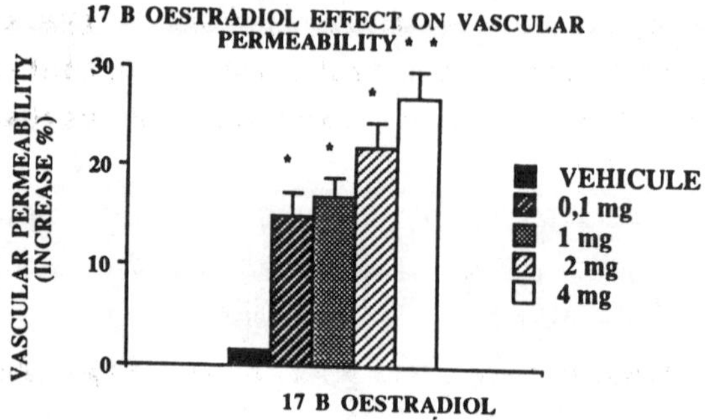

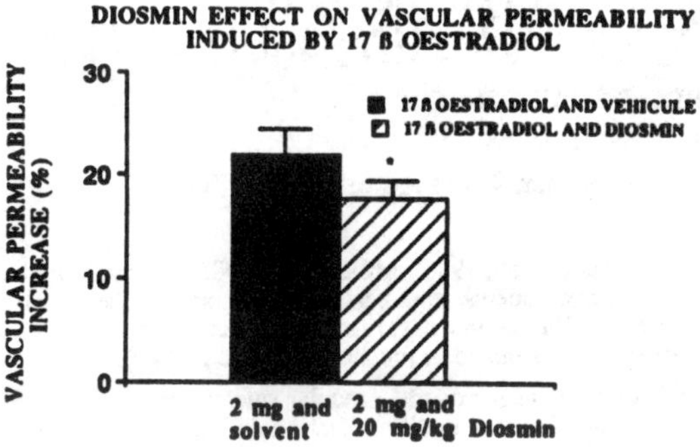

CONCLUSION

These results suggest that high doses of 17 ß oestradiol administrated sub-cutaneously increase local vascular permeability. This effect could be observed at women treated by hormonal patch, known to be strongly dosed with hormone.

It appears also that Diosmin, which is a strong antiedema drug in vascular hyperpressure and inflammatory conditions, can also inhibit vascular hyperpermeability induced by high local doses of 17 ß oestradiol. These observations suggest an interaction of 17 ß oestradiol with the microvascular processus implicated in the regulation of the vascular permeability. The mechanism of action had to be studied to better understand the relation between sexual hormone and vascular permeability.

REFERENCES :

Beach V. and Steinetz B.G., (1961), J. Pharmacol. Exp. Therap., 131, 400-406.

Merlen J.F and Sarteel A.M., (1979), J. Mal. Vasc., 184-185.

EFFECTS OF OESTROGEN TREATMENT ON NORADRENALINE AND CACL2 CONTRACTILE RESPONSES ON RABBIT SAPHENOUS VEIN AND FEMORAL ARTERY

C. DACQUET, F. MARDON, P. LUCE, M. FINET

Dpt. of Pharmacology, INNOTHERA

10, avenue Paul-Vaillant-Couturier, 94111 Arcueil Cédex, France.

Oestrogen treatment can influence vascular tone (Gisclard et al., 1986 ; Miller et al., 1988) and could be implicated in women venous insufficiency. The present experiments were performed to compare the effect of prolonged administration of diethylstilbestrol (100 µg IM for ten days) on the noradrenaline and CaCl2 contractile responses of saphenous vein and femoral artery from adult female rabbit (2,5 to 3 kg).

The endothelialized saphenous vein and femoral artery were removed ; vascular rings were suspended for isometric force measurement in vitro. Tissues were bathed with a modified Krebs solution at 37°C and aerated with a gas mixture of 95 % O2 and 5 % CO2.

Diethylstilbestrol pretreatment significantly shifted to the right the noradrenaline (10^{-9} to 10^{-5} M) dose-response curves on both saphenous vein and femoral artery. ED50 (- log M) values were modified respectively from 8.67 ± 0.15 to 6.53 ± 0.20 ($p<0.001$, n=5-8) and from 7.29 ± 0.15 to 6.49 ± 0.18 ($p<0.001$, n=5-8). CaCl2 (0.01 to 5 mM) cumulative dose-response curves were similar on treated and untreated female rabbits. ED50 (- log M) values on saphenous vein were respectively equal to 3.80 ± 0.70 and 3.82 ± 0.90 (n=8-21) and on female artery to 3.93 ± 0.42 and 3.63 ± 0.50 (n=4-2).

These results show that oestrogen treatment reduces particularly noradrenaline contractile response without affecting CaCl2 response. This effect was more important on saphenous vein than on femoral artery. This work confirms the existence of an oestrogen effect on noradrenaline response (selective compared to CaCl2). This could play a role in women venous insufficiency, noradrenaline being the neuromediator of venous tone.

REFERENCES : Gisclard V. et al., J. Pharmacol. Exp. Ther., 1986, 240, pp. 466-470 ; Miller et al., Phlebology, 1988, 3, pp. 63-69.

Phlébologie 92. Eds P. Raymond-Martimbeau, R. Prescott, M. Zummo.
John Libbey Eurotext, Paris © 1992, pp. 723-725

Comparison of hemisynthetic diosmin effect on $CaCl_2$ contractile response on rabbit saphenous vein and femoral artery

C. Dacquet, C. Rouvreau, S. Richard, M. Finet

Innothera, Department of Pharmacology, 10, avenue Paul-Vaillant-Couturier, 94111 Arcueil Cedex, France.

INTRODUCTION

Hemisynthetic Diosmin (Diovenor®) is a flavone derivative indicated in chronic venous insufficiency. Its venotonic property on women has been attributed to an indirect mechanism, which is an inhibition of the noradrenaline metabolism (Araujo and Osswald 1989, Araujo et al., 1991). In vitro, we have shown that Diosmin accelerates the filling of the intracellular calcium store mobilized by noradrenaline (Dacquet and Finet, 1990) suggesting an effect on calcium movements at cellular level. The aim of this work is to study Diosmin venoselectivity by comparing its effects on $CaCl_2$ contractile responses on both female rabbit saphenous vein and femoral artery.

MATERIALS AND METHODS

The saphenous vein and the femoral artery were dissected from female New Zealand White rabbits (2,5-3 kg). Isometric contractions of endothelialized rings were recorded. Tissues were bathed with a modified Krebs solution at 37°C and aerated by a gas mixture of 95 % O2 and 5 % CO2 to maintain the pH at 7.4. The presence of vascular endothelium was tested by the relaxation caused by acetylcholine (1-10 µM) on KCl 100 mM precontraction.

Responses of the vascular smooth muscles to extracellular $CaCl_2$ were studied on rings bathed with a $CaCl_2$ free EGTA (0.5 mM) solution for 10 min, followed by a second period of 10 min in a $CaCl_2$ free and KCl 40 mM solution. Then, a cumulative concentration response to calcium (0.01 to 5 mM) was determined.

The effect of Diosmin (10^{-9} to 10^{-6} M) was studied on response to cumulative doses of $CaCl_2$ after 20 min of incubation on calcium free solution.
Data were expressed as means + s.e.m. of $CaCl_2$ maximal response control. Statistical evaluation of the data was made using the Student's t test for paired and unpaired comparisons of vascular responses in presence of Diosmin or its solvent. P values < 0.05 were considered as significant. n represented the number of experimentations.

RESULTS

Dose-response curves to $CaCl_2$ were potentiated in presence of Diosmin (10^{-9}, 10^{-8} and 10^{-7} M) on saphenous vein but not on femoral artery. Venous contractile responses were significantly increased by about 45 to 200 % ($p < 0.05$, $n = 4-5$), compared to control responses, especially at low calcium concentrations (0.01 to 0.3 mM). Maximal venous contractile responses were also increased (from 4.38 ± 0.20 g with control solvent to 5.24 ± 0.28 with Diosmin 10^{-7} M). ED_{50} (- log M) of $CaCl_2$ cumulative curve was not significantly modified in presence of Diosmin (3.60 ± 0.5, n=4-5). This effect on contractile response was no more observed with high Diosmin concentrations (10^{-6} M).
On femoral artery, Diosmin has no significant effect on $CaCl_2$ contractile response. The Diosmin effect at low $CaCl_2$ doses (0.01 to 0.3 mM) was not modified (3.70 ± 0.2 to 3.50 ± 0.3, n=4-5) on the vein. Moreover, maximal contractile response to $CaCl_2$ on femoral artery was not changed in presence of Diosmin (10^{-8}, 10^{-7} and 10^{-6}). Its values was equal to 8.33 ± 2.12 g (n=5).

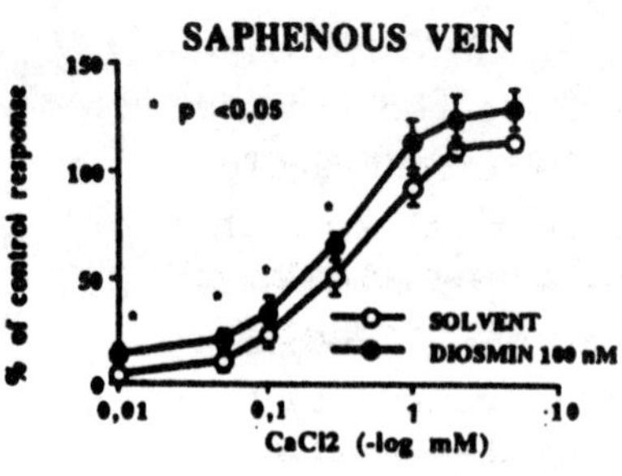

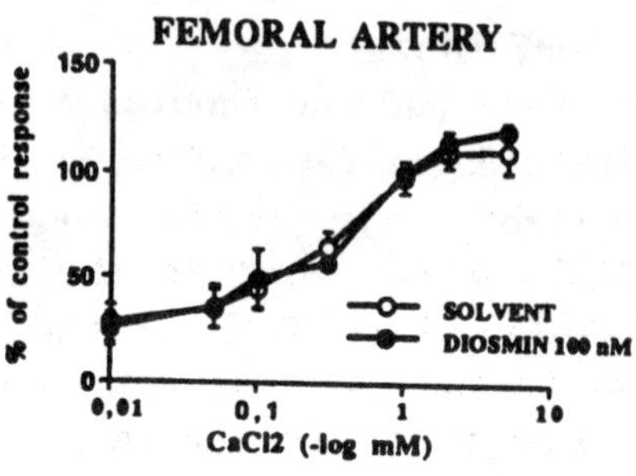

DIOSMIN EFFECT ON CACL2 (0.3 mM) CONTRACTILE RESPONSES

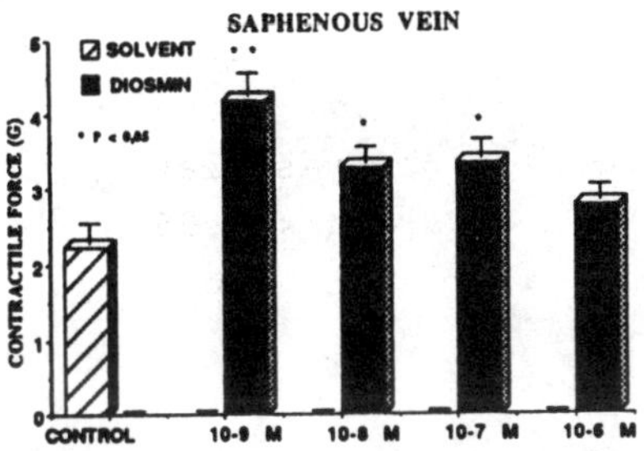

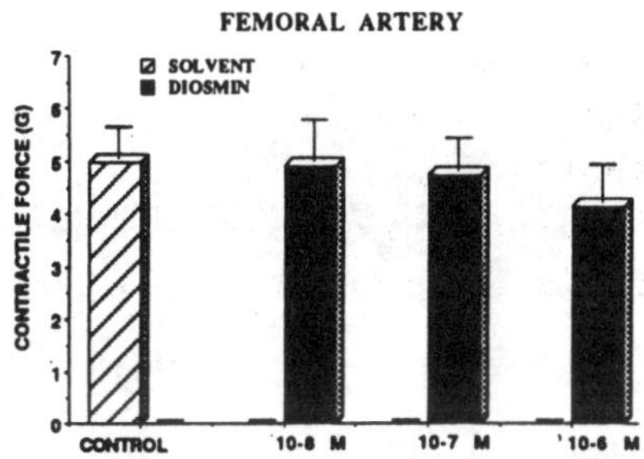

CONCLUSION

These results suggest that low concentrations of Diosmin (10^{-9} to 10^{-7} M) can act specifically on $CaCl_2$ venous contractile response without affecting arterial response.Diosmin produced a two fold increase of contractile force at low calcium doses. This positive effect of Diosmin is not competitive on $CaCl_2$ contractile response, suggesting an indirect mechanism on $CaCl_2$ mobilization. It confirms the study realized on rabbit saphenous vein (Dacquet and Finet, 1990) that showed an increase of contractile response to noradrenaline when only intracellular calcium concentration is mobilized. At low concentrations of extracellular calcium, the contraction is relatively more dependent of intracellular calcium stores than at high extracellular calcium. This Diosmin interaction with the calcium movements and their consequences on contractile responses of the venous vascular cell could be a new pathway to understand better the potential mechanism of action of this molecule prescribed on venous insufficiency.

REFERENCES :

Araujo D., Osswald W. (1989) : Phlébologie, Davy and Stemmer Eds, John Libbey Eurotex, 666-668 ;

Araujo, Viana & Osswald (1991) : Diosmin therapy alters the in vitro metabolism of noradrenaline by the varicose human saphenous vein, Pharmacological Res., 24:3, 253-256

Dacquet C., Finet M. (1990) : Effect of Diosmin on the noradrenaline sensitive intracellular store in isolated saphenous veins, Eur. J. Pharmacol., 183, 1248-1249.

Phlébologie 92. Eds P. Raymond-Martimbeau, R. Prescott, M. Zummo.
John Libbey Eurotext, Paris © 1992, pp. 726

Protective action of hemisynthetic diosmin against hyperpressure and etacrynic acid induced hyperpermeability on rat isolated vena cava

C. Escot, C. Dacquet, M. Finet

Innothera, Department of Pharmacology, 10, avenue Paul-Vaillant-Couturier, 94111 Arcueil Cedex, France.

INTRODUCTION

Chronic venous insufficiency is characterized by hyperpressure on venous and capillary systems, leading to edema. The vascular endothelium plays a central role in controling edema by the regulation of the exchange of fluid, proteins and cells between the blood and the extravascular tissues (Grega et al. 1981, Crone 1986 and Blumberg et al. 1989). It could be modulated by a physical effect of the perfusion pressure, and by a chemical effect induced with Etacrynic acid perfusion that is reported to damage the endothelial cells and consecutively increased vascular permeability.

The aim of this study was to explore the effect of hemisynthetic Diosmin (Diovenor®), a venotonic and antiedema flavonoid, on a simple in vitro model, where hyperpermeability is induced by increasing pressure and by perfusing Etacrynic acid on isolated large veins.

MATERIALS AND METHODS

Segments of rat vena cava (length of 2.5 cm) are canulated on both sides and bathed with a modified Krebs solution at 37 °C and aerated with a gas mixture of 95 % O_2 and 5 % CO_2. The tissues are perfused with a constant flow (8 ml/min) with this solution containing Evans blue ($3.9 \; 10^{-5}$ M) for a stabilisation period of 60 min. The perfusion pressure is maintained at 30 cm H_2O.

Permeability is estimated by measuring Evans blue in the extravascular compartment in function of time (Beach and Steinetz method, 1961). This model is modified from the one reported by Honig & Felix (1989).

Change in perfusion pressure (30 cm to 60 cm or 90 cm) is realized after a period of 60 min at constant pressure (30 cm H2O) where permeability is measured every ten minutes. After this pressure variation the venous permeability is controled for an hour.
Etacrynic acid (0.1 %) is added to the physiological solution when the pressure is increased from 30 to 60 cm of H2O. Its effects are compared with those of the solvent.
Diosmin effects are studied on basal venous permeability (30 cm H2O pressure), on the induction of hyperpressure (30 cm to 60 cm H2O) and finally on the Etacrynic acid action.
Results are expressed in percentage of the maximal Evans blue concentration obtained in the extravascular compartment at the end of the experimentation, or directly in µg of Evans blue. They are presented as the mean + s.e.m. and comparisons are made with the Student's t test.

RESULTS

The results showed a significant increase of rat vena cava permeability when the perfusion pressure was increased from 30 cm to 60 cm of H2O. This effect appeared 20 min after the pressure change ; after one hour of perfusion at 60 cm, the venous permeability was increased by 4 ($p<0.001$, $n=5$).
When the perfusion pressure was directly increased from 30 cm to 90 cm H2O the augmentation was equal to 9 ($p<0.001$, $n=5$).
The basal venous permeability was reduced by 60 % ($p<0.05$, $n=5$) in presence of 1 µM of Diosmin after one hour of perfusion at 30 cm H2O pressure.
Diosmin perfusion (0.1 and 1 µM) significantly reduced the effect of hyperpressure (30 cm to 60 cm H2O) on venous permeability (-70 and -50 % $p<0.001$, $n=5$). The venous permeability was maintained at the same level in presence of Diosmin (0.1 µM) in time function and was only represented by 30 % of those measured without Diosmin.
Etacrynic acid (0.1 %) perfusion increased significantly vascular permeability from 10 min of perfusion (+63 % $p<0.05$, $n=4$) when the imposed pressure was equal to 60 cm H2O. This effect was maximal after 20 min of perfusion and reached +74 % ($p<0.05$, $n=4$).
Diosmin (1 µM) decreased the effect of Etacrynic acid by about 50 % ($p<0.01$, $n=4$) after 10 min. This effect was maintained for the time of experimentation (60 min).

DIOSMIN EFFECT ON VASCULAR PERMEABILITY INDUCED BY HYPERPRESSURE (60 cm)

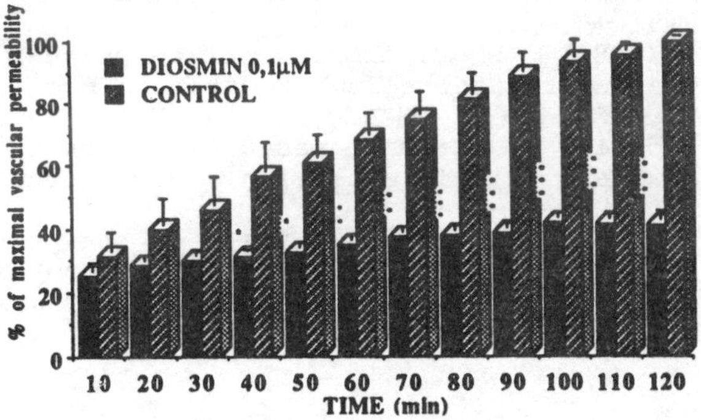

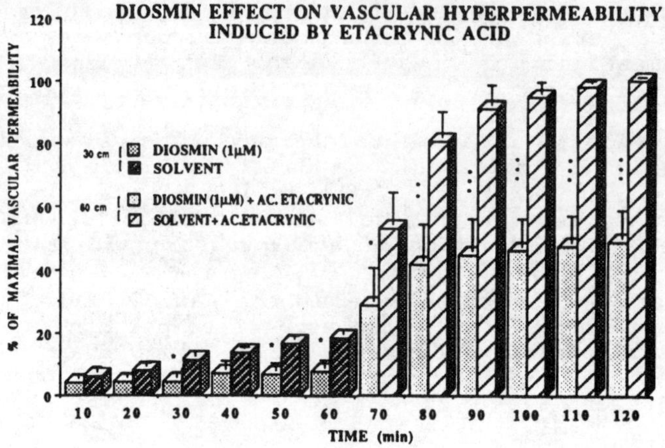

CONCLUSION

The protective effect of Diosmin against the augmentation of venous permeability induced by hyperpressure was very marked. Diosmin reduced the increase of permeability and maintained those at a stabilized level.
Moreover, when vascular endothelium was damaged with Etacrynic acid, Diosmin preserved the passage of Evans blue through the vein. This effect was dependent on the perfusion time of Diosmin and it rapidly reached a maximal value.
This showed that Diosmin could protect also large veins against the increase of permeability.
This simple model appears to be an interesting in vitro screening test to study the protective properties of drugs against hyperpressure-induced edema, as suggested by the effects of Diosmin which is reported to be an antiedema reference drug in vivo.

REFERENCES

Beach V. and Steinetz B.G. (1961) : Quantitative measurement of Evans blue space in the tissue of the rat : Influence of 5-Hydroxytryptamine antagonists and phenelzine on experimental inflammation. J. Pharmacol., 131, 400-406

Blumberg S., Clough G., Michel C. (1989) : Effect of hydroxyethyl rutosides upon the permeability of single capillaries in the frog mesentery. Br. J. Pharmacol., 96, 913-919

Crone C. (1986) : Modulation of solute permeability in microvascular endothelium. Federation Proc., 45, 77-83

Grega G.J., Svenjö E., Haddy F.J. (1981) : Macromolecular permeability of the microvascular membrane : physiological and pharmacological regulation., Microcirculation, 1, 325-341

Höning I., Felix W. (1989) : Effect on the permeability of the isolated eat vein of the pig ; a comparison between flavonoids and saponins., Phlebologie, Eds A. Davy, R. Stemmer, 680-682

"EFFICACITÉ PHARMACOLOGIQUE DANS L'INSUFFISANCE VEINEUSE: VARIABLES HEMATIQUES ET VEINE-PROTECTEURS"

Marinello,J: Alós,J.
Unitat d'Angiologia i Cirurgia Vascular
Consorci Hospitalari de Mataró. Barcelona. Espagne.

Introduction: De nombreuses références bibliographiques donnen son aval sur l'effet déterminant des certaines variables hematiques dans les manifestacions cliniques de l'Insuficance Veineuse des Membres Inferieurs (IVMI). Raisonablement, cettes alterations il doit viser a leur normalité sous l'influence des substances aceptès comme veine-protecteurs. **Materiel et Mèthodes:** Nous avont sélectionné(Doppler et Pletismography),55 malades avec IVMI ou Syndrome Variqueux, dans 5 groupes, chacun de 11 malades.Du maniere aléatoire, nous avont donnè une de les suivantes substances, a la dose terapeutique et par groupe: Dobesilate de Ca.; Hidrosmina; Melilotus Oficinalis; Rutina et Placebo. pendant 8 semaines. Le bilan hematique a eté efectué au début et a la fin du 2,4,6,et 8 semaines moyen punction (Venocath 21),de la veine saphene interne malléolaire, avec la suivante sistematique dans touttes les determinations: avec la jambe dans position de décubitus et aprés 10 minutes en pente.Dans chaque bilan hematique, nous avont valoré les suivantes parametres: hematocrite, rapport hématies/leucocytes, fibrinogène et agregabilité plaquetaire. **Resultats:**On observe correlations statistiquement significatives entre les determinations basal et après estasis, ainsi que entre les cinc groupes.Dans les groupes traités avec Hidrosmina et Melitotus Oficinalis, nous avont observé un plus rapide retour du rapport hématies/leucocytes.

"SINGULETT-OXYGEN" THERAPY (S.O.T.) IN PHLEBOLOGY

G. QUARTO, MD, N. TURCO, MD, M. GARGIULO, MD

II Department of Surgery, II Faculty of Medicine, University of Naples (Italy)

Singulett-oxygen (SO) is an achromic, inodorous, not penetrating gas obtained from therapeutic oxygen, irradiated by 253.7 nm ultraviolet light. It has an oxidative capacity between oxygen and ozone.

SO is a physiologic product of some human cell ractions, particularly it is involved in lipoxigenase reaction.

Because of its oxidative capacity and high affinity with unsaturated organic compounds, singulett-oxygen, by activation of NADH and NADPH, and production of acetil-CoA, affects metabolism of proteins, carbohydrates and lipids. These biochemical effects cause an antiphlogistic, eucoagulative action, with decrease of blood viscosity.

SO is administered by inhalation, by intramuscular, intradermal and intravenous injection, and by topical contact.

By this technique we treated various venous diseases (venous ulcers, varicous eczema, superficial thrombophlebitis), meaking a quicker recovery compared to conventional treatments.

Phlébologie 92. Eds P. Raymond-Martimbeau, R. Prescott, M. Zummo.
John Libbey Eurotext, Paris © 1992, pp. 730-732

Comparative effects of NOLA on the perfusion pressure of rat mesenteric arterial and venous beds in basal and stimulated condition

F. Le Marquer, M. Finet

Department of Pharmacology, Innothera, 10, avenue Paul-Vaillant-Couturier, 94111 Arcueil Cedex, France.

1. INTRODUCTION

The endothelium releases a potent vascular relaxing factor, which is similar to nitric oxide (NO) (Palmer et al. 1987). In vivo, this factor plays an important role, as demonstrated by the hyperpressure induced by inhibitors of endothelial NO biosynthesis (Rees et al., 1989). In vitro, the EDRF release can depend on localisation, diameter of arterial or venous rings and whole vascular beds. It can also depend on different stimuli : flow, pressure, depolarisation and agonists.

The purpose of this study was to investigate the effects of NO inhibitor (N-nitro-L-arginine (NOLA)) on both basal and agonists EDRF release in the isolated perfused mesenteric arterial and venous beds of the rat. This preparation allows a direct comparison between the responses of perfused arterial and retrogradely perfused venous beds (Warner, 1990). In this model, Warner showed that acetylcholine (Ach) and bradykinin (BK) produced dose-dependent relaxations on the arterial and venous beds.

2. MATERIALS AND METHODS

Surgical preparation

The superior mesenteric arterial and venous beds were prepared as described by Warner et al. (1990). Male Wistar rats (250-350g) were anaesthetized (urethane, 1,5g/kg), and their abdomens opened. The superior mesenteric vein and artery were separated from connective tissues and then cannulated (Biotrol, external diameter 1,27mm, internal diameter 0,86mm). Heparinized Krebs buffer (50 UI/ml) were slowly perfused via the artery before cutting the intestinal border to separate the mesentery.

Separated mesenteric arterial and venous beds were perfused independently at 2ml/min with a warmed (37°C) and gassed (95% O_2 and 5% CO_2) modified Krebs solution containing indomethacin (5µM) and composed as follows (mM) : NaCl: 118, KCl:5, $MgSO_4$:1,2,

$CaCl_2$:2,5, KH_2PO_4:1,7, $NaHCO_3$,25,Glucose:5.

Perfusion pressures were measured with Gould transducers (P23XL) and recorded on a Linseis physiograph (L6534).

To test the preparation, a solution of Krebs containing KCl 100mM were perfused twice during 10min with a delay of 20min between each perfusion. Presence of endothelium was tested on the steady contraction with a bolus injection (10µl) of acetylcholine (10^{-3}M).

Materials

Heparine (Leo), Urethane(Sigma) NOLA (Novabiochem),Bradykinin (Sigma) and acetylcholine (Sigma) were dissolved in saline, indomethacin (Sigma) was prepared as a stock solution (10^{-2}M) in dimethylsulfoxide.

3. RESULTS

Effect on basal tone

NOLA (0,1-100µM) increased basal perfusion pressures on the two beds. The maximum effect was similar on the arterial and venous beds (about 14% increase of the basal pressure) and observed at 100µM, but arterial bed was more sensitive than venous bed, ED 50(-log(M)) being respectively equal to 5.83±0.12 and 5.22±0.14 (n=5, $p<0.001$) (Fig.1).

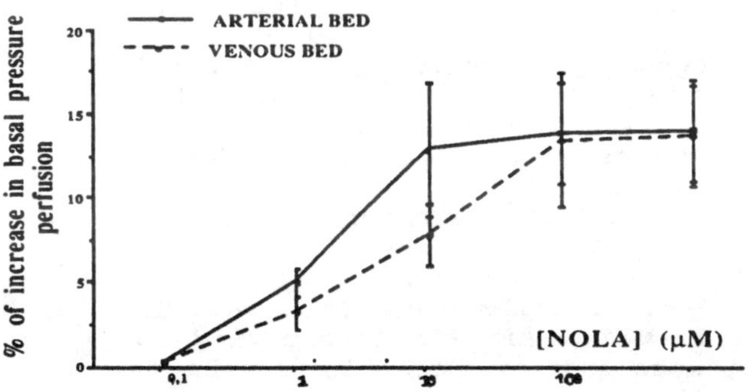

Fig.1. Effect of NOLA on the basal tone of arterial and venous beds of the perfused mesentery of the rat.

Effect on depolarisation

Depolarisation with KCl (100mM) produced a maximal increase of the pressure on the arterial and venous beds, respectively equal to +35.1±2.9mmHg and +7.15±0.69mmHg (n=8). NOLA (1-100µM) produced a dose dependent pressure increase of the two beds preconstricted by KCl 100mM, and this effect was more important on arterial than venous bed (respectively 210±9 and 106±20% increase). The ED 50(-log(M)) being equal to 5.1±0.1 (n=5) on the two beds.

Effect on agonist -induced relaxation

After a basal pressure increase produced by depolarisation (KCl 100 mM), ACh and BK (0.01-10nmole) produced an important fall in pressure of the two vascular beds. ACh was more active on arterial than on venous bed , the response to ACh 10-7M being respectively -58.2±4.2 and -40.5±4.7% of KCl response (100mM). BK was equiactive on the two beds.L-NOLA 10µM abolished totally the relaxation produced by BK and partially but at the same extent the relaxation of different ACh concentrations producing a similar effect on arterial and venous beds. However, NOLA 100µM abolished the ACh-induced relaxation (Fig.2.)

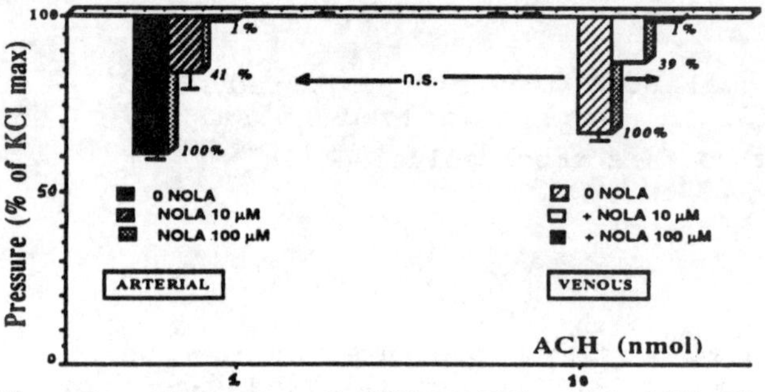

Fig.2. Effect of NOLA (10 and 100µM) on the ACh-induced relaxation, on the arterial and venous beds.

3. DISCUSSION

Our results show that when the cyclooxygenase pathway is inhibited :

- NOLA increases basal tone suggesting the existence of a basal liberation of NO induced by the flow or the pressure, the arterial bed being more sensitive than the venous bed.
- NOLA increases the response to depolarisation (KCl 100 mM) suggesting the existence of a liberation of NO induced by depolarisation, which is more important on the arterial bed than the venous.
- NOLA inhibited relaxation-induced by ACh and BK, suggesting that those agonists responses were totally mediated by NO. In this condition, the two beds showed a similar sensitivity to NOLA. However, ACh response was more resistant to NOLA than BK on the two beds.

REFERENCES

PALMER, R.M.J. FERRIGE, A.G. MONCADA, S. (1987):Nitric oxide release accounts for the biological activity of endothelium-derived relaxing factor. *Nature* 327, 524-526.

REES, D.D. PALMER, R.M.J. MONCADA, S. (1989):Role of endothelium-derived nitric oxide in the regulation of blood pressure. *Proc. Natl. Acad.Sci.USA* 86, 3375-3378.

WARNER, T.D.(1990):Simultaneous perfusion of rat isolated superior mesenteric arterial and venous beds : comparison of their vasoconstrictor and vasodilator responses to agonists. *Br. J. Pharmacol.* 99,427-433.

Phlébologie 92. Eds P. Raymond-Martimbeau, R. Prescott, M. Zummo.
John Libbey Eurotext, Paris © 1992, pp. 733-735

Haemodynamic effects of sulodexide in post-thrombophlebitic syndromes

M. Cospite, G. Milio, F. Ferrara, V. Cospite, E. Palazzini*

*Department of Angiology of the University of Palermo, Italy. * Alfa-Wassermann s.p.a., Medical Department, Bologna, Italy.*

It is well known that sulodexide, glycosaminoglycan containing fast moving heparin (80%) and dermatan sulphate (20%) (SILBERT, 1982) provide excellent anti-thrombotic protection and reduce the risk of deep vein thrombosis in recurrent thrombophlebitis in post-surgical patients and in other conditions (COSPITE, 1985 and ALEDORT, 1982).
This drug, in fact, have positive effects on factors influencing the fluidity of blood (LOWE, 1986) and rheological properties such as plasma fibrinogen level (ERNST, 1990 and AVOGARO, 1977) and whole blood or plasma viscosity (NGUEYEN, 1988), on fibrinolysis and platelets aggregation (PALAZZINI, 1981), on plasma lipoproteins (CIUFFETTI, 1989) and on endotelial cell protection. It therefore appears that sulodexide might be clinically useful in venous thrombosis and thrombophlebitic syndrome.

The aim of this study is to identify the effects of oral sulodexide on haemodynamics parameters related to venous micro- and macro-circulatory characteristics in patients with recurrent deep vein thrombosis and post-thrombotic syndrome.

Following a double-blind study protocollo, 30 patients (10 males, 20 females, age range 21-63 years) suffering from the post-thrombophlebitic syndrome for at least 1 year, were enrolled. After a 20 days wash-out period, patients were randomly allocated to two equinumerical groups (Group 1: 7 males and 8 females; Group 2: 3 males and 12 females); Group 1 was administered sulodexide, 2 capsules of 250 Lipoproteinlipase Releasing Units (LRU) twice a day, for total of 1000 LRU orally/day for 3 months; Group 2 received identical placebo (2 capsules b.i.d.).
During both wash-out and sulodexide/placebo therapy, no other vasoactive, antithrombotic, antiaggregant or fibrinolitic drugs were prescribed.

Before the start of therapy and 1 month and 3 months after treatment, the following parameters were evaluated by means of strain gauge plethysmography and CW doppler, using a 4 MHz probe:
- MVIV (40 or 60): maximal venous incremental volume (index of venous capacitance), evaluated after cuff insufflation at 40 and 60 mmHg;
- tMVIV: time required to reach the maximal venous incremental volume;
- MVO: maximal venous outflow (expression of venous emptying capacity);
- tTE: total emptying time;

- dV/dP ratio: venous distensibility;
- dP/dV ratio: venous tone;
- CFC: capillary filtration coefficient (index of microcirculatory flow);
- PTVP: posterior tibial vein pressure, both in standing and lying positions.

At the same checking times, a series of symptoms and signs (pain, itching, oedema, dyschromic alterations of skin, alterations in cutaneous sensitivity and parestesia) were also monitored and recorded using an arbitrary score from 0 to 3.

Statistical analysis of results whose performed using Student's paired or unpaired "t" test (for intra- and inter-group comparisons respectively) and by the chi-square test on m x n contingency tables (for dichotomous variables).

Patients in both groups completed the study with good adherence to therapy and no major complaints or side-effects.

Analysis by the Chi-square test for homogeneity of the two groups showed no significant differences between them (always $p>0.1$).

TABLE 1 shows the overall results. MVIV measured at two pressures (40 and 60 mmHg) in the two patients groups, evidenced a clear decrease of both measurements in sulodexide treated patients: from 2,85 to 1,91 for MVIV 40 and from 4.08 to 2.57 for MVIV 60 (both $p<0.001$, intra-group analysis). The comparison versus the placebo group also revealed statistically significant differences at the end of the study ($p<0.01$ for MVIV 40 and $p<0.05$ for MVIV 60).

On the contrary, the time taken to reach the maximal venous incremental volume (tMVIV) remained unchanged during both sulodexide and placebo administration (in the sulodexide group from 245" at baseline to 230" after 90 days).

As to the dV/dP and dP/dV ratios, expressing venous distensibility and tone respectively, while non significant variations were found in the placebo-treated subjects, a net change was observed at the end of the study in the sulodexide group. These changes were obviously in the opposite direction and one almost mirrored the other. Inter- and intra-group analysis were highly significant ($p<0.01$).

No significant changes were recorded in maximal venous outflow (MVO) or in total emptying time (tTE), either on the 30th or on the 90th day after sulodexide administration (38.5, 37.7 and 38.1 for MVO and 58, 65 and 59 for tTE; p always >0.1).

Unlike the other parameters, a statistically significant change in CFC values was already apparent by the 30th day of therapy and was more evident at the end of the study ($p<0.01$ after 30 days and $p<0.001$ after 90 days).

Also the checked symptoms and signs evidenced a reduction in severity, also detectable, with an exception for oedema, in the placebo group. This is probably an expression of a placebo effect and/or of casual variations. The reduction was, however, significantly greater in the sulodexide than in the placebo group for pain, itching and paresthesiae ($p<0.05$ with the Chi-square test on the absolute values of severity).

The results of our study clearly emphasize the improvement of the micro- and macro-circulatory efficiency of the limb venous system, induced by oral sulodexide. The capillary filtration coefficient seems particulary sensitive to the action of the drug, with changes already apparent after the first month of therapy.

The effects of Sulodexide on microcirculation may be mediated by its well known effects on plasma viscosity and on the fibrinolytic system. It seems more difficult to explain the drug's mecchanism of action on the macrocirculatory flow, since at that level only a direct interaction of the active principle with the venous wall could induce favourable results. It therefore seems possible that orally administered sulodexide can concentrate in the arterial wall, with a consequent modification of its functions. A recent pharmacokinetics study on C-radiolabelled sulodexide, showing a rapid gastro-intestinal absorption, a peek blood level within 1 hour and a subsequent vascular distribution of the drug, could support this theory.

The results of our study ultimately justify the use of oral sulodexide in patients with post-thrombophlebitic syndromes of the lower limbs, both for its antithrombotic effects and its beneficial influence on venous circulation.

Parameters	Sulodexide			Placebo			p
	T 0	T 30	T 90	T 0	T 30	T 90	
MVIV 40 ml/100 ml	2.85±1.02	2.35±0.79	1.91±0.84	2.80±1.24	2.70±1.30	2.56±1.42	<0.05
MVIV 60 ml/100 ml	4.08±1.58	3.25±1.29	2.57±1.74	4.10±1.86	4.09±2.04	4.00±1.89	<0.01
tMVIV sec.	245±52	235±48	230±57	243±44	238±42	231±50	n.s.
MVO ml/100ml/min	38.5±4.4	37.7±6.1	38.1±4.3	38.3±3.9	38.1±4.0	38.0±4.7	n.s.
tTE sec.	58±14	65±17	59±15	60±14	61±15	59±18	n.s.
dV/dP ml/mmHg	0.075±0.019	0.069±0.021	0.055±0.017	0.073±0.030	0.070±0.025	0.070±0.024	<0.01
dP/dV mmHg/ml	11.23±3.74	13.25±3.82	15.48±4.01	11.35±3.74	12.00±4.05	12.10±3.84	<0.01
CFC ratio	0.013±0.009	0.008±0.0035	0.007±0.0029	0.013±0.005	0.013±0.002	0.013±0.008	<0.01
PTVP mmHg$_a$	51±29	50±32	46±28	55±34	56±27	56±31	n.s.
PTVP mmHg$_b$	94±40	85±43	78±37	95±35	95±40	99±41	<0.05

TABLE 1. - Evolution of the various haemodynamic parameters during sulodexide or placebo treatment.

REFERENCES

ALEDORT L.M. (1982): Principles of anticoagulant therapy: Guidelines for prophylactic and therapeutic use. In: Recognition and Management of Thromboembolic Disorders, ed. Gorlin R., Aledort L.M., p.8. New York: Professional Postagraduate Service Inc.

AVOGARO P., BITTOLO BON G.C., et al. (1977): Effects of the extractive heparinoid, glucuronoglycosaminoglycan sulfate on human plasma lipids. Pharmacology Research Communications, 9, 977-982.

CIUFFETTI G., MERCURY M., et al. (1989): Effects of 3-Glucosaminiglycan Sulfate on haemorheologic parameters in hyperlipidemic vascular desease patients. Angiology, 40, 255-259.

COSPITE M., MILIO G., et al. (1985): Double-blind study of the pharmacological effects of sulodexide in patients with multiple atherosclerotic vascular desease. Eur. Revue of Pharm. Med. Sci., 7, 97-104.

ERNST E. (1990): Plasma fibrinogen: an indipendent cardiovascular risk factor. J. Int. Med., 277, 365-9.

LOWE G.D.O. (1986): Blood rheology in arterial desease. Clinical Science, 71, 137-142.

NGUEYEN P., ADJIZAIN J.C., et al. (1988): Rheology of hemodialysed patients: erythrocyte population studies. Clinical Hemorrheology, 8, 415-419.

PALAZZINI E., VERARDI S. (1981): Effect of naturally occurring mucopolysaccharide 3-GS on coagulative parameters in patients and chronic haemodialytic treatment. Current Ther. Research, 29, 678-683.

SILBERT J.E. (1982): Structure and metabolism of proteoglycans and glycosaminoglycans. Journal of Investigative Dermatology, 79, 31-36.

Phlébologie 92. Eds P. Raymond-Martimbeau, R. Prescott, M. Zummo.
John Libbey Eurotext, Paris © 1992, pp. 736-738

Sulodexide and microcirculatory component in macrophlebopathies

Michele Cospite, Filippo Ferrara, Glauco Milio, Valentina Cospite

Department of Angiology, University of Palermo, Italy.

PURPOSE OF RESEARCH

We carried out, through the evaluation of C.F.C. (Capillary Coefficient of filtration), an analysis on the efficacy of oral sulodexide on the treatment of microcirculatory changes of chronic venous insufficiency owing to idiopathic varices.

Sulodexide is a highly purified preparation of extractive glucosaminoglycans, containing an endogenous heparin-like fraction by about 70% and a dermatan fraction by anout 20%.
Sulodexide exerts hoth a clear antithrombotic effect (due to Xa factor inhibition), a fibrinolytic activity (due to interaction with the endothelial production of TPA and PAI) (Andriuoli,1984; Bianchini,1985; Fiore,1991) and an hypoviscosimetric activity (due to reduction of plasma tryglicerides and fibrinogen) (Castelluccio 1991, Crepaldi 1990). Recently Busutti (1991) pointed out the pharmacokinetic pattern of Sulodexide after oral admnistration.

METHOD

We involved in this research 36 patients (29 females and 7 males) aged 30 to 50 years, suffering from chronic venous insufficiency due to idiopathic varices.
The study was conducted according to the double-blind, placebo controlled method. An informed consent was obtained from all patients After a wash-out period of two weeks, patinte were divided, following a randomization list, in two groups:
GROUP A: patients were treated by oral route with Sulodexide, 500 Lipoproteinolipase Releasing Units (LRU), twice daily for 45 days (each Sulodexide capsule contained 250 LRU).
GROUP B: patients were treated with placebo, 2 indistinguishable capsules, twice daily for 45 days.

The Capillary Coefficient of filtartion (C.F.C.) was calculated for both legs of each patient before the beginning of the treatment (TO), after 30 days (T30) and 45 (T45) of treatment.

The statistical evaluation of the data was performed by means of the ANOVA test.

RESULTS

After the randomization, the two groups resulted comparable as to age and sex.
The mean values of CFC for the Sulodexide group and for the placebo group are reported in Table I. As it can be osserved, while in the treated group the coefficient of capillary filtration undergoes a clear-out reduction as time goes on, in the placebo group on the contrary is slowly increases.
These results are confirmed also by the statistical analysis performed (Table II): a net significance was detectable as for the "between drugs" comparison also, within the Sulodexide group, as to the "between control times" comparison, thus clearly underlining the effective changes induced by therapy on the microcirculatory level.

CONCLUSION

The data obtained suggest that Sulodexide is efficacious for the treatment of microcirculatory changes induced by chronic venous insufficiency. This is demonstrated by significant reduction of CFC already obtained after 30 days of therapy and kept also after 45 days. In our opinion these results are due to the numerous effects of Sulodexide: a reduction of platelets aggregation, a shift towards fibrinolysis in the balance between fibrinolysis and fibrinogenesis; moreover, an interference with the Xa factor and with AT III, wich results in a clear influence on the haemocoagulative parameters and on haemorheology.

TABLE I- Mean CFC values (± S.E.) in the 18 Sulodexide Treated and in the 18 placebo treated patients at each control time.

	SULODEXIDE GROUP	PLACEBO GROUP
n.	18	18
0 Time	0,196 (± 0,032)	0,240 (± 0,043)
after 30 days	0,085 (± 0,006)	0,241 (± 0,043)
after 45 days	0,075 (± 0,005)	0,255 (± 0,042)

TABLE II - Results of statistical analysis of the CFC data in the groups of patients.

ONE-WAY ANOVA: SIMPLE CONTRAST BETWEEN CONTROL TIMES:		
	F value	p value
SULODEXIDE GROUP	12.737	<0.001
PLACEBO GROUP	0.040	n.s.
ONE-WAY ANOVA BETWEEN GROUPS:		
0 Time	0.660	n.s.
30 days	12.915	<0.001
45 days	18.011	<0.001

REFERENCES:

Andriuoli et al (1984): Antithrombotic activity of a glycosaminoglycan (Sulodexide) in rats. Thromb. Res., 34: 81-85.

Bianchini P. (1985): Lack of correlation between in vitro and in vivo antithrombotic activity of heparin fractions and related compounds. Heparan sulphate as an antithrombotic in vivo. Thromb. Res. 40: 597-601.

Busutti L., Breccia A. (1991): Pharmacokinetics of Sulodexide af ter single oral administration in man. Eur. J. Res. 1: 25-37.

Castelluccio A., Bologna A. (1991): Effect of Sulodexide on blood viscosity in patients with peripheral avscular disease. Curr. Med. Res. Opin., 12: 325-331.

Crepaldi G. et al. (1990): Double-blind multicenter trial on a new medium molecular weight glycosaminoglycan. Current therapeutic effects and perspectives for clinical use. Atheros., 81: 223-43

Fiore G. et al.(1991): Inhibition of plasminogen activator inhibitor (PAI-1) by Sulodexide in post-thrombophlebitic patients. J. Drug Develop, 3: 173-78.

Phlébologie 92. Eds P. Raymond-Martimbeau, R. Prescott, M. Zummo.
John Libbey Eurotext, Paris © 1992, pp. 739-743

Red blood cell rheologic characteristics during venous insufficiency and therapeutic implication : Cyclo 3 fort®*

C. Le Devehat, T. Khodabandehlou, M. Vimeux

Unité de Recherches d'Hémorhéologie clinique, Service de Diabétologie-Nutrition-Maladies Métaboliques, Centre Hospitalier, 58000 Nevers, France.
** Laboratoire Pierre Fabre, France.*

INTRODUCTION

Venous insufficiency is usually associated with multiple blood rheological abnormalities (4,9,11). In consequence, particular benefits are to be expected from hemorheological therapy. Indeed, the precocious use of an hemorheological therapy should improve the blood flow properties and avoid by consequence the development of severe functional or structural damages. A certain number of hemorheological treatment such as hemodilution, plasma defibrination (12,16) and use of flavonoids (10,15), are already tested. The aim of this work is to evaluate the hemorheological actions of CYCLO 3 FORT in patients suffering from a venous insufficiency. The clinical interest of CYCLO 3 FORT, whose major active principle is the extract of Ruscus, is already pointed-out in different pathological circumstances (1,7,8,13,14). The extract of Ruscus was suggested to stimulate the pumping activity of lymph vessels and thus to improve the veno-lymphatic return which is reduced in peripheral oedema (13). Morover, CYCLO 3 FORT is shown to act as a venoconstrictor stimulus. But up to date, there is no data about its hemorheological action.

MATERIALS AND METHODS

1:Patients

Patients recruited for this study were 40 females aged from 43 to 83 years old (mean = 60+-9 years). They suffered from a venous insufficiency with varicose at lower limbs. Patients presenting any other pathology were not included. They had no medication known to modify the hemorheological properties. 5 healthy volunteers, aged from 24 to 46 years (mean = 32+-8 years), without venous insufficiency, have also participated in this study.

2:Experimental trial

The experimental protocol was based on a double blind randomised treatment with CYCLO 3 FORT and Placebo. 20 patients received the CYCLO 3 FORT et 20 others were treated by Placebo. Both CYCLO 3 FORT and Placebo were administrated at a daily dose of 2 pills during 4 weeks. Hemorheological properties were investigated either before (B) and after (A) a venous occlusion (100 mmHg during 10 minutes), before (Day 0) and at the end of a 4-week medication (Day 28).Blood samples for hemorheological studies were obtained from a foot vein with patients remaining at supine position.

3:Hemorheological investigations

Investigations consisted of red blood cell (RBC) aggregation and deformability measurements. RBC aggregation was evaluated by the Sefam erythroaggregometer (3) which is based on the analysis of the backscattered light through the blood suspension. The derived parameters are RBC aggregation time, expressed in seconds and corresponding to the rate of rouleaux formation and also the disaggregation shear rate. RBC aggregation measurements were performed at a hematocrit of 40 % and T = 37°C. RBC deformability was evaluated via filtration measurements made by using an initial flow rate method as described by Hanss (5). Red cells suspended in TRIS buffer (Ht = 9%), are filtered through the nucleopore membrane with a pore diameter of 5 µm and T = 37°C. Results are expressed in terms of a rigidity index. Other factors such as plasma viscosity in mPa.s by a KSPV 4 capillary viscometer (6), and fibrinogen level in g/l by a thrombin clotting time technique (2) were also determined.

4:Statistical analysis

Either before and after treatment, differences between before and after venous occlusion were analysed by Student "t" test for paired data. Effect of a 4-week medication has been assessed by comparing the relative variations, obtained between before and after venous occlusion, between before and at the end of treatment by Student "t" test for unpaired data in each group.

5:Results

Before treatment and before venous occlusion, fibrinogen level and plasma viscosity were significantly higher in patients, than those in the controls (Fig.1a,1b). Before treatment, these parameters were found to be increased after venous occlusion in both groups of patients whilst they remained unchanged in the controls. After treatment, increases in both parameters caused by venous occlusion persisted only in the group of patients treated by placebo.

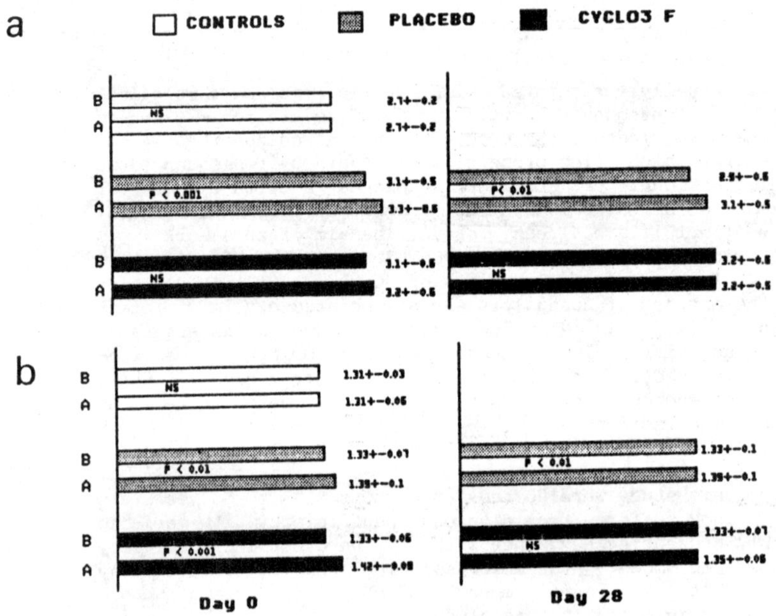

Figures 1a, 1b : Fibrinogen level and plasma viscosity before (B) and after (A) venous occlusion, before (Day 0) and at the end (Day 28) of treatment.

In regard to RBC aggregation, patients showed before treatment and before venous occlusion, significant lower RBC aggregation time than that obtained in the controls (Fig.2a). This result means a more accelerated kinetic of RBC rouleaux formation in patients and is confirmed by the higher values of RBC disaggregation shear rate (Fig.2b), indicating that forces necessary to disperse the RBC aggregates are more important in patients. Before treatment, disturbances in both parameters were found to be significantly increased as a result of venous occlusion in patients;By contrast, venous occlusion had no effect on these parameters in the controls. The effect of venous occlusion persisted on both parameters after treatment by placebo while it disappeared in patients treated by CYCLO 3 FORT (Fig.2a,2b). Relative variations of parameters between before and after venous occlusion, were also calculated for both groups of patients before and after treatment (Fig.3). One can notice significant decreases in relative variation of parameters after treatment by CYCLO 3 FORT whereas they remained unchanged in the group of patients treated by placebo. Rigidity index was not significantly different between patients and the controls. Before treatment, this parameter was found to be slightly increased as a result of venous occlusion in the group CYCLO 3 FORT ; this effect was disappeared after treatment by CYCLO 3 FORT.

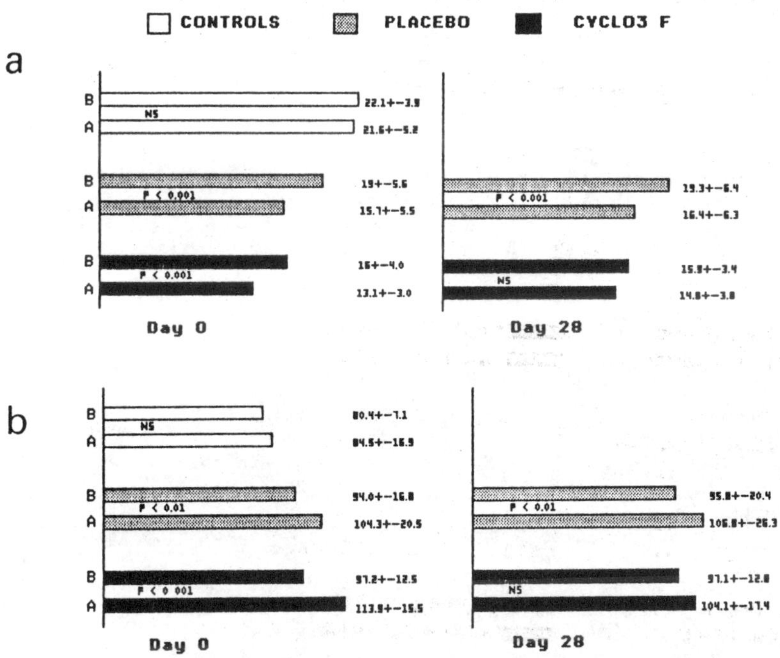

Figures 2a, 2b : RBC aggregation time, RBC disaggregation shear rate before (B) and after (A) venous occlusion, before (Day 0) and at the end (Day 28) of treatment.

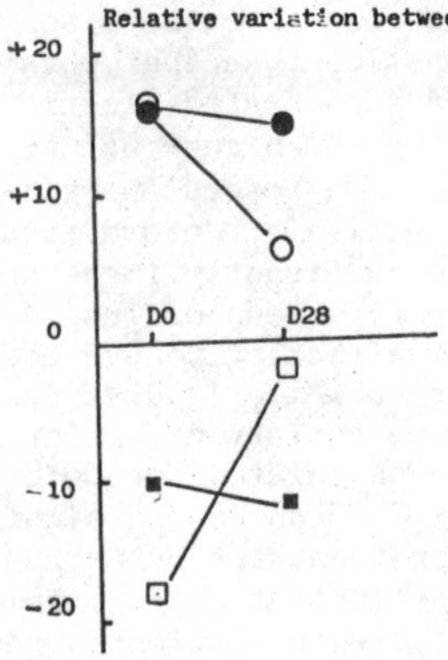

Figure 3 : Relative variation between before and after venous occlusion of hemorheological parameters (O ● RBC aggregation time ; □ ■ RBC disaggregation shear rate), before (DO) and at the end of treatment (D28) for patients treated by Cyclo 3 Fort (O □) and by placebo (● ■).

CONCLUSION

Three points can be noticed from our findings :

- Venous insufficiency is accompanied by hemorheological disturbances
- Hemorheological disturbances are significantly more important after venous occlusion in patients suffering from venous insufficiency. This shows the deleterious effect of venous stasis on hemorheological parameters in patients while there is no effect on hemorheological parameters of normal subjects.
- CYCLO 3 FORT is found to inhibite the deleterious effect of venous stasis in patients.

REFERENCES

1. Baudet J., Collet D., Aubrard Y.(1990) Essai thérapeutique du Cyclo 3 Fort chez la femme enceinte : évaluation de la tolérance foetale par la technique du Doppler pulsé du cordon. Precepta Medica, N°6, 26-28.

2. Caen J. Larrieu MJ. Samama M. (1975) L'hémostase : méthode d'exploration et diagnostic pratique. L'expansion scientifique, Paris.

3. Donner M. Siadat M. Stoltz JF (1988) Erythrocyte aggregation : approach by light scattering determination. Biorheology 25, 367-375.

4. Dormandy JA. Nash G. (1986) L'importance de l'agrégation des hématies dans la pathologie veineuse. Hémorhéologie et agrégation érythrocytaire Ed.EM Inter 1, 151-154.

5. Hanss M. (1983) Erythrocyte filtrability measurement by the initial flow rate method. Biorheology 20, 199-211.

6. Jung J. Roggenkamp HG, Schreiber R. H. Keisewetter (1983) Ein neues gerät zür quantifizierung der blut plasma-viskosität. Biomed. Tech. 28, 249-252.

7. Kiesewetter H. Blume J. Jung F. Spitzer S. (1990) Efficacité de l'extrait de Ruscus dans le traitement de l'insuffisance veineuse chronique. Preceptia Medica N°6, 74-77.

8. Lagrue G. Behar A. Laurent J. (1990) Oedèmes induits par les inhibiteurs calciques : action du Cyclo 3 Fort sur les paramètres cliniques et biologiques. Precepta Medica N°6 44-47.

9. Le Dévéhat C. Boisseau M. Bertrand A. (1988) Signification physiopathologique des paramètres microrhéologiques dans l'insuffisance veineuse. Hémorhéologie et agrégation érythrocytaire Ed EM Inter 2, 181-189.

10. Le Dévéhat C. Vimeux M. Bondoux G. (1989) Hemorheological effects of oral Troxerutin treatment versus placebo in venous insufficiency of the lower limbs. Clin. Hemorh 9(4) 543-552.

11. Lowe GDO (1984) Blood rheology and venous thrombosis. Clin. Hemorh 4(6), 571-588.

12. Lowe GDO. (1984) Defibrination, blood flow and blood rheology.Clin. Hemorh. 4(1) 15-28.

13. Marcelon G. Pouget G. Tisne-Versailles J. (1988) Physio-pharmacology of the veno-lymphatic system : comparative activity of Ruscus extract. Angiology. Ed. H. Boccalon, John Libbey Eurotext, Paris 415-416.

14. Monteil- Sevrin J. Ladure P. (1990) Etude de l'efficacité du Cyclo 3 Fort

dans le traitement du syndrome prémenstruel. Precepta Medica n°6, 18-21
15. Robin RC. (1971) Effect of phenylbenzopyrone derivatives (flavonoïds) on blood cell aggregation : basis for concept of mode of action. Clin. Chem. 17, 433-437.
16. Schmid-Schonbein H. Weiss HJ. Volger E. Klose HJ. (1978) Microhemorheology and defibrination. ZFA (Stuttgart), 54, 1635-1643.
17. Schmid-Schonbein H. Volger E. Weiss J. (1975) Effect of O-(-Hydroxyethyl) rutosides on the microrheology of human blood under defined flow conditions. Vasa 4, (3), 263-270.

Modifications capillaroscopiques périunguéales des insuffisances veineuses pariétales avant et après traitement par Troxérutine

J.R. Dumas, P. Radier, M. Cloarec

Laboratoire d'explorations fonctionnelles vasculaires. Service du Pr Cloarec M.
Hôpital Tenon - Paris

Dans le cas d'insuffisance du tonus pariétal veineux on note:

1) à la pléthysmographie digitale, une hyperdialatabilité veineuse lors de la manoeuvre d'occlusion veineuse (pouvant doubler le Δ V usuel). En cas d'insuffisance valvulaire, ceci n'existe pas ou peut-être associé en cas d'hypertonie pariétale associée, uniquement.

2) à la capillaroscopie périunguéale il existe également des modifications

- existence d'un oedème péricapillaire intense, blanc opalescent, redressant les anses capillaires vers la verticale.

- tendance nette à l'égalisation des branches de l'anse capillaire et de la boucle sans coloration hyperchrome de celle-ci (comme dans le diabète non insulino-dépendant).

Après Troxérutine 4g/j 20 jours par mois il faut attendre au minimum deux mois pour voir disparaître ces signes dans 62% des cas et ce n'est qu'au bout de quatre mois qu'ils ont disparu totalement chez les 45 patients explorés.

Phlébologie 92. Eds P. Raymond-Martimbeau, R. Prescott, M. Zummo.
John Libbey Eurotext, Paris © 1992, pp. 745-746

Efficacy and tolerance of « cloricromene » in phlebopathies

Giuseppe Riccio, Salvatore Riccio, Annamaria Cretella*, Rosaria Paterni**

*Divisione di Chirurgia, Ospedale S. Maria di Loreto, USL 44, Napoli, Italy. * Divisione di Chirurgia, Ospedale Loreto Crispi, USL 37, Napoli, Italy. ** Divisione di Chirurgia Vascolare, Ospedale Pellegrini, USL 44, Napoli, Italy.*

SUMMARY

The authors report results given by use of cloricromene (PROENDOTEL) in forty cases (30 females, 10 males; aged 21 - 75). These patients had lower extremity venous diseases, so divided: 20 stasis ulcers, 12 DVT, 8 patients undergoing phlebological operation.

INTRODUCTION

Chronic venous insufficiency (CVI) is a syndrome characterized by valvular incompetence and venous stasis, reduced perfusion, topic hypercoagulation and thrombotic risk. If the stasis lasts, pressure in the venous system increases. Venous hypertension is the most significant of CVI. The increase in pressure results in a disorder in capillary permeability, leakage of mostly high molecular weight proteins, and later also leads to to pericapillary fibrin deposits. The clinical expression of these disorders are oedema, phlebitis, thrombosis, dermatosclerosis, stasis pigmentation, eczemas and ulcers. Stasis on microcirculation causes a thining of endothelium bed and a change of cell structure; at this level we can see white blood cells becoming "trapped". According to new knowledges, the "kidnapped" white cells are the most liable of the haemodinamic microvascular disorders and the skin lesions.

Then, we need to remove the leucocytes and to stimulate endothelium activity to therapeutic purposes.

Our work studies the action of a new drug: cloricromene. This acts on endothelium increasing its activity, and on white blood cells, which loose their adhesive capacity.

METHODS

Forty patients were observed; among them there were 30 females and 10 males, aged 45 years (range 21 - 75). These patients had venous diseases so divided: 20 stasis ulcers, 12 DVT, 8 patients nominated for phlebologic surgery. They told that their symptoms were: itching legs (70%), pain (80%), sensation of leg weight (92%), parestesies (45%). We saw surely more or less oedema (87%), stasis pigmentation and florid leg ulcers (55%).

During the clinic exam, the patients were undergone to Doppler ultrasound and measurement of venous pressure; in ten subjects we carried out capillaroscopy, while in four of them it was necessary a phlebography. In all patients we wanted to test these parameters: Hct, PT, PTT, thromboxane, β-thromboglobulin, PFA, fibrinogenum and FDP. These assays were repeated in twenty ulcer patients and in twelve DVT, after 30 treatment days. In these cases, cloricromene was given as 300 mg/die/os for a month. In this period, our patients wore a compressive aid, if they needed. In the persons undergoing surgical operation (we use to do it in day-hospital), cloricromene was given as 200 mg/die/i.v. for one preoperative week. The same haematic parameters were valued in these patients. As surgery, we carried out one short saphenous vein stripping, four short strippings of the long saphenous, three phlebectomies by Muller.

RESULTS

The use of cloricromene results in a very important reduction of pain and oedema (90% of treated patients). All the trialed patients underwent follow up weekly. After a 30 days treatment, Hct, thromboxane, β-thromboglobulin, PFA and fibrinogenum values were reduced to less than 40% from initial values. PT and PTT remained unchanged. Venous pressure was lovered in 95% of cases, meaningfully. We subjected ten patients to capillaroscopy before the cloricromene therapy. This showed abnormalities of the capillaries and presence of fibrin cuffs. After treatment, we saw a reduction of fibrin cuffs and a pink picture of capillary bed. The observed florid leg ulcers curtailed their healing time. In patients nominated for surgery, Hct, PFA and fibrinogenum were reduced too.

DISCUSSION

The use of cloricromene in forty patients greatly satisfied us. The drug tolerance has been very good; anybody hadn't collateral results. These data confirm the hypotesis in which leucocytes become "trapped" in capillary endothelium producing ischaemia and become activated causing damage to the endothelium.

Cloricromene acts on endothelium restraining tromboxane synthesis. This effect stimulates production of prostacyclin by endothelium cells. Cloricromene has anti-inflammatory action, it moves away white cells and improves microcirculation. Besides, it restrains phospholipase A_2; this freezes leucocytes adhesive capacity. Because of these properties, cloricromene has, in our opinion, a proper antithrombotic action too. In observed cases, it allowed a reduction of healing time; in patients undergoing phlebologic operation, it allowed to perform surgical operation without thrombotic risk and coagulation alterations.

REFERENCES

Browhe N. L., Burnard K. G. (1982): The cause of venous ulceration *Lancet* 243-5.

Michel C. (1989): Microcirculation in the limbs in venous hypertension *Medicographia* Vol. XI, n. 2.

Moyses C. et al. (1987): Haemoconcentration and accumulation of white cells in the feet during venous diseases *Int. J. Microcirc. Clin. Exp.*, **5**, 311-320.

Scott H. J. et al. (1991): Histological study of white blood cells and association with lipodermatosclerosis and venous ulceration *Br. J. Surg.*, vol. 78 February, 210-211.

Thomas P. R. S. et al. (1989): Accumulo di leucociti nelle porzioni declivi degli arti inferiori di pazienti con aumento della pressione venosa; un possibile meccanismo per spiegare le modificazioni del trofismo cutaneo. *British Med. J. Ed. Ital.*, vol. XI, 30-33.

Phlébologie 92. Eds P. Raymond-Martimbeau, R. Prescott, M. Zummo.
John Libbey Eurotext, Paris © 1992, pp. 747-749

The effect of nifedipine on capillary filtration rate in lower limb of man

Karel Roztočil, Ivo Přerovský, Marie Gebauerová

Clinic of Cardiology, Institute for Clinical and Experimental Medicine, Vídeňská 800, 140 000 Prague 4, Czechoslovakia.

While commonly well tolerated, treatment with calcium antagonists may be associated with some side effects including limb swelling. The mechanism of oedema formation is poorly understood. The oedema is not believed to be due to overall natrium and water retention in the body (Opie,1986), or to be related to changes in central hemodynamics (Ježek et al.,1990). The aim of our study was to try to determine whether nifedipine administration does not lead to alterations, at the level of microcirculation, which might possibly be related to oedema formation.

MATERIAL AND METHODS :
Patients were examined in the supine position at an ambient temperature of 23°C. To determine capillary filtration rate, the method of venous occlusive plethysmography was used. Changes in the limb circumference were registered using a mercury-in-rubber strain gauge plethysmography (Whitney,1953). Venous occlusion at a height of 60 mmHg for 10 minutes was induced by means of a cuff placed on the thigh. The magnitude of capillary filtration rate was determined from the slope of plethysmographic curves between 5 and 10 minutes of occlusion and expressed in ml/100 ml/min.

Capillary filtration was measured three times before and, then, three times in the interval between 45 and 90 minutes following oral single dose of nifedipine (20 mg). Mean values of capillary filtration rate in both parts of the examination were statistically compared.

Measurement was performed in a group of 14 patients aged 49-73 years (12 M, 2 F). They were patients with ischaemic heart disease, six patients had concomitant arterial obliterative disease involving periferal arteries. Eight patients had been previously treated with nifedipine, and limb oedema was noted in four subjects provided nifedipine therapy.

RESULTS:

Tab.1 shows the mean values of capillary filtration rate in both parts of the examination. Baseline capillary filtration rate averaged 0.07 ml/100 ml/min; the value rose after nifedipine administration by a mean 30%; this difference was statistically significant.

In addtition to the rate of capillary filtration, the amount of filtrate remaining in the extravascular space following the application of venous occlusion was assessed by means of baseline limb volume. Under normal circumstances, the increment is zero or absolutely negligible. As can be seen from the figure, it was a mean 0.1 ml/100 ml. The value almost tripled after nifedipine administration, and this difference is statistically significant.

Tab.1 Mean values of capillary filtration (ml(100 ml/min) and fluid accumulation (ml/100ml) before and after administration of nifedipine

	initial		after nifedipine
capillary filtration	0.07 ± 0.03	$p < 0.01$	0.09 ± 0.02
fluid accumulation	0.10 ± 0.12	$p < 0.01$	0.35 ± 0.21

DISCUSSION:

Signs of increased filtrate transport and accumulation in the interstitium were observed following nifedipine administration. One of the possible reasons for the enhanced filtration rate may be qualitative changes in the capillary bed, and its increased permeability. However, as nifedipine exerts potent hemodynamic effects manifesting themselves by dilatation of both precapillary and postcapillary vessels, another likely mechanism is an effect on forces involved in the processes of filtration and absorption. Previous experimental findings suggest primarily an increase in capillary filtration pressure due to the different vasodilatory action of nifedipine on precapillary and postcapillary vessels (Gustafsson, 1987). In our view, the formation of oedema assooiated, in some cases, with treatment with calcium antagonists may be related to this mechanism leading to an effect on capillary transport functions.

REFERENCES:

Gustafsson, D. (1987): Microvascular mechanisms involved in calcium antagonist edema formation. J.Cardiov.Pharmacol. 10 (Suppl.1) S 121-131

Ježek,V., Ježková,J., Michaljanič,P., Niederle,P., Feureisl,R.(1990): Long-term effect of isosorbide dinitrate and nifedipine,singly and in association, in patients with chronic heart failure. Europ. Heart J. 11, 1059-1064

Opie, L.H. (1986): Fluid retention with nifedipine in antihypertensive therapy. Lancet ii, 1456
Whitney, R.J. (1953): Measurement of volume changes in human limbs. J.Physiol. (London) 121, 1.

Calcium dobesilate (doxium) in the treatment of venous insufficiency a pharmacological and clinical study

Prof. E. Altmann Canestri, O.G. Leouizamon, C. Sanchez, M. Cuocarese, O. Martin

San Fernando Hospital

In a previous experimental work on dogs the authors showed that calcium dobesilate (doxium) promotes the flow of lymph (lymphagogue action) through the thoracic. The new study has confirmed this action. Concomitantly a statistically significant increase of serum neuraminic acid and glycoproteins was noted in experimental thrombophlebitis induced in dogs by local injection of turpentine after ligation of the external iliac veins.

In man, the effect of calcium dobesilate (DOXIUM) on oedema was confirmed by measuring the ankle perimeter and with the use of a Doppler ultrasound device.

Phlébologie 92. Eds P. Raymond-Martimbeau, R. Prescott, M. Zummo.
John Libbey Eurotext, Paris © 1992, pp. 751

Result of short term antibiotic therapy with Teicoplanina in ambulatory venous and limphatic surgery

Maurizio Valeriani, Sandro Lalle

Department of Plastic Surgery, St. John Hospital, 00184 Rome, Italy.

The aim of our work was to test the efficiency of short term antibiotic therapy with Teicoplanina to prevent infections due to Gram + pathogens.
The types of operations included:

1) stripping of long and/or short saphenous vein.
2) vasectomy of the anterior group of the spermatic veins in young infertile men affected by varicocele.
3) liposuction in young women with mild limphedema of lower extremitiies.

All the patients were free from hematologic and immunitary disorders.
400 mg. of Teicoplanina was administrated intraveinously 1 hour prior to surgery and at the end of operation 80 mg. of Gentamicyn was administrated subcutaneously at the sites of the wounds.
On eighty two patients we did not observe any kind of surgical infection due to Gram + pathogens.

REFERENCES

Greenwood,D. (1988): Microbiological properties of Teicoplanin. J.Antimicrob.Chemother. 21 :1-13.

Johnson, J.D. (1980) : Antibiotic uptake by alveolar macrophages. J.Lab. Clin. Med. 95 (3):373.

Ratto,G.B. (1990): Antibiotic prophylaxis in lung cancer surgery. Lung Cancer.5 : 1-8.

Phlébologie 92. Eds P. Raymond-Martimbeau, R. Prescott, M. Zummo.
John Libbey Eurotext, Paris © 1992, pp. 752-754

Intérêt thérapeutique dans le domaine veino-lymphatique de molécules pharmacologiquement actives extraites de *justicia pectoralis Jacq*

Pierre Sainte-Luce, Henry Joseph, Régine Ramdine

Angéiologie, 26, rue Maurice Marie-Claire, 97100 Basse-Terre, Guadeloupe, France.

En médecine populaire, Justicia pectoralis Jacq (Acanthacées) possède de nombreux usages: la plante entière est utilisée pour la fabrication d'un sirop pectoral (Wong, 1976; Morton, 1977) et les feuilles fraîches entrent dans l'élaboration de cataplasme cicatrisant (Ayensu, 1981).
A Cuba et en Amérique latine, les feuilles sont utilisées pour ses propriétés sédatives.

La première étape de ce travail a consisté en l'isolement et l'identification des molécules contenues dans cette plante. Les travaux d'extraction et de purification du docteur H. JOSEPH ont permis d'identifier ces molécules.

STEROL	TRITERPENE	COUMARINE	C-GLYCOSYLFLAVONE
B-Sistérol	Lupéol	Coumarine simple	Swertisine
Stigmastérol		Ombelliférone	Swertiajaponine
		Acide Ortho-coumarique	O-Rhamnosyl-2"-Swertisine
			O-Rhamnosyl-2"-Swertiajaponine

Les flavonoïdes et les coumarines sont des molécules connues pour leurs propriétés anti-oedémateuses et anti-inflammatoires et entrent dans la composition de plusieurs spécialités pharmaceu-tiques pour ces indications.

INTERDEPENDANCE DES CIRCULATIONS D'ECHANGE ET DE RETOUR
Il existe entre les quatre secteurs impliqués dans la circulation de retour une véritable interdépendance fonctionnelle, au sens où l'équilibre fonctionnel de chacun des éléments est déterminant pour l'équilibre fonctionnel de l'ensemble.
Ce système implique des fragilités multiples qui peuvent transformer l'interdépendance fonctionnelle en interdépendance physiopathologique.

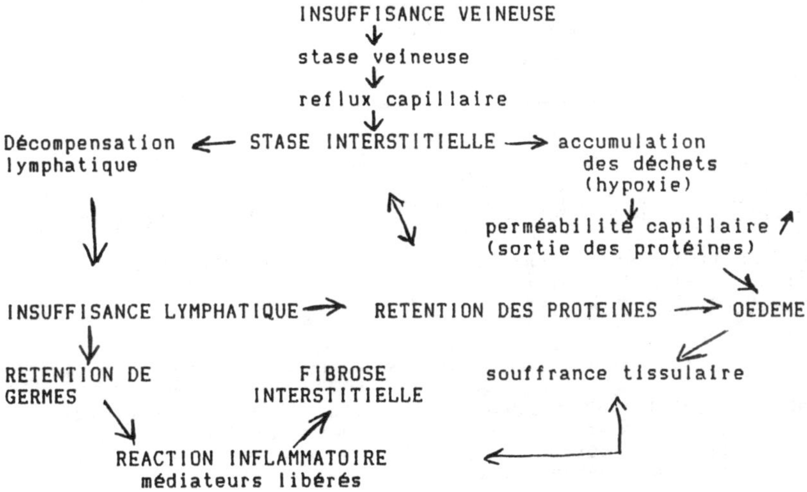

Il apparait du point de vue clinique que le mélange de coumarine et de rutine montre les meilleurs effets sur la circulation lymphatique.

On a pu montrer chez le chien que la coumarine (5,6-benzo-alpha-pyrone) entraîne au niveau du canal thoracique une importante augmentation du débit lymphatique; la coumarine ajoutée à un milieu de survie contenant un lymphangion régularise les contractions de celui-ci et augmente l'amplitude et la fréquence de celles-ci.

Ces données ont été confirmées chez l'homme (Bartos et Brzek,1970) Des études faites chez l'animal et chez l'homme (Krajnovic, 1969; Sandmann, 1971) ont permis de montrer que, lors de lymphographies, le liquide de contraste était plus rapidement transporté si l'on injectait en même temps(de façon endolymphatique, intra-veineuse ou intra-artérielle) de la coumarine.

De plus Boillot et ses collaborateurs ont observé que la coumarine augmente le retour veineux au niveau des cuisses et des pieds; il existe en effet une action vaso-dilatatrice de la coumarine , ce qui provoque une diminution des résistances périphériques (Kovack, 1960).

Une action de la coumarine est liée à la fonction des macrophages. En milieu de culture, la coumarine augmente le pouvoir de dégradation du macrophage sur les protéines de haut poids moléculaires (Bolton et Casley-Smith, 1975).

Dans les spécialités pharmaceutiques existant on peut trouver un mélange de coumarine et de rutine. De nombreux effets pharmacologiques sont attribuables à la coumarine mais il faut noter que la rutine en tant que diflavonoïde présente également une activité pharmacologique. En effet , testée seule, la rutine a montré un effet positif sur le débit lymphatique.

Nous connaissons l'importance du traitement manuel de la lymphostase: l'apport médicamenteux ne représente qu'un complément du traitement physique du lymphoedème.

Les molécules actives (coumarines et flavonoïdes) sous forme de gel, crème ou pommade associées au drainage lymphatique manuel correspond au traitement le plus rationnel et le mieux indiqué dans les pathologies de la circulation d'échanges et de retour.

Ces formes (gel, crème ou pommade) présentent un avantage : Les flavonoïdes, de part leur caractère polaire, se mélangent aisément à une phase aqueuse de type "gel" ou à une émulsion de "type" crème.

Les coumarines, au contraire sont apolaires et se mélangent au milieu huileux de type "pommade".

L'absorption de la coumarine par voie transcutanée a été vérifiée. Aussi retrouve-t-on la 7-hydroxycoumarine, principal métabolite de la coumarine dans les urines 30 minutes après l'application locale d'une préparation à base de coumarine.

Ces avantages sont résumés dans le tableau suivant :

GEL	PHASE AQUEUSE	FLAVONOIDES, coumarines
CREME	EMULSION	FLAVONOIDES, COUMARINES
POMMADE	PHASE HUILEUSE	flavonoïdes, COUMARINES

Ainsi selon que nous utiliserons une de ces trois formes, nous disposerons d'un produit dont la composition sera différente et mieux adaptée au cas traité.

LES MEDICAMENTS

Les molécules extraites de Justicia pectoralis montrent des effets positifs sur la contractilité du lymphangion et possèdent une composante anti-inflammatoire non négligeable.

De toute ces substances naturelles, les coumarines et les flavonoïdes sont les seules à présenter un profil pharmacologique leur permettant d'être actives aussi bien sur l'inflammation, la lutte anti-microbienne, la régulation de la perméabilité capillaire et la contractilité du muscle lisse veineux et lymphatique.

Aussi Justicia pectoralis, jusqu'ici utilisée pour ses propriétés cicatrisantes, nous apparait comme une plante aux potentialités nombreuses qu'il serait intéressant d'inclure dans les thérapies anti-oedèmateuses compte tenu des coumarines et de flavonoïdes identifiées chez cette Acanthacée.

Safety and Efficacy of Sodium Tetradecyl Sulphate

Wayne M. Marley, M.D.

Sodium Tetradecyl Sulphate is one of the few FDA approved sclerosants in the United States. Recently, there has been much concern about necrosis and pigmentation from use of this agent, causing many American physicians to prefer to use other sclerosants, particularly Aetoxysclerol. To evaluate the safety and efficacy of Sodium Tetradecyl Sulphate, the records of 100 patients with varicose veins and/or reticular veins and small vessel telangiectasias were reviewed. Patients were treated according to the "French school", big vein to small vein, top to bottom, after abolishing the point of maximum reflux. The diameter of veins treated ranged from 1.5 cm's to 0.05 cm's. There were no ulcerations. The incidents of pigmentation immediately post-sclerotherapy was 20 %. After six months, pigmentation was noted only in 8 1/2 % of patients. Three patients had dose related side effects that were eliminated using a lower dosage. There was one case of reported delayed urticaria six hours after injection. In summary, Sotradecol is an extremely safe and effective agent when used properly, its chief advantage being reproduceability, and the ability to treat a wide variety of vein sizes.

Phlébologie 92. Eds P. Raymond-Martimbeau, R. Prescott, M. Zummo.
John Libbey Eurotext, Paris © 1992, pp. 756-758

Pharmacokinetics of sclerosing iodine injections

Élise Bernier*, Chantal Savoie**, Emanuel Escher**

** Clinique Médico-Esthétique, 80 Vimy N., Sherbrooke (Québec) J1H 1MA, Canada, and ** Department of Pharmacology, Faculty of Medicine, University of Sherbrooke, Sherbrooke (Québec) J1H 5NA, Canada.*

Iodine is one of the most commonly used agents in the sclerotherapy of varicose veins. Its standing in time and good experience have permitted this drug to go almost unchallenged by modern research and to stay in clinical use, although the exact mode of action and the pharmacokinetics of it are poorly documented in recent literature. Sclerosing iodine (e.g. Sclerodine) is always a solution of molecular, diatomic iodine (I_2) in aqueous sodium iodide in about equal portions (w/v) at variable strength (6% to 1%). The sclerosing action of this solution on varicose veins is through the irritating, inflammation causing action of molecular iodine alone; the content of sodium iodide is needed to solubilize the molecular iodine which otherwise is not soluble in water. Molecular iodine produces iodinated proteins and, upon dilution in the blood stream, the redox-potential of blood is rapidly converting the remaining molecular iodine to its reduced iodide form which is devoid of any sclerosing action. The pharmacokinetics of inorganic iodide are quite well known in the low concentration range because of its importance to thyroid status. The toxicology of ingested high doses of iodine is also known and doses of 2g are reported to be lethal according to Gosselin et al (1976). On the other hand, the immediate and long-term pharmacokinetics of peripherally injected iodine in the concentrations needed for sclerotherapy has never been specifically addressed and therefore merits some attention.

In our contribution, we have carried out on an animal model the nuclear imaging of a i.v. injected iodine-iodide bolus and its pharmacokinetics (distribution and excretion) in time.

MATERIAL AND METHODS

For imaging purposes, male mongrel dogs of 14 kg were anesthetized (pentobarbital, 15 mg/kg i.v.) and provided with an urinary catheter. The left external saphenous vein was fitted with a butterfly catheter and the animal was placed on a γ-camera (Picker Dynacamera 4/15). A Sclerodine solution (1 ml, 1 % free iodine) was labeled with 111 MBq. of ^{131}I and immediately injected into the animal. Picture accumulation was 60/min for 1 min, further pictures were taken at every 15 min and the animal was sacrificed after 1 h. For the pharmacokinetic evaluation of iodine distribution and excretion, an identical approach was chosen but with 7.2 μCi of ^{125}I as label. The animal was kept normovelumic by an infusion of 300 ml/4 h of physiological saline for the duration of the experiment. Urine was collected at regular intervals and blood samples were drawn (cephalic vein) every 15 min or longer during 4 hours. Radioactivities were determined in a γ-counter (LKB 1271 RIA-Gamma). Thereafter, the animal was left to recover with blood, urine and stool sampling continued for up to 6 days. At the end of the experiment, the animal was sacrificed and the iodine content of target organs was analyzed by γ-counting.

RESULTS

γ-camera experiments: The iodine bolus migrated within seconds from the injection site to the general circulation. After 1 min, no measurable iodine was visible above background at the injection site and a distribution pattern typical to vascular space was obtained. This vascular distribution of the first minutes gradually changed to a more important localization in liver and at 15 min, a predominant liver localization was visible. Pharmacokinetics: The first post-injection measurement was taken at 5 min and indicated a blood concentration of 25[μM] for iodide. This corresponded to a volume of distribution of 3.15 l. During the first hour, a rapid reduction of blood iodide concentration was visible, which was then followed by a slower, linear decrease (see fig. 2). Urine iodine concentration was roughly constant throughout the experiment at 64 ± 11 [μM] until 48 h post-injection, whereupon a decrease was observed. Tissue radioactivities (liver and thyroid) were below detectable levels after autopsy.

DISCUSSION

Renal clearance of iodide has been described in the past at several occasions, however with rather contradictory results and mostly on concentrations far from those encountered during sclerotherapy (Bricker and Hlad (1955), Giebisch et al (1956), Childs et al (1950)). The generally accepted fact of pure renal excretion of iodine was however followed by disputes over active or passive glomerular filtration and about tubular reabsorption (Williamson et al (1962)). This was illustrated by an incredibly large range for the renal clearance of iodide which varies from as small as 0.05 ml/min to as large as 18 ml/min in the dog but not in man according to Giebisch et al (1956). In man, renal clearance of tracer amounts of iodide has been well studied because of its importance in thyroid function. In those cases low nanomolar ranges of iodide were examined and no oxidized i.e. molecular iodine was considered. The iodine injected during sclerotherapy is however in a good part of this latter, molecular form, capable to react with proteins to form iodinated proteins with a different pharmacokinetic for total iodide.

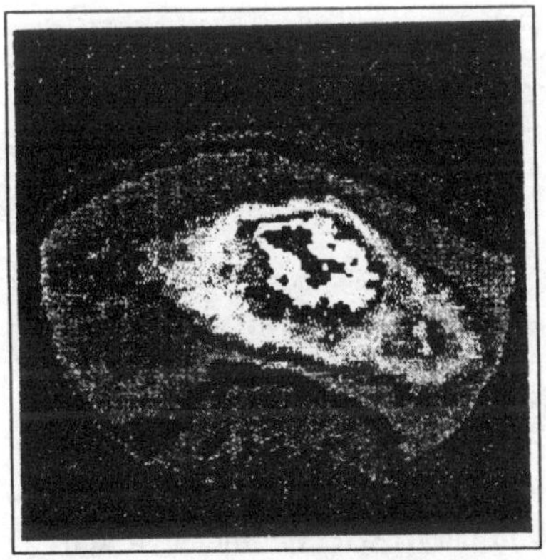

Fig. 1. *Gamma camera picture of 15 min post-injection. The animal is placed in lateral position with its shoulder at the right side, the pelvis at the left side and the back is on top of the picture. The most important radioactivity concentration is visible in the hepatic area, other areas are the heart on the right and the mesenteric bed on the left.*

The fast γ-scanning sequence (0-1 min) reveals a rapid, blood-borne distribution, closely resembling the total vascular space and, at the end, no above-background radioactivity on the injection site. The body distribution thereafter (15 min - 1 h) indicates an important liver accumulation. The rapid blood concentration decrease observed in the blood iodide content during the first hour (fig. 2) is probably this hepatic redistribution, because no increase is visible in the urine. The γ-scan confirms this behaviour with no or almost no kidney and bladder radioactivity (fig. 1). A partial reason for this is probably the presence of iodinated proteins (e.g. serum albumin) which are retained progressively in the liver and released slowly afterwards. This is in good agreement with the observed volume of distribution of more than 3 l, almost the triple of the normal blood volume (1.12 l for a 14 kg dog), and the hepatic "hot spot" in the image at 15 min (fig. 1).

The literature reports normal first order kinetics and a constant renal clearance for iodide secretion (Childs et al, 1950 and Bricker et al, 1955), others proposed variable clearance kinetics. In our experiments, the linearity of blood iodide decrease between 1 and 4 hours is however strongly suggestive

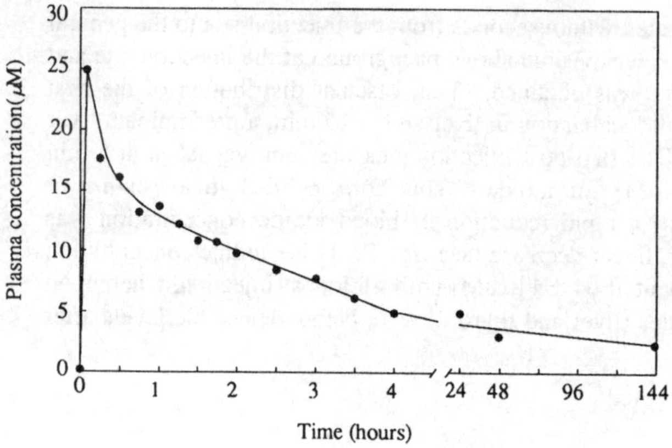

Fig. 2. *Time-course of blood iodine concentration. Blood iodide concentration is assessed from 0.3 ml samples and a specific radioactivity of 92 mCi/mol for iodine.*

of apparent zero-order kinetics with glomerular transporter saturation. This is further supported by the constant urine concentration in the first 24 hours.

The blood concentration range in which apparent zero-order kinetics occur is above 5[μM], a surprisingly low concentration for transporter saturation by a simple ionic species like iodide. Such a prolonged zero-order kinetic may have important consequences for iodide excretion after sclerotherapy with high-strength solutions for major vessels. In particular, prolonged thyroid saturation has to be considered for patients undergoing repetitive, short-interval treatments, for patients with questionable thyroid status and for patients with renal insufficiency.

ACKNOWLEDGEMENTS

We would like to thank Mr J. Rousseau for the operation of the γ-camera and Mrs L. Dionne for secretarial help. This work was supported in part by funds from the Medical Research Council of Canada.

REFERENCES

Bricker, N.S., and Hlad, C.J. Jr. (1955): Observations on the mechanism of the renal clearance of I^{131}. J. Clin. Invest. 34: 1057-1072.

Childs, D.S. Jr., Keating, F.R. Jr., Rall, J.E., Williams, M.M.D., and Power, M.H. (1950): The effect of varying quantities of inorganic iodide (carrier) on the urinary excretion and thyroidal accumulation of radioiodine in exophthalmic goiter. J. Clin. Invest. 29: 726-738.

Giebisch, G., MacLeod, B. and Kavaler F. (1956): renal excretion of radioiodide in the dog. Am. J. Physiol. 187: 529-535.

Gosselin, R.E., et al (1976): Clinical toxicology of commercial products. Sect. III, pp. 181-182. Baltimore: Williams & Wilkins, 4th edition.

Williamson, H.E., Scranton, J.R., Marshall, F.N., and Halmi, N.S. (1962): Stop flow analysis of renal tubular site of reabsorption of radioiodide in dogs. Proc. Soc. Exp. Biol. 109: 23-28.

Phlébologie 92. Eds P. Raymond-Martimbeau, R. Prescott, M. Zummo.
John Libbey Eurotext, Paris © 1992, pp. 759-761

Infectious considerations in diluting sclerosant solutions

Neil S. Sadick

772 Park Avenue, New York 10021, USA.

The objective of this study was to determine whether dilution of sclerosant is associated with an increased risk of bacterial contamination and subsequent bacterial phlebosepsis. As sclerotherapy becomes a more sophisticated discipline, different sclerosant concentrations are employed for different vessel diameters; (MSC)--minimal sclerosant concentration. With these considerations in mind, the present study was undertaken.

The study was conducted with dilutions of 23.4% NaCl to 11.7% NaCl, employing both bacteriostatic water and 0.9% normal saline. 0.5% aethoxysklerol was diluted to 0.25% utilizing bacteriostatic water; 22 gauge needles and 5 cc syringes (Smith-Kline) were employed. Cultures for aerobic, anaerobic bacteria and fungi were taken at time 0, day 1, day 7, day 14, day 28, day 56. Each solution was utilized an average of 5.5 times/week.

The results showed there were no positive cultures for bacteria or fungi in any of the aforementioned sclerosant subgroups.

In conclusion, dilution of sclerosing agents under sterile conditions is not associated with solution contamination. For hypertonic saline, utilization of normal saline or bacteriostatic water may be utilized, while with Polidocanol, bacteriostatic water is the dilutant of choice. Solvents might be screened for benzoate sensitivity when bacteriostatic water is employed.

Diluted saline, i.e., 11.7% N.S. is associated with decreased morbidity, i.e., pain, sclerotherapy pigmentation and extravasation necrosis, while producing comparable vascular obliteration comparable to 23.4% NaCl.

Dilution of sclerosing agents is safe and may produce excellent cosmetic results, while producing less morbidity then sclerosing agents of higher concentrations.

TABLE: CULTURE RESULTS OF DILUTED SCLEROSANTS

(Each sclerosant solution was utilized 10 times over given time interval)

SCLEROSANT SOLUTION	TIME INTERVAL	CULTURE RESULTS BACTERIA	CULTURE RESULTS FUNGAL
23.4 HS	Day 1	--	--
	Week 1	--	--
	Week 2	--	--
	Week 3	--	--
	Week 4	--	--
	Week 8	--	--
11.7 HS diluted with bacteriostatic water	Day 1	--	--
	Week 1	--	--
	Week 2	--	--
	Week 3	--	--
	Week 4	--	--
	Week 8	--	--
11.7 HS diluted with 0.9%NS	Day 1	--	--
	Week 1	--	--
	Week 2	--	--
	Week 3	--	--
	Week 4	--	--
	Week 8	--	--
0.5% POL	Day 1	--	--
	Week 1	--	--
	Week 2	--	--
	Week 3	--	--
	Week 4	--	--
	Week 8	--	--
0.25% POL diluted with bacteriostatic water	Day 1	--	--
	Week 1	--	--
	Week 2	--	--
	Week 3	--	--
	Week 4	--	--
	Week 8	--	--
1.0%STS	Day 1	--	--
	Week 1	--	--
	Week 2	--	--
	Week 3	--	--
	Week 4	--	--
	Week 8	--	--
0.5% STS diluted with bacteriostatic water	Day 1	--	--
	Week 1	--	--
	Week 2	--	--
	Week 3	--	--
	Week 4	--	--
	Week 8	--	--

REFERENCES

Graham, D.R., Keldermasz, M.M., Klemm, L.W., Demenza N.J., Shafer, M.L. (1991): Infectious Applications Among Patients Receiving Home Intravenous Therapy with Peripheral Control or Peripherally Placed Central Venous Catheters. Am J Med. 91 (Supplement 3B) 955-1005.

Mesotherapy its application in phlebology

César F. Sanchez, Prof. E. Altmann-Canestri, R. Barcelo, N. Rosli, U.Tropper

Mesotherapy is a new and simple therapeutic concept that introduces the medication into the area of the pathology by means of minimum and regional intradermic doses.

The equipment used to administer the mixtures is quite varied, but their purpose is always the same: to introduce medication into the dermis at about 4 mm depth. This may be performed with complex devices (Den Hub, Pistormatic, Dermojet, Mesoflash, etc.) or simply with a syringe and a label needle.

The mesotherapeutic mixtures are made of a constant substance, i.e., procaine or lidocaine, and variable substances, according to the pathology to be treated. All the substances used appear in the dictionary of pharmaceutical specialities. This dependence tightly ties the mesotherapy to the allopathy.

As an example, some of the mixtures used in France and those currently used in our country appear below.

French Mixtures

PERIDIL-HEPARINE (R)	1 ml
ESSERIVEN (R)	1/2 amp
Thiomucase	2 vials
MADECASSOL (R)	1 amp
Procaine 1%	1 ml

Phlébologie 92. Eds P. Raymond-Martimbeau, R. Prescott, M. Zummo.
John Libbey Eurotext, Paris © 1992, pp. 763-764

Mesodermal treatment by calcic heparin in recurrent lymphangitis due to post-thrombotic syndrome : two years follow-up

R. D'Alterio, R. Gloria, E. Marchitelli, R. Pepe, R. Musso

Service of Angiology, S. Eugenio Hospital, USL RM/7 Rome, P. le dell' Umanesimo n° 10,00144, Rome, Italy .

INTRODUCTION

Lymphangitis is a frequent complication of the Post Thrombotic Syndrome above the chronic dermo hypodermitis;it is secondary to the microvascular alterations subsequent to the chronical venous hypertension.
Generally the clinical characteristics of this kind of patology are rapresen- -ted by red,hot,painful plaques or striations which induces a faster evolu- -tion of the sclerotic dermitis.
The difficult in the treatment of this patology is well known,specially during the phases of phlogistic recidivations,moreover the fibrin cuff limits the diffusion of the pharmacological substances to the connectivum and to the interstitial spaces,but also the collateral effects due to the topical subministration of drugs limits routine clinical use of this kind of terapy.
Among the drugs normally used,the Calcic Heparin,for its properties (antithrombotic,antiinflammatory,profibrinolitic,anticoagulant),seems to have some advantages.
The aim of the study was to control the long-term efficacy of a single mesodermal treatment by Calcic Heparin in a group of ten patients affected by recurrent lymphangitis in chronic post thrombotic dermo-hypodermitis.

MATHERIAL AND METHODS

Ten patients,female,medium age 48 years were submitted once a week for ten times to a mesodermal treatment by Calcic Heparin,at dosage of 5000-10000 I.U.,mixed with Xylocaine HCl 1 ml.and bidistilled Water,using a linear multiinjector,27 G needles,Luer Cone.
The clinical evaluetion was made giving an arbitrary attribute(from 0 to 4 in ascending value) to the most characteristical symptoms:pain,phlogosis (plaques and striations extension,cutaneous temperature),degree of the basal fibrosis and the cutaneous pigmentation.
The treatment consisted in two phases,in the first the subministration of Calcic Heparin was made once a week for ten weeks;after this phase of treatment were registered the results obtained and the patients entered in second phase of follow-up,which consisted in clinical controls every six

months for two years,evaluating:the eventual recidivations,the time after the treatment in which appeared,and the persistance of the clinical results.

CLINICAL RESULTS

During the first phase only one patients (10%) stopped the treatment for allergical complications.

In two cases (20%) wasn't necessary to end the treatment for the early diseappering of the clinical symptoms.

The 70% of the subjects showed a relevant improvement of all the clinical parameters considered.

The follow-up has shown a good long-term maintenance of the clinical results;only two patients referred a recurrence of lymphangitis,all the others refferred a persistance of the amelioration of the clinical results obtained after the first phase of therapy.The two patients affected by clinicall recidivation (one after 18 months,the other after 24 months from the endig of first phase) were again treated by subministration of Calcic Heparin (three times for each,once a week) and the symptoms quickly disapperead .

CONCLUSIONS

The relevant clinical amelioration,the very low incidence of collateral effects,the relative simple tecnique used,in confrontation with the well known difficulties of treatment of this kind of patology make us continuing to use this method on a larger casistic.

We must understrike the persistance of the clinical improvement perhaps for the long term action of Calcic Heparin in the targed zone.

REFERENCES

-BRONCHI G.F.,CARINI A.:Trattamento topico delle ulcere venose degli arti inferiori con eparina calcica somministrata per via mesodermica.

-MERLEN J.F.,COGET J.,SARTEEL A.M..:Pigmentation et stase veineuse . Phlebologie,36(4),307-314,1983.

- SCHMIDT C.,SCHMIDT J. et al.: Haemodynamics of the post phlebitic syndrome.Angiology 1987 6(2),187-192.

- SOPIN G.:Traitement classique des troubles trophique des syndrome post phlebitique.Phlebologie,37(4),483-489,1984.

B.
SCLÉROTHÉRAPIE
SCLÉROTHERAPY

a. Varices technique et résultats / *Varices technique and results*

Phlébologie 92. Eds P. Raymond-Martimbeau, R. Prescott, M. Zummo.
John Libbey Eurotext, Paris © 1992, pp. 769-770

Sclerotherapy versus surgery in the treatment of varicose vein in Poland (1991) in various age groups

Krystyna Twardowska-Saucha, Dariusz Czaczka, Monika Moniuszko*

*Varicose Vein Clinic-Medservice, 44-100 Gliwice, Konstytucji St. 10/2, Poland and * Mayfield Square Medicenter, 10 456 Mayfield Road, Edmonton, Alberta T5P 4P4, Canada.*

INTRODUCTION

Literature coming from America, Japan, Africa and Europe supply us with data concerning different frequency of varicose vein occurrence in the above mentioned parts of the world (Belcaro, 1986),(Hirai at al., 1990), (Quaile,1986), (Thelsius et al.,1986).
There is not much data describing the varicose vein occurrence in different age groups. Consequently, the analysis of the specific methods of treatment depending on the age of the patients is not presented either.
Sclerotherapy and day surgery for varicose veins are exciting therapeutic options offered to our patients in the Varicose Vein Clinic in Zabrze, Poland. It is the first one in our country in operation since January, 1991.

METHODS

Our treatment protocol is based on history, physical examination of venous system and noninvasive venous Doppler reflux studies.We pay particular attention to the saphenofemoral and saphenopopliteal junctions (SFJ and SPJ, respectively). We recommend surgery (ligation and limited stripping) as an initial treatment to the patients with saphenous incompetence, and sclerotherapy for treatment of nonsaphenous and residual veins.

RESULT

We examined and treated 836 patients between age 10-89 (93.1% were female and 6.9% were male). 43.4% of the patients (93.1% were women) were treated by sclerotherapy. Surgery was carried out on 48.8% of the patients (85.2% were women).
The majority of our patients (66.4%) were in the 30-49 age group. Sclerotherapy was most often applied on young women in the 10-29 age bracket. Between ages 30-39 both methods were applied almost equally, with slight predomination of surgery (50.1% versus 49.9%).

In the age group past 40, we observed a significant increase in the number of patients with incompetent SFJ and SPJ which required surgical treatment (Table 1).

Table 1. Frequency of varicose veins treatment by means of sclerotherapy versus surgery in various age groups.

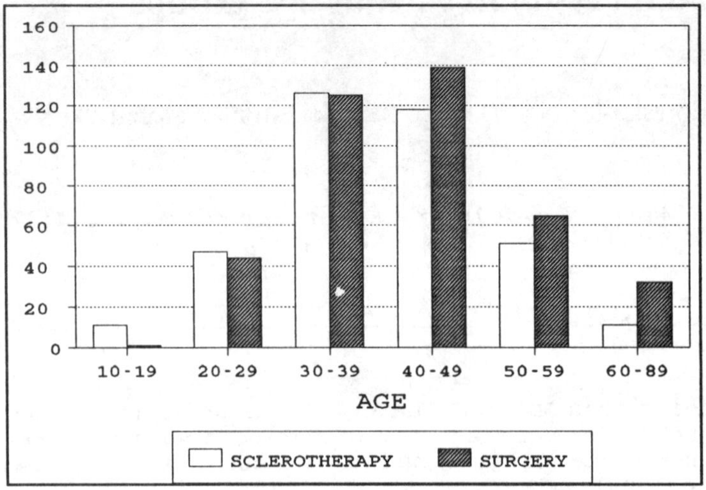

CONCLUSION

Varicose disease is an ongoing process progressing with time and age of the patient. The age of the patient is a good indicator of the type of initial treatment they will need.
Questions that arise, are the dynamics of hemodynamic deterioration of venous system in other countries comparable with our findings.
What is the significance of the age factor as compared with nationality,race and lifestyle factors?
What is the frequency of saphenous versus nonsaphenous primary pathology in other countries.

REFERENCE

Belcaro, G.V. (1986):Saphenofemoral incompetence in young asymptomatic subjects with a family history of varices of the lower limbs. In *Phlebology 85*, ed. D. Negus & G. Jantet, pp. 65-79. John Libbey & Co. Ltd.

Hirai, M. at al.,(1990): Prevalence and risk factors of varicose veins in Japanese Women. *Angiology*. 3:228-232.

Quaile, A. (1986): A retrospective study of the epidemiology and treatment of varicose veins. In *Phlebology 85*, ed. D. Negus & G. Jantet, pp.85-91. John Libbey & Co. Ltd.

Thelsius, D. et al. (1986): Incidence of venous disease in Kuwait (1984).In *Phlebology 85*, ed. D. Negus & G.Jantet, pp.99-103. John Libbey & Co. Ltd.

SCLEROTHERAPY BASING ON VEIN PERCUSSION TEST AND TPM /TOE-PLETHYSMOMETRY/

S. Fontányi, Z. Fontányi

Department of Surgery "A", Péterfy S. Hospital and Military Health Service, Budapest, Hungary

The popularity of sclerotherapy is more and more increasing. The usual indications extend recently to the truncular typs. Method: In screening the vein percussion test modified by us in detection deep lying truncs and injections site during the treatment as well as the TPM to examine deep vein patency, measuring venous pressure non-invasively, proved to be useful. In horizontal position eliminating hydrostatic pressure, even a slight rise referrs to flux insufficiency.
Material: 322 limbs of 221 patients /male 36, female 185; mean age 54, ranges 20-80; previous surgery 56, sclerotherapy 42/.
Technique: For the 3018 injections /foot 295, leg 2103, thigh 687/ 4059 ml of Sclerovein /%: 0,5: 313, 1: 496, 2: 624, 3: 1428, 5: 1198 ml/ have been consumed, placed at our disposal by AG Resinag, Zürich, to gain experiences. The presclerotherapeutic venous state displaying sketches /laid out on plain-surface/ completed by marking injections sites represent the sclerotherapeutic map, serving for documentation of carrying out therapy and for base in follow-up.
Result: After 9 injections/limb /ranges 1-48/ 17 limbs underwent repeated sclerotherapy, 1 surgery for recurrency.

Phlébologie 92. Eds P. Raymond-Martimbeau, R. Prescott, M. Zummo.
John Libbey Eurotext, Paris © 1992, pp. 772

Sclerotherapy and digital photoplethysmography (D-PPG)

Jaroslav Strejček

Dermatological Clinic I, Charles University, Prague 12800 Prague 2, Vyšehradská 49, Czechoslovakia.

We are presenting the results of the clinical use of D-PPG, before, during and after sclerotherapy with a group of 237 persons treated in 1989 - 1991. We emphasize especially the importance of the D-PPG examination to differentiate the patients with so-called "non improvable" chronic venous insufficiency (19,8 %) by the test with tourniquet. In this type of CVI any active treatment of varices is without hemodynamic importance.

The treatment of now reduced group of patients (190) by means of sclerotherapy was finished according to the at present used criteria (the clinical and ultrasonic ones). Using D-PPG we, however, found out that 23,1 % of patients do not show sufficiently improved functional venous parameters so far. The results of the D-PPG examination become a new impulse for a continuation in sclerotherapy, that the resulting hemodynamic effect - beeing the main expected result of the treatment - would be as good as possible. That is why the Digital Photoplethysmography shows as a necessary and useful method in all outpatients, where the examination and treatment of varices is performed.

REFERENCES

Strejček, J. (1992): Die Kontrolle des hämodynamischen Effekts der Sklerotherapie mit Hilfe der D-PPG. In Fortschritte in der computerunterstützten nichtinvasiven Gefässdiagnostik. Berichte des 3. Internationalen Symposiums CNVD´91, eds. V. Blazek und U. Schultz-Ehrenburg, pp. 29-33. Düsseldorf: VDI Verlag.

Phlébologie 92. Eds P. Raymond-Martimbeau, R. Prescott, M. Zummo.
John Libbey Eurotext, Paris © 1992, pp. 773-775

Can duplex be useful in the choice of the sclerotherapy technique ?

P. Pavei, A. Gongolo, P. Sorrentino, P. Borelli, G. Sovernigo, E. Tiso, U. Baccaglini

Clinica Chirurgica I, University of Padova, Italy, Presidio Ospedaliero Dolo, Venezia, Italy.

The scope of the study, carried out from 1988 to 1991 on 90 patients suffering from great saphenous vein varices, was the identification by means of Duplex of morphological and fluxmetrical elements, useful for the choice of the sclerotherapy treatment to be used.

PATIENTS

Between 1988 and 1991 we have selected 90 patients, treated with sclerotherapy in order to study them with Duplex.
All the patients had great saphenous vein varices and they were: 69 women and 31 men between 25 and 68 of age (47 on average).

MATERIALS AND TECHNIQUES

All the 90 patients were studied with Duplex equipped with real-time probe of 7.5 MHz frequency and doppler of 5 MHz. The Duplex test has been performed with patient in orthostatism position and it has been carried out both an ultrasound study with transversal and longitudinal scannings of the great saphenous vein and fluxmetrical mappings by means of the classical dynamic tests of compression and relaxation, the Valsalva manoeuvre and a cough.
In our study we considered: the morphology and the diameter of the saphenous-femoral junction (3), the vein morphology (tortuous or straight), the kind of venous wall (thick or thin) and the presence/entity of the reflux.
Considering these characteristics, the patients have been subdivided in two groups:

a) 43 patients with saphenous-femoral junction and tortuous veins with slight and medium reflux have been treated with a sclerotherapy starting from the top;
b) 47 patients with ampullary or straight junction and rectilinear vein in the thigh have been treated with sclerotherapy starting from the bottom.

The patients with rectilinear vein, thick wall and high reflux have been operated and not included in this study.
For the sclerotherapy we used the iodine-potassium iodide solution with variable concentration from 2 to 8% and the sodium tetradecil-sulphate with variable concentration from 1 to 3%.

The substance type and its concentration depend on the capacity and caliber of the vein to be treated. The treatment has been performed with a number of sittings included between 3 and 6 (4 on average).
The Duplex test has been performed at the end of the therapy. The patients have been re-examined with Duplex test within a period of six months, one year and two years to verify the effectiveness of the therapy. The presence of reflux and sclerosis effects (thick walls, reduction of vein caliber, disappearance or reduction of the reflux, endolumen thrombosis) have been observed (1, 4, 5, 6).
The patients follow-up was 12-36 months (24 on average).

RESULTS

At the post-sclerotherapy Duplex examination, we observed:
42 complete sclerosis with total obliteration and incompressibility of the vasal lumen, absence of internal flux and reflux, with evident endolumenal echoes and iperhecogenicity of the vein wall. (6).
Obviously the echographic success is connected to a good clinical result.
Echographic sclerosis signs in the vein wall with lumen incompressibility and presence of flux without reflux in 33 cases.
Successful clinical results but with lumen compressibility and flux and reflux in 15 cases.
Total therapy failure in 10 cases.
Therefore, the sclerosing therapy results, performed on 90 patients in accordance with the morphological and functional data pointed out with Duplex, are the following:

- 75 successful sclerosis, even if a venous flux has been noticed in 33 patients;
- 15 sclerosis with good clinical result, i.e. with disappearance of vein varices and presence of a fibrous cord but instrumental confirmation of poor sclerosis effects with reflux.
- Sclerosis failure in 10 cases.

DISCUSSION

The sclerotherapy of the great saphenous vein is still considered an insufficient and dangerous technique. (2)
Such opinion is certainly due to the fact that this therapy depended upon the phlebologist, without the possibility to base the choice of drug and its concentration on objective elements.
The Duplex utilization in the study of the venous desease has allowed new openings because it is possible to perform a suitable follow up of such therapy and to obtain exact data about the morphology and the fluxmetry of the vein to be treated (1,2,4,5).
In the patients with varicose veins and slight or medium reflux a scleroterapy technique starting from the saphenous-femoral junction has been performed.
On the contrary, for the rectilinear veins in the thigh, always with slight-medium reflux, we choose a sclerotherapy starting from the bottom (according to the technique of Sigg) in order both to reduce the speed and the reflux entity and to avoid the "washing" effect of the drug injection in the thigh.
On the basis of Duplex data we excluded from sclerosing treatment the patients with rectilinear veins, straight junction or with a diameter higher than one centimeter and high grade reflux.
So in 83% of cases we have been able to obtain good results and to complete the treatment in 15 patients with relapse to Duplex control.

CONCLUSIONS

Most Authors consider now that the clinical evaluation of the varicose disease is inadequate for a correct diagnosis and, as per our opinion, for a correct choice of the therapy.
The Duplex examination, thanks to its innocuity and its repeatability, has to be utilized in the study of the varicose disease in order to supply the morphologic and fluxmetrical elements which are necessary for the phlebologist in order to choose the most suitable sclerotherapy technique.
Moreover its repeatability allows an adequate follow-up of the therapy, mentionning the progressive results that have been obtained and the moment in which the sclerotherapy can be considered complete.

REFERENCES

Avramovic A., De Simone J.C., Avramovic M., Brizzio E. (1989): Evaluation de la sclerose de la crosse et du tronc de la saphene interne grace a l'echotomographie. Phlebologie 89, A. Davy, R. Stemmer eds. John Libbey Eurotext Ltd, 834-835.

Bishop C.C.R, Fronek H.S., Fronek A. et Al. (1991): Real time color duplex scanning following Sclerotherapy of the great saphenous vein. J. Vasc. Surg., 13-16.

De Simone J.G, Brizzio E. (1988): Etude du confluence veineux sapheno femoral par echotomographie. Phebologie 41, 449-460.

Schadeck M.: Etude par doppler et echotomographie de l'evolution des saphenes sous traitement sclerosant. Comunication au XIX Congres de Pathologie Vasculaire: Paris, 16 Mars 1985

Schadeck M. (1987): Doppler and echotomography in sclerosis of the saphenous veins. Phebologie 2, 221-240.

Schadeck M., Allaer F. (1991): Echotomographie de la sclerose. Phlebologie 44;1, 111-130.

DUPLEX RESULTS AFTER SUCCESSFUL GREAT SAPHENOUS VEIN SCLEROTHERAPY

*A. Gongolo, *E. Giraldi, *G. Spreafico, P. Pavei, G. Sovernigo, P. Sorrentino e U. Baccaglini
Clinica Chirurgica I, Universita' di Padova
*Presidio Ospedaliero Dolo -Venezia, Italy

The Authors evaluate the late results of the sclerotherapy of the great saphenous vein with Duplex. The evaluation (average follow-up 22 months), on 90 patients, clinically healted after the sclerosing treatment, shows a wide range of results: a) persistence of relux without ecographic signes of sclerosis of the vein (12/90); reduction of the lumen with parietal thickness both endo and extraluminal but with persistence of reflux (35/90); c) incomplete sclerosis because of the uninvolvement of the saphenous femoral junction and presence of phisyological flux (20/90); d) complete sclerosis with vasal lumen occlusion (23/90). Du[plex investigation is therefore used as an instrumental support to the clinical evaluation of the sclerotherapy effect. Patients with a good clinical sclerotherapy presentec different Duplex situations and only 23/90 patients had a complete sclerosis of the long saphenous vein.

Modern Indications of Sclerotherapy

Dr.med. H.E.Gerlach

Office of Vascular Deseases,
T 6,25 6800 Mannheim, Germany

Today indication of Sclerotherapy must not only focus on apparent external outcomes of a venous desease but a complete up-to-date and not invasive diagnostic with Doppler Ultrasound and Duplexsonography, completed by tests of venous function, has to clarify if larger transfasciale insufficiencies exist.
Those are mostly the starting-points of a so-called Recirculationcircle which should be removed surgically for a better long-term result. Clinical examples will be shown.

Afterwards small varicous veins can be treated by sclerotherapy. Various absolute and relative contraindications exist for a sclerotherapy.

Principles and Treatment of Sclerotherapy

Dr.med. H.E.Gerlach

Office of Vascular Deseases,
T 6,25 6800 Mannheim, Germany

To do the sclerousing injection only at an oedema free leg is the first principle.
While the injection is done the patient is lying. Make injections first to lager and then to smaller varicous veins, from proximal to distal. The concentration of sclerousing medication depends on the size of the vericous veins.
Treatments may take place every other day.

The aftertreatment is extremely important for the result of the sclerotherapy.
A compression bandage is applied after the sclerotherapy.
The duration of the compression therapy depends on the size of the atrophied varicous veins: it needs only a few hours after sclerotherapy of spider veins up to maximally two weeks for lager superficial veins.
For the patint it is more convenient to use a compress stocking together with a bloodstaunching tape right after sclerotherapy.
This statement is base on ten years of practice with more than 10,000 annual sclerotherapies following this treatment.

"COMPRESSION - SCLEROTERAPY"

Dr.Hans R. Bernbach, Ch-6900 Lugano-Viale Carlo Cattaneo 25- Switzerland.

Basing on Karl Sigg's principles this injection-compression technique is shown in detail.
The safety-mechanisms to prevent serious complications are listed. Wuppermanns theory of wall-destruction is explained.
The economical point of view in treating varicose veins is stressed upon.

NOTRE OPINION SUR LA SCLEROTHERAPIE COMME METHODE DE TRAITEMENT DES VARICES DES MEMBRES INFERIEURS.

Dr.Serban Radulescu,Prof.Dr.Aurel Andercou,Dr.Clara Mironiuc

CLINICA CHIRURGIE Nr.II, UNIVERSITATEA DE MEDICINA CLUJ, ROMANIA.

La sclérothérapie a son lieu bien défini dans le traitement des varices des membres inférieurs, s'adressant aux varices simples, disséminées, sans incontinence ostiale et un système nerveux profond perméable.

En Roumanie la phlébologie n'existe pas encore en tant que spécialité indépendante, et la sclérothérapie est effectué par un chirurgien vasculaire exercé.

Dans la 2e Clinique Chirurgicale de l'Université de Cluj nous avons employé la sclérothérapie dans trois circonstances: traitement indépendant, traitement adjuvant postopératoire et traitement associé intraopératoire.

Sur un groupe de 1000 patients avec varices, chez 252 on a appliqué la sclérothérapie avec solutions hypertoniques, détergents ou substances caustiques.

Les meilleurs résultats ont été obtenus dans les cas bien selectionnés et dans ceux où on a employé l'aetoxysclérol.

Safety angle in sclerotherapy

César F. Sánchez, MD, E. Canestri, MD, O. Leguizamon, MD, U. Tropper, MD

"Dr. César F. Sánchez" Phlebology clinic

The authors show by means of phlebographies and cinephlebographies the behavior of a radiopaque substance when injected in the surface venous system in a varicose patient, in standing position, lying down, lying down with the lower member at 90° and 45° in relation to the stretcher level. They demonstrate the benefits of sclerotherapy when observing the Safety Angle of 45° described by them.

La sclerothérapie cathéter dans le traitments des varices les mémbres inférieures.

M.Yu.Bogachev,G.D.Constantynova,S.M.Ignathenko, N.G.Gordadze.

L'univèrcité de medecin de Russia.

La venèctomie traditionnelle a quelques insuffisances:le traumades nerfs adjacents,le trauma des collèctores lymphatiques,qui accompagnent la vena saphena magna et vena saphena parva,et outre cela insuffisant cosmetique d'intervention,qui a déterminé d'indispensabilité d'incisio complémentaire.En alternative de methode traditionnelle nous employons la sclerothérapie cathéter des veines subcutanées par la méthode suivante:après de la réalisation d'opérations d'opération d'isolement,qui insére crosséctomie avec l'incision des veines perforantes insuffisantes,nous introduisons,rétrogradement,le cathéter vasculaire dans la veine et emplissons dans le tronc et l'affluents principales les solutions de 1-2% aethoxysklerolі où 3% decilati.La compressios élastique se réalise pendant deux semaines.L'expérience dans le traitment des 152 malades /184 membres inferieures/ a l l'aide de cette méthode,qui nous proposons,témoigne de la grande effectivité de ces moyen dans le traitment des varices les membres inferieures.

Phlébologie 92. Eds P. Raymond-Martimbeau, R. Prescott, M. Zummo.
John Libbey Eurotext, Paris © 1992, pp. 779

Sclerotherapy-16 years of experience

Angelo Scuderi

« Inspecmoc », Inst. Soroc. de Pesq. de Molestias Circulatorias, Caixa Postal 493, Sorocaba 18001 SP, Brasil.

The author refers his experience in the last 16 years working in a small city. During this period he made more than 15000 applications of sclerotherapy. In our country, due to the hot climate the main indication of sclerotherapy is aesthetical in the small veins or telangectasies. Rarely this treatment is made in great or dilated veins. In these cases he normaly prefers the surgical procedures. Lately, with the new sclerotherapic agents,(Polidocanol-Aethoxysklerol, Varigloban, and the Monoetanolamina-Ethamolin) he can also make sclerotherapy in big veins, mainly when the surgical procedures do not have good indications as old age, other pathologies and if the patient doesn´t want to be submitted to the surgery. The telangiectasies requires special attention due to the complications, principally the ulcers. In all groups of patients and procedures, the author refers only 5 (five) cases of these complications. These complications were due to tecnical error in the begining of the profession-high pressure and high speed of injection-. For more than 12 years the author doesn´t have this type of complication. Another type of complication refered by many authors is the hiperpigmentation. In the experience of the author this fact ocurred in only 18 cases. The author never had cases of Deep Venous Thrombosis. However, the superficial thrombosis in the specific vein is commom specially when the sclerotherapy was made in great veins. The pain of this therapic procedure was reduced a lot with the the new sclerotherapic agents and with the new combinations of the drugs. The conclusion of the author is that the scleroterapy is a very important way of treatment when well indicated and practically without complications.

Phlébologie 92. Eds P. Raymond-Martimbeau, R. Prescott, M. Zummo.
John Libbey Eurotext, Paris © 1992, pp. 780

The non-surgical treatment of varicose veins

Louis A. Ivey, D. Brian McDonagh

Vein Clinics of America, 5454 Wisconsin Avenue, Suite 1625, Chevy Chase, Maryland 20815, USA.

Twenty-five patients with 2 cm or greater varicose veins are presentedin three year follow-up to treatment using refined compression sclerotherapy. These patients range in age from 25 to 58. All were symptomatic, and their veins obvious at the start of treatment, and are all asymptomatic and cosmetically improved at the completion of treatment.

Materials: 1% and 3% Sodium Tetradecyl Sulfate
Three inch compression wraps

Methods: The anatomy of the pathologic vein was identified and proposed sites of injection were marked. Initial injections were from the highest point of incompetency to the distal most position, emptying the vein by gravity first. Compression was then applied and maintained over a seven week period.

Conclusion: Compression sclerotherapy for varicose veins is excellent.

LA SCLEROTHERAPIE SELON SIGG ET TOURNAY: LES DEUX METHODES EN COMPARAISON DANS NOTRE EXPERIENCE

Farina M.A., Aversano V., Paternosto D., Consiglio L.*

I Divisione di Chirurgia Generale - Sez. Agg. di Chirurgia Vascolare
Ospedale Multizonale di Caserta - *Div.Chir. Ospedale di Cortona (AR)

Abstract

Les auteurs presentent leur casuistique personelle de sclérothérapie exécutée dans la période comprise entre janvier 1981 et avril 1990, en illustrant les téchniques utilisées (école française et allemande) et les résultats obtenus sur 900 patients (731 f. et 169 m.) âgés de 18 à 71.

Pour un très bon traitement de la insuff'isence veineuse des membres inf'érieurs dans ses phases évolutives, une approche clinique et instrumental est sans doute la meilleure présupposition.

Au point de vue thérapeutique, la sclérothérapie a un rôle fondamental dans les différentes méthodes surtout après l'opération de saphènectomie.

Les patients sous notre observation dans la période susdite ont été soumis à traitement sclétothérapique par les deux méthodes avec prédilection pour la méthode française.

On n'a pas remarqué les complications décrites en littérature.

Selon les résultats obtenus dans le groupe des patients traités par la sclérothérapie, on peut conf'irmer la validité de la méthode française et ses avantages sur la téchnique de Sigg, soit sur les varices restantes, récidives et évolutives, soit surtout comme complétement de la intervention de saphènectomie.

En outre le bas prix et la simplicité d'exécution dans les deux méthodes se placent à côté des avantages esthétiques et fonctionnels en comparaison du traitement seulement chirurgical traditionnel.

Phlébologie 92. Eds P. Raymond-Martimbeau, R. Prescott, M. Zummo.
John Libbey Eurotext, Paris © 1992, pp. 782-785

Sclerotherapy techniques - video text

Pauline Raymond-Martimbeau, Jean-Luc Dupuis

Dallas Non-Invasive Vascular Laboratory, 8226 Douglas, suite 609, Dallas, Texas 75225

Various injection techniques and sclerosing agents are used to induce permanent sclerosis in the saphenous veins - the greater and lesser saphenous veins - the perforating veins, which unite the superficial and deep venous systems, the reticular and feeder veins and the telangiectasias.

How to recognize greater saphenous incompetence

The existence of greater saphenous incompetence can be determined through clinical examination using visual inspection, palpation, and percussion. Percussion is used to obtain a tactile impression of the blood rebounding at the site of valvular incompetence. This clinical examination makes it possible to identify the main points of reflux. To objectively assess these points of reflux, it is absolutely essential to visualize them with Duplex ultrasound.

We can observe a transverse view of the superficial and deep femoral arteries, as well as the common femoral vein being compressed with the probe. Doppler signals are used to determine venous patency.

The imaging shows a sapheno-femoral junction with the ostial valve in motion. Malfunction of this valve causes an inversion of blood flow and dilation of the greater saphenous vein. In the assessment of the greater saphenous vein with Duplex ultrasound, it is imperative to locate the external pudendal arteries, so that they are not accidentally injected later on. Here we can see these arteries on either side of the greater saphenous vein.

Tributaries must also be evaluated, as some types of terminations can cause post-sclerotherapeutic relapses.

After the complete clinical and non-invasive examinations have been carried out, the highest point of reflux of the greater saphenous vein must be injected. We can now see the incompetent sapheno-femoral junctional valve.

How to treat sapheno-femoral incompetence

When treating sapheno-femoral incompetence, the risk of complications can be reduced by injecting below the sapheno-femoral junction, away from the risky arterial zone.

Appropriate major sclerosing agents, disposable syringes and needles, and bandaging material should be used for this treatment.

An emergency kit containing epinephrine, local anaesthetics, anti-coagulants, corticoids, antihistamines, I.V. perfusion and a resuscitator must always be readily available. The patient may be in either standing or sitting position when the sapheno-femoral junction is injected.

Percussion should be used to ascertain the site of injection, a little dabbing with alcohol is all that is required before the vein is punctured.

In a standing position, a 25-gauge, 5/8 inch butterfly needle is used to give an injection below the sapheno-femoral junction. Digital compression is applied at the junction and below the site of injection. The right index finger must always be positioned so as to relieve the left finger if necessary.

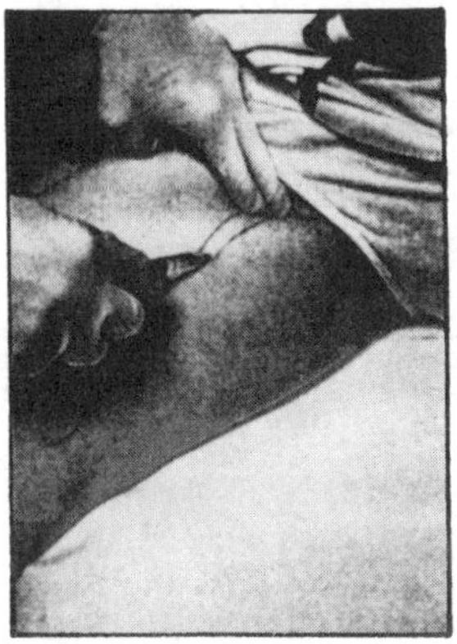

Fig. 1 - Injection below the junction in a sitting position.

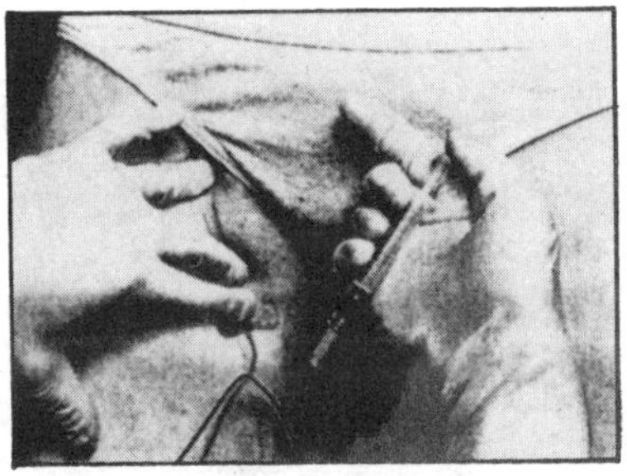

Fig. 2 - Injection below the junction in a standing position.

In the sitting position, while digital compression is applied at the junction only, the greater saphenous vein is injected below the junction with a 25-gauge, 5/8 inch standard needle.

When using the standing position technique, the junction can also be compressed with the right hand.

Once the injection is completed, the limb is elevated to ensure that the sclerosing agent makes complete contact with the junction. A local compressive dressing is applied for 48 hours and an elastic bandage for 2 weeks.

We will now discuss the injection of the sapheno-femoral junction with the patient in the standing position. The leg is abducted and rotated externally. Percussion is continued until there is perfect tactile perception of the site of injection.

If there is any doubt about the feeling of the site of injection, the injection should not be administered.

When the patient's stability and the site of injection have been ascertained, the fingers are placed so as to apply compression in order to sequester the saphenous trunk.

The puncture must be brisk and without hesitation so as to prevent venous spasm. The needle used must not be too thin or too long, in order to ensure that the arteries or the deep veins are not accidentaly punctured.

After the needle has been inserted, it is necessary to check the color of the blood and for signs of arterial pulsation. The injection should be made very slowly, and must be stopped whenever the patient experiences pain.

At mid-injection, it is important to check the stability of the needle in the vein.

The last cc of liquid must be injected rapidly so as to increase contact with the junctional intima and prevent spasm.

Once the injection has been completed, the needle should be withdrawn quickly. A drop of medication on the skin could induce skin necrosis at the site of injection.

While compression is still being maintained at the junction, the patient should lie down immediately and elevate the limb. A compressive dressing is then applied with wide tape.

A 4" tensor elastic bandage must be applied from the toe to the knee for daywear, and walking is prescribed.

Injection protocol

The injection protocol will now be described. For this treatment it is important to master the use of at least two major sclerosing agents.

When iodine solution is used, the concentration is increased progressively at each of the first three visits: however, the volume is always the same. If no sclerosis occurs, distal injections are added during the fourth and fifth visits.

The protocol for STD is similar to the one for iodine. If a 5% solution is unavailable, the iodine protocol should be followed during the third visit.

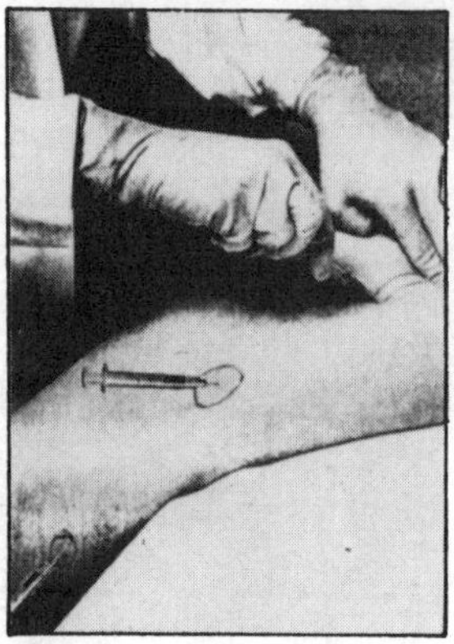

Fig. 3 - Sommation technique

A Duplex ultrasound post-sclerotherapy assessment is essential for the localization and assessment of venous changes.

This transverse ultrasound image demonstrates an echocharacteristic sclerotic reaction brought on by the presence of heterogeneous material within the lumen of the non-compressible greater saphenous vein, as well as a specific increase in the density of the venous walls. In this longitudinal image, we now see definitive sclerosis and a reduction in the diameter of the greater saphenous vein.

Pre and post-sclerotherapy images will show a patient's lower limb with sapheno-femoral incompentence and distal varicosities before treatment, and a visible sclerotic reaction in the greater saphenous vein two months after treatment.

When sclerosis has occurred, palpation should reveal an indurated sapheno-femoral junction, and an indurated saphenous segment of varying diameter and length.

A fibrotic cord is present 6 months after treatment, although it is not usually visible.

How to recognize and treat lesser saphenous incompetence

As there are many possible variations in the terminations of lesser saphenous veins, it is sometimes difficult to locate the main point of incompetence.

Clinical examination techniques are the same as for the greater saphenous vein. The highest point of reflux should be injected first, even when the visible varicosities are in the lower part of the leg.

Duplex ultrasound is indispensable in assessing incompetence. In this particular case, we have a perforating vein incompetence at mid-calf, and another incompetence at the saphenous-popliteal junction. These valve leaflets at the perforating vein site are very badly damaged.

Here, we can observe an enlarged incompetent lesser saphenous vein and the sapheno-popliteal junction with the popliteal vein and artery. In this case, the sapheno-popliteal junction should be injected first. Otherwise, inflammation and recanalization can occur. The injection can be made while the patient is in a prone position, or in a standing position with the knee flexed.

The percussion technique is used to locate and feel the vein. After the sapheno-popliteal junction, the gastrocnemius veins and arteries, and the small saphenous or Dujarrier artery have been located, it is safe to make the injection.

It is recommended that the injection be made slowly to avoid potential problems. If you cannot feel the site of the injection properly when wearing gloves, it is advisable to remove the gloves.

The injection of the sapheno-popliteal junction can once again be observed. The injection protocol for the lesser saphenous vein is 1 cc of a 1% iodine or STD solution during the first visit, with the concentration increasing by 1% at every subsequent visit, but the volume remaining the same.

The summation technique, which consists of additional injections of distal points, can also be used in the case of the lesser saphenous vein.

When the sapheno-popliteal junction is injected first, and the perforating veins second, complete sclerosis of the sapheno-popliteal junction, saphenous trunk perforating veins and varicosities below the perforating vein incompetence will result.

Giacomini's vein, which links the greater and lesser saphenous vein, is one of the most important anastomotic veins. A major sclerosing agent is used to inject Giacomini's vein. The dosage and volume must be adjusted according to the degree of incompetence. In this particular case, one injection was made at the site of incompetence at the point where Giacomini's vein branches out from the greater saphenous vein, and a second injection in the perforating vein on Giacomini's trajectory. When this vein is incompetent, failure to inject it can cause recanalization of the sclerosed greater or lesser saphenous veins.

Strange as it may seem, I have found that wearing gloves one size larger than my usual size give me a better tactile impression of the veins.

The next step is injecting the perforating vein on Giacomini's trajectory.

How to treat perforating vein incompetence

There are four groups of perforating veins linking the greater saphenous vein to the deep venous system. If they are all incompetent, they should be injected in the following order: first, the Hunter; second, the Geniculate; third, the Boyd; and fourth, the Cockett.

The perforating veins in the Hunter group are often indirect, and their incompetence can cause substantial reflux.

The geniculate perforating vein incompetence will cause tortuous varicosities in the knee area.

Incompetence of the Boyd perforating veins, a group of 5 or 6, does not usually cause significant reflux.

Incompetence of the 3 or 4 Cockett perforating veins can cause considerable reflux and is often responsible for venous stasis ulcer.

We will now describe the injection of a Boyd perforating vein. When the injection is made at the perforating vein site, a brisk puncture is made with a syringe held at an angle of at least 45 degrees. To treat the perforating vein, an injection can also be made a few centimeters below the perforating vein site. In both cases, the injection should be made with one hand so that the needle may be held in place with the index finger of the other hand.

Major sclerosing agents are also used to inject the perforating vein. Their concentration and volume will depend on the site of injection and the seriousness of the incompetence.

How to treat reticular veins and telangiectasias

When treating these veins, it is useful to have pre-filled syringes containing varying concentrations of sclerosing agents ready on the treatment table. The syringe used will depend on the size of the reticular veins and telangiectasia. Injecting different points on the axis of the reticular veins is recommended.

For more aesthetic results, the site of injection of the telangiectatia should be carefully chosen. The sclerotherapist should personally remove the cap of the needle and hold the syringe in such a way as to permit easy puncture and avoid extravasation.

There are several kinds of reticular veins and telangiectasias. Minor sclerosing agents such as folidocanol hypertonic solutions, chromated glycerine, weak concentrations of iodine and STD should be used for these veins.

For these injections, my personal preference is a 3 cc disposable syringe and a 26-g, 1/2-inch Terumo needle, as opposed to the 3O-g needle. The bevel is more elongated, which makes it easier to perform the puncture when you hold the needle face up. This type of needle is also less flexible and seems to cause less bruising.

Cotton balls are applied at injecting sites with 1/2-inch tape and kept on for 2 hours.

For clustered telangiectasiae, the injection is made in the deeper vein, which normally lies behind the point of confluence.

In conclusion, one can safely say that successful sclerotherapy involves meticulous preparation, patience, and vigilance.

Sclerotherapy of the Greater Saphenous Vein with Incompetence of the Sapheno-femoral Juncture.

Kurt M. H o e r d e g e n

Studio of Vein Diseases, Basel, Switzerland

Even taking into account the advantage of surgery of the sapheno-femoral juncture one has to consider the number of patients who dislike it or where is a contraindication for a surgical intervention. For this reason we must be able to offer an alternative treatment in the form of a reliable injection technique which yields good results and prevents the so feared complications of intraarterial injections and deep venous thromboses if the puncture is executed high up in the groin.
With our technique (developed with K. Sigg) the above mentioned complications have never been seen.
The puncture is done in upright position, the injection is made in lying position with the leg elevated. As sclerosant we use a sodium iodide solution of 8% or 12% concentration. No more than 0,5 ccm of solution is given per injection to avoid painful local reactions, ascending thrombophlebitis and the flowing off of large amounts of the sclerosant into the deep venous system.
A strong compression bandage including the groin must be applicated immediately after injection.
As preliminary examinations and for the control of further progress we use the Doppler and the Light-Reflection-Rheography.

Phlébologie 92. Eds P. Raymond-Martimbeau, R. Prescott, M. Zummo.
John Libbey Eurotext, Paris © 1992, pp. 787-792

Principe, technique et résultats du traitement rapide des saphènes internes incontinentes par sclérothérapie

F. Vin

Hôpital Notre-Dame de Bon Secours, Paris, France.

Les varices de la face interne de cuisse et de jambe sont souvent secondaires à une incontinence ostiale et tronculaire de la saphène interne.
La sclérothérapie pratiquée en Europe depuis plusieurs décenies a fait la preuve de son efficacité.L'injection des jonctions saphèno-fémorales a été critiquée par de nombreux auteurs car elle pouvait exposer à des risques d'injection intra-artérielle accidentelle et surtout à des récidives avec recanalisation. Cette technique nécessite un apprentissage et une grande prudence lors de l'injection pour éviter ces accidents. Par ailleurs, plusieurs travaux ont déjà montré que les récidives in-situ après injection des jonctions saphèno-fémorales étaient possibles mais que dans un grande nombre de cas il s'agissait de traitements incomplets (1).

La sclérothérapie de la jonction et du tronc de la saphène interne telle qu'elle est exposée ci-dessous permet d'obtenir une occlusion plus rapide et plus efficace du segment variqueux traité.

PRINCIPE DU TRAITEMENT

La sclérothérapie des varices du territoire de la saphène interne se fait le plus souvent en deux temps.
Le premier temps consiste à injecter la solution sclérosante au niveau de la jonction saphèno-fémorale afin de supprimer le reflux long.
Lorsque la sclérose complète est obtenue, il est alors possible dans un deuxième temps de traiter les collatérales variqueuses résiduelles avec des concentrations de solution sclérosante peu élevées compte-tenu de l'absence de reflux sus-jacent.
Aucune compression élastique n'est appliquée après les séances.

Cette technique permet d'obtenir des résultats esthétiques meilleurs compte-tenu des faibles réactions inflammatoires observées. Lorsque la maladie veineuse est évoluée, la methodologie exposée ci-dessus nous paraissait insuffisante car elle laissait en place un tronc saphenien souvent perméable et succeptible d'être réalimenté par une perforante sous-jacente exposant à une récidive.

Nous proposons une technique plus rapide inspirée du traitement sclérosant accéleré de GRELLETY-BOISVIEL(2). L'indication est représentée essentiellement par les insuffisances ostiales et tronculaires entrant dans le cadre de varices essentielles avec dilatations étagées de la saphène interne associées ou non à des perforantes incontinentes et des dilatations variqueuses jambières. L'injection de la saphène interne est pratiquée en trois sites différents au cours de la même séance (jonction saphèno-fémorale, tiers moyen de cuisse, tiers inférieur de cuisse).

Au niveau du tronc saphènien, cette injection est le plus souvent réalisée dans les dilatations cliniquement palpables. Elle est souvent guidée par l'échographie (écho-sclérothérapie)(3) (4) compte-tenu de la difficulté rencontrée pour cathétériser cette veine dans ces régions ou elle est située dans la profondeur de l'hypoderme.

MATERIEL ET METHODES

Avant d'entreprendre un traitement sclérosant de varices dépendant du territoire saphène interne, un examen clinique est indispensable pour rattacher les dilatations variqueuses au tronc saphènien. Il permettra également de mettre en évidence l'incontinence saphènienne. L'examen écho-doppler est devenu indispensable (5) (6) pour confirmer le reflux, mesurer les calibres de la saphène à 3 cm de l'ostium et à différents sites au niveau du tronc.
Il localisera des différents collatérales ainsi que le niveau des perforantes et leur éventuelle incontinence. Cette cartographie est devenu nécessaire si l'on veut éviter les traitements incomplets ou les récidives précoces.

L'écho-doppler permettra d'éliminer les reflux profonds, ou séquelles de thromboses veineuses qui sont le plus souvent sources de récidives après traitement.

La technique d'injection en trois sites est indiquée pour les saphènes présentant des dilatations tronculaires étagées supérieures à 3-4 mm.

INJECTION AU SITE A : JONCTION SAPHENO-FEMORALE

Pour l'injection au niveau de la jonction saphèno-fémorale, le sujet est assis, le membre en abduction, rotation externe et jambe pendante (7).
La saphène est repérée cliniquement par la palpation éventuellement à l'écho-doppler.
La ponction est réalisée à la liminte inféro-interne du triangle de SCARPA au niveau du tendon du moyen adducteur loin du carrefour vasculaire fémoral.
Parfois, guisé par l'échographie, cette injection sera faite en deux temps et toujours après avoir constaté la présence d'un reflux franc dans la seringue.

INJECTION AU SITE B : TIERS MOYEN DE LA CUISSE

L'injection de la saphène interne au tiers moyen de la cuisse est pratiquée là ou elle est cliniquement la mieux palpée chez le sujet assis jambe allongée en légère rotation externe. Elle est souvent guidée par l'échographie.

INJECTION AU SITE C : TIERS INFERIEUR DE CUISSE

L'injection au tiers inférieur de la cuisse est réalisée dans la région condylienne, là ou la saphène est très souvent visible, dilatée et aisément palpable.

En présence d'une perforante incontinente au tiers moyen ou au tiers inférieur, l'injection sera préférentiellement faite au niveau de la zone de reflux (8).

Les dosages et concentrations sont résumés dans le tableau 1.
Une compression par bande élasto-adhésive est recommandée lorsque les dilatations du tronc saphènien et leurs calibres échographiques sont importantes > 4-5 mm.

Les séances sont répétées toutes les deux à trois semaines jusqu'à obtention du résultat attendu.

RESULTATS

Les résultats seront appréciés cliniquement et par écho-doppler à chaque séance.
Sur le plan clinique, la palpation-percussion du tronc saphènien peut réveler la persistance d'un signe du flot témoignant d'une inefficacité du traitement en rapport avec un dosage insuffisant. Dans d'autres cas, elle permet de percevoir une induration du tronc saphènien avec parfoir rougeur et sensibilité à la palpation. Rarement on observera une importante réaction inflammatoire avec rougeurs et douleurs au niveau de l'axe saphènien fémoral.

Seul l'écho-doppler est capable d'affirmer l'efficacité de la sclérothérapie en confirmant l'absence de reflux et de flux avec incompressibilité de la veine, épaississement du mur intimal et échogénicité endopariétale(9).

On vérifira également la perméabilité et la compressibilité de la veine fémorale.

En cas d'échec complet, les injections seront répétées avec augmentation des dosages au niveau des trois sites (tableau 2).

En présence d'un échec partiel (occlusion du tronc avec perméabilité de la jonction ou inversement), les injections seront répétées au niveau de la zone non sclérosée en augmentant le dosage jusqu'à obtenir une occlusion complète de l'axe saphènien;

Ultérieurement le traitement des collatérales peut être entrepris selon le protocole classique: injection des varices, veinules et varicosités avec des agents sclérosants de force moyenne ou faible à concentration basse et dosages élevés.

Les contrôles cliniques et écho-doppler représentent une étape importante de la sclérothérapie qui conditionne le résultat final et l'efficacité. Ils seront réalisés selon les critères précedemment décrits en fin de traitement, à 6 mois et chaque année.
Toute récidive implique la réinjection du segment reperméabilisé en utilisant comme concentration celle employée lors de la dernière séance.

DISCUSSION

La sclérothérapie des jonctions et des troncs saphèniens internes permet de supprimer des reflux et évite la crossectomie avec événage chirurgical.
Elle peut être utilée quelque soit le calibre saphènien en s'aidant d'artefacts comme des injections de bas en haut (10) et compression élastique pour les saphènes de gros calibre (11). Néanmoins, il est raisonnable de ne l'utiliser que pour des calibres saphèniens inférieurs à 8-9 mm (12) compte-tenu de la rapidité et de son efficacité à cours et moyen terme.

Avec cette technique d'injection en trois sites, les résultats obtenus sont plus rapides et plus durables. Dans la majorité des cas, la compression élastique n'est pas indispensable, mais elle est recommandée lorsque les dilatations du tronc sont supérieurs à 4 -5 mm.

En présence d'une réaction inflammatoire, il n'existe aucun retentissement cutané au niveau de la cuisse comme pigmentations et télangiectasies qui peuvent être rencontrées dans la même situation lorsque l'injection est réalisée à l'étage jambier.

En supprimant le reflux au niveau de l'ostium et du tranc saphènien, il est possible de traiter les collatérales de cuisse et de jambe en utilisant des agents sclérosants de force moyenne et à concentrations faibles toujours sans contention et en l'absence de réaction inflammatoire excessive.

L'inconvénient de cette technique est la répétition des injections à chaque séance jusqu'à l'obtention du résultat souhaité, c'est à dire la suppression complète des reflux.
Il est toutefois possible de laisser un flux sans reflux à condition de surveiller plus régulièrement l'état du réseau veineux superficiel du patient. Dans de rares cas on observe une importante réaction inflammatoire sur tout le trajet saphènien avec rougeurs et douleurs qui sont secondaires à la potentialisation du produit sclérosant injecté en différents sites.

Pour certaines raisons encore indéterminées, (insensibilité de l'endothelium de la paroi, succeptibilité individuelle du sujet ...), certaines saphènes même de calibre moyen ne réagissent pas à la sclérothérapie ou se recanalisent précocement.
Dans ces cas d'insuccès, la cure chirurgicale avec crossectomie et stripping peut être envisagée, le tronc saphènien restant toujours perméable et cathétarisable par le stripper.

CONCLUSION

La sclérothérapie de la veine saphène interne avec injection d'agent sclérosant à la jonction, au tiers moyen et au tiers inférieur de jambe permet d'obtenir une occlusion plus rapide du segment veineux traité. Elle est réservée aux varicoses évoluées avec dilatations tronculaires étagées découvertes à l'écho-doppler et dont le calibre est supérieur à 4-5 mm et nécessite souvent une compression localisée pour éviter les réactions inflammatoires.

En supprimant le reflux ostial et tronculaire, il est possible d'entreprendre ultérieurement la sclérothérapie des varices collatérales de cuisse et de jambe avec des concentrations de produit sclérosant peu élevées et un résultat esthétique satisfaisant.

La maladie veineuse étant chronique et évolutive, il est parfois difficile de distinguer les récidives des formes évolutives, des contrôles cliniques et écho-doppler sont toujours nécessaire ceci quelque soit le type de traitement, qu'il soit chirurgical ou médical.

TABLEAU 1

TETRADECYL SULFATE
DE SODIUM

Site A	3 %	1 cc
Site B	1 %	1 cc
Site C	0,50 %	1 cc

Concentrations et dosages lors de la 1ère séance.

TABLEAU 2

	2 éme séance		3 éme séance		4 éme séance		5 ème séance	
	Tétracylate sulfate de sodium				Ina			
Site A	3%	2cc	3%	3cc	3%	3cc	6%	3cc
Site B	1%	2cc	1%	3cc	1%	3cc	3%	2cc
Site C	0,50%	2cc	0,50%	3cc	0,50%	3cc	1%	2cc

BIBLIOGRAPHIE

1 - VIN.F
Contrôle d'efficacite des traitements sclérosants en phlebologie.
Phlebologie, 1990,43,n°4,673-680.

2 - GRELLETY-BOISVIEL J.P., HUTINEL.B.
Le traitement sclérosant acceléré dans " la sclérose des varices" par R.TOURNAY et Coll.
Expansion scientifique 1 volume 215-223

3 - KNIGHT.R.M, VIN.F, ZYGMUNT.J.A.
Ultra sonic guidance of injections into the superficial venous system
Phlébologie '89 A.DAVY, R.STEMMER
1989 JOHN LIBBEY EUROTEXT Ltd P.P.339-341

4 - MISEREY.G, REINHAREZ.D, ECALARD.P.,
Sclérose sous échographie dans certaines zones à risques.
Phlébologie,1991, 44, n°1,85-86

5 - BLANCHEMAISON.P, MOUREN.X, CAILLARD.P, ELBEZE.Y, CLOAREC.M.
Qu'attendre d'un bilan écho-doppler veineux superficiel des membres inférieurs en 1989.
Phlebologie'89 A.DAVY, R.STEMMER
1989 JOHN LIBBEY EUROTEXT Ltd P.P. 309-311

6 - RAYMOND-MARTIMBEAU.P.
Duplex ultrasound colour fluw doppler and magnetic resonance imaging in phlebology.
Phlébologie '89 A.DAVY, R.STEMMER
1989 JOHN LIBBEY EUROTEXT Ltd P.P.347

7 - DAVY.A, OUVRY.P.
Incontinences ostiales ; sclérose de crosse ou crossectomie
Phlébologie 1986,39, P.P 35-45

8 - VIN.F.
Perforantes et varices isolées.
Phlebologie, 1986,39(2) 227-232

9 - SCHADECK.M, ALLAERT.F
Echotomographie de la sclérose
Phlebologie 1991,44,n°1,111-130

10 - BERNBACH.H.R.
Le traitement sclérosant selon SIGG
Phlebologie 1991,44,n°1,31-36

11 - STEMMER.R.
Sclérose des varices et compression
Phlebologie 1991,44,n°1,49-67.

12 - SCHADECK.M.
Doppler and echotomography in sclerosis of the saphenous veins
Phlebology, 1987n2,221-240.

Phlébologie 92. Eds P. Raymond-Martimbeau, R. Prescott, M. Zummo.
John Libbey Eurotext, Paris © 1992, pp. 793-795

Statistical evaluation of sclerotherapy of the long saphenous vein and the sapheno-femoral junction

Aurora Avramovic, Miguel Avramovic

Centro Flebologico Privado, Riobamba 747, 1045 Buenos Aires, Argentina.

Introduction

The aim of this study was to perform a clinical and statistical evaluation of the sclerotherapy of long saphenous vein and the sapheno-femoral junction in a group of 564 patients, with a flollow up period of 4 years.

Material:

1) For injection:
   a) Disposable needles, 0,50x16;
   b) Disposable syringes 5 cc.
   c) Elastic bandages.
2) Sclerosing substances:
   a) Variglobin 8 % y 12 %;
   b) Hypertonic glucosed solution 25 %

Method:

In the first place, a semiological study to determine the degree of incompetence is carried out. This study may be complemented by a Doppler and an echotomographic study. Then, it is decided in which position the sclerosing treatment will be performed, preferently in semiseated position: semiseated patient with elevated leg in out ward rotation, trying to achieve the sclerosis of long saphenous and sapheno-femoral junction at a distance, so as not to interfere with the neurovascular bundle. If the arch sclerosis is not achieved, after 15 days a second session is performed, with the direct puncture technique. The interval between sessions was 15 or 20 days because it is necessary to wait until the sclerosing reaction takes place.
If some technical impediment is found in the semiseated position, the injection is made with the patient standing.

Plan of treatment:

First session: 2 ml. Variglobin 8 % , 2 ml hypertonic glucosed solution 25 % (distributed along the course of internal saphena).
Second session: 1 ml Variglobin 8 %, 1 ml hypertonic glucosed solution 25 % (in the sapheno-femoral junction).
Third session: idem.

RESULTS:

The sclerosis of long saphenous vein and the sapheno-femoral junction was achieved in 80 % of patients, 20 % of patients did not respond to the treatment (scleroresistance or intolerance to the drug). From the 80 % that reacted positively, 51% had a favourable evolution. 29 % presented recanalization between 8 and 18 months after treatment and had to be reinjected, showing then a positive evolution.

CONCLUSION:

The above mentioned results show that a good sclerotherapeutic technique makes possible the sclerosis of long saphenous vein, with good clinical and esthetical results, in 80 % of cases.

BIBLIOGRAPHY

1. A. Avramovic, J. G. De Simone, M. Avramovic, E. Brizzio; Evaluation de la sclérose de la crosse et du tronc de la saphéne interne gracé a l'echotomografie; ACTS. 10º Cong. Mondial. Vol. 2, pág. 834. 1990.
2. Hordegen K. M., Sigg K.; Sclerotherapy of the long safhenous vein with incompetence of the femoral junction; Abstract 9º Congress of Phlebologie W. S. 1-10-1986 Kyoto-Japan.
3. P. A. Ouvry, P. A. G. Ouvry; La Sclérotherapie des perforantes; ACTS. 10º Cong. Mondial, Vol 2., pág. 786.
4. P. Vallois; Suppresion del reflux saphéniens par sclerotherapie; Techniques et resultats; Phlebologie 30,15, 1986.

Sclérothérapie, techniques et résultats

Never Rosli, Raul Lapid, Eduardo Rodi

Centre de Flebologia Dr. Never Rosli

Il est obligatoire chez tout phlébologue de perfectionner les techniques sclérothérapeutiques pour obtenir de meilleurs résultats fonctionnels et esthétiques: le développement de ce travail s'est effectué dans notre Centre Phlébologique avec une vingtaine d'années d'expérience dans le perfectionnement et hiérarchisation de la Sclérothérapie. Dans une projection de disponibilités on pourra observer les résultats par rapport à l,emploi de la sclérothérapie et les différents cas, à savoir:

- Télangiectasies et veinectasies simples
- Varices essentielles
- Syndrome post-phlébitique non ulcérés
- Syndrome post-phlébitique ulcérés

Cette grande méthode thérapeutique phlébologique donne d'extraordinaires résultats quand elle est appliquée suivant les strictes règles qu'exigent ses techniques d'application. Pour finir, n'oublions pas que toutes les thérapeutiques phlébologiques chirurgicales ou non, même la sclérothérapie, peuvent se complémenter entre elles selon les circonstances phlébopatiques.

Nous mettrons les techniques et résultats les plus dépurées pour le traitement de: télangiectasies, veinectasies, varices essentielles, varices post-phlébitiques et perforantes insuffisantes.

Phlébologie 92. Eds P. Raymond-Martimbeau, R. Prescott, M. Zummo.
John Libbey Eurotext, Paris © 1992, pp. 796-798

Télangiectasies et sclérothérapie

Paul A. Ouvry, Pierre A.G. Ouvry

Service d'Angéiologie, Clinique Saint-Pierre, 38, rue Thiers, 76200 Dieppe, France.

Introduction

19 % des patients traités par un phlébologue, le sont uniquement pour des télangiectasies.
51 % pour des varices et des télangiectasies.
30 % uniquement pour des varices.

C'est à dire que le traitement des télangiectasies concerne 70 % des patients.

Terrain

Il s'agit de femmes.
Il peut s'agir de télangiectasies associées à des varices.
Il peut s'agir de télangiectasies sans varices décelables.

- Télangiectasies associées à des varices : (51 % des cas).

Les varices peuvent être plus ou moins évidentes. Le traitement des varices doit précéder celui des télangiectasies. Il peut suffir à les faire disparaître partiellement ou complètement. Le traitement des varices dans un premier temps facilite toujours le traitement des télangiectasies dans un second temps. Certains phlébologues qui ne pratiquent la sclérothérapie qu'au niveau des télangiectasies exposent par conséquent leurs patients à des résultats moins satisfaisants.

- Télangiectasies sans varices : (19 % des cas).

Elles s'expliquent par une diminution de l'élasticité pariétale, une atonie. Dans ces anomalies interviennent des facteurs héréditaires, hormonaux et des facteurs aggravants tels les stations debout prolongées, la chaleur, les inflammations locales.

Clinique

Le siège des télangiectasies varie selon qu'elles sont

associées ou non à des varices.

Leur aspect est variable. Il dépend du trajet, du calibre, de la couleur des télangiectasies.

Elles peuvent apparaître dès l'enfance, subir des poussées à l'occasion de grossesses, de la prise d'O.P.S..

Elles sont le plus souvent purement inesthétique mais peuvent parfois entraîner des douleurs de caractères particuliers.

Explorations complémentaires

Les explorations angiographiques permettent d'identifier plusieurs modes de drainage. La capillaroscopie confirme qu'il s'agit d'une dilatation du plexus veinulaire sous papillaire. L'anatomie pathologique montre une structure cellulaire de type veineux.

Diagnostic

Il s'agit d'une affection commune qui ne pose pas de problèmes. Les télangiectasies secondaires ou congénitales s'inscrivent dans des tableaux cliniques plus complexes et bien différents.

Traitement

La sclérothérapie est le traitement le plus efficace. Les premiers essais datent de 1933 mais c'est l'apparition de produits plus adaptés dans les années 50 qui a permis l'essor de la sclérothérapie. Les produits les plus employés en Europe sont la glycérine chromée, le polydocanol et le salicylate de soude. Le mode d'action est comparable à celui des varices plus souvent étudiées.

Les résultats d'une étude prospective sont rapportés.

- Matériel :

Seringue de préférence à embout de verre excentré.

Aiguilles 26 G et même 30 G ½ pour les télangiectasies les plus fines.

Lunettes loupe X 2 pour les télangiectasies les plus fines.

- Méthode :

A - Commencer par les vaisseaux les plus gros, les plus haut situés et continuer par les vaisseaux plus petits, plus bas situés :

C'est à dire commencer par les varices, puis les varicosités, puis les télangiectasies bleues et enfin les télangiectasies rouges. L'injection se pratique dans un plan très superficiel. La peau est tendue entre le pouce et l'index de la main gauche.

B - Injecter peu à la fois. Multiplier les points d'injection :

Ce nombre peut atteindre plusieurs dizaines. L'intervalle entre les injections varie de 2 à 4 semaines. Une contention est toujours bénéfique. Les résultats sont rapidement favorables dans plus de 80 % des cas. Les complications surtout thromboses excessives et pigmentations résultent de doses trop fortes. Des échecs sont possibles.

Conclusion

La sclérothérapie des télangiectasies est une méthode efficace qui nécessite un apprentissage et une pratique suffisante.

Références

Arlaud R, Ouvry PA. Les télangiectasies acquises des membres inférieurs. Phlébologie 32:359-364, 1979.

Ouvry PA, Arlaud R. Le traitement sclérosant des télangiectasies des membres inférieurs. Phlébologie 32:365-370, 1979.

Davy A, Ouvry PA. Possible explanations for recurrence of varicose veins. Phlebology 1:15-21, 1986.

Griton P. Conceptions étiopathogéniques des télangiectasies. In Davy A, Van der Stricht J : Phlébologie, Tome 1. Brussels, Ars Medici, 1983, pp 686-687.

Kuiper JP, Jagtman BA, Brakkee AJM. Mechanical properties of skin in venous lower limb syndrome. Phlebology 1:7-14,1986.

Bihari I. In Davy A, Van der Stricht J : Phlébologie, Tome 1. Brussels, Ars Medici, 1983, p 686.

Merlen JF. Télangiectasies rouges, télangiectasies bleues. Phlébologie 22:167-174, 1970.

Ouvry PA, Davy A. Réflexions sur 16 cas de strippings abusifs pour varices essentielles. Phlébologie 35:835-841, 1982.

Tournay R. Traitement des télangiectasies. In : Journées angéiologiques de langue Française. Paris, Expansion Scientifique Française, 1972.

Moraes IN. Tableau clinique et radiologique des télangiectasies Ann Brasil Derm 1:40, 1965.

Coget J. Quel est l'apport de la capillaroscopie dans le diagnostic des télangiectasies ? In Davy A, Van der Stricht J : Phlébologie, Tome 2. Brussels, Ars Medici, 1983, pp 689-690.

Shelley WB. Essential progressive telangiectasia : Successful treatment with tetracycline. JAMA 216:1343-1344, 1971.

Goor W. Que doit-on penser de l'histopathologie des télangiectasies du point de vue dermatologique ? In Davy A, Van der Stricht J : Phlébologie, Tome 2. Brussels, Ars Medici, 1983, p 688.

Phlébologie 92. Eds P. Raymond-Martimbeau, R. Prescott, M. Zummo.
John Libbey Eurotext, Paris © 1992, pp. 799

La slcérothérapie des télangiectasies

Michel Schadeck*, Jean-Louis Salomon**, Serge Mako***

* *École Européenne de Phlébologie, 6, rue Giordano Bruno, 75014 Paris, France.* ** *89, av. de Wagram, 75017 Paris, France.* *** *31, rue d'Arras, 92000 Nanterre, France.*

La télangiectasie est le plus petit vaisseau de l'épiderme visible à l'oeil nu. Dans l'insuffisance veineuse superficielle, son rôle n'est qu'esthétique. Pourtant, l'importance des désordres de ce type qu'il entraîne en fait un des principaux motifs de consultation.

De couleur rouge ou bleue voire violette suivant sa profondeur ou la pression veineuse qu'elle subit, la télangiectasie mérite d'être traitée de façon rigoureuse.

La suppression des principaux points de fuite, d'abord saphèniens puis secondaires représentés par les branches restantes puis le "sous-sol" se révèle indispensable pour l'obtention d'un bon résultat.

L'utilisation de seringues en verre ou en plastique est essentiellement liée à la pratique du phlébologue. le choix de l'aiguille va osciller entre une 4,5/10 et une 3/10, cette dernière permettant d'éviter, surtout pour les débutants, l'injection à chaque fois d'une trop grande quantité de produit sclérosant. Celui utilisé ici, le POLIDECANOL, peut être dilué avec du GLUCOSE à 60% ou du sérum physiologique. Les injections seront multipliées afin d'éviter un surdosage et ses conséquences.

Bien réalisée en évitant les injections extra-vasculaires, cette sclérothérapie se fera sans douleur et sans complications.

La sclérothérapie des télangiectasies est un traitement qui nécessite donc attention, prudence et rigueur, seuls critères pour satisfaire médecins et surtout patients.

VIDEO-CLIP SUR LA SCLEROTHERAPIE DES TELANGIECTASIES

André CORNU-THENARD Hôpital Saint-Antoine Paris
Frédéric VIN Hôpital Américain Neuilly/Seine

- INTRODUCTION

Les télangiectasies sont un motif fréquent de consultation. Elles sont souvent considérées à tort par les patientes, comme les témoins du vieillissement. EN fait, il ne s'agit que d'un problème esthétique, n'engendrant aucune complication. Malgré cela, elles peuvent et doivent être traitées si les patientes le demandent. La sclérothérapie est le traitement de choix. Elle donne la plupart du temps d'excellents résultats.

- DEFINITION

Les télangiectasies sont des dilatations des plexus veineux sous papillaires. Le drainage du sang se fait soit dans le réseau veineux profond, soit dans le réseau veineux superficiel, parfois dans les deux réseaux à la fois.

- PHYSIOPATHOLOGIE

Les télangiectasies apparaissent le plus souvent de façon progressive au cours des années. Elles sont souvent alimentées par un reflux sanguin provenant d'une veinule. Ce reflux entraine une dilatation de ces plexus veineux sous-papillaires.

- ASPECTS CLINIQUES

Plusieurs aspects cliniques peuvent être rencontrés :

- les télangiectasies peuvent être uniques et rectilignes, ou prendre l'aspect caractéristique de feu d'artifice. Elles peuvent être en araignées, avec une partie centrale d'où rayonnent de fines branches. Dans d'autres cas, elles sont diffuses, sans aspect particulier. Enfin, elles peuvent être ponctiformes, comme celles rencontrées au cours des atrophies blanches.
- Elles peuvent siéger au niveau de la cuisse ou de la jambe. Sur la face externe, comme sur la face interne. Parfois, elles siègent au niveau de la face interne du pied : c'est la couronne phlébectasique de VAN DER MOLEN. Dans tous les cas la pression les fait disparaitre, l'arrêt de la pression les fait réapparaitre.
- Elles sont bleues ou rouges. Les bleues sont plus volumineuses et plus profondes que les rouges. Les rouges sont filiformes.

- DIAGNOSTIC A VISEE THERAPEUTIQUE

Trois situations cliniques sont possibles : Dans certains cas, les télangiectasies sont isolées : il n'existe pas de varice à l'examen clinique et l'examen doppler confirme cette impression. A l'inverse, l'examen clinique met en évidence une varice responsable. En général, les télangiectasies sont situées à son extrémité. Le doppler confirmera la présence d'un reflux. Enfin, varices et télangiectasies peuvent coexister sur le même membre inférieur, mais être totalement indépendantes.

- CONDUITE DU TRAITEMENT

La conduite du traitement est simple : lorsque les télangiectasies sont isolées, ou totalement indépendantes des varices présentes, elles peuvent être traitées d'emblée par la sclérothérapie. Celles qui siègent au niveau des atrophies blanches ne seront, bien évidemment, pas injectées. Enfin, lorsqu'elles sont secondaires à une saphène incontinente ou à toute autre varice, il faut commencer par supprimer les sources de reflux, puis entreprendre la sclérothérapie des varices, des veinules et enfin des télangiectasies.

- MATERIEL

Le matériel pour les injections comporte : des seringues en verre ou en plastique, des aiguilles 26 G ou 30 G. Les produits sclérosants sont nombreux et le choix d'utilisation dépend de leur disponibilité.

- TECHNIQUE

Pour obtenir de bons résultats, quelques règles simples sont à respecter : il faut toujours commencer par des injections de produits, de faible concentration. On utilisera par exemple du scléremo dilué au 1/3, de l'aétoxisclérol à 0.3% ou du trombovar à 0.1%. En fonction des résultats obtenus les doses, lors des séances suivantes, seront soit augmentées, soit diminuées, soit identiques. Ces injections doivent être strictement intra-veineuses. Il est nécessaire de commencer par les télangiectasies les plus grosses, car elles sont le plus souvent responsables des plus petites. La vitesse d'injection sera lente. Le volume injecté ne dépassera pas 0.3cc par injection. Si l'on se réfère à une surface cutanée, il faudrait éviter de blanchir une zone supérieure à 5cm de diamètre. Dix à 20 injections pourront être faites à chaque séance. Enfin, un délai de quinze jours sera nécessaire pour apprécier l'efficacité.

- RESULTAT

Les résultats seront appréciés au moment de l'injection et à distance :

Au moment de l'injection de la substance sclérosante, on observe souvent un blanchiment de la zone traitée. Dans certains cas, un discret érythème du derme peut apparaître. Si l'érythème est trop important, il est recommandé d'utiliser une compression locale, faite d'une bande élasto-adhésive, circonférentielle mais non serrée.
A distance, lors des séances suivantes, on observe le plus souvent une importante diminution des télangiectasies, avec parfois persistance de certaines d'entre elle qui nécessiteront d'être réinjectées pour disparaitre à leur tour. Parfois quelques complications peuvent apparaitre : pigmentations, télangiectasies supplémentaires, voire ulcérations. Ces complications sont en général dues à des doses trop élevées de substances sclérosantes.

- CONCLUSION

Un diagnostic clinique complet est indispensable avant d'entreprendre cette thérapeutique. Il est impératif de traiter dans un premier temps toutes les sources de reflux, puis les varices, les veinulectasies, avant d'entreprendre la sclérose des télangiectasies. Comme il s'agit d'une demande esthétique, il faut absolument éviter les complications locales. Pour cela, il ne faut pas hésiter à utiliser en début de soins, des produits dilués. La sclérothérapie lorsqu'elle est bien conduite, représente encore aujourd'hui, le meilleur traitement des télangiectasies des membres inférieurs.

La microscléroélectrothérapie (Miesel) pour le traitement des télangectasies des membres inférieurs

Eugenio Oscar Brizzio

Escuela Argentina de Flebologia de la Asociacion Medica Argentina

La microscléroélectrothérapie est une méthode qui associe la microsclérothérapie traditionnelle à la diathermocoagulation programme en utilisant des électrodes isolées, ce qui permet d'optimiser la sclérothérapie en améliorant le résultat esthétique et en diminuant les risques de récidive.

Phlébologie 92. Eds P. Raymond-Martimbeau, R. Prescott, M. Zummo.
John Libbey Eurotext, Paris © 1992, pp. 803-804

A comparative study of two sclerosing agents in the treatment of telangiectasias

Robert Prescott

1490 Sherbrooke St. West, Montreal, P. Quebec, H3G 1L3, Canada.

Choice of patients:

All patients treated in this study had been treated for their underlying varicose desease prior to treating their telangiectasias. All were female under 60 years of age. They were randomly separated in two groups, the first to be treated with an hypertomic dextrose solution at 10% and the second with sodium tetradecyl sulfate at a concentration of 0.15%.

Method:

36 patients were treated with the hypertonic solution while 24 have been treated with sodium tetradecyl sulfate. Treatment was stopped either at the request of the patient or when completed, some patient being satisfied with a partial disappearance of their telangiectasias and wanting to postpone any further treatment.

Results were then compiled using four criterias: 1- pictures before and after 2- subjective evaluation of over all disappearance by the patient 3- subjective evaluation of overall disappearance by the operator 4- complications.

Results:

a) Quantity of telangiectasias: patients in group A (hypertonic solution) appeared to have 20% more telangiectasias at the beginning of treatment than patients in group B (sodium tetradecyl sulfate).

b) Number of sessions:
Group A (hypertonic sol): 2 to 8
Average 4.2
Group B (sod. tetrad. sulf.): 2 to 5
Average 2.6

c) Disappearance:

	Group A (hypertonic sol.)	Group B (sod. tetrad. sulf.)
According to patient	25 to 100% Average 75%	25 to 90% Average 70%

According to operator	25 to 90% Average 70%	25 to 85% Average 70%
Pictures before and after	25 to 90% Average 72.5%	30 to 85% Average 70%

D) Complications:

	Group A (Hypertonic sol.)	Group B (sod. tetrad. sulf.)
Pain	mild 28% of pats. (10)	mild 17% of pats. (4)
echymosis	mild to moderate	mild
Matting	2 patients 6%	1 patient 4%
Postsclerotic pigmentation	light 1 patient 3%	light to moderate 2 patients 8%

Discussion:

a) Number of sessions:
Although the group A presented 20% more talangiectasias, it took 61% more sessions to give 70% of overall disappearance.

b) Disappearance:
In both groups, we had 70% of disappearance of the telangiectasias in a small number of sessions.

Pictures before and after and evaluation by operator and patient do not show big discordances.

c) Complications:
Pain at the time of injection is reduced with sodium tetradecyl sulfate. Echymosis are a matter of technic rather than of the medication used. Matting is rare (3 patients) in these groups, probably due to the fact that all perforators and tributories (>2mm) had been treated prior to their telangiectasias (<2mm). Postsclerotic pigmentation seems more important with sodium tetradecyl sulfate.

Conclusion:

There are signs in this study that sodium tetradecyl sulfate at 0.15% is more effective (less sessions needed), less painful to inject but gives more postsclerotic pigmentation than the hypertonic dextrose solution. The concentration chosen (0.15%) evolves from our experience through the years with different concentrations. Superior concentrations had been abandonned for giving too many complications.

Phlébologie 92. Eds P. Raymond-Martimbeau, R. Prescott, M. Zummo.
John Libbey Eurotext, Paris © 1992, pp. 805-807

Traitement comparé des varicosités par le polidocanol à 0,5 % et par la glycémie chromée

Gérard Zemmour

48 Bd Voltaire, 75011 Paris, France.

Notre experience du traitement des varicosites par le Polidocanol à 0,5%depuis une dizaine d'années nous a conduit à tenter de confirmer nos résultats par une étude sur 20 cas.

MATERIEL ET METHODE

-Seringues plastique 3 pièces de 2 ml

-Aiguilles 3/10 èmes de mm de diamètre

-Traitement des varicosités des faces externes des cuisses (varicosités le plus souvent isolées dans cette région) chez 20 patientes avec pour chacune à gauche, utilisation de Polidocanol à 0,5%, et à droite glycérine chromée non diluée. On fait de chaque côté pour chaque patiente une dizaine de piqûres à chaque séance pendant 10 séances. On n'injecte que lorsqu'on est sûr de cathétériser la varicosité. L'absence de blanchiment de la varicosité, une sensation de résistance à l'injection, le début d'une formation de papule au point d'injection doit faire cesser immédiatement l'injection. On arrête l'injection lorsque l'on obtient un blanchiment de la ou des varicosités sur 1,5 cm à partir du point d'injection.

RESULTATS

-Efficacité :

Au bout de 10 séances

Le résultat est meilleur à gauche dans 14 cas.

Le résultat est équivalent des 2 côtés dans 4 cas.

Le résultat est ininterprétable dans 2 cas du fait d'une efficacité réduite après 10 séances.

Le plus grand pouvoir sclérosant, la plus grande fluidité et par conséquent, la plus grande maniabilité du Polidocanol injecté avec les aiguilles les plus fines (3/10 èmes de mm de diamètre) permet d'atteindre et de traiter un plus grand nombre de varicosités.`

-Risques liés à la microsclérose :

Dans les 20 cas étudiés, nous n'avons pas observé d'incidents liés à la sclérose (absence d'eschares, de pigmentations, de varicosités iatrogènes).

Nous avons observé de micro-hématomes aux points d'injection (qui disparaissent en 10 à 15 jours) de façon équivalente des 2 côtés.

Les conditions de traitements font que les risques liés aux injections ne sont pas plus grands à gauche avec le Polidocanol qu'à droite avec la glycérine chromée réputée pour son moindre pouvoir escharifiant.

En effet, la maniabilité du Polidocanol associée à la finesse des aiguilles permet un moindre débit et une moindre pression intravaricositaire du liquide sclérosant et donc une bonne maîtrise de l'injection ce qui permet de limiter les risques liés au surdosage et à l'injection extravaricositaire - en mettant à profit le meilleur pouvoir sclérosant du produit.

Une bonne expérience du traitement des varicosités est toutefois indispensable.

On peut envisager d'utiliser dans un premier temps des dilutions plus grandes de Polidocanol, mais ces dilutions ne sont pas disponibles en préparations commerciales et les solutions réalisées au cabinet sont assez souvent instables.

Par ailleurs, si le pouvoir sclérosant de la glycérine chromée peut être suffisant dans certains cas, son manque de maniabilité limite son utilisation.

REFERENCES :

R. Tournay et collaborateurs : La sclérose des varices
P. Wallois : Le choix du sclérosant; la conduite du traitement sclérosant; incidents et accidents de la sclérose.

Phlébologie 92. Eds P. Raymond-Martimbeau, R. Prescott, M. Zummo.
John Libbey Eurotext, Paris © 1992, pp. 808-810

Sclerotherapy of leg teleangiectasia : chromated glycerin versus polidocanol : a retrospective study

Michael Georgiev

Via Lombardia, 40, 00187 Rome, Italy.

Chromated glycerin at 72% (Sclérémo, Laboratoires E. Bouteille, France) (SCL) is a milder sclerosing agent than Polidocanol at 0.5% (Aethoxysklerol, Kreussler, Germany) (POL) and is reported to cause less post-sclerotherapy hyperpigmentations (PSH) (2). This paper presents the results of a retrospective study of 134 clinical records with the scope to investigate how and to what extent SCL can replace POL in order to lower the incidence of PSH.

Materials and Methods

Patients. The records of 217 patients treated for leg teleangiectasia during 1990-91 were reviewed; 134 of them provided useful information which is reported and discussed in this article. All patients were female, mean age 38.5 years (range 17 - 82). Fifteen of the patients (11%) had venous teleangiectasia only, i.e. red/blue tiny vessels 0.1-1.0-mm diameter. In the remaining 119 patients (89%), venous teleangiectasia were accompanied by larger, Doppler incontinent, blue/green dermal veins, 1.0-3.0-mm diameter. The latter are often refered to in the literature as "nurturing", "drainage" or "reticular"veins; it is the last definition that is used in the present article.

Sclerosing solutions. Prior to use, to the 5 ml vial of SCL was added 0.5 ml of 2% mepivacaine with 1:100 000 epinephrine (10% dilution). Pol was used at 0.5% and 1.0% without further dilution or intermediate concentrations; 0.5% was injected into the teleangiectasia and 1.0% into the reticular veins.

Injection technique. All-glass syringes and Terumo 26G½, 0.45x12 mm disposable needles were used. With a proper technique one can successfuly inject with the n.26 needle - and without a magnifying lense - even teleangiectasia which diameter is inferior than the calibre of the needle. Reticular veins are injected in a way similar to a common EV injection. The technique of injecting teleangiectasia is different. No attempt is made to incanulate the vessel, but only the beveled tip of the needle is entered into the teleangiectasia; when the tip is correctly positioned, its opening transpares under the thinned epidermis that covers the teleangiectasia and is clearly seen in the teleangiectasia. As reccomended by Sigg (3), only a small amount (0.05 - 0.2 ml) of the sclerosant is given per injection, while as many injections as needed may be given at each session. As a rule injections are given at a weekly interval; in case of extremely numerous teleangiectasia, in the beginning of the treatment the patient may be conveniently injected at a shorter interval, even every day, in order to shorten the duration of the treatment.

Any blood retained in the injected vessels - especialy if there is a visible inflammatory reaction with brownish perivenous staining - is promptly evacuated through a needle or blood lancet incision.

Compression. Immediately after the injections, elastic stocking is applied to every patient and worn during the daytime for the entire duration of the treatment. 114 of the patients (85%) in this series had a 30 - 40-mm graduated (Sigvaris 504) stockings, and 20 patients (15%) a 15 -18-mm graduated panty hose. Some of the patients were advised to sleep for 1 -3 nights after the injections with a 15 - 18-mm stokings.

At the first session all the patients were injected with SCL. From the second session on, treatment was continued - according to the reaction to the SCL injection - either with SCL or with the stronger POL.

Results

In 36 patients (27%) treatment was carried out with SCL only. These patients had a strong reaction to SCL. All (or majority) of the injected teleangiectasia/reticular veins were visibly damaged and many had blood clots with or without a visible perivenous inflammatory reaction. Three of the patients in this group (8%) had few PSH at the end of the treatment (one persisting after one year).

In 98 patients treatment was continued and finished with POL.(73%).

In 55 of these patients (41%) POL was started at the second session, since there was no (or very little) vessel damage and no inflammatory reaction after the SCL injection.

In the remaining 43 patients (32%) there was some vessel damage but no (or very mild) inflammatory reaction, so that a clear-cut decision was difficult to make after only one session. In these patients treatment was first continued with SCL, but when after few more (average of three) sessions it became evident that many repeated SCL injections were needed, treatment was continued with the stronger POL.

In the group treated with POL there were no PSH at the end of the treatment.

Considered separately, red/blue teleangiectasia (0.1-1.0-mm diameter) and reticular veins (1.0-3.0-mm diameter) were treated successfuly with SCL in respectively 32% and 30% of the cases.

In 7 cases teleangiectasia were treated with SCL while the reticular veins with 1.0% POL, and in 8 cases the reverse happened: teleangiectasia were treated with 0.5% POL and the reticular veins with SCL. Thus both teleangiectasia and reticular veins were treated successfuly with the same agent - SCL or POL - in respectively 8 out of 10 and 9 out of 10 cases. These figures suggest that - for the types of veins object of this study - the sensibility to the sclerosing agent varies considerably from patient to patient, but does not depend much on the size of the vessel.

In few cases it was found convenient to inject SCL and POL to the same patient, usually in vessels of different size: interestingly there were 8 cases in which POL was prefered for the teleangiectasia and the milder SCL for the reticular veins.

Discussion and Conclusions

POL and other sclerosing agents different from SCL are reported to cause from 48% of early to 1 - 30% of late (over one year) PSH (1). This difference (1-30%) is probably due to different sclerosing techniques. In author's experience, the use of all-glass syringe, low concentration and very small amount of a sclerosant per injection, prompt evacuation of the retained blood and, in particular, adequate and continuous compression, all contribute to the reduction of the incidence of PSH (and of teleangiectatic matting as well).

While PSH are best avoided by an adequate sclerosing technique, this study shows that the incidence of PSH may be further reduced with the use of a milder sclerosing agent, which seems to "select" the patients with a stronger sclero-inflammatory reaction. In this series, at the end of the treatment only 2.2% of the patients - all treated with SCL only - had PSH. This figure is much lower than the 15% previously reported with POL and iodine/Na iodide (1).

It appears that a single session with SCL is sufficient for the selection of the patients to be treated with SCL only (strong reaction - 27% in this series) and this may reduce the incidence of PSH. In the remaining part of the patients (absent or mild reaction - 73% in this series) SCL is conveniently substituted with the stronger POL in order to shorten the duration of treatment.

This simple approach proved so effective in avoiding excessive inflammatory reactions and PSH, that it is now adopted by the author as a routine procedure.

References

1. Georgiev M. (1990) Postsclerotherapy Hyperpigmentations: A One Year Follow-Up. J Dermatol Surg Oncol; 16:608.
2. Martin DE and Goldman MP. (1990) A Comparison of Sclerosing Agents: Clinical and Histologic Effects of intravascular Sodium Tetradecyl Sulfate and Chromated Glycerin in the Dorsal Rabbit Ear Vein. J Dermatol Surg Oncol; 16:18.
3. Sigg K. (1976) Varizen Ulcus Cruris und Thrombose. Berlin; Springer Verlag.

Phlébologie 92. Eds P. Raymond-Martimbeau, R. Prescott, M. Zummo.
John Libbey Eurotext, Paris © 1992, pp. 811-812

Evaluation of results of any curative treatments of varicose veins

André Cornu-Thénard, Pierre Boivin

4, rue de Lyon, 75012 Paris, France.

In order to be able to evaluate the results of any curative therapy of varicose veins, a quantification of the disease is required. In fact, it is necessary to establish a "score" in order to compare the pre-therapeutic state to the post-therapeutic state. Of course, such a system would also allow us to reach an important goal : to compare the results of the different techniques actually used.

Clinical examination, doppler examination and ultrasonography (echography) examination are the three principal means to quantify the disease. For each mean, some parameters have to be selected and defined. They will enable one to establish a clinical score, a doppler score and an echography score.

The different clinical scores have been already studied. A recent work [1] has proved that the simplest score was the Maximum Diameter (MD) of varicose veins determined by palpation. This MD must be given for the Long Saphenous, the Short Saphenous and the No Saphenous Varicose veins. (No Saphenous varicose veins means varicose veins which are present when the Long Saphenous and the Short Saphenous veins are normal or treated).

The doppler and echography scores are much more difficult to establish. Calculating the score should be easy because of the presence of curves given by doppler and photographies given by echography. Unfortunately, doppler examination is not easily reproducible if the technician is not the same.
However, a doppler study [2] has proved that, after the squeezing-releasing-manouver, longer is the time of the reflux, smaller is the diameter of the varicose vein where is the probe. Conversely, shorter is the time, larger is the diameter.
For echography there is a difficulty as well : the compression by the probe of the superficial veins, even light, can vary the diameter considerably.

In conclusion, it seems that the clinical examination is actually the only way to quantify the disease. The best criterion is the MD found by palpation. In order to establish more reliable doppler and echogrpahy scores, it is necessary to carry out profound research.

[1] - CORNU-THENARD André, MD ; DE VINCENZI Isabelle, MD ; MARAVAL Max, MD
- Evaluation of different systems for clinical quantification of varicose veins.
- J.Dermatol.Surg.Oncol.1991 ; 17 : 345-348

[2] - CORNU-THENARD André, MD ; VALTY Jean, MD
- Valeur diagnostique des ondes de flux et de reflux obtenues au doppler lors de la manoeuvre de compression-décompression des veines du mollet.
- Angiologie, 1988, 5, N°69 p29.

Results of sclerotherapy

César F. Sánchez, MD, R. Barcelo, MD, A. Pedrazzoli, MD, E. Tkach, MD, and U. Tropper, MD
"Dr. César F. Sánchez" Phlebology clinic

A series of photographics comparing the varicose veins of a patient at the time of consultation and the results obtained after therapy will be submitted. The patients chosen present various varicose pathologies in order to demonstrate the extension and benefits of this method.

Phlébologie 92. Eds P. Raymond-Martimbeau, R. Prescott, M. Zummo.
John Libbey Eurotext, Paris © 1992, pp. 8814-816

La compression immédiate en sclérothérapie. Un nouvel instrument

R. Bisacci, A. Colasanti, G. Genovese

Istituto di Clinica Chirurgica Generale, Università degli Studi di Perugia, Italia.

La compression représente une aide essentielle de la sclérothérapie. Son utilisation change selon l'école, les habitudes et l'expérience du flébologue. On peut distinguer une compression immédiate et une compression élastique ou rigide permanente qui varie d'après le type de sclérose, le type de produits sclérosants et le calibre de la varice.
La compression immédiate est pratiquée par le médecin ou par l'infirmier assistant, après chaque injection sclérosante, pour comprimer les points d'injection: actuellement cette compression est réalisée par un tampon d' ouate et après par d'autres tampons fixés par un sparadrap hypoallergique ou recouverts d'un bandage élastique ou rigide (compression permanente).
Cette procedure de compression manuelle est souvent difficile et labourieuse, en particulier si le médecin travaille tout seul, il s'ensuit que, parfois, le resultat n'est pas tout à fait satisfaisant.
Pour dépasser ces difficultés, nous avons réalisé un procédé plus rapide et en même temps plus efficace, en créant un instrument, dont la structure et le fonctionnement sont très simples, et qui remplace, d'une façon valable et fonctionnelle, la compression immédiate manuelle dans la sclérothérapie.

MATERIELS ET METHODES

L'instrument que nous avons conçu comprend un support qui sert d'appui au segment du membre qu'on doit scléroser et qui comprend un châssis rectangulaire (mais qui pourrait avoir n'importe quelle forme convenant à ce fin) en métal pour être facilement stérilisé (fig. 1-1).
Sur le côte extérieur longitudinal du support on a fixé des couples équidistants de petits pivots cylindriques, à l'extrémité plus grosse (fig. 1-2) préparés pour être accrochés par des couples correspondants de trous faits sur l'extrémité d'une bande élastique en caoutchouc.
Le membre du patient est appuyé sur le support et donc, anfur et à mésure qu'on pratique les injections sclérosantes, les parties traitées sont immédiatement comprimées en tendant sur chacune d'elles la bande élastique en caoutchouc correspondante qui a été déjà fixée sur une côté de l'instrument et qui est accrochée

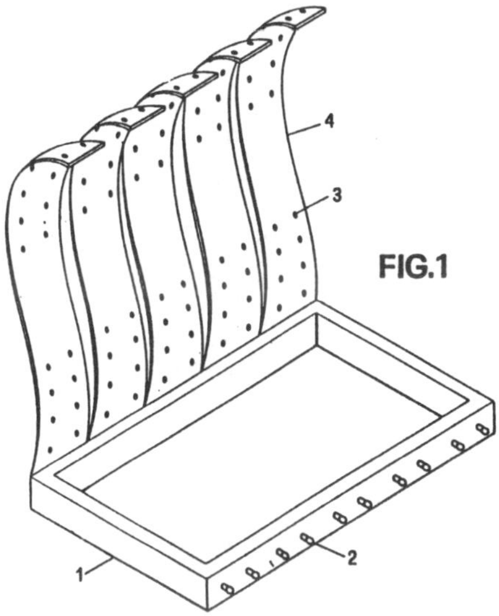

FIG.1

de l'autre côté, en bloquant les couples de trous dans les pivots correspondants. Après avoir terminé la sclérose, les parties traitées sont toutes parfaitement comprimées et le médecin, après avoir enlevé les bandes en caoutchouc, peut procéder au bandage pour la compression permanente.

DISCUSSION

Nous pratiquons la sclérothérapie dans les varices de moyen et petit calibre et dans les telangiectasée en utilisant la thérapie chirurgicale pour les grandes varices saphéniques et pour la crosse saphéno-fémorale.
Nous utilisons constamment la compression élastique permanente par des méthodes et des temps defférents d'après le calibre de la veine traitée.

Nous considérons essentielle la compression immédiate soit pour favoriser un plus grand contact du liquide sclérosant avec l'endothélium, soit pour réduire le reflux du sang à l'intérieur de la lumière de la veine et la formation de caillots intravariqueux.
L'utilisation de ce nouvel instrument a beaucoup amélioré la réalisation de la sclérothérapie soit en ce qui concerne les résultats.
Son emploi s'est averé essentiel dans la réduction des temps pour l'exécution de la sclérose, notamment si elle est pratiquée sans l'aide de infirmier assistant. Il faut encore remarquer une réduction importante du sangnement des points d'injection avec réduction des risques pour le médecin.

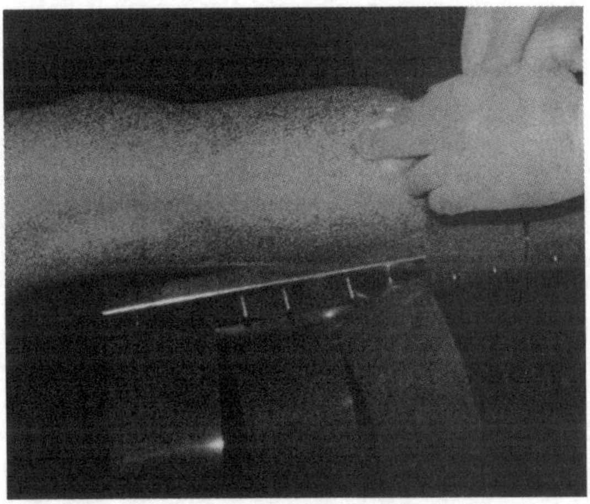

BIBLIOGRAPHIE

1) G.L. Bassi, R. Stemmer: Traitemens mécaniques fonctionnels en phlébologie.
2) G.L. Bassi, R. Stemmer: Compendio di terapia flebologica. Ed.Min.Med.,Torino
3) A. Cornu-Thenard, I. De Vincenzi, J. Valty: Sclérothérapie des varices: intêret de la mesure clinique de leur diamètre avant les premières injections. Actes du 10° Congrès Mondial Union Internationale de Phlébologie. Strasbourg 1989.
4) W.G. Fegan, D.E. Fitzgerald: A histologic assessment of continous compression sclerotherapy. Angiologie 16: 433, 1965.

5) P. Wallois: La compression en phlébologie. Actes du 10° Congrès Mondial Union Internationale de Phlébologie. Strasbourg 1989.
6) Haid-Fischer: Malattie delle vene. Ed. Sagraf, Napoli 1989.
7) R. Fisher: Surgical treatment of varicose veins, the bloodless limb technique. Actes du 10° Congrès Mondial Union Internationale de Phlébologie. Strasbourg 1989.

Phlébologie 92. Eds P. Raymond-Martimbeau, R. Prescott, M. Zummo.
John Libbey Eurotext, Paris © 1992, pp. 817-819

Apport de l'écho-sclérose dans le traitement de l'insuffisance veineuse superficielle

B. Cales, O. Creusot

G.R.A.C.I.A., Groupe de Recherche en Angéiologie Clinique Interventionnelle Ambulatoire, Ile-de-France, Paris, France.

L'échographie-doppler véritable 6 ème doigt de l'angio-phlébologue a permis d'établir des cartographies variqueuses trés précises autorisant une plus grande rigueur dans les indications thérapeutiques est d'être le plus conservateur possible au niveau saphénien interne, sauvegardant ainsi le capital veineux pour d'éventuelles chirurgies de revascularisation artérielle.

L'écho-doppler a de plus mis en évidence la naissance souvent complexe, loin du point d'émergence visible ou palpable de la varice, dont la profondeur rend impossible une sclérose classique ou une phlébectomie ambulatoire.

Dans ces situations où la varice se situe à 1 cm, 1, 5 cm sous la peau, zone d'excellente définition pour une sonde d'écho de 7,5 /10 MHZ, la sclérose écho-guidée a tout son intérêt.

LA TECHNIQUE :

Après repérage au crayon en orthostatisme du segment variqueux, on installe le patient en décubitus. Le matériel pour effectuer la sclérose ne differe pas d'un geste classique, les aiguilles doivent être les mêmes, celles de 16 mm permettent d'effectuer la plupart des actes réservant celles de 25 mm pour des patients adipeux. Une main tient la seringue et l'autre ne palpe plus la varice elle tient la sonde d'échographie, l'idéal étant une sonde dite à barette beaucoup plus facile à utiliser qu'une sonde sectorielle pour ce geste. Le mieux est qu'elle soit dans l'axe longitudinal du vaisseau qui est cependant en général flexueux et souvent vu en coupe transversale.

L'echographie voit l'aiguille, ou la devine du fait :

- de la modification de l'échogénicité des tissus qu'elle traverse,
- de la dépression qu'elle produit sur la paroi veineuse en la transfixiant,

La position endoluminale de la pointe est en général signalée pratiquement immédiatement par l'apparition d'un point hyperéchogène traduisant l'agrégation érythrocytaire sur la goutte de produit sclérosant présente au niveau du biseau.

Le reflux atteste de la bonne position, l'injection peut-être effectuée de la même façon que pour une sclérose ordinaire visualisant des turbulences au passage du produit et trés souvent deux phénomènes en fin d'injection : soit un spasme du vaisseau, soit une hyperéchogénicité de toute la lumière traduisant l'agrégation érythrocytaire.

Parfois on ne peut obtenir de reflux mais la visualisation du biseau attestant de la position endoluminale.

Après ce geste une contention de 24 heures par une bande à varices cohésive est nécessaire, un simple pansement n'étant pas assez compressif vu la profondeur des varices concernées.

PLACE DE L'ECHO-SCLEROSE DANS L'ARSENAL THERAPEUTIQUE

Elle découle de la cartographie initiale et ne sera jamais le traitement unique de la maladie variqueuse d'un patient.

Elle s'adresse à tous les segments variqueux non chirurgicaux ou séquellaires d'une chirurgie n'ayant pas donné tous les résultats escomptés, profonds au voisinage de l'aponévrose sous-cutanée dans la graisse ou dans un dédoublement aponévrotique.

Cette situation rend difficile ou impossible une phlébectomie ambulatoire, gestes qui seront par contre utilisés dés l'apparition cutanée de la varice avec d'excellents résultats compte tenu de la disparition du reflux d'amont, elle permet de traiter des vaisseaux de petit calibre jusqu'à 2 mm de diamètre dont la somation aboutit souvent à l'alimentation d'un plus gros.

Laisser en place un segment variqueux expose à une récidive par effet de siphon.

L'échographie doppler veineux permet de surveiller les résultats de la sclérose écho-guidée objectivant l'absence de résultat où le caractère partiel de celui-ci, une veine sclérosée se présente dans un premier temps comme un vaisseau à la lumière pleine d'un matériel à l'échogénicité soutenue incompressible sous la sonde d'échographie. Le doppler permet d'attester de l'absence de chenal résiduel circulant aux différentes manoeuvres de compression d'amont et d'aval.

L'écho-sclérose permet une reprise même sur une zone trés segmentaire du geste. Le reflux sanguin dans la seringue est en général minime, ou absent mais cette façon de procéder renseigne parfaitement sur la position endoluminale de l'aiguille et l'injection intra-variqueuse.

LES CONTRAINTES

Pour le praticien habitué à une sclérothérapie classique la mise en oeuvre d'une telle technique pour un tel geste peut sembler lourde. En fait, trés vite, le temps passé n'est pas beaucoup plus long, ce n'est plus le doigt qui palpe la varice à scléroser manoeuvre essentielle et difficile sur ces varices profondes c'est l'oeil qui surveille échographiquement le positionnement de l'aiguille. Il y a évidemment la contrainte financière de l'achat de l'appareil mais celui-ci semble de plus en plus incontournable pour la prise en charge du variqueux.

Pour le malade il n'y a pas de contrainte, il suit le geste avec le praticien dans la plupart des territoires ce qui a pour effet de le sécuriser. Le geste est par ailleurs parfaitement indolore même quand plusieurs déplacements de l'aiguille sont nécessaires pour cathétériser.

LES INCIDENTS

Il n'y en a pas si l'on respecte les mêmes règles que celles qui président à toute sclérose classique : dose et injection strictement intra-variqueuse ce qui est encore une fois l'avantage absolu de l'apport de l'échographie. Aucune complication infectieuse n'est survenue, malgré la présence du gel d'échographie.

LES RESULTATS

Après trois ans et probablement une dizaine de milliers d'injections écho-guidée les résultats sont excellents permettant d'améliorer ceux de l'association chirurgie sclérose classique :

- en traitant des territoires variqueux à leur naissance en particulier chez l'adipeux, en limitant les réactions inflammatoires, en garantissant un résultat plus durable, la sclérose prenant tout le corps de la varice,

- autorisant la correction de résultats chirurgicaux imparfaits

- rendant phlébectomisable une grosse branche variqueuse qui ne l'était pas au départ vu son origine profonde.

Arme thérapeutique de plus en terme de conservation des troncs saphéniens peu incontinents non ectasiques.

permettant ainsi de mieux tendre à ces trois buts de notre pratique phlébologique quotidiennne :

- être radical,
- être indolore,
- être esthétique

Pressé par nos patients d'utiliser du matériel à usage unique devant la peur de contamination par le virus H.I.V, l'écho-sclérose est le moyen technique d'assurer une garantie absolue injection intra-variqueuse en particulier au voisinage des crosses.

A la condition sine qua non cependant d'une formation phlébologique et écho-doppleriste rigoureuse.

BIBLIOGRAPHIES

MISEREY G., REINHAREZ D., ECATARD P.
Sclérose sous échographie dans certaines zones à risque.(Phlébologie, 1991, 44-1, 85-96)

SCHADECK M.
Doppler et Echotomographie dans la sclérose des veines saphènes.(Phlébologie, 1986, 39,37, 697-716)

VIN F.
Echo-sclérothérapie de la saphène externe.(Phlébologie 1991, 44-1, 79-84)

Phlébologie 92. Eds P. Raymond-Martimbeau, R. Prescott, M. Zummo.
John Libbey Eurotext, Paris © 1992, pp. 820-821

La sclérose échoguidée

S. Ermini*, M. Cappelli**, A. Turchi***, G. Bono**

** Studio flebologico, via Tizzano 18, Grassina, Firenze, Italy. ** Studio flebologico, via Datini 46, Firenze, Italy. *** 1° UO Chirurgia generale, Ospedale S.M. Annunziata, USL, 10/H Firenze, Italy.*

La sclérothérapie échoguidée consiste dans l'utilisation de la guide échographique pour effectuer l'injection sclérosante. Les avantages de cette tecnique sont tous ceux dus à une vision directe de la pointe de l'aiguille et de la veine et de réaliser de cette façon une recherche guidée par la lumière vasale. Nous pourrons choisir à volontée la tecnique à utiliser et le point précise ou' effectuer injection sans se soucier des problèmes tecniques liés à la "palpabilité du vaisseau". Nous aurons moins de risque d'injection extravasculaires ou intraarterieuses, et il n'y aura aucune limitation dans le traitement des patients obèses ou nous serons toujours certains d'avoir piqué le vaisseau voulu. Les traitement est plus precis et par conséquent plus sur.(Vin 1991,Miserey 91)

<u>La sclérothérapie réalisée sous guide échografique est plus efficace de celle traditionelle ?</u>

L'emploi de l'échographie permet l'injection du vaisseau à son calibre minimum possible, de façon à réduire la dilution ématique du liquide sclérosante. Tel accorgement peut etre appliqué soit à la tecnique française qu'à celle de Cloutier employée pour augmenter le temps de contact du liquide sclérosant avec la paroi du vaisseau (Zummo 1990).

L'étude échographique du traitement sclérothérapeutique à mis en evidence que la recanalisation veineuse advient à calibre inférieur et avec épaississement de la paroi.

Dans cette phase la reprise sclérothérapeutique devient fondamentale pour progrédire dans la reduction du calibre vasale jusq'à son éventuelle disparition (Ermini 1991).

La persistance d'un vaisseau fibreux avec un calibre inférieur à 3 mm. même si refluant rapresente un très bonne résultat sclérothérapeutique s'il n'est pas associé à la réapparitios des varices ou de la sintomatologie. L'emploi del-l'échographie dans les reprises sclérothérapeutique devient donc fondamentale en rapport à la difficulté tecnique de piqué un vaisseau de petit calibre avec épaississement parietal.

Dans un point de vue pratique, cette tecnique est réalisé tenant dans une maine la sringue et dans l'autre la sonde, controlant sur l'écrain que l'aiguille reste toujours dans le plan de scansion.

Il peut arriver que la point de l'aiguille semble à l'interieur du vaisseau mais non s'aspire le sang: il s'agit d'un artefact appellé "épaisseur de couche altéré " pour le quel les structures à coté du vaisseau et donc aussi la point de l'aiguille située ùn proximité de la veine, semblent, dans l'image échographique contenues dans la lumière du vaisseau étant celle-ci non entierément comprise dans l'épaisseur du plan de scansion.

Les indications de la méthode sont le memes que la sclérothérapie traditionnelle meme si vient considérablement augmentéé la potentialité applicative e l'efficacité.

Avec cette technique ont été traité 105 saphènes internes (25 avec un calibre superieur a 10 mm) 60 saphènes externes(5 avec un calibre superieur à 10 mm) 73 récidives post stripping et 12 varices non systématisées. La tecnique de Cloutier a été utilisé dans 130 cas et celle français dans 120 cas.On a du utiliser en moyenne 3 séances pour traiter la saphène interne, 2 pour la saphène externe et 4 pour le récidives.

Les controles des malades traités ont été effectués a 6 mois à 12 mois et plus et nous avons fait un nouveau traitement sous guide échographique meme pour les recanalisations partielles.

A 6 et à 12 mois nous avons rencontrés le 30% de récidives tandis qu'après 12 mois la pourcentage rencontré était seul de 10%. La disparition échographique du vaisseau à été vu dans 21 cas sur 127 controles a 12 mois (15 récidives post stripping, 5 varices non systematisées, 1 saphène interne).

CONCLUSIONS

Le numéro des cas et le temps de controle (2 ans) et tel de ne pas pouvoir trair aucune conclusion.

Cependant l'expérience acquise et les résultats obtenus font entrevoir avec cett tecnique un supérament des problèmes rencontrés dans le traitement sclérothérapeutique traditionelle augmentant énormement l'efficacité.

BIBLIOGRAPHIE

1. ERMINI S. CAPPELLI M. TURCHI A.: La scleroterapia ecoguidata della safena interna. Atti del III° Congresso Internazionale di Flebolinfologia - Ferrara - San Marino settembre 1991 pag 4.1- 4.3

2. MISEREI G. REINHAREZ D. ECATARD P.: Sclérose sous écographie dans certaines zones à risques. Phlébologie 1991, 44 - 1, 85-96.

3. Vin F.:Echosclérothérapie de la saphène externe. Phlébologie 1991 44-1, 79 -84.

4. Zummo M.: Sclérose des saphènes internes selon G. Cloutier. Réunion de la societé française de phlébologie 20/10/1990.

Phlébologie 92. Eds P. Raymond-Martimbeau, R. Prescott, M. Zummo.
John Libbey Eurotext, Paris © 1992, pp. 822

A single treatment protocol for sapheno-femoral or sapheno-popliteal incompetence by duplex guided sclerotherapy

Mark D. Forrestal, Deborah P. Foley

Vein Clinics of America, 1101 perimeter Drive, Suite 615, Schaumburg, Illinois 60173, USA.

Two hundred patients were selected who demonstrated sapheno-femoral or sapheno-popliteal insufficiency by Duplex ultrasound.
All patients were treated with a single session of ultrasound guided injection sclerotherapy with 3% Sotradecol® (Elkins-Sinn, Inc., Cherry, Hill N. J.) followed by external compression. The therapeutic goal was obliteration of reflux from the sapheno-femoral or sapheno-popliteal junctions. Short term assessment of results was made by physical examination and Continuous Wave (CW) Doppler. At three months—87% of the patients were found to be CW Doppler negative for reflux at either junction.

Treatment protocol via video, number and selection of injection sites, and all complications will be reviewed. Ongoing one year follow-up with Duplex ultrasound evaluation will be presented.

A rationale for one year follow-up will be given in the form of a literature review of previous long term follow-up studies. The authors feel that the conditions responsible for most long term treatment failures could have been identified at one year with the current available technology of Duplex color ultrasound.

Treatment of Superficial and Perforator Venous Disease with Accurate Sclerotherapy: an Update on Echosclerotherapy®

Robert M. Knight, M.D.

VeinCare® of Florida, Boca Raton, FL USA

Abstract

Echosclerotherapy, a treatment protocol for performing extremely precise sclerotherapy for superficial and perforator venous disease has been described by the author in prior publications. The protocol utilizes real-time B-mode ultrasound to guide needle placement into truncal saphenous veins and all involved branches and tributaries. The procedure was developed to be analogous to complete surgical saphenectomy. The treatment concept assumes the saphenous system in its entirety to be the etiological target in varicose disease- hence the need for its ablation. The importance of color-flow will also be discussed. Updated results will be presented.

Phlébologie 92. Eds P. Raymond-Martimbeau, R. Prescott, M. Zummo.
John Libbey Eurotext, Paris © 1992, pp. 824-825

Duplex-echo-sclerotherapy : the quest for the safe technique

Louis Grondin, Jeannette Soriano

Circulatory Disease Center, Calgary, Alberta, Canada.

Surgery as a treatment for varices has been in existence at least since Galen, and there are anecdotal reports that Hippocrates may have been the first to apply sclerotherapy to the treatment of varices by repeated puncture with green willow wood splinters. In 1851 Charles Gabriel Pravaz fashioned the modern syringe with the apparent intent to inject arterial aneurysms, his disciples later applied the technique to the treatment of varices, thus he both started modern sclerotherapy as a treatment for varices, and uncovered one of its most serious complications: accidental arterial injections (1).

In the century that followed both the European and North American Schools (2) clearly identified the pitfalls and complications of both surgery and sclerotherapy, and admonished careful and prudent practice of the art as a safeguard against failure and against complications.

Since 1945 with the development of endovascular surgery (3), it was inevitable that the aid of modern technology was soon to be requested in the performance of either surgery or sclerotherapy. Endoscopic-sclerotherapy has been described but can only be applied to rather large and tear-resistant varices (4). More recently ultrasound guided injections have been described (5), but are accompanied, however, with a surprisingly high level of complications (6).

A review of these complications will prove timely and useful as in our case, where it lead us to the development of a safer and more precise technique.

REFERENCES

1. Browse, Norman L., Arnold, Edward. (1988): Milestones, Pebbles, and Grains of Sand. *Disease of the Veins.*

2. Tournay, Raymond. (1985): La Sclerose Des Varices. *Expansion Scientifique Francaise.*

3. Moore, Wesley S., Saunders, W.B. (1989): *Endovascular Surgery.*

4. Biegeleisen, Ken. (1989): Use of A Venoscope For Accurate Injection of Sites of Deep-to-Superficial Reflux in Varicose Veins. *Proceedings of the Phlebology Scoeity of America.*

5. Knight, R.M., Zygmunt, J.A. (1989): Echosclerotherapy. *Proceedings of the Phlebology Scoeity of America.*

6. Knight, R.M. (1991): Treatment of Superficial Venous Disease With Accurate Sclerotherapy. *Proceedings of The Canadian Society of Phlebology, Whistler.*

Phlébologie 92. Eds P. Raymond-Martimbeau, R. Prescott, M. Zummo.
John Libbey Eurotext, Paris © 1992, pp. 826

L'échosclérose, la nouvelle donnée

Michel Schadeck

École Européenne de Phlébologie, 6, rue Giordano Bruno, 75014 Paris, France.

La sclérothérapie guidée dans le même temps par l'examen échographique a pour but de permettre ou de faciliter l'accès de l'aiguille et donc à la sclérose d'un axe variqueux peu ou non palpable car trop petit ou trop profond
Mais toute varice nécessite que son reflux soit authentifié et localisé avec précision. L'utilisation du duplex scann s'impose donc, l'objectif n'étant pas de traiter une image échographique mais une anomalie hémodynamique représentée par le reflux.
L'échosclérose nécessite donc un bilan anatomique, morphologique et hémodynamique très précis réalisé par le phlébologue. Le repérage ed la varice et sa ponction se font en coupe transversale avec une aiguille de longueur appropriée. L'injection peut être unique ou répétée.
La première indication de cette technique concerne les récidives post-chirurgicales dont l'origine des reflux est très souvent difficile à dépister. Les axes saphèniens peuvent également bénéficier de l'échosclérose, surtout après les premières réactions de thrombose ou de fibrose, afin que les injections soient effectuées juste en dessous des zones sclérosées.
Mais l'abord, par cette méthode, des régions dites délicates comme le triangle de Scarpa et le creux poplité n'est pas synonyme de sécurité. L'utilisation, pour la petite saphène en particulier, d'un mini catheter ou d'un "butterfly" pour les plus superficielles facilite grandement les conditions de sécurité et donc de l'injection.
Nous devons toujours conserver notre rigueur d'examen, notre prudence et toute notre vigilance.
Les résultats obtenus à partir de scléroses réalisées à l'origine des reflux sont très sensiblement supérieurs à ceux générés par la sclérothérapie uniquement clinique. En outre l'accès aux récidives majore encore plus le succès de ce type de traitement.
Il reste toutefois un acte thérapeutique qui engage la responsabilité du médecin et non pas celle de la " machine ".

Echosclerotherapy of recurrent varicoses veins after surgery

F. Vin

Notre Dame de Bon Secours 750:4 Paris

Many papers have shown the importance of Echo-sclerotherapy in dangerous areas as Scarpa area, popliteal fossa to avoid intra-arterial injection of sclerosing agent.

After surgery, ligation division or ligation division with long or short stripping, recurrence is possible.

The anatomical connections after this kind of surgery make difficult palpation of the new reflux at the sapheno-femoral junction or at the level of perforators.

We have performed sclerotherapy with ultrasonic guidence to identify the leaking point and to have the best sclerosing effect of the vessel responsible of recurrence without complications.

The technique is described with a video.

Phlébologie 92. Eds P. Raymond-Martimbeau, R. Prescott, M. Zummo.
John Libbey Eurotext, Paris © 1992, pp. 828-831

Echosclerotherapy, a canadian study

Louis Grondin, Jeannette Soriano

Circulatory disease Center, Calgary, Alberta, Canada.

I.INTRODUCTION:

Surgery as a treatment for varices has been in existence at least since Galen, and there are anecdotal reports that Hippocrates may have been the first to apply sclerotherapy to the treatment of varices by repeated puncture with green willow wood splinters. In 1851 Charles Gabriel Pravaz fashioned the modern syringe with the apparent intent to inject arterial aneurysms, his disciples later applied the technique to the treatment of varices, thus he both started modern sclerotherapy as a treatment for varices, and uncovered one of its most serious complications: accidental arterial injections (1).

In the century that followed both the European and North American Schools (2) clearly identified the pitfalls and complications of both surgery and sclerotherapy, and admonished careful and prudent practice of the art as a safeguard against failure and against complications.

Since 1945 with the development of endovascular surgery (3), it was inevitable that the aid of modern technology was soon to be requested in the performance of either surgery or sclerotherapy. Endoscopic-sclerotherapy has been described but can only be applied to rather large and tear-resistant varices (4). More recently ultrasound guided injections have been described (5), but are accompanied, however, with a surprisingly high level of complications (6).

A review of these complications will prove timely and useful as in our case, where it lead us to the development of a safer and more precise technique.

II.TECHNIQUE AND METHODOLOGY.

1.For the sapheno-femoral junction:

Under local anaesthesia and after skin disinfection, a 20 G, 44 mm Teflon/Radiopacque catheter is used to penetrate and canalise, under ultrasound guidance the Greater Saphenous Vein 6 cms to 8 cms distal to its termination. Spontaneous venous return must be observed prior to proceeding with the injection. Subsequently a pulse doppler window is opened within the vein distally to the catheter, and both venous flow and reflux is ascertained. A modified "cloutier technique" is then performed by compressing the most proximal part of the sapheno-femoral junction, and sufficient pressure is applied to suppress the valsalva reflux. Then 2 cc 0.1% diluted iodine is then injected and recuperated under ultrasound and doppler monitoring, and painlessness is ascertained. Finally once all the above steps have been successfully completed 2.5 to 3 cc of iodine 3% is injected slowly and under ultrasound and doppler monitoring.

The patient is seen on follow up 3 weeks later and is re-examined clinically, and by doppler and ultrasound, to determine the presence or absence of proximal saphenous sclerosis. If sclerosis is present conventional sclerotherapy is applied if needed to the distal truncal varices or to the incompetent perforators veins.

On the other hand if proximal sclerosis is absent the above described procedure is repeated using 3 cc of 6% iodine as sclerosant. A Junctional assessment is repeated 3 weeks later. If proximal sclerosis is again absent the patient is sent for a stripping of the greater saphenous vein.

2. For the sapheno-popliteal junction:

Under local aesthesia and after skin disinfection a 20 G, 44 mm. Teflon/Radiopacque catheter is used to penetrate under ultrasound guidance the Lesser Saphenous Vein 6 cms to 8 cms distal to its termination. Spontaneous venous return must be observed prior to proceeding with the injection. Subsequently a pulse doppler window is opened within the vein distally to the catheter, and both venous flow and reflux is ascertained. Then 2 cc 0.1% diluted iodine is then injected and recuperated under ultrasound and doppler monitoring, and painlessness is ascertained. Finally once all the above steps have been successfully completed the sclerosant consisting of 2 cc of iodine 3% is injected slowly and under ultrasound and doppler monitoring.

The patient is seen on follow up 3 weeks later and is re-examined clinically, by doppler and by ultrasound, to determine the presence or absence of proximal saphenous sclerosis. If sclerosis is present conventional sclerotherapy is applied if needed to the distal truncal varices or to the incompetent perforators veins.

On the other hand if proximal sclerosis is absent the above described procedure is repeated using 2 cc of 6% iodine as sclerosant. A Junctional assessment is repeated 3 weeks later. If proximal sclerosis is again absent the patient is sent for a ligation of the sapheno-popliteal junction.

III.RESULTS:

Patients with a personal or family history of hyper-coagulability or lupus were not treated with sclerotherapy. Cases where for technical reasons the procedure could not be completed were not considered in this study. Our first 500 injections performed were compiled and distributed as follows:

327 injections were performed on the Greater saphenous vein.

- 214 were single successful injections (65%).
- 113 were repeated injections (35%).
  - Of these 52 were successful (overall 81,3%),
  - and 61 were failures (overall failures 18.7%).

173 injections were performed on the Lesser Saphenous vein.

- 131 were single successful injections (75.7%).
- 42 were repeated injections. (24.3%).
  - Of these 19 were successful (overall 86.7%),
  - and 23 were failures (overall failures 13.3%).

Complications:

Allergic reactions:	none were observed.
lipothymia :	11 cases. (2.2%).

post injection pain: 97 cases. (19.4%).
superficial phlebitis: 32 cases. (6.4%).
deep venous thrombosis: none were observed.
Pulmonary emboli: none were observed.
intra-arterial injections: none were observed.
extravasation of sclerosant: none were observed.

In conclusion we find that for junctional superficial venous incompetence, sclerotherapy performed by ultrasound guided "open ended" catheter technique is both an effective and safe alternative to surgery. The use of iodine rather than sodium tetradecyl sulfate offers both a safety advantage and a more definite sclerosis. Long term studies are needed however to compare the efficacy of the technique with that of standard surgery. Nevertheless the low cost and ambulatory nature of the procedure make it a very attractive alternative for the time being.

V.REFERENCES:

1. Milestones, Pebbles, and Grains of Sand, Diseases of The Veins, Norman L. Browse & Coll., Edward Arnold, 1988.

2. La Sclerose Des Varices, Raymond Tournay et coll. Expansion Scientifique Francaise. Paris, 1985.

3. Endovascular Surgery, Wesley S. Moore. W.B. Saunders. 1989.

4. Use of A Venoscope For Accurate Injection of Sites of Deep-To-Superficial Reflux in Varicose Veins. Ken Biegeleisen. Proceedings of the Phlebology Society of America, 1989.

5. Echosclerotherapy, Robert M. Knight & Joseph A. Zygmunt Jr. Proceedings of the Phlebology Society of America, 1989.

6. Treatment of Superficial Venous Disease With Accurate Sclerotherapy, Robert M. Knight. Proceedings of The Canadian Society of Phlebology. Whistler, 1991.

b. Pathologies diverses / *Various disorders*

Phlébologie 92. Eds P. Raymond-Martimbeau, R. Prescott, M. Zummo.
John Libbey Eurotext, Paris © 1992, pp. 835-836

The effect of sclerotherapy on restless legs

Alan H. Kanter, D. Brian McDonagh

Vein Clinics of America, 19800 MacArthur Boulevard, Suite 270, Irvine, California 92715, USA.

Restless Legs Syndrome (RLS) may be defined as the irresistible urge to move the legs due to dysesthesiae of the legs at rest (Ekbom, 1950). Temporary relief is obtained only by leg movement or walking, graphically illustrated by the name a national self-help support group has chosen—"RLS Nightwalkers" (Orange Park, Florida). Nocturnal myoclonus and leg cramps may be associated with RLS, but are separate and distinct entities as defined by Sleep Disorder Medicine specialists. (Clough, 1987; Montplaisir et. al., 1985).

In patients with nocturnal awakening, resultant daytime somnolence and associated sleep deprivation symptoms impair cognitive performance and cause mood disturbance. Despite a plethora of studies including numerous drug trials, the etiology, pathogenesis, and an effective treatment all remain elusive. While Levodopa maintenance therapy seems to be the most efficacious form of treatment to date (Clough, 1987; Walters & Hening, 1987), symptoms return after discontinuing the medication.

Although RLS has been recognized in association with vein disease by the European literature (Tournay, 1948), there has been no systematic investigation of this connection. In our experience, RLS commonly improves after sclerotherapy for varicose vein disease. Therefore, a prospective study was undertaken to determine the incidence of RLS in a population seeking treatment for varicose veins, both with and without saphenous trunk reflux, and to assess the therapeutic response of RLS to sclerotherapy.

Data analysis revealed that the incidence of RLS was approximately 20%, typically females ages 30-50. The vast majority exhibit non-truncal posterior 3-6 mm venules. The affected patients usually experience daytime symptoms when stationary, and often lack the classical nocturnal awakening which has been an integral feature helping to define this syndrome. Over 90% experience resolution of symptoms after sclerotherapy. Post-treatment follow-up at 12-18 months demonstrates good durability of "cure" thus far.

Thus, RLS is easily treated when associated with vein disease. While non-truncal veins appear to be associated with RLS more commonly than saphenous trunk disease, it was also found that RLS waking-hours symptoms occur more commonly in the absence of nocturnal symptoms.

It is the responsibility of the Phlebology field to alert our primary care colleagues to this common treatable condition, presently underrecognized in general medicine. Cooperation between Phlebology and Sleep Medicine specialists will help to elucidate the pathogenesis that may explain the connection between RLS and vein disease. To this end, the authors have begun a collaborative study with a certified sleep disorder center.

References

Clough C., (1987): Restless legs syndrome. *Br. Med. J.* 294, 262-262.
Ekbom K.A., (1950): Restless legs. A report of 70 new cases. *Acta. Med. Scand.* [Suppl.]. 246, 64-68.
Montplaisir J. & Godbout R. & Boghen D., (1985): Familial restless legs with periodic movement in sleep. *Neurology.* 35, 130-134.
Tournay, (1948): *In Les varices de la grossesse et leur traitement principalement par injection sclérosants*, ed. R. Tournay, P. Wallois, Paris: L' Expansion Scientifique Française.
Walters A.S. & Hening W., (1987): Clinical presentation and neuropharmacology of restless legs syndrome. *Neuropharmacol.* 10, 225-237.

Phlébologie 92. Eds P. Raymond-Martimbeau, R. Prescott, M. Zummo.
John Libbey Eurotext, Paris © 1992, pp. 837-838

Treatment of facial telangiectasias by sclerotherapy

Robert Prescott

1490 Sherbrooke St. West, Montreal, P. Quebec, H3G 1L3, Canada.

Choice of patients:

All the patients in this study were female between 20 to 45 years of age. All complained of facial telangiectasias that appeared at an adult age and none had any significant underlying desease. The treated telangiectasias were all on the nose and cheeks.

Method:

30 patients were treated with an hypertonic dextrose solution at a concentration of 10%. We used microdrops, through a needle gauge 30, creating 1 to 3 blanching of the telangiectasias according to response to sclerotherapy.

Results were then compiled using four criterias: 1- pictures before and after 2- subjective evaluation of overall disappearance by the patient 3- subjective evaluation of overall disappearance by the operator 4- complications.

Results:

A) Number of sessions:

2 to 7 sessions
Average 3.2

B) Disappearance:

According to patient: 40 to 100%
Average 71%
According to operator: 40 to 90%
Average 66%
Pictures before and after: 30 to 90%
Average 68%

C) Complications:

1- Pain: mild to moderate: 40% of patients (12)
2- Echymosis: mild: 6.6% of patients (2)

3- Postsclerotic pigmentation: none
4- Others: none

Discussion:

A- Number of sessions:
Around 70% of disappearance of telangiectasias was obtained with a small number of sessions (3.2).

B- Overall disappearance:
Pictures before and after and evaluation by operator and patient do not show big discordances.

C- Complications:
Very few complications are reported. This is probably due to a good technique and extreme caution with the dosage of sclerosing agent, using a progressive dosage (1 to 3 blanching) with consecutive sessions.

Conclusion:

With a good technique, sclerotherapy of facial telangiectasias seems a very effective and safe method of treatment. Our twenty years of experience with this technic have proved very satisfactory and we beleive it is at the moment favorably comparable to electrocoagulation or laser therapy.

Phlébologie 92. Eds P. Raymond-Martimbeau, R. Prescott, M. Zummo.
John Libbey Eurotext, Paris © 1992, pp. 839-840

Sclerotherapy for multiple angiomata

Edward P. Gould

W. 105 8th Avenue, Suite 650, Spokane, Washington 99204, USA.

INTRODUCTION

Several different tumors are composed of multiple masses of vascular compartments; hemangiomata, lymphangiomata, and glomangiomata, are all characterized by extensive vascular development. Surgery remains the primary means of managing these tumors, but sclerotherapy may, under certain circumstances, be a very valuable adjunct. The establishment of an accurate tissue diagnoses and complete resection of bulky vascular lesions, is essential in tumor management. However, sclerotherapy may be preferable in the management of multiple small lesions or in lesions in which surgery may cause an unsatisfactory cosmetic result. Sclerotherapy may also make a valuable contribution in palliation of massive lesions which defy resection.

Several cases will be presented which illustrate the combined use of surgery and sclerotherapy in the management of angiomata.

CASE I.

23 Year old presented with a lifelong history of "varicose veins in the hand". She had a painful lesion of the right ring finger, the left thigh, and the left flank. There were also multiple tumors of her arms which were non-tender. Excisional biopsy of the thigh revealed presence of a glomangioma. The lesion of the ring finger was resected primarily in order to avoid the possibility of damage to the neurovascular bundle. However, the lesion on the left flank was treated with two (2) injections of Sodium Tetradecol Sulphate. The patient stated that she was pain free within twelve (12) hours. The mass has shown no evidence of recurrence after an eighteen (18) month period of follow-up.

CASE II.

A 21 year old female with a congenital hemangioma/lymphangioma of the right thigh, hip and abdominal wall was evaluated because of chronic pain. She had extensive involvement of the skin from her right knee to the right rib cage, and MRI revealed extension into the retroperitoneum with probable involvement of the uterus and the liver. This lesion had been slowly expanding since childhood. It had a massive area of erythema, induration and chronic weeping of proteinaceous fluid. Multiple lymphoceles had been previously drained, but all fluid appeared to be sterile.

Two extensive resections had been undertaken to control the tumor mass, but there was immediate recurrence. The massive extension of the tumor precluded further curative surgical attempts. The patient complained of severe pain, and there were several areas in the groin which were indurated and very tender. Three of these areas were injected on two occasions with small quantities of 0.5 cc STD. The patient reported a rapid pain reduction; there was visible tumor regression after one week. Although the patient's prognosis is grim, it is hoped that sclerotherapy may ameliorate some of her symptomatology.

CASE III

28 Year old female presented with a lifelong history of multiple subcutaneous hemangiomata. She had numerous previous resections for painful hemangiomas, but recurrence had been rapid. Physical examination revealed multiple tender grayish subcutaneous masses of the buttocks and the inner aspect of the right arm and hand. All lesions were injected with 0.5% STD. After two weeks the majority of lesions were obliterated, and none were painful. Visible tumors were injected with 0.33% STD, there has been no evidence of recurrence to date.

CASE IV

A 17 year old female presented with a life long subcutaneous tumor of the left cheek, lip, and eyelid. The lesion had been stable for the past five years; it was felt to be unresectable. The patient received a series of sclerotherapy treatments to all tumor areas. The mass tumor lesions were obliterated, and the patient is pleased with her cosmetic results.

DISCUSSION

Surgery will always be the primary method for management of bulky, solitary tumors. However, sclerotherapy is a wise choice in the management of multiple vascular tumors. It is effective management for difficult anatomical areas and relatively small tumor mass. It can be effectively employed to obliterate small lesions and palliate the discomfort of large ones.

Phlébologie 92. Eds P. Raymond-Martimbeau, R. Prescott, M. Zummo.
John Libbey Eurotext, Paris © 1992, pp. 841

The corona phlebectatica before and after treatment

Walter P. de Groot

Swedish Hospital Medical Center, Seattle, USA.

Patients with large varicose veins often show numerous fine vessels on the medial or lateral aspect of the ankle and foot. H.R. van der Molen[1] coined the term "Corona phlebectatica paraplantaris" for these vessels and pointed out that they are not simple spider veins, but rather an expression of the venous stasis in the whole leg. Accordingly, the best treatment of the corona phlebectatica is treatment of the clinical varicose veins.

We have taken photographs of the corona phlebectatica of patients with large varicose veins before treatment and later again after treatment had taken place, which usually consisted of a surgical ligation and division, followed by sclerotherapy. We noticed a definite improvement of the corona phlebectatica after treatment of the proximal varicose veins.

Following the above improvement, direct sclerotherapy of the remaining corona phlebectatica often accomplished considerable additional cosmetic improvement.

1. van der Molen HR. Taches de stase, corona phlebectatica et autres signes de stase veineuse. Folia Angiologica, 1961. Vol.VIII.nr.3

Phlébologie 92. Eds P. Raymond-Martimbeau, R. Prescott, M. Zummo.
John Libbey Eurotext, Paris © 1992, pp. 842-847

Two cases of Klippel-Trenaunay syndrome treated by sclerotherapy with 3 % sotradecol

Robert W. Dole

301 W. Huntington Drive Suite, Arcadia, CA 91007, USA.

Klippel-Trenaunay Syndrome is a congenital angiodysplasia consisting of a port wine stain, hypertrophy of the involved limb, and massive varicose veins. The first patient is a 38 year old male who presented with the classic symptomatology. He was evaluated at the Mayo Clinic in 1981. He was told nothing could be done surgically and he would have to wear compression hose the rest of his life. He was next evaluated in 1987 when he began to show massive enlargement of his right lower extremity including an increase of three shoe sizes. Arteriographic studies showed a normal arterial system, two venograms were read as massive venous prefusion into superficial varicosities. Again, the recommendation was to wear 50mm surgical compression hose.

On August 7, 1989 traditional injection, compression, ambulation sclerotherapy was begun. Initially he was treated twice weekly with 8 to 10 injections of 1 to 2 cc of 3% sotradecol. On four occasions to close huge incompetent perforators he received 8% variglobin. He received intensive treatment for nine months to March, 1990. His clinical response exceeded our expectations. Fig. 1 shows the anterior view before treatment, Fig. 2 nine months later. The leg has decreased two inches in circumference. His gait is normal, and he no longer carries around an extremity full of edema and stagnant blood. Fig. 3 shows the posterior aspect of the leg before treatment, Fig. 4 after 9 months. Fig. 5 and 6 show the lateral aspects of the thigh and lower leg and the massive varicosities and perforators. Fig.7shows the lateral aspect of the leg nine months later. The patient the last two years has been treated for newly opened varicosities about every four to six months.

The second patient is a 15 year old girl who moved from Boston to California and was first seen in consultation in March 1991. She had been worked up in Boston and her ultimate treatment was wearing a 30-40 mm surgical compression hose. She did not complain of pain, just extreme heaviness and edema of the left leg. She has a port wine stain from gluteus down the thigh and calf to the foot and toes. There were massive varicosities of the left thigh, calf, and foot. In addition she had a multiplicity of various sized phlebectasias all through the port wine stain which hemorrhaged frequently both spontaneously and with minimal friction trauma.

This patient was diagnosed with Duplex Ultra-Sound scanning and then received duplex ultra-sound guided injections of the deep perforators. The deep venous system appeared intact, including the sapheno-femoral junction into the superficial femoral and popliteal veins. The popliteal and posterior tibial veins are within normal limits. As in many Klippel-Trenaunay Syndromes, there is a massive lateral vein down the entire leg with huge varicosities in the lateral thigh and especially the lower leg. Fig. 8 shows this vein in its longitudinal axis which measured 3.4 X 1.89 cm. Fig. 9 shows this same vein in cross section measuring 1.77cm X 1.37 cm. There was a huge bulging perforator in the posterior thigh just below the gluteus. The entire extremity was a mass of varicosities and cavernous hemangioma. The Duplex scan showed no A-V malformations.

The patient commenced treatment Sept. 17, 1991 and was first seen on a weekly basis, now bi-monthly as of April 1992. She usually received 6 to 8 injections of 1-2cc 3% sotradecol.

Fig.10 shows the leg prior to treatment, Fig.11 the leg as of March of 1992. Clinical and subjective improvement include the following. The leg overall has decreased 1.5 inches in circumferance, is not edematous, and of particular note are the port wine stain and phlebectasias. The port wine stain has decreased markedly from a deep purple red to a pale white pink. The phlebectasias, which in the past would sometimes hemorrhage, the blood shooting several feet through the air, are now shrinking in size, disappearing as they are absorbed into the skin. A recent scan showed a complete absence of abnormal deep perforators, and treatment will be continued on the yet considerable superficial venous insufficiency on a periodic basis. Subjectively the patient, now 16 yrs. old, has a whole new demeanor and social life enhanced. The ultimate outcome has yet to be determined.

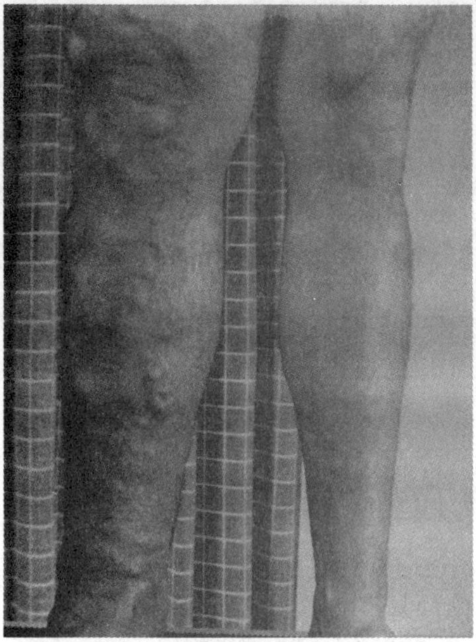

FIG. 1

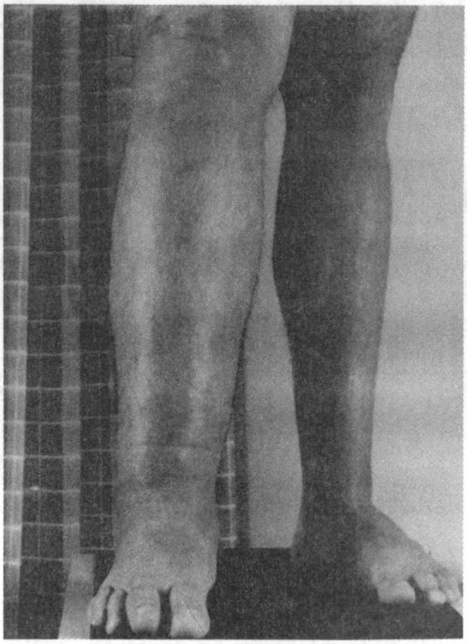

FIG. 2

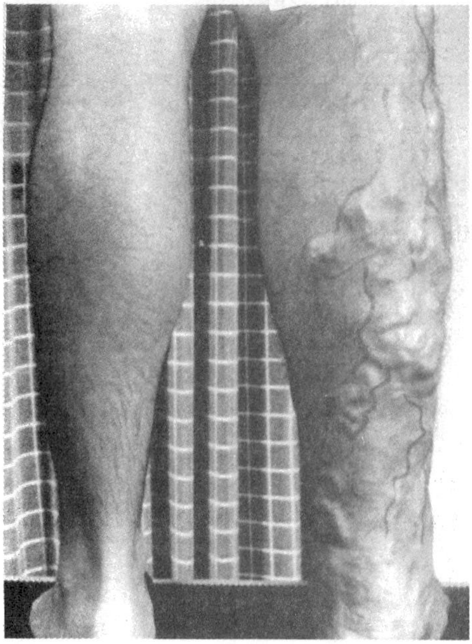

FIG. 3

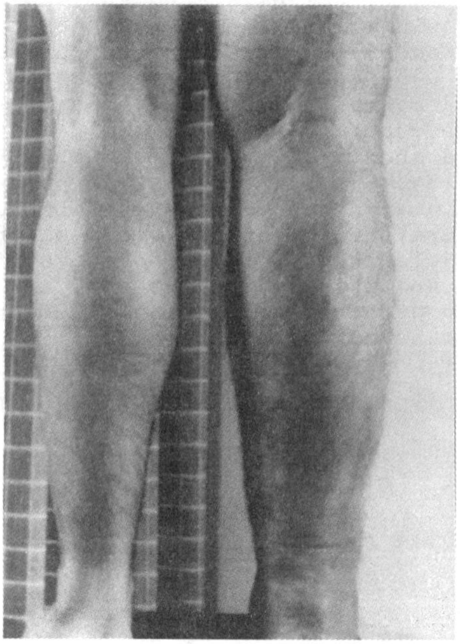

FIG. 4

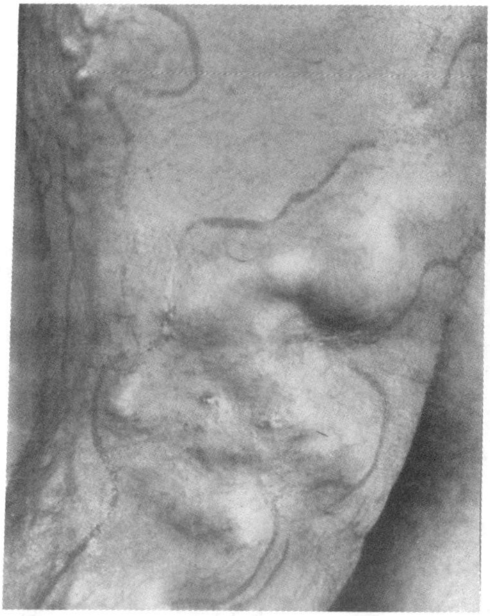

FIG. 5

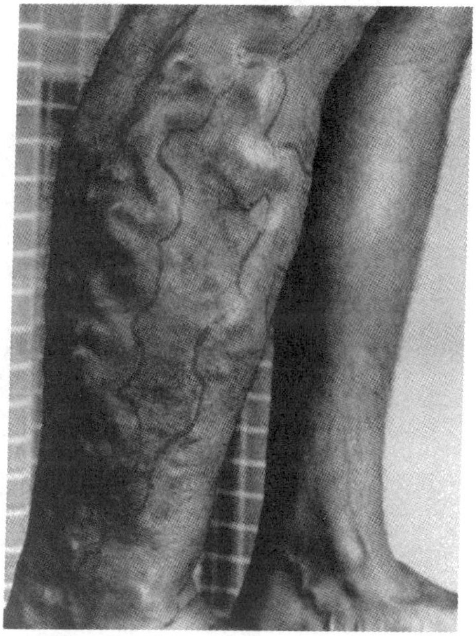

FIG. 6

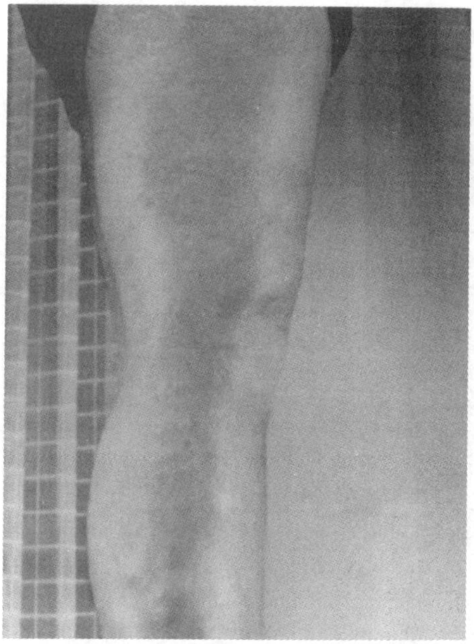

FIG. 7

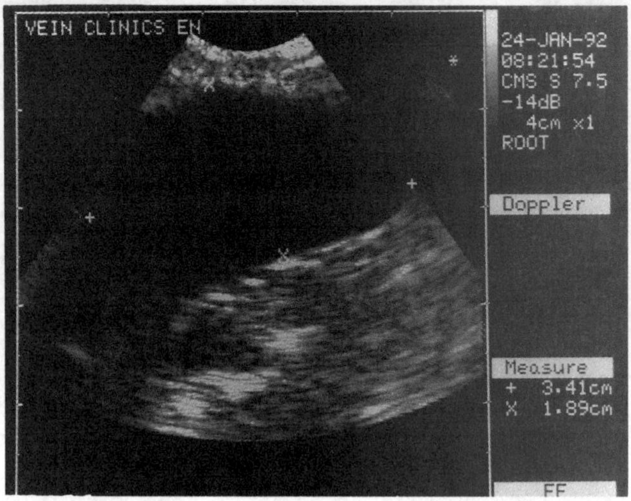
VEIN CLINICS EN
24-JAN-92
08:21:54
CMS S 7.5
-14dB
4cm x1
ROOT
Doppler
Measure
+ 3.41cm
X 1.89cm
FF

FIG. 8

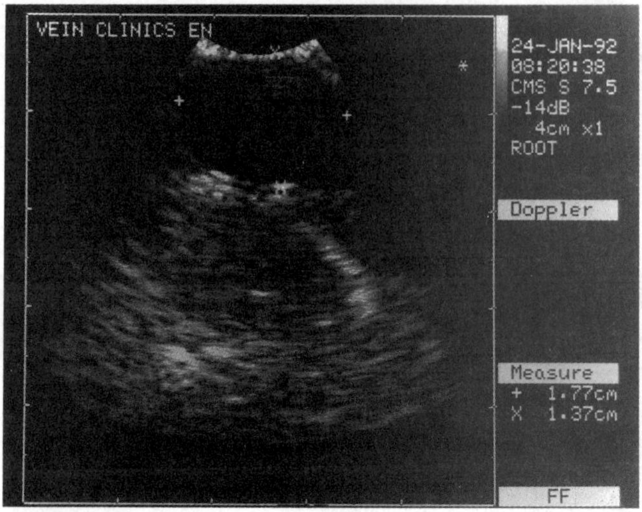
VEIN CLINICS EN
24-JAN-92
08:20:38
CMS S 7.5
-14dB
4cm x1
ROOT
Doppler
Measure
+ 1.77cm
X 1.37cm
FF

FIG. 9

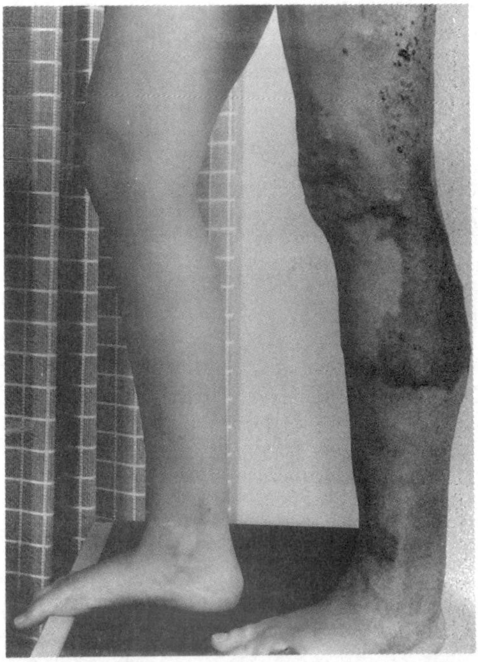

FIG. 10

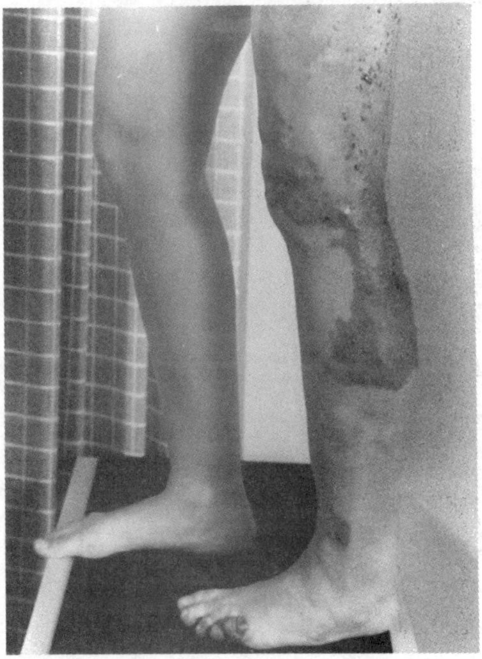

FIG. 11

The black and white reproduction of the color slides that are shown do not show the dramatic changes in this leg.

Phlébologie 92. Eds P. Raymond-Martimbeau, R. Prescott, M. Zummo.
John Libbey Eurotext, Paris © 1992, pp. 848

A case of leiomyosarcoma of the thigh diagnosed during injection sclerotherapy treatment

Mark D. Forrestal

Vein Clinics of America, 1101 perimeter Drive, Suite 615, Schaumburg, Illinois 60173, USA.

A 58 year old woman presented for evaluation of symptomatic bilateral extensive varicose veins of the lower extremities. These varicosities had been present for thirty years. The patient had undergone a series of injection treatments with good results and no complications. Over a three day period the patient developed severe edema, erythema, tenderness, and pain of the right thigh. Duplex ultrasound evaluation revealed a mass with flow characteristics of an A-V malformation. Biopsy of the mass showed Leiomyosarcoma.

The patient's clinical course will be detailed. A literature review of Leiomyosarcoma of the lower extremities will be provided.

PHENOLIZATION OF HAEMORRHOIDS

Skřička T., Veverková L., Růžička M.,
Melicharová M., Robek O.,
I.st Surgical Clinic, Masaryk University, Brno
Czechoslovakia

Within the period from 1986 - 1990 altogether 205 phenolizations were performed in 78 patiens at the Ist surgical clinic These were mostly the haemorrhoids of the Ist and IInd stage / 62 patiens/ In 16 older persons with severe accompanying affection the phenolization was applied even in haemorrhoids of the IIIrd stage. In 16 patients the improvement was not achieved and the operation was necessary within 2 years. Complications were experienced in 2 cases/ ulceration of mucosa to Ø 4mm./
We use 5ml 5% suspension of phenol in sun-flower oil applied strictly submucously, always to one predilection spot. After one week the second node and, after the next week, the last main node are injected.

c. Complications / *Complications*

Phlébologie 92. Eds P. Raymond-Martimbeau, R. Prescott, M. Zummo.
John Libbey Eurotext, Paris © 1992, pp. 853-855

Les complications de la sclérothérapie dans le traitement des varices

Jean Natali

Département de chirurgie vasculaire, American Hospital of Paris, 92202 Neuilly-sur-Seine, France.

La sclérose des varices est dans notre pays une des procédures thérapeutiques les plus répandues,et plusieurs centaines de milliers d'injections sont effectuées chaque année, sans qu'aucun accident ou incident ne se produise. Cependant, même s'ils sont très rares, des accidents se produisent.

MATERIEL ET METHODE :

Il convient de distinguer les accidents locaux et les accidents généraux . Les accidents locaux surviennent lorsque le produit sclérosant est injecté ,

-soit dans une artère , 39 cas
-soit dans le tissu cellulaire sous cutané, 46 cas .

Les accidents généraux sont beaucoup plus rares

- 2 morts pendant la sclérose
- 2 septicémies
- 4 réactions allergiques graves
- Il convient enfin de noter 3 cas de thrombo-phlébites .

LES INJECTIONS INTRA-ARTERIELLES

En l'espace de 16 ans , de 1975 à 1991 , nous avons observé 39 lésions de ce type dont les conséquences ont été :

- 7 amputations majeures, dont 2 au dessus du genou et 5 au dessous du genou
- 6 amputations périphériques mineures de un ou plusieurs orteils,
- 26 séquelles graves consistant essentiellement dans la rétraction ischémique du muscle triceps sural .

Le tableau clinique est pratiquement toujours le même . Immédiatement, lors de la fin de l'injection, plus rarement quelques instants après , se produit une douleur extrêmement vive à distance du point où la peau a été pénétrée , se propageant ensuite distalement vers l'extrémité du membre .
Dans tous les cas, la douleur entraîne rapidement une incapacité fonctionnelle presque absolue, le patient étant dans l'impossibilité de poser le pied par terre . Dans les heures qui suivent, malgré les différents traitements entrepris, la douleur demeure toujours très vive et elle n'est calmée ni par le repos,

ni par la mise du membre en position déclive, ni par la marche. Elle est réellement insupportable . Dans trois de nos observations, il a fallu recourir à une anesthésie péridurale pour soulager le patient .

EVOLUTION : A l'examen effectué dans les minutes ou dans les heures qui suivent cette injection, on note des modifications de la coloration de la peau, qui apparaît livide ou cyanique . Les éléments sous-jacents sont également modifiés; après l'injection au niveau de la crosse saphénienne externe, le mollet apparaît tendu ,atrocement douloureux, spontanément et au moindre contact . Les pouls périphériques peuvent demeurer présents dans les premières heures, parfois plus longtemps, dans d'autres cas, au contraire, ils peuvents disparaître . Au bout de 48 ou 72 heures, on peut commencer à se faire une idée de l'évolution des lésions . Dans certains cas, il persiste des phénomènes ischémiques qui intéressent des groupes musculaires très étendus, voire la totalité d'un membre . Dans ces cas , une amputation devra être discutée . Dans d'autres cas, les lésions seront plus limitées , pouvant intéresser soit la peau, soit les éléments musculaires plus profonds, et, le plus souvent , les deux . L'atteinte cutanée se traduit par une escarre noirâtre, la nécrose musculaire se manifeste sous forme d'une tuméfaction douloureuse dont on peut apprécier l'importance par différentes méthodes : échographie, mais de façon plus précise, tomo-densitométrie-Scanner ou imagerie par résonance nucléaire . Dans certains cas, l'atteinte cutanée peut être minime et sous une peau presque indemne apparaissent cependant des phénomènes de rétraction du mollet . La lésion nécrosante du triceps, la plus fréquente, évolue vers une fibrose rétractile qui entraîne un pied en équin en même temps que l'atrophie de la jambe

DISCUSSION : La pathogénie de ces lésions nous apparait univoque, elles sont provoquées par la pénétration du produit sclérosant dans le système artériel. Les autres étiologies évoquées : spasme artériel d'origine veineuse , fistule artérioveineuse, ne peuvent être retenues .

Dans la pluspart des cas, l'injection n'a pas été faite dans un gros tronc veineux tel que la veine poplitée, mais dans une de ses branches, en particulier au niveau du mollet ; des études anatomiques ont montré que des artères très superficielles, branches des artères jumelles pouvaient être situées au contact même de la crosse de veine saphène externe ou de ses branches, et pouvaient donc être cathétérisées par mégarde lors de l'injection sclérosante . Des travaux expérimentaux (W. Mac Gowan 1) ont tenté de préciser l'action de certains produits en particulier le tétra-décyl-sulfate de Sodium (T.D.S.S.)lorsqu'il est injecté en intra-artériel . Cet auteur a observé, après injection dans les artères de chiens, l'absence de thrombose du vaisseau principal mais la formation d'un agrégat par altération des globules rouges lorsque le produit se mélange au sang . Cet agrégat est propulsé par le débit artériel vers l'aval, et provoque une obstruction embolique dans le territoire irrigué par l'artère . Les nécroses musculaires et cutanées en sont la conséquence . Ces accidents sont connus depuis longtemps, mais il semble qu'actuellement ils soient plus fréquents, avec l'augmentation des de tentatives de sclérose de crosses . COCKETT (2) indique que, dans son expérience , les accidents de sclérose apparaissent plus fréquents que les accidents après chirurgie . Il rapporte 18 cas avec deux amputations de jambes, deux amputations trans-métatarsiennes, 4 séquelles douloureuses invalidantes .

TRAITEMENT : Le traitement de ces lésions apparaît difficile . Immédiatement , on fait appel aux moyens classiques, injections intra-artérielles de vasodilatateurs et de corticoïdes, mais la pathogénie des accidents explique que bien souvent l'efficacité en est limitée . Il faut également insister sur l'intérêt de vaso-dilatateurs très puissants , type NITROPRUSSIATE DE SOUDE, associés à un traitement par HEPARINE. On prendra toujours soin de calmer la douleur, et la mise en place d'une anesthésie péridurale peut s'avérer nécessaire. Après le traitement effectué en urgence , le bilan lésionnel comporte essentiellement des échographies, ou mieux des examens tomodensitométriques ou par I.R.M. qui permettront d'évaluer l'importance des lésions musculaires . Si l'atteinte cutanée est rapidement visible ,le degré de l'atteinte musculaire ne peut être déterminé avant plusieurs semaines . Par ailleurs, il convient de ne faire aucun geste intempestif au niveau du mollet et surtout aucun curage ni aponévrotomie de décompression. Ce n'est qu'après une étude attentive en poursuivant la rééducation qu'on pourra juger de l'importance des rétractions musculaires, en particulier du muscle triceps sural qui est le plus souvent touché . A ce stade des séquelles, on pourra avoir recours à une libération musculaire qui donne de bien meilleurs résultats que les allongements du tendon d'Achille qui avaient d'abord été proposés . La prophylaxie de ces accidents a été à plusieurs reprises évoquée, en particulier on a proposé de ne faire ces injections au niveau des crosses que sous échographie. Mais même avec cette précaution, nous avons observé des accidents . La précaution essentielle réside dans la nécessité d'une injection extrêmement lente qui permet à la douleur de se manifester avant que la totalité du produit ne soit injecté . (NATALI .3)

LES INJECTIONS SOUS CUTANEES

Ce sont les injections effectuées dans le tissu cellulaire sous-cutané qui vont aboutir soit à une simple réaction inflammatoire, soit à une nécrose cutanée avec escarre . 46 cas de ce type ont été observés, pouvant aller de lésions très minimes ne dépassant pas quelques millimètres de diamètre, jusqu'à des lésions extrêmement étendues d'une longueur ou d'une largeur de plusieurs centimètres . Il convient là aussi d'être très conservateur sur le plan du traitement et d'attendre l'élimination de l'escarre en ayant au besoin recours à une greffe cutanée .

Lorsque l'injection extra-artérielle et extra-veineuse a été effectuée de façon plus profonde, on peut observer des lésions nerveuses (4 cas) . Il s'agit de troubles neurologiques dus à l'atteinte directe du nerf par le produit sclérosant . Dans certains cas, les troubles seront uniquement sensitifs avec atteinte de la branche cutanée du nerf sciatique poplité externe; dans un cas une lésion tronculaire importante du nerf sciatique poplité a été observée avec troubles moteurs.

LES ACCIDENTS GENERAUX

Les accidents allergiques et anaphylactiques apparaissent fort heureusement rares . Cependant, nous avons observé deux cas de mort survenus pendant la sclérose sans étiologie retrouvée . 4 réactions allergiques graves, mais guérissant sans séquelle ont également été observées . Il faut aussi citer deux cas de septicémie, dont une après incision d'une veine sclérosée . Enfin, 3 thrombo-phlébites affirmées par phlébographie ont été observées avec un cas de mort par embolie pulmonaire .

CONCLUSION

Les accidents liés à la sclérose des varices sont fort heureusement rares, en regard du très grand nombre d'actes réalisés ,mais ils sont, dans certains cas, dramatiques, et ils peuvent aboutir à la mutilation d'un membre . Le phlébologue ne se départira jamais d'une technique rigoureuse, n'injectant le produit que progressivement, prêt à arrêter son geste si une douleur est signalée par le patient . Il n'oubliera pas qu'il existe des zones dangereuses, comme la gouttière rétro-malléolaire interne, le triangle du Scarpa, le creux poplité, à tel point que certains phlébologues renoncent à s'y aventurer .
(COCKETT. 2)

Bibliographie

1 GOWAN W.A.L. : Comment éviter les accidents de la sclérose . Phlébologie 1985 ;38 : 205-208

2 COCKETT F.B. : Arterial complications in treatment of varicose veins , Phlébology ;1986 , 1 : 3-6

3 NATALI J. : L'expertise en Phlébologie . Phlébologie 1989 ,A. DAVY , R. STEMMER Eds 1989 John LIBBEY Eurotext LTA : 1209-1219

Phlébologie 92. Eds P. Raymond-Martimbeau, R. Prescott, M. Zummo.
John Libbey Eurotext, Paris © 1992, pp. 856-858

Sclerotherapy of varices : complications and their treatment

Gabriele Tombari, Vicenzo Gasbarro*, Dino De Anna*, Antonio Morri, Davide Rosa, Paolo Piva, Giovanni Fuga, Ippolito Donini*

*Divisione di Chirurgia, Ospedale di Stato Rep. San Marino, * Istituto di Clinica Chirurgica Generale, Università di Ferrara, Italia.*

Introduction

The use of sclerotherapy, alone or combined with the surgical therapy, has a greater and greater importance in the treatment of varices of the lower limbs.

In order to practice it, it is necessary to have not only a perfect knowledge of venous pathophisiology, but also to know well the technique and the complications that it may cause. The troubles that may derive from sclerotherapy are caused either by the inexperience of the surgeon or by some factors that, influencing each other, may invalidate the results. The complications in sclerotherapy may be general or local.

General complications

In our 5 years experience of out-patient treatment (500 cases), we had no pneumonic embolism.

The allergic reactions can be avoided through an exact anamnesis of the patients.

We had 5 cases (1%) of allergic reaction caused by the injection of hidroxy-polyetoxysodium at 3%, during the treatment of big varices of saphenic collateral veins. One patient had an anaphylactic shock and we immediately treated him with hydrocortison at high dosage, and with antihistaminics. Three patients, who showed minor reactions, as urticaria, were succesfully treated with oral intake of antihistaminics.

Digestive problems, like nausea and vomiting, scotomes, acuphenes, abdominal pain, sweating, were found in 6 neurolabile patients with allergic diathesis. The treatment of these patients was easy, and the problems disappeared few hours after adequate symptomatic therapy with antispasmodics and antiemetics.

Local complications

These represent the largest and the most frequent group of complications in sclerotherapy. A rare complication and, without doubt, a very dangerous one is represented by the intra-arterial injection of the sclerosant substance: the consequence is an acute ischemia the degree of which depends on the nature and uantity of the injected substance and on the type of the artery nterested. During our experience we met no trouble like that. nother dangerous complication is the necrosis. It shows itself n the area of the injection of the sclerosant substance and it s caused either by an high concentration or excessive quantity f the substance, or by the extravascular injection.

he formation of a phlyctene is followed after about 24-72 hours y the appearance of a brown, blackish, painfull eschar with a arge hyperaemic reaction at the edges of it. The cicatrization rocess is extremely slow and it takes about 1-3 months to ecuperate.

nfortunately 10 patients suffered from this consequences. The reatment consisted in the removal of the eschar and in periodic edications with local disinfectants.

he ascending phlebitis is an inflammatory hyperreaction of the reated vein, with the implication of a larger distal tract. This omplication may be caused by the use of a too high concentration f the sclerosant substance in venous rectilinear tracts; as a onsequence of this, an excessive individual reactivity must not e underevalued. Its prevenction consists of an immediate eambulation after the therapy, an elastocompressive bandage and ome injection of little quantities of the sclerosant substance, voiding the bolus or using the "air block" technique. The use of n elastic bandage associated to some hot packs, to some anti-nflammatoric and some fibrinolytic mesotherapically permitted us o resolve very well the only case observed.The intra venous ematoma shows itself throgh very large varixes with some thin arieses.

he best prevention is a good compression. Otherwise it is ecessary to proceed to a dumping of the hematoma, with a little hlebectomy made after 10-20 days, provided that a post phlebitic tate doesn't coexist.

egarding the 11 cases we met, we preferred to empty the intra-enous hematoma with an aspiration with needles n. 19 or 21 or ith a little trocar.

he discovery of residual subcutaneous pigmentation in the reated areas are very frequent. This type of problem is always aused by an overdosage of the utilized fluid or by the uperficiality of the sclerosis veins.

e found this complication in 68 patients (16,5%). We considered seful an intracutaneos injection of a little dose of sodic eparin and the use of pomades with heparin wich shorten the very ong period of resorption of the hemosiderinic deposits. It is ossible to reach good results using a pomade composed by ssential oil of orange, vegetable oils, ascorbic acid, distilled ater of hamamelis, fatty of mono and diglycerides fatty acids mulsified

he secondary teleangiectasis are often caused by unskilfulness r by a condition of venous hypertension due to the first session of therapy. The 50 patients (10%) observed were treated by the isual sclerotherapy.

Results and conclusions

The complications we recorded during the last five years, brought s not to undervalue their therapeutic aspects. The period of ecovery was variable according to the importance of the omplications. The allergic reactions and the subjective troubles lisappeared after two hours. The average period of the necrosis recovery, according to our therapeutic protocol, varied from 10 days (lesions of 1 cm. max.) to 4 weeks (3 cm. max.). The ascending phlebitis, cured with fibrinolytic mesotherapeutically, recovered in 13 days. The intravenous hematoma took place in 11 patients who recovered in 15/325 days. The residual pigmentations, treated with our protocol, took 30/105 days. The long period of recovery is caused by the lacking efficacy of pharmacological remedies. The secondary teleangiectasias, treated with sclerotherapy, had very brief periods of recovery (7/21 days).

To sume up, sclerotherapy is a sure and efficacious method: it's value is reduced by the troubles that may occur and that are caused principally by inexperience. For this reason, sclerotherapy must be exercised by specialists who have a long experience.

References

Bassi G.(1966): Les varices des membres inferieurs, Doiu, Paris.

Goot W.(1982): Tecknik der Skleretherapie. Ein Rundtischgesprach. Swiss Med, 4a:41.

Hobbs J.T.(1977): The treatment of venous disorders. MTP. Press Limited. Lancaster.

Sarteel A. M., Merlen J. F.(1985): Incidents et Accidents dus a la sclerotherapie. Prevention de la pigmentation. Phlèbologie, 33 (3), 383-387.

Steemmer R.(1969): Bases théoriques de la sclerose des varices. Conclusions pratiques. Phlèbologie, 22/77.

Tournay R. e coll.(1984): Terapia sclerosante delle varici. III Ed. R. Cortina.

Wallois P. (1985): Varicositès post-sclèrose. Phlèbologie, 33 (4), 669-672.

Wallois P. (1981): Pour une meilleure prèvention des accidents en pratique sclèrosante. Phlèbologie, 34 (1), 77-80.

Phlébologie 92. Eds P. Raymond-Martimbeau, R. Prescott, M. Zummo.
John Libbey Eurotext, Paris © 1992, pp. 859-860

Complications of sclerotherapy : a statistical study

Aurora Avramovic, Miguel Avramovic

Centro Flebologico Privado, Riobamba 747, 1045 Buenos Aires, Argentina.

Introduction

A retrospective study of 7200 case histories of or phlebologic center has been performed. The complications produced during the sclerosing treatment have been observed and statistically analyzed.

Material:

The following sclerosants were used:

1) Monoethanolamine oleate
2) Hydroxypolyethoxydodecane
3) Iodine-iodide solution

Clasification and statistics:

Local complications:

Residual pigmentation	35,0 ‰
Secondary Teleangiectasies	16,0 ‰
Hypertrichosis	4,4 ‰
Necrosis	2,9 ‰
Indurative Plaque	2,08 ‰
Focal Allergy	1,5 ‰

General complications:

Atypical Allergy	→ Dizziness, hypotensión, asthenia	4 ‰
	→ Vomiting, epigastric ache	1,7 ‰

1) Minor
10,4 ‰

Neurovegetative	→ Troubles oculaires	3,3 ‰
	→ Paresthesia	0,8 ‰
	→ 5 th. lumbar ache	0,6 ‰

2) Major 2,5 ‰

Severe allergic reaction (anaphylactic shock)

To improve the practical understanding, the statistics is presented as number of cases ‰.

Conclusion:

From the above mentioned data, it is concluded that the probability of a major allergic reaction is 2,5‰. The other general complications are transitory. In respect of the local complications, each one has a specific treatment.

BIBLIOGRAPHY

1. Benhamon et Natali. Les accidents des traitements sclérosant et chirurgical des varices des membres inférieurs. Phlebologie. 34-41, 1981.
2. García Méndez. Iusen. Flebopatías, estudio y tratamiento. Buenos Aires. Pág. 223, 1986.
3. Mac Gowan. Comment éviter les accidents de la sclérose. Phlebologie. 38-205, 1985.
4. Raymond Tournay y Coll. La sclérose de Varices. París. Pág. 274, 1975.
5. M. Vigoni. Phlebologie. Pág. 81. Maloine Edit. París. 1983.
6. Wallios P. Pour une meilleure prevention des accidents et incidents en practique sclérosante. Plebologie, 34-77, 1981.

Phlébologie 92. Eds P. Raymond-Martimbeau, R. Prescott, M. Zummo.
John Libbey Eurotext, Paris © 1992, pp. 861-862

Complications of Sotradecol® sclerotherapy with and without heparin

Alan H. Kanter

Vein Clinics of America, 19800 MacArthur Boulevard, Suite 270, Irvine, California 92715, USA.

The addition of Heparin Sodium (Norbrook America, Inc., Walnut, California) to sclerosing solutions has been purported to decrease the risk of thromboembolic phenomenon, as well as local thrombus formation at the injection site. Reduction of post-injection intravascular hematoma and angioneogenic "matting" are theoretical advantages of the latter.

Although current PDR guidelines indicate that Heparin and Sotradecol® (Elkins-Sinn, Inc., Cherry Hill, New Jersey) are incompatible, this is being actively reviewed and will soon be updated due to the tenuous anecdotal basis for this original recommendation (Foley, 1965).

The only systematic reported study to date compared hypertonic saline with and without Heparin (Sadick, 1990). In 800 patients, Sadick concluded there were no significant differences between the control and experimental groups with regard to post-treatment hyperpigmentation, matting, thrombophlebitis, and microthrombi. Unfortunately, this large-scale study was not double-blind, and did not control separately for the two variables of compression and Heparin use.

The purpose of this study was to determine what effect the addition of Heparin would have on certain complications of sclerotherapy with Sotradecol®. Patients treated had non-truncal "small vein disease," and served as their own controls. One leg was treated without Heparin and the other with Heparin solution combined with 0.1% and 0.2% Sotradecol®, with immediate post-treatment compression and ambulation.

Three to eight days following treatment, 100 patients were evaluated in a double-blind fashion on a four-point scale with regard to degree of bruising, intravascualr hematoma, and matting. Evidence for matting was further sought three months later by examination. No advantage could be found by the addition of Heparin to Sotradecol®. By deleting Heparin, significantly less bruising was noted, and there was less subjective discomfort on injection. There was no difference with regard to either intravascular hematoma or matting. No precipitation or discoloration of solution was observed.

Thus, despite chemical compatibility, the theoretical advantages of adding Heparin to Sotradecol® were not observed in this study limited to "small vein disease."

References

Foley W.T., (1965): Office treatment of veins and ulcers. *GP*. 31, 90-99.

Sadick N.S., (1990): Treatment of varicose and telangiectatic leg veins with hypertonic saline. *J. Dermatol. Surg. Oncol.* 16, 24-28.

Phlébologie 92. Eds P. Raymond-Martimbeau, R. Prescott, M. Zummo.
John Libbey Eurotext, Paris © 1992, pp. 863-865

Local complications in course of the sclerotherapy

Vincenzo D'Agata, Dàrio Danieli, Paola Marzotto, Leonarda Perrone, Nizar Sacran, Francesco Dall'Antonia

Dipartimento di Chirurgia Generale I, Ospedale Civile di Vicenza, Italia.

Sclerotherapy can cause serious damage if carried out by surgeons who are not very experienced in the appropriate technique or in the choice of product. A regular and carefull analysis of the possible complications is extremely important; in order to evaluate whether the complications were a question of a mistaken choice between sclerotherapy or surgery, or badly applied sclerotherapy techniques.
The pathology, the products used and the techniques are illustrated in the to be seen at the end of the report.
It is possible to decide, acconrding to the size of the vein, which technique to applay, and the quantity, percentage and choice of the product to be used and the number of injections to be given.
However there are general outlines which must be borne in mind quite apart from the pathology to be trated as was noted in our 600 cases.
As far as complications are concerned there are general ones and local ones. The general ones are created by an allergy to the product and appeared as pallor, extreme disconfort, and nausea and difficulty with vision. Such symtoms arise during treatment.
Whereas a temperature and pains in the back appear between eight and twelve hours after the sclerotherapy. All those symptoms disappear by themselves and affect respectively 1% of the patients. The local complications which appear in a higher number of patients were bruising 20%, muscular cramps 10%, rising flebitis 10%, clots inside the vein 5% and dark permanent scaring 3%.
The bruising appears two weeks after the therapy and the cause could be attributed to an excess of pressur during the injection which causes the breahage of the vein, however it disappears naturally by itself.
There the muscular cramps appear during therapy due to an intolerance to the product and disappear on their own.
The risig fleabitis from the injected area appears after a week or two and is due to either an excess of quantity or density of the product or an incorrect bandaging of the leg.

The advised treatment consist of binding with an oxide zinc bandage and an elastic adesive bandage all around the entire leg. The clots inside the vein can appear as a result of the fleabites after a week. It is necessary to empty the clot. If the clot is not emptied, permanent dark scaring after 4 or 8 weeks appears. It disappears by itself over a period of two years or sooner if treated with scraping surgery or injections of heparine just below the surface of the skin. Another complication which affects a minimum number of patients about 1% is the swelling of the foot; wich appears after four weeks caused by an injection in the ankle or the foot with too much of the product. It disappears with lengthy elastic bandaging. Complications: pain,inflamation of the skin,blistering,and scabs are the result of the quantity of the product injected and can be predicted by the extreme pain suffered at the moment of the injection. Patients should be informed.They must say if they feel pain. In this case it is essential not to complete the injection as there is a risk that the product injected in larger doses will enter the microarteric circulation causing the above mentioned problems varying in the area. Teleangectasy, or the new appearence of reddened minute veis in the surrounding areas, of the site already treated with sclerotherapy appear one or two weeks later. I presume because of the non closure of the principal vein trunk which fed the formerly treated area. Other authors presume that the phenomena is caused by the proliferation of new veins stimulated by the product.
The only form of treatment is more sclerotherapy.
In conclusion for a patient to undertake sclerotherapy,the advantage aesthetically and functionally must out weight the time required,the pain and the risk of complications.

METHODS OF TREATMENT

Teleangiectases and Reticular varices 0.5 - 3.0 mm.
-The patient is laying on his back - Direct Injection - Air Block
-Injection till the capillaries are filled in area of 2 cm.diameter
-Elastic compression after the injection.

Varices 3 - 15 mm.
-The patient is standing up - Injection with butterfly needle 25
-Check the color and the pulsation of the blood running in the cannula. -Injection while the patient is laying on his back after washing with physiologic solution. -Elastic compression with zinc oxide bandage and with elastic adhesive bandage, or only elastic stocking Varisma 20-30 mm.Hg., product by Basel. -First medication after 7 days and new elastic compression with minimun elasticity bandage. Walk 2 km. every day for the entire period of the sclerotherapy. Begin the sclerotherapy a month after possible crossectomy or saphenectomy. Never begin the sclerotherapy immediately before surgery. Begin the sclerotherapy from the bigger varices to the smaller ones from the top to the bottom.

From 1986 to 1992: 500 - 100 from 15 to 70 years old. Teleangiectases 60%. Reticular Varices 1-3 mm. 25%. Extra Truncus Saphenous Varices 3-8 mm. 20%. Extra Truncus Saphenous Varices 8-15 mm. 5%. Patients who already underwent crossectomy or saphenectomy 80%. Patients with proven cross or great saphena continence 20%.
Chromate Glycerol 1.1% 4.5cc and Xilocaina 2.0% 0.5cc: Teleangiectases and Reticular Varices 0.5-1 mm.
Idrossi Polietossi Dodecano 1% 2cc Varix Size 1-3 mm., 3% 2cc Varix Size 3-5 mm.
Variglobin 2-4% 1cc Varix Size 5-15 mm.

REFERENCES

Fegan,W.G.,(1967): Varicose veins. Heinemann, London
Hobbs,J.T.,(1985): A new approach to short saphenous vein varicosities.Chap.23 (p 301-321) in Surgery of the veins,ed.Bergan
Stemmer,R.,(1974): Bases theoriques de la sclerose des varices.Conclusions Pratiques. Phlebologie, 27:77
Tourney,R.,e coll.,(1984):Terapia sclerosante delle varici. Ed.R. Cortina, Milano
Van Der Stricht, J.,(1982):Le traitment des varices essentielles en 1981, phlebologie 1982, 35:403

Phlébologie 92. Eds P. Raymond-Martimbeau, R. Prescott, M. Zummo.
John Libbey Eurotext, Paris © 1992, pp. 866-868

Residual chromatoses

Vincenzo D'Agata, Dario Danieli, Paola Marzotto, Leonarda Perrone, Nizar Sacran, Francesco Dall'Antonia

Dipartimento di Chirurgia Generale I, Ospedale Civile di Vicenza, Italia.

There is no doubt that sclerotherapy is a method that can be conside red most effective in all cases where indication,technique and produ ct to be used have all been previously evaluated with great care and have been judget to be compatible with the condition to be cured.
In some instances sclerotherapy could represent an alternative to the surgical treatment, e.g. in cases of extra trunk saphenous insuf ficiency of the collateral veins. In other instances - and for certain subjects- it would be preferable to the surgical treatment as any hazard inherent in the latter would be avoied.
However,having recourse to sclerotherapy is something that should be pondered over adequately,because if practised by unskilled hands or by operators little or inadequately familiar with the injection technique,the modalities connected with the products and their effects, the nature of the condition,serious damage could easily be caused, sometimes even worse than the condition which was expected to be cured.
Such damages can be seen in the residual chromatosis caused by the formation of a substance haemosiderin which is deposited excessively and which is absorbed very slowly by the organism even taking up to a Year. This complication can appear initially after sclerotherapy or as a consequence of other pathologies consequences of sclerothera py. Like: Blistering necroses, which heals leaving a chromatosis scar; This complication takes place because of an excessive amount of scle rosantis is agent injected in one single point. The patient at the time of the injection feels a very strong burning pain as in that ca se it is advisable to stop the injection even though the burning has taken place.
An other cause of residual chromatosis is ascending phlebites which is an inflamation of the trunk vein further away than the point at which the injection is given. This injury manifests itself one or two days after the removal of the elastic compression bandage. The most evident manifestation of this complication inthe swelling of

the leg,the reddening and heat of the leg and clearly difficulty in walking. As soon as these symptoms disappear,inner vein brusing remains and causes the residual chromatosis right down the vein. The cause of these complications is due to insufficient binding after Sclerotherapy and since it is impossible to establish exactly how long binding should remain for each individual person.

In order to avoid those complication it is necessary to carry out multiple injections not close to each other using a minimum amount of the agent. It would alse be advisable to walk for 3 kilometres a day. Another cause of residual chromatosis is the appearance of close knitted tufts of tiny fine veins brought about after sclerotherapy of large size veins with insufficient elastic bandaging. A partial occlusion of the scleroticized trunk causes in order to compensate the dilation of the smalles veins,which lead of from the trunk vein. This frequently occurs when the preassure of the bood inside is higher than normal. The mistake in the sclerotherapy is caused by not having used the most snitable agent and appropriate quantity. The treatment of this last cause of chromatosis consists of more sclerotherapy.

The therapeutic strategy carried out at the Centre for the treatment of vein diseases care of Surgery I^ Civil Hospital Vicenza consists of the use of Mesotherapy with weekly sessions using agents which are: Durochinasi in1100.000 U.I. injected just below the skin. With this system the chromatosis colourin is lightened until it disappears. The explanation of all this in words or with photoes is very difficult even whit years of experience in this field. In order to avoid and treat this injury as for as I'm concerned requires constant practice and first hand experience. To carry out this art it is necessary to attend for a considerable time phlebologistic surgeries where colleagues who have a great deal of experience and excellent results.

REFERENCES

Bartoletti,C.A.,(1983): Mesoterapia e Cellulite. In Ed, Salus, Roma

Bassi,G., Stemmer,R.,(1983): Traitements mecaniques foncitionelles ed phlebologie. In Piccin, Padova

Curri, S.B.,(1990): L'istogramma da stasi. Giorn.Flebologiche Algheresi,Alghero 1-4 Giugno 1989, CIC ed. Int.

Dutot,F.,(1983): Traitement des escarres par Mesotherapie. In Mesoterapia 1982.,Atti del III Congresso Internazionale di Mesoterapia, ed. Salus, Roma

Hobbs, J.T.,(1985): A new approach to short saphenous vein varicosities. In Surgery of the veins, Ed. Bergan, J.J.and Jao, J.S.T. Grune and Stratton

Kluken, N.,(1991): Streptochinasi versus Urochinasi nella tromboflebite profonda. In Flebologia, Giugno 1991
Pistor, M.,(1979): Un défi mésothérapie thérapeutique. In Ed.Maloine Paris
Piumi, J.M.,(1988): Le drainage et la régénéuscense du terrain. In Atti del V Congresso Internazionale di Mesoterapia, Parigi, 1988
Tomaselli,F., Bartoletti,C.A.,(1985): Farmaci flebotonici per via intradermica e sottocutanea superficiale sec. Pistor. In Abstr., IV Congresso Internazionale di Mesoterapia 3-6 ottobre 1985
Tourney,R., e coll.,(1984): Terapia sclerosante delle varici. Ed. R. Cortina, Milano
Wenner, L.,(1984): Zum heutigen stand der Sklerotherapie der Saphenenstamme. Phlebol. 13:1
Wuppermann,Th.,(1986): Varizen, Ulcus cruris und Thrombose. In Springer-Verlag, Berlin.

Post-sclerotherapy pigmentation: Hemosiderin or Melanin?

César F. Sánchez, MD, E. Canestri, MD, N. Rosli, MD, U. Tropper, MD

"Dr. César F. Sánchez" Phlebology clinic

The authors have carried out an exhaustive histopathologic study in order to demonstrate the presence, location, and pathogenic role of hemosiderin and melanin involved in hyperchromia after sclerotherapy at 3, 6 and 9 months of evolution. From the results obtained the authors suggest treating this unesthetic complication with cryotherapy or chemical methods. Iconography together with the results achieved will be submitted.

Étude et traitement de la tache hémosidérotique

Never Rosli, Raul Lapid, Eduardo Rodi

Centre de Flebologia Dr. Never Rosli

L'extrême importance de l'étude et traitement des taches hémosidérotiques en Phlébologie se doit surtout au pourcentage très élevé de celles-ci comme séquelles de phlébopathies et souvent comme iatrogénie résiduelle post-sclérothérapique.

Ayant fait une étude anatomopathologique préalable de la tache, nous exposons les différents traitements que nous avons réalisés:

1) Application de substances quélantes
2) Épidermiectomie avec instrumental de Finochietto
3) Tatouage avec des pigments dont la coloration soit similaire à la peau du patient.

Par rapport aux différentes thérapeutiques appliquées: 1) amélioration légère, 2) légèrement positif, 3) résultat positif (méthode aléatoire, très peu de cas à présent. Actuellement nous travaillons d'une manière intense avec cette technique).

Les résultats obtenus tout récemment nous poussent et encouragent à continuer à travailler avec les méthodes énumérées, et la finalité de ce travail c'est aussi que d'autres centres phlébologiques du monde puissent approfondir les études et traitement de cette affection phlébologique inesthétique par excellence.

Phlébologie 92. Eds P. Raymond-Martimbeau, R. Prescott, M. Zummo.
John Libbey Eurotext, Paris © 1992, pp. 870-872

Therapeutic interventions in the prevention of extravasation necrosis

Steven E. Zimmet

Austin Regional Clinic, 3708 Jefferson St., Suite 103, Austin, Texas 78731, USA.

ABSTRACT
Extravasation is the most common cause of cutaneous necrosis occuring as a complication of sclerotherapy. A variety of treatments have been recommended in the event of extravasation. This prospective, blinded and randomized study utilized Sprague-Dawley rats to evaluate various treatments in the prevention of necrosis following extravasation of 23.4% hypertonic saline (Study I) and 3% sodium tetradecyl sulfate (Study II). In Study I, hyaluronidase treated groups had significantly fewer and smaller mean surface area of necrosis compared to those treated with normal saline (p=0.004), sterile water (p=0.004) and no intervention (p=0.002). This protective effect of hyaluronidase closely approached significance vs. a 1% procaine treated group (p=0.08). In Study II, only 1/15 S's (7%) in the hyaluronidase group developed necrosis. This was significantly fewer than the normal saline treated group (7/15, 47%,p=0.013). However, the hyaluronidase group was not significantly different from other groups, including no treatment. Larger group sizes would have been necessary to achieve significance. In conclusion, in the model studied, hyaluronidase was particularly efficacious in the prevention of extravasation necrosis.

INTRODUCTION

The burgeoning interest in sclerotherapy in recent years has given rise to a large number of inexperienced phlebologists. A recent survey conducted by the North American Society of Phlebology found that inexperienced practitioners (less than 500 treatments) reported approximately a 5% incidence of post-sclerotherapy necrosis(Butie & Goldman,1991). Hypertonic saline(HS), widely used by U.S. dermatologists, was found in the survey to be the most common sclerosant associated with necrosis. Sodium tetradecyl sulfate (STD) is known to be painless when extravasated, which increases the risk for signficant extravasation. In an attempt to prevent extravasation necrosis, most authors have recommended injecting normal saline or procaine into the extravasated area. A controlled study regarding the efficacy of various treatments in the prevention of necrosis following extravasation of hypertonic saline and sodium tetradecyl sulfate seemed worthwhile.

Study I was designed to evaluate the efficacy of equal volumes of normal saline (NSS), sterile water (H2O), 1% procaine (Novocain®, Winthrop®), and hyaluronidase (Wydase®, Lyophilized, 150 USP units/cc, Wyeth®) in the prevention of necrosis following extravasation of HS (Concentrated Sodium Chloride®, American Regent®). In Study II NSS, 1% procaine and hyaluronidase were evaluated as protectants following extravasation of 3% STD (Sotradecol®, Elkins-Sinn®).

MATERIALS AND METHODS

Female Sprague-Dawley rats (150-200 grams) were utilized as subjects. S's were housed 2-3 per cage under identical climate-controlled conditions. The study protocol was approved by the University of Texas Animal Use and Care Committee. On the day before the study protocol was to be carried out, all subjects had the dorsum of their trunk shaved. The following day, after induction of halothane anesthesia, each Study I subject was given an intradermal injection of 0.25cc of 23.4% hypertonic saline in the shaved area. Care was taken to try to inject all subjects at the same level. Immediately following the hypertonic saline injection the subjects received, in a blinded and randomized way, either 3.0cc NSS, 3.0 cc H2O, 1.5 cc NSS plus 1.5 cc 2% procaine (1% procaine), 1.5 cc NSS plus 1.5 cc hyaluronidase (NSS/hyaluronidase), 1.5 cc sterile water plus 1.5 cc hyaluronidase (H2O/hyaluronidase) or no intervention (No Rx). Subjects were then re-housed according to groups with 2-3 S's per cage and were placed back in their normal climate-controlled conditions. There were 20 S's per group. Three days later, all subjects who developed necrosis were noted and, under anesthesia, had their ulcers traced onto tracing paper. The surface area in mm2 of each ulcer was then determined utilizing a Targa digitizing pad, Javelin camera and Java software (Jandel Scientific). Study II subjects underwent a similar protocol as utilized in Study I. The day after being shaved, subjects were anesthetized and given 0.5 cc of 3% STD intradermally. Immediately following this injection subjects were given, in a blinded and randomized fashion, either 3 cc NSS, 1.5 cc NSS plus 1.5 cc 2% procaine (1% procaine), 1.5 cc NSS plus 1.5 cc hyaluronidase(NSS/hyaluronidase) or no intervention (No Rx). There were 15 S's per group. Three days later each subject who developed necrosis was noted, and under anesthesia, ulcers were traced onto tracing paper. The surface area for each ulcer was determined as in Study I.

RESULTS

Study I

Eighty-five per cent of the S's in the No Rx group developed necrosis, while 80 per cent of the NSS group and H2O group, seventy-five per cent of the procaine group, 60 per cent of the H2O/hyaluronidase group and 40% of the NSS/hyaluronidase group developed necrosis. The mean surface area of necrosis for the No Rx, NSS, H2O, procaine, H2O/hyaluronidase and NSS/hyaluronidase groups respectively was 25.07 mm2, 22.17 mm2, 21.3 mm2, 19.73 mm2, 9.26 mm2 and 7.26 mm2. Statistical analysis was accomplished using SPSS software. In Study I, chi square analysis compared the number of subjects developing necrosis between groups. An overall significant difference between the groups for this parameter was found (p=0.017). Individual comparisons, made with certain groups being logically combined to increase the n per group, are listed in Table 1.

Table 1. Individual comparisons between groups regarding percentage of subjects developing necrosis in Study I.

			Pearson	
No Rx	vs	NSS + H2O	.637	NS
No Rx	vs	NSS/hyaluronidase + H2O/hyaluronidase	.009	
No Rx	vs	procaine	.429	NS
NSS+H2O	vs	NSS/hyaluronidase + H2O/hyaluronidase	.005	
procaine	vs	NSS/hyaluronidase + H2O/hyaluronidase	.064	(approach significance)
NSS/hyaluronidase	vs	H2O/hyaluronidase	.206	NS

Regarding lesion size, ANOVA revealed an overall significant difference between groups (p<.004). Planned multiple comparisons are presented in Table 2.

Table 2. Planned multiple comparisons (Dunn's test) of mean surface area of necrosis between groups in Study I.

No Rx	vs	NSS + H2O	p=2.29	NS
No Rx	vs	NSS/hyaluronidase + H2O/hyaluronidase	p=0.002	
No Rx	vs	procaine	p=0.33	NS
NSS+H2O	vs	NSS/hyaluronidase + H2O/hyaluronidase	p=0.004	
procaine	vs	NSS/hyaluronidase + H2O/hyaluronidase	p=0.08	(appr. significance)
NSS/hyaluronidase	vs	H2O/hyaluronidase	p=.71	NS

Study II

Twenty percent of the No Rx group, 47% of the NSS group, 27% of the procaine group and 7% of the hyaluronidase group developed necrosis following intradermal 3% STD. The mean surface area of necrosis for the No Rx, NSS, procaine and hyaluronidase groups respectively was 0.22, 3.37, 1.14 and 0.12 mm2. Chi square analysis of the percentage necrosis between groups approached significance (p=0.08). Deleting the no treatment group, individual comparisons revealed no significant difference between NSS and procaine or between procaine and hyaluronidase groups. However, the NSS group developed necrosis significantly more frequently than the hyaluronidase group (p=0.013). Looking at size of necrosis, ANOVA revealed a significant difference between groups (p=0.011). A Least Significance Difference test found the NSS group as having significantly larger necroses than other groups (p=0.05). No other statistically significant differences were found.

Discussion

Following intradermal HS (Study I) the NSS/hyaluronidase group clinically seemed to clearly have fewer and smaller ulcers than other the groups. The NSS/hyaluronidase group developed ulcers roughly at 50% of the frequency as non-hyaluronidase groups. The non-hyaluronidase groups (NSS, H2O, procaine, No Rx) did not vary by more than 10% in the incidence of necrosis. The mean surface area of necrosis in the non-hyaluronidase groups was 200%-300% larger than those that developed in the hyaluronidase groups. Non-hyaluronidase groups did not vary among themselves by more than 30%.

Statistical analysis, done with certain logical combinations of groups (NSS+H2O, NSS/hyaluronidase + H2O/hyaluronidase, procaine and no treatment), found that only the hyaluronidase group had significantly fewer and smaller ulcers than the no treatment group. The hyaluronidase group also had significantly fewer and smaller ulcers than the NSS+H2O group, and approached significance vs. the procaine group. No other significant differences were found.

Following intradermal 3% STD (Study II), the hyaluronidase group developed only one small necrosis. Even though the hyaluronidase group developed one-third the number of ulcers as the second "best" group, this did not reach statistical significance. Given the relatively low rate of ulcer formation in the no treatment group, larger group sizes would have been necessary to demonstrate significance. Paradoxically, the NSS and procaine groups developed the most largest ulcers. Perhaps this was because it spread the sclerosant without adequately diluting or "inactivating" it. Three cc of diluent added to 0.5cc 3% STD yields 3.5cc of 0.5% STD. The hyaluronidase group did have significantly fewer ulcers than the NSS group and the NSS group had significantly larger mean surface area of necrosis than other groups.

Hyaluronidase is an enzyme that breaks downs hyaluronic acid in ground substance.This disrupts the normal interstitial fluid barrier and is thought to rapidly diffuse extravasated solutions through tissues, thereby increasing the effective absorption(Zenk,1981). Hyaluronidase has been used to treat extravasation of nafcillin (Zenk & Dungy,1981), 10% dextrose injection, calcium salts, potassium salts, contrast media, sodium bicarbonate, and aminophylline (Zenk,1981). It has also been recommended following extravasation of vinca alkaloids (MacCara,1983). There have been several controlled studies which demonstrated the effectiveness of hyaluronidase in reducing necrosis following calcium chloride, hyperalimentation solution, and adriamycin (Laurie et al.,1984;Raszka et al.,1990). Hyaluronidase is remarkably free of side effects(Britton & Habif,1953;Schwartzman,1951). It rarely causes allergic reactions, which are primarily urticarial. It should not be injected into infected or cancerous areas, which might otherwise promote the spread of those conditions. Wydase® Lyophilized is reconstituted with normal saline, usually in the proportion of 1 cc per 150 USP units of hyaluronidase, and is stable for two weeks after reconstitution if stored below 30 C° (86 F°). Wydase® Stabilized Solution (Wyeth®) is an injection solution ready for use. Refrigeration is recommended.

In conclusion, one should always strive for excellent technique in order to minimize complications such as extravasation. However, at least in the model studied, hyaluronidase proved superior to normal saline, sterile water, and 1% procaine in the prevention of necrosis following extravasation of HS and STD.

References

Britton, RC & Habif, DV. (1953): Clinical uses of hyaluronidase. A current review. *Surgery*, 33, 917-942.

Butie, A. and Goldman, M.(1991): Preliminary results from the North American Society of Phlebology. In *Phlebolgoica:Houston '91*, pp 257-259. Dallas: PRM Editions.

Laurie, SW, Wilson, KL, et al. (1984): Intravenous extravasation injuries: The effectiveness of hyaluronidase in their treatment. *Ann Plastic Surg*, 13, 191-194.

MacCara ME. (1983): Extravasation: A hazard of intravenous therapy. *Infusion*, 17, 713-717.

Raszka, WV, Kueser, TK, et al. (1990): The use of hyaluronidase in the treatment of intravenous extravasation injuries. J. Perinat, 10, 146-148.

Schwartzman, J. (1951): Hyaluronidase: a review of its therapeutic use in pediatrics. *J Pediatr*, 39, 491-502.

Zenk, KE. (1981): Management of intravenous extravasation. *Infusion*,5, 77-79.

Zenk, KE, Dungy,CL, et al. (1981): Nafcillin extravasation injury: Use of hyaluronidase as an antidote. *Am J Dis Child*, 135,1113-1114.

Phlébologie 92. Eds P. Raymond-Martimbeau, R. Prescott, M. Zummo.
John Libbey Eurotext, Paris © 1992, pp. 873

The risk of transmission of blood-borne infection via needle stick in a busy sclerotherapy practice

Deborah P. Foley, Lori Notowitz

Vein Clinics of America, 1101 perimeter Drive, Suite 615, Schaumburg, Illinois 60173, USA.

The risk of exposure to Hepatitis B virus and HIV (AIDS virus) in clinical practice is increasing as the incidence of these diseases in the patient population increases. Practitioners of sclerotherapy are at increased risk due to their extensive use of needles.

Fifteen physicians and fifteen nurses whose full time practice is devoted exclusively to sclerotherapy were monitored for six months. The incidence of accidental needle stick exposure per treatment session was calculated. The total number of needle sticks was low but was increased among practitioners with less experience. A full review of the large scale United States and European needle stick exposure studies will be given.

Recommendations will be made for appropriate universal precautions for sclerotherapy practice. A Hepatitis B vaccination protocol will be recommended. The OSHA regulations regarding transmission of blood-borne infections will be presented.

In conclusion this study found that there is a small but real risk for exposure to blood borne infectious disease in a sclerotherapy practice. Review of current infectious disease literature reveals that universal precautions are currently the only effective protection available to the health care practitioner

Phlébologie 92. Eds P. Raymond-Martimbeau, R. Prescott, M. Zummo.
John Libbey Eurotext, Paris © 1992, pp. 874-876

Pentoxifylline in the sclerotherapeutic arterial accident

Jacques Romeo

Clinique Médic-Ami, Rouyn-Noranda, Québec, J9X 4X8, Canada.

We present a case of obliteration of the external pudendal artery following a paraarterial injection of iodine 6 % solution, during a trial sclerosis of the great saphenous vein. Pentoxifylline 400mg three times a day has been prescribed starting on third day (initial consultation) and daily until the end of tissue cicatrising process. Pentoxifylline has controlled the pain associated with the scarifying process. The ischemic and cyanotic initial zone of 9 X 8 cm with subcutaneous adipose necrosis of 4 X 2 cm has been reduced with this treatment to a remaining pigmented zone of 2 X 6 cm with a not very noticeable cutaneous remodelling. There has been no scar formation. Pentoxifylline seems to be an effective adjuvant for healing and reduction of the initial ischemic zone after an accidental obliteration in sclerotherapy. It should deserve a more exhaustive investigation in arterial phlebologic accidents. Its use in the treatment of small scarifying process following a paravenous subcutaneous injection could be evaluated being given its efficacy in ischemic cutaneous process as venous ulcers and accidental arterial obliteration (see table 1,2,3).

Table 1

Pentoxifylline mecanism of action

- reduction of blood viscosity (white blood cells)
- increase deformability of red blood cells
- inhibition of platelets aggregation
- reduction of fibrinogen
- increase of tissular PO 2

Then a global improvement of tissular nutrition

Table 2

Contraindications to pentoxifylline

Absolute

- children
- pregnancy
- acute myocardial infarction
- severe coronary disease

Relative

- increases the effect of antihypertensive drugs
- stimulates central nervous system when given with sympathicomimetic drugs or xanthines
- increases risk of hypoglycemia when given with oral hypoglycemic drugs

Table 3

Side effects of pentoxifylline

Usual dosage is 400mg three times a day with meals
generally well tolerated - side effects are transitory

- dyspepsia 2.8 %
- nausea 2.2 %
- vomiting 1.2 %
- dizziness 1.9 %
- headache 1.3 %

decreasing the dosage decreases side effects
antacids can control dyspepsia

BIBLIOGRAPHIE:

Angelides N.S.,(august 1989),Effect of oral pentoxifylline therapy on venous lower extremity ulcers due deep venous imcompetence , Angiology vol. 40 no.8

Arenas R, Atoche C, avril -(juin 1988), Post-thrombotic leg ulcers: safety and efficacy of treatment with pentoxifylline (double - blind study in 30 patients),Dermatologia, segunda epoca, volumen XXX II no.2

Brenner Mare A,(novembre 1987), Nonhealing venous stasis ulcers, pentoxifylline as adjunctive therapy. Journal of American Podiatric Medical Association, vol.77 no.11

Colgan M.P.,Dormandy J. and al,(may1989), The efficacy of trental in the treatment of venous ulceration Venous Forum, Manchester.

Conseil consultatif de pharmacologie,(juillet1989), Information medicament

Harris R.B.,févrièr - (mars 1989), Canadian Journal of Dermatology Benefits of oral therapy in management of leg ulcers. vol.1 no.1

Herger R.,(septembre 1986), The significance of the micocirculation in the treatment of leg ulcers no.38

Lenoble-Giovaximangeli,(septembre 1988), Du globule rouge au globule blanc, laboratoire Hoechst,

Ward A., Clissold S.,(juillet 1987), Drug, focus on pentoxifylline vol. 34 no.1

Weitgasser H.,(1983), The use of pentoxifylline(trental 400) in the treatment of leg ulcers (result of a double - blind trial pharmatherapeutica vol.3 suppl.1

C.
TRAITEMENT COMPRESSIF
COMPRESSIVE TREATMENT

Phlébologie 92. Eds P. Raymond-Martimbeau, R. Prescott, M. Zummo.
John Libbey Eurotext, Paris © 1992, pp. 879-880

Mechanism of action of external compression in venous disease

S. Sarin, J.H. Scurr, P.D. Coleridge Smith

Department of Surgery, University College and Middlesex School of Medicine, The Middlesex Hospital, London, W1N 8AA, UK.

There remains considerable controversy over the mechanism of action of external compression therapy despite the widespread acceptance of the benefits of this form of treatment. Compression stockings and bandages may act by reducing venous reflux. The aim of this study was to assess the mechanism of action of compression therapy on venous function and to determine whether this treatment may correct valvular incompetence.

Both the lower limbs of 36 patients (median age 59yrs interquartile range (IQR) 45-65) were assessed by Duplex Scanning (Acuson128, Acuson Inc, Mountain View, California). There were 17 limbs with popliteal vein (PopVn) reflux, 19 with long saphenous vein reflux (LSV), 21 with short saphenous vein reflux (SSV) and 15 normal lower limbs. An adjustable pressure, water filled, external compression cuff was applied around the knee. The cuff was then inflated gradually, while continuously assessing the vein for reflux using ultrasound imaging, until reflux was abolished or the vein completely occluded, and the pressure noted.

RESULTS	**Pop Vn**(n=17)	**LSV**(n=19)	**SSV**(n=21)
Reflux Abolished (n=15)	4	8	3
Pressure: mmHg median(IQR)	62(60-64)†	31(22-83)✤	58(50-85)✞
Reflux Not Abolished (n=42)	13	11	18
Occlusion Pressure: mmHg median(IQR))	89(67-96)†	87(70-108)✤	75(65-93)✞

Wilcoxon's Rank Sum Test-unpaired samples: †$p<0.05$, ✤$p<0.01$, ✞p=ns

We have been able to show that external compression does restore valvular competence in a proportion of cases, both in the superficial and deep venous systems. The external pressure required to achieve restoration of valvular competence was far higher than that produced by Grade 3 stockings at the knee. However, direct comparison to graduated compression stockings may not be appropriate. Though the static pressures achieved at the knee by stockings are much lower than the pressures required in our study, it has been shown that dynamic pressure measurement with stockings (eg with the patient walking) may be higher. In addition, we have investigated the effect of compression on valvular function at the knee only and it is possible that external compression from the ankle to the knee restores competence in a larger number of veins thereby improving venous function in a greater proportion of limbs. These results suggest that the mechanism of comprssion therapy may be by allowing better apposition of valvualr cuffs and so improving venous function.

Venous pressure as base of compression therapy

S. Fontanyi, Z. Fontanyi,

Department of Surgery "A", Péterfy S. Hospital and Military Health Service, Budapest, Hungary

The venous pressure as reliable hemodynamic parametermay be convenient base of a dosaged, graded compression therapy.

Method: TPM /Toe-Plethysmometry/ non-invasive technique has been used for venous pressure measurement. The horizontal position eliminates hydrostatic pressure, so, even a slight rise demonstrates the flux insufficiency.

Material: 739 limbs of 369 patients has been investigated

Result: 3 severity classes were established by mean values in /mmHg/:

1. Healthy limbs 213 /22/
2. Primary varicose vein 383 /24/
3. CVI without DVT 109 /54/
4. Post thrombotic syndrome 37 /68/

Practical consequence: The severity classes may be considered as **compression classes** and the individualized, dosaged, graded compression has been exerted by:

1. Light - 30 mmHg: 1 layer of elastic bandage EB
2. Medium - 30-60 mmHg: 2 layer of EB
3. Heavy - 60 mmHg: 2 layer of EB + compression stocking

Special bandage technique for crural ulcer: if crust adherent cutting around, swabbing, 10% Aluminiumchloride-hydroxide gel, sterile gauze, elastic compression bandage.

Phlébologie 92. Eds P. Raymond-Martimbeau, R. Prescott, M. Zummo.
John Libbey Eurotext, Paris © 1992, pp. 882-884

The effect of using high compression elastic stockings on oedema and skin oxygenation

P. Rashid, M.C. Stacey, Y. Vandongen, S.E. Hoskin

University Department of Surgery, Fremantle Hospital, Alma Street, Fremantle, Western Australia.

INTRODUCTION

Venous ulceration and the skin changes of lipodermatosclerosis have been associated with reduced transcutaneous oxygen (Tcp02) measurements in the skin [Byrne, et al - 1984; Clyne, et al - 1985]. Several studies have shown that treatments aimed at reducing venous ulcer recurrence result in improvement of the skin Tcp02 (Stacey, et al 1987; McMullin, et al 1991).

The improvement of Tcp02 has been proposed to result from an improvement in the underlying abnormality within the leg. This could be a reduction in pericapillary fibrin (Stacey et al 1987) or an improvement in the physiological changes which result in white cell accumulation [Coleridge-Smith, et al - 1988]. However, it has been suggested that Tcp02 may be due to oedema within the legs and that the Tcp02 impairment is a direct result of oedema [Mani, et al -1989].

This study was conducted as part of a long term study on the effectiveness of elastic compression stockings in preventing venous ulcer recurrence. The aim was to determine whether skin Tcp02 readings were related to changes of oedema in the legs of patients with recently healed venous ulcers.

METHOD

Patients with a recently healed ulcer that was due to venous disease alone, were considered for this trial if they were able to put stockings on and off. Patients were randomised into stockings (VENOSAN[R] 2003, Salzman AG, St Gallen, Switzerland) or no-stockings. Stocking patients were informed that the stockings were to be worn at all times except when in bed and in the shower.

After healing, using outpatient compression bandaging, the patient's legs were kept in bandages until initial measurements were performed 2 weeks later. They were then randomized into the study and were reviewed at 2 weeks, 3 months and 6 monthly intervals thereafter.

At the initial assessment, foot volume was measured using a water displacement method. Tcp02 was measured TCM2 (TCM3, Radiometer, Copenhagen), in lipodermatosclerotic skin of the affected leg, and a standard site on the chest.

The leg/chest Tcp02 ratio was used in this study. The probe temperature was set at 45oC and, readings were taken after a 15-20 minute acclimatisation period in a quiet, darkened room at a constant temperature (25°C). Repeat readings were not performed in patients with recurrent ulceration since they were being treated by compression bandaging.

RESULTS

79 patients (84 limbs) entered the trial. In the stocking group there were 20 males (median age 71.5, range 38-87 years) and 18 females (median age 76, range 48-86 years). In the no stocking group there were 22 males (median age 62, range 33-84 years) and 19 females (median age 75, range 52-84 years). Of the total number of limbs entered into the trial, 41 were in the stocking group and 43 in the no stocking group.

7 limbs were considered as withdrawals from this study in the stocking group and one from the no stocking group. The reasons for withdrawal from the stocking group were - unable to wear stockings (3), refused to continue wearing stockings (2), allergy to stockings (1) and death (1). One patient refused to continue in the no stocking group for personal reasons.

Patients who came out of bandages and were randomised into the no stocking group had a significant increase in leg volume in the first 2 weeks (Wilcoxon rank test paired, p<0.01) but, there was no further increase in volume when re-measured at 3 months (p=0.31). The patients who came out of bandages and into stockings showed no significant change in volume measures (p=0.84) at 2 weeks or at 3 months (p=0.58), (Fig. 1).

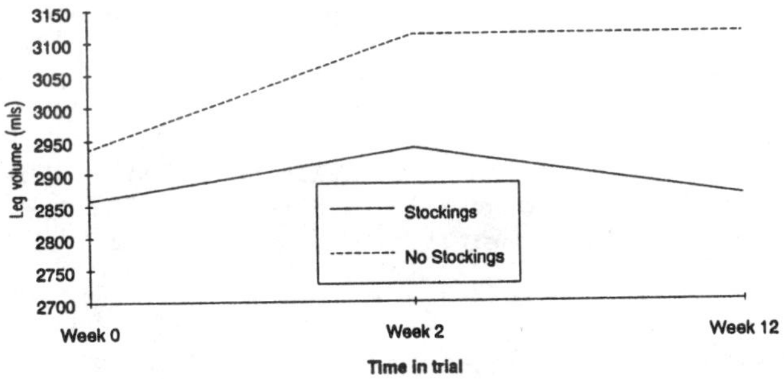

Figure 1. Leg Volumes from the Stocking and No Stocking Groups (median values)

Tcp02 measurements were not statistically altered at the 2 week or 3 month follow-up in either group. There appeared to be an increase in Tcp02 at 3 months compared to 2 weeks in the stocking group but this was not significant (p=0.66) (Fig. 2).

All patients were asked to keep a diary of the number of hours in a day, as well as, the number of days per week the stockings were worn. Those included in the study informed us that the stockings were worn for at least 8 hours a day for 5 or more days a week. At 3 months, 8 limbs (26%) had reulcerated in the stocking group and 14 (38%) in the no stocking group.

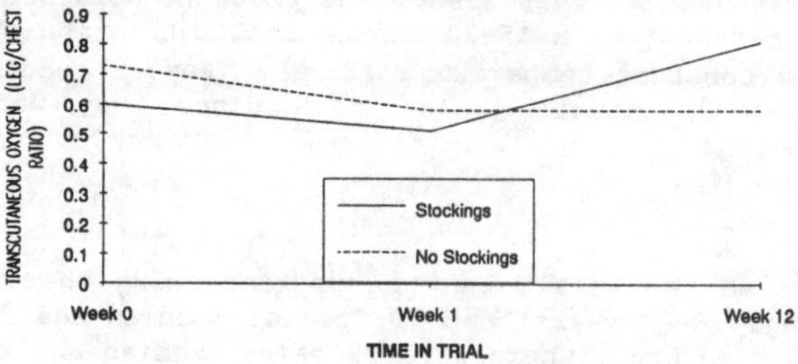

Figure 2. Tcp02 Ratios from Stocking and No Stocking Groups (median values)

DISCUSSION

The current follow-up period in this study is short. At 3 months, however, certain findings were apparent. Compression stockings did assist in the control of oedema in these venous patients. In the no stocking group, removing compression bandages without further use of compression therapy did increase the oedema in the leg within a short period of time. This increase in oedema, however, did not appear to reduce skin oxygenation. Using an external pneumatic compression device to reduce oedema has been shown to reduce oedema but not improve skin oxygenation (Nemeth, et al 1989).

In this study Tcp02 was not significantly increased at 3 months by the use of elastic stockings, McMullin et al (1991) found that stockings did increase Tcp02. This discrepancy may be due to the short follow up to date in this study and review after a longer follow up will be subsequently performed. The results of this study would tend to indicate that Tcp02 ratio increases found by previous workers are unlikely to be due to reduction in oedema and are more likely to be due to alterations in the leg as a result of using compression stockings.

The influence of elastic stockings on recurrent ulceration can not be assessed at this early stage of the study, and we will need to wait until the follow up is closer to the planned before any conclusions can be made.

REFERENCES

Byrne P, Naughton P M, O'Higgins N J 1984: Transcutaneous oxygen tension in the lower limbs with venous disease. *Br J Surg* **71(12)**: 990.

Clyne C A C, Ramsden W H, Chant A D B, Webster J H H 1985: *Oxygen tension on the skin of the gaiter area of limbs with venous disease*. *Br J Surg* **72**: 644-647.

Coleridge-Smith P D, Thomas P R S, Scurr J H, Dormandy J A. 1988: Causes of venous ulceration: a new hypothesis. *Br Med J* **296**: 1726-1727.

Mani R, White J E, Barrett, Weaver P W. 1989: Tissue oxygenation, venous ulcers and fibrin cuffs. *J Roy Soc Med* **82**: 345.

McMullin G M, Watkin G T, Coleridge-Smith P D, Scurr J H. 1991: Efficacy of fibrinolytic enhancement with Stanozolol in the treatment of venous insufficiency. *Aust N Z J Surg* **61**: 306-309.

Nemeth A J, Falanga V, Alstadt S, et al.1989: *Ulcerated edematous limbs: Effect of edema removal on transcutaneous oxygen measurements*. *J Am Acad Dermatol* 20(2i): 191-197.

Stacey M C, Burnand K G, Layer G T, Pattison M.1990: *Transcutaneous oxygen tensions in assessing the treatment of healed venous ulcers*. *Br J Surg* **77**: 1050-1054.

Phlébologie 92. Eds P. Raymond-Martimbeau, R. Prescott, M. Zummo.
John Libbey Eurotext, Paris © 1992, pp. 885-888

Quantification of therapeutic effects in legs with various venous disorders

M. Emter[1], D.P. Pretschner[2], H. Hundeshagen[2], K. Alexander[1]

Medizinische Hochschule Hannover, Abteilung Angiologie[1], Abteilung Nuklearmedizin und spezielle Biophysik[2], Karl-Weichert-Allee, D 3000 Hannover 61, Germany.

INTRODUCTION

The determination of blood volume and velocitiy of venous flow (1, 7) in the leg has always been of great interest in phlebological research (4, 6). The differentiation between the edema induced increase of volume and an increase caused by hemodynamic changes was not possible with simple volumetric or plethysmographic methods (5).
Because of methodic complications a continuous measurement for a period of time which would have opened the view of kinetic connections between blood compartment and edema space was not possible.
The engymetric double radionuclide method offers a new chance to differentiate between the two above-mentioned compartments. With this method the two compartments can be selected not only for a short time and locally fixed but over time periods that can be almost freely determinated. This method offers the chance to quantify therapeutic interventions on a leg, for example compression therapy on postthrombotic legs (2, 3).

MATERIALS AND METHODS

Measurement of the intravascular space is archieved by in vivo labelling of erythrocytes. By labelling the extracellular space, the measurement of changes in edema volume is given after subtraction of the intravascular fraction. Edema space is defined as extravascular and extracellular .
Engymetry, from the Greek "engys", which means "nearby", stands for measuring directly at the patient; in contrast for other methods this one is mobile.
3 uCi Br-82 and 3 mCi Tc-99m are used for the investigation. The total body quantity of radiation for the patient is relatively small with 2 mrad/uCi for Br-82 and 9 mrad/mCi for Tc-99m.
The energy of Tc-99m is 140 keV and 768 keV for the Br-82.
Discrimination of the nuclides in vivo can be achieved by a special detector system. Impulses are counted by miniaturized Geiger-Müller-tubes in lead chambers. The separation of the tubes and the use of "windows" in the counting area ensure the discrimination of the nuclides .
The short wave bromide can penetrate the lead, the long wave technetium cannot do so.
Channel 1 counts impulses of technetium and bromide, channel 2 nothing but bromide impulses.
The Geiger-Müller-tubes are run with a voltage of 600 V. The voltage is reached by a miniaturized amplifier.
Impulses are stored in MIESSY by cable (Medical Information Extraction and Storage SYstem). The weight of the apparatus is approximately 350 g and therefore it is easily to be carried by a patient. The electronics of the apparatus consist of highly integrated CMOS electronics with four independent counting channels (5).
The "integration" time (that means the time during which impulses are counted) and "interval" (time between two integrations) can be chosen. Time is variable from 0.25 sec up to 2.5 hours per place in the memory. In one MIESSY with 64 places it is possible to store data gathered between 10 minutes and 160 hours.
The digitally stored data are fed directly to a computer for further evaluation.

The physical investigations concerning the geometry of the apparatus and the loss of counts guarantee valid data; in the used zone loss is negligible. Many investigations have been performed by other authors concerning the nuclides in vivo.
There are some problems that have to be considered while using the double radionuclide method. The Br-82 must be applied early enough before starting the investigation in order to guarantee a good distribution. In a long-term investigation the loss by urine must be taken into account (3% in 24 hours).
The in vivo labelling of the erythrocytes is reached by the IV application of non radioactive pyrophosphate (SN - PYP) with the following application of the Tc-99m pertechnetat. A steady state in distribution is reached in approximately 15 minutes. This is nearly constant up to 8 hours. We saw 98 % of the activity after 6 hours.
24 hours before the start the patient gets the IV injection of 3 uCi Br-82. At the day of the measurement the patient is in a lying position and a blood sample is taken.
After 30 minutes the detectors which are put in the desired positions (for example on the calf or on the foot) are connected with the storage unit.
After references have been obtained on both channels, pyrophophate and Tc-99m are given IV. A second blood sample is taken after the Tc-99m has reached a steady state.
After that the wanted investigations can be started (for example during walking, standing lying or sitting). At the end of the investigation stored date are fed into a computer.

Blood samples at the beginning of the investigation and after Tc-99m application do not only guarantee the correct application of the nuclides, but also allows quantification of the intravascular share of bromide.
In the blood apparatus 1 ml blood is exactly fixed at same distance from four GM-tubes. Two of these are packed in 4 mm thick lead, the other two are free; so discrimination of the nuclides in blood is achieved in the same way as in the detector .
It is nessesary to have the continuous control of the impulses emitted at the patient in order to determine the false application of nuclides or wrong placement of the detectors.

It is necessary to fix a standard value initially:
1. because of the non-paired number of GM-tubes and the individual counting of each of them,
2. to find out coefficient of absorbance under the given circumstances,
3. to take into account the difference of counting in various places of detectors of the patients.
With these data, constants, half-life periods of nuclides and time shifts first of all discrimination of nuclides in patient and in blood is reached.
Changes of the intravascular volume represented by Tc-99m induced impulses are directly proportional to the adjusted countrates.
Since Br-82 is a marker of the extracellular compartment, the intravascular share must be subtracted to get an impression of the edema space. The intravascular share can be figured out using the countrates in the blood apparatus and the quantity of changes seen in the Tc-99m channel.

To get valid data the following essentials must be fulfilled:
- correct application of nuclides
- adequate time for distribution of nuclides
- obtaining standard values
- detection of nuclides in the blood
- adequate time for the investigation.

The engymetric double radionuclide method offers new aspects of getting informations from an angiological or phlebological point of view. Especially therapeutic interventions, which should have effects on the above-mentioned compartments, can be looked at critically. Mobility of equipment, the possibility of continuous counting over longer periods and with all wanted therapies offer a good basis for answering many questions.
Without doubt this method is not one for everyday practice because of the complicated technical equipment. This method should be used to answer special questions put concerning angiological respectively phlebological problems.

RESULTS

In a study with 20 patients having primary varices and were treated with adequate compression stockings (class II) and 10 patients having a postthrombotic syndrome which was verified by phlebography and

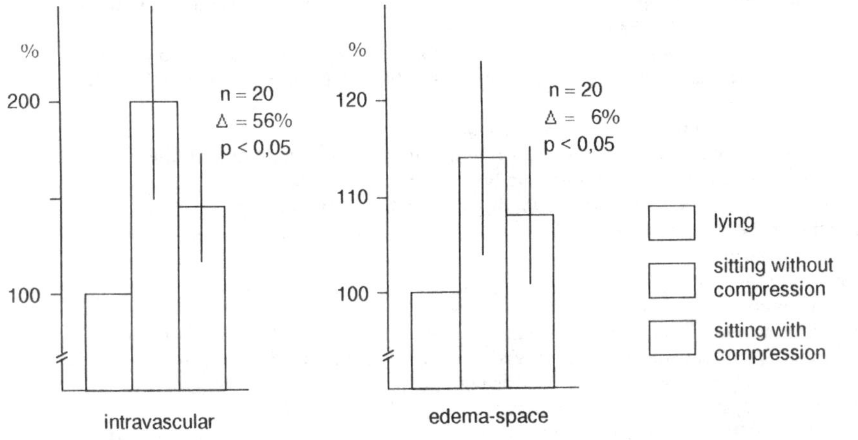

Changes in the calf during one hour sitting without and with compression (class II compression stockings) in patients with primary varicose veins (lying = 100%)

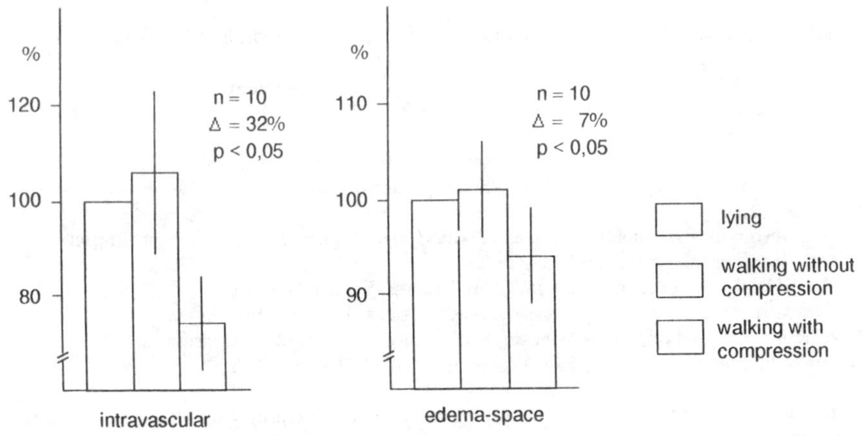

Changes in the foot during half an hour walking without and with compression (zinc paste bandage) in patients with postthrombotic syndrome (lying = 100%)

was treated by a zinc paste bandage, the effects on intravascular and extravascular compartments were measured with and without compression therapy.
Lying was used as standard value and was put 100 % in comparison to sitting in the group with primary varicosity with legs put in an angle of 90 degrees and in comparison to half an hour walking in the group with a postthrombotic syndrome.
One day before investigation the edema was removed by bandaging the legs.
The investigation was done first without compression during one hour of sitting. After that, the investigation was repeated with compression under exactly the same conditions.
In order to obtain valid and reproducible data the following conditions were fulfilled:

- standardization of time of the day
- constant temperatur in the room
- adequate compression therapy
- adequate time for investigation.

In the group with primary varicosity from lying to sitting an increase of 100 % + 50% took place in the intravascular space of the calf without compression. It was possible to reduce this increase to 44 % + 27% with a compression stocking (class II). The difference was significant on the $p<0.05$ level. The extravascular increase of initially 14 % + 10% was reduced to 8 % + 7% ($p < 0{,}05$).
In patients with a postthrombotic syndrome the intravascular increase was 6% + 17% in the foot, this increase was reduced to a decrease to 74% + 10% using a zinc paste bandage during walking ($p<0.05$). The edema space could be reduced in the first thirty minute for 7 % + 5% ($p<0.05$).
These data showed that compression therapy induces the wanted effects on the compartments. A decrease of intravascular volume in the lower limb with the following consequences for congestion and pressure is responsible for a lower increase of edema volume in the leg having a venous disorder.
Up to now quantification of the shifting has not been possible with other methods. With engymetric double radionuclide equipment a good evaluation of the therapy was obtained.

References

1. Bollinger, A. Flußgeschwindigkeit in der Vena saphena magna und der Vena femoralis mit und ohne Kompressionsverbände. SWISS Med. 2: 61, 1980.
2. Emter, M., K. Alexander und D. P. Pretschner. Methode zur Beurteilung von Veränderungen des intravasalen und extravasalen Kompartiments am Bein: Die engymetrische Doppelradionuklidmessung. SWISS MED. 10(4a): 17 - 21, 1988.
3. Emter, M., D. P. Pretschner, H. Hundeshagen und K. Alexander. Determination of changes in the intravascular and extravascular compartment in the leg - The engymetric double radionuclide method -. Nuklearmedizin. 26: 265-269, 1987.
4. Fröhlich, M. and T. Wuppermann. Verhalten der venösen Hämodynamik unter Kompressionsstrümpfen bei ausgeprägter primärer Varikosis. medita. 3a: 7 - 13, 1978.
5. Haid-Fischer, F. and H. Haid. "Venenerkrankungen." 1980 Thieme-Verlag. Stuttgart.
6. Molen, H. R. v. d. Gummistrumpfprobleme. Ergebnisse d. Angiologie. 4: 169 - 180, 1970.
7. Partsch, H. and O. Lofferer. Untersuchungen des venösen Rückstroms aus der unteren Extremität mit einem direktionalen Ultraschalldetektor. Wiener Klin Wochenschr. 83: 781 - 789, 1971.

Authors address: Dr. Michael Emter, Medizinische Hochschule Hannover, Abteilung Angiologie, Karl-Wiechert-Allee, D 3000 Hannover 61, Germany

Phlébologie 92. Eds P. Raymond-Martimbeau, R. Prescott, M. Zummo.
John Libbey Eurotext, Paris © 1992, pp. 889-890

Objectivisation of the long term effect of various types of compression bandages with digital photoplethysmography

Jaroslav Strejček

Dermatological Clinic I, Charles University, Prague 12800 Prague 2, Vyšehradská 49, Czechoslovakia.

The effect of various types of compression bandages used after the sclerotherapy was compared by means of Digital Photoplethysmography (D-PPG ELCAT).

Three groups, each consisting of 25 patients treated with a different type of bandage were used. The first group had an elastic cohesive bandage (Medirip 2000, KOB KG), the second group a new type of semirigid plastic compression, the third group had the "classic" elastic bandage (Idealtex, Rico).

All three groups of patients with these three types of bandages show just after the application using a standard overlapping spiral technique from toes to the knee (in the case of Medirip 2000 an overlapping criss-cross method was used) a good improvement of the muscle-venous pump through D-PPG screening.

However classic elastic bandages controlled after 5 - 24 hours after aplication partially slipped down and the initial positive improvement of the venous hemodynamics diminished 43 % after 24 hours.

On the other hand, the other two types of bandages tested on the second, fourth and sixth day after application stayed nearly in its initial position and the parametres of venous hemodynamics didn´t change significantly.

Therefore, we can conclude, that the elastic cohesive bandage the same as the new type of a semirigid plastic compression are more convenient in situation, where a longterm compression therapy is desired.

REFERENCES

Strejček, J. (1992): Die Kontrolle des hämodynamischen Effekts der Sklerotherapie mit Hilfe der D-PPG. In Fortschritte in der computerunterstützten nichtinvasiven Gefässdiagnostik. Berichte des 3. Internationalen Symposiums CNVD´91, eds. V. Blazek und U. Schultz-Ehrenburg, pp. 29-33. Düsseldorf: VDI Verlag.

Phlébologie 92. Eds P. Raymond-Martimbeau, R. Prescott, M. Zummo.
John Libbey Eurotext, Paris © 1992, pp. 891-893

Compression of the lower limbs by elastic stocking : a morphological study of the peripheral veins with T.A.C.

Sergio Mancini, Luca Volterrani*, Giuseppe Botta, Simonetta Massi, Carla Ruggieri

*Institute of General Surgery and * Institute of Radiology, University of Siena, Bracci Avenue, 53100 Siena, Italy.*

ABSTRACT

Fifteen phlebopathic patiens (6 with varicose veins and 9 with SPF) were morphologicaly evaluated carring out T.A.C. of the veins of the lower limbs, both before and during appropriate elasto-compression. T.A.C. sections were carried out on various areas of the lower limbs. The most important superficial and deep veins were studied. Computerized elaboration of the images obteined allowed the evaluation of centre, dimention, morphology and contrast medium distribution of the blood vessels, examined before and during compression with elastic stocking. The results showed a notable increase in the velocity of the venous flow during compression, while the major peripheral arteries showed no apparent change.

KEY WORDS: Varicose veins, T.A.C., Elastic stocking.

INTRODUCTION

Compressive action on the lower limbs of phlebopathic patients has been greatly studied by large number of Authors, using various methods as phlebographic, radioisotopic, ecographic, plethismographic and anatomopathological (Schoop 1964, Fischer 1972, Lofferer 1970-1972, Partsch 1979, Wilkins e coll. 1972, Stemmer 1976, Altenkamper e coll. 1983, Curri e coll. 1989, Emter e coll. 1989, Brizzio 1990, etc.).

From those studies the following was concluded:

A) "Compressive action on venous and lymphatic microcircles of the lower limbs"
   1) Calibre reduction of deep and superficial veins;
   2) Reduction by up to 30-40% in pathological refluxes;
   3) Reduction of the venous pool;
   4) Overloading of the valve edges, mainly in the deep venous system;
   5) Increase in the velocity of flow by up to 5 times;
   6) Increase in fibrinolytic activity;
   7) Acceleration of lymphatic transport.

B) " Compressive action on the microvascular tissue unit"
   1) Decrease of capillary-venous ectasia;
   2) Reactive thickening of the basal membrane;
   3) Decrease in interstitial oedema;
   4) Improvement in the phisio-chemical conditions of the interstice.

From the research carried out, however, we cannot define with clarity the in life action of the elastic stocking on both venous and arterial microcircles of the lower limbs

There are the technical reasons (we still cannot provide an unfailing method for the study of the pressure exerted at rest and above all in the dynamic study of the illness) and the objective difficulties in the manifacture of the "ideal" elastic stocking suitable for every patient.

On the other hand, clinical evaluation of the effectiveness of compression with elastic stocking is positive in the majority of cases, even if there is a small percentage of patients who without apparent reasons show an intollerance to the elastic stockings.

Data obtained from on experimental physical study of the compression exerted by an elastic stocking, carried out in collaboration with the Institute of Medical Physics of Siena University, further stimulated us to try new parameters in the evaluation of the compressive action in peoples.

Until now T.A.C. had not been used in the study of elasto-compression and for this reason it seemed appropriate to start this research by establishing the validity of the known data and to possibly obtain new data.

The only drawbach of T.A.C. is the position in which the patients have to lie, which itself can be an invalid factor.

We have tried to rule this out as much as possible, allowing the patients to lie down only a few minutes before the examination and getting then to make feet dorso-flexion movements as if to simulate walking throughout the investigation.

If this, one more hand, is the methodical limitation, then the results obtained, on the other hand, are presumably better than those which would have been obtained with patients in the orthostatic position, and can therefore be considered as realistic.

MATERIALS AND METHOD

Fifteen patiens were examined: 6 had essential varicose veins and 9 were affected with post-phlebitic syndrome.

All had worn for some time elastic stockings appropriate to their illness.

The patients were subjected to T.A.C. with T.C. General Electric 9800 apparatus, administering a contrast medium into arm's vein by means of the automatic injector.

Four scans were carried out:

1) on the upper malleolar region
2) on the widest part of the calf
3) on the region between the two regions mentioned above
4) on the upper side of the tibia

Every region was studied either in the early or late stages, and only for the pathological limb on which the patient had worn the elastic stocking.

The most important comparison throughout the study was that made between the scans carried out in the late phase and those carried out with the elastic stocking in place.

The early phase served to locate the arteries (popliteal, anterior tibial, posterior tibial, peroneal) used as landmark for later scans.

The parameters taken into consideration throughout the study were as follows:

1) diameter of the limb
2) thickness of the subcutaneous tissue
3) diameter of the superficial blood vessels
4) diameter of the deep blood vessels
5) evaluation of eventual varicose ectasia
6) evaluation of the eventual incontinent perforants.

RESULTS

1) The diameter of the limb was noticeably reduced and the calf reassumed its normal conformation.

2) The subcutaneous tissue, particularly if sclerotic, seemed not to be affected by compression. In these cases we noted the disappearance of some phlebectasies and the appearance of others neighbouring areas, as if compression was greater in normal areas and less in the hardened areas, redistributing the stagnant blood into superficial circulation.

3) The diameter of the superficial blood vessels (saphenous veins), in the majority of cases, decreased significantly.

4) The deep blood vessels (peroneal, anterior and posterior tibial veins) tend to significantly reduce in actual diameter and in some cases disappear.

5) The phlebectasies generally reduce until theyr eventually disappear.

6) The perforants (in the few scans in which they can be seen) seem to be beneficially affected by elasto-compression, with a clear reduction in surface flow.

REFERENCES

ALTENKAMPER H.: "Effects de la compression forte intermittente sur les activateurs du plasminogene dans la saphene interne" Atti del Congresso Mondiale dell'Unione Internazionale di Flebologia, Bruxelles 2-6 maggio 1983,489-491.

BASSI G., STEMMER R.: "Traitments mecanique fonctionelles en phlebologie ".Piccin Ed.Padova 1983.

BOLLINGER A. et al.: "Transcapillary and interstitial diffusion of Na-Fluorescein in chronic venous insufficiency with white atrophy". Int. J. Microcirculation Clin. Exp. 1982,1,5-17.

COGET J.M., MERLEN J.F., DUPUIS-CUNY C.: "Influence de la compression sur la microcirculation". Phlebologie 1986,39,3,509-516.

COLERIDGE SMITH P.D. et al.: "Intermittent pneumatic compression improves venous ulcer healing".Atti del X Congresso Mondiale dell'Unione Internazionale di Flebologia, Strasburgo 1989,1146-1148.

CURRI S.B. et all.: "Changes of cutaneous microcirculation from elasto-compression in chronic venous insufficiency". Atti del X Congresso Mondiale dell'Unione Internazionale di Flebologia, Strasburgo 1989,852-854.

KOLARI P.J., PEKANMAKI K.: "Foot transcapillary filtration in patients with severe chronic venous insufficiency". Vasa 1988,17,2,92-96.

MERLEN J.F.: "Retentissement de la stase sur le segment capillaro-venulare". Phlebologie 1982,35,53-60.

Does medical therapy exist for calf vein insufficiency?

Dr. I. Staelens

Flebology AZ VUB Brussels B 1090, Belgium

The venous circulatory insufficiency of the calf seldom results in visible disturbances of the superficial venous circulation of the leg in young patients.

Compression is most of the time the only possible therapy that can be offered to these patients.

Certain precise condition have to be fulfilled so that compression is efficient on the deep veins. These conditions are very different from those met in compression therapy of the superficial venous insufficiency.

The compression for muscular vein insufficiency needs also the support of good muscular activity of the calf region to obtain real emptying of the deep muscle veins.

Medicamental therapy needs still more fundamental research.

Phlébologie 92. Eds P. Raymond-Martimbeau, R. Prescott, M. Zummo.
John Libbey Eurotext, Paris © 1992, pp. 895-897

The effect of training using feedback from a pressure monitor on nurses bandaging techniques

E.A. Nelson[1,2], J.C. Barbenel[1], C.V. Ruckley[1], D. Queen[3]

[1] *Lothian and Forth Valley Leg Ulcer Study Royal Infirmary Edinburgh, Scotland, UK.* [2] *Bioengineering Unit, University of Strathclyde, Glasgow, Scotland, UK.* [3] *Convatec WHRI, Deeside, Wales, UK.*

Aim

The purpose of this study was to answer the following questions.

1) How well do registered nurses apply a compression bandage, as measured using a pressure monitor?
2) Can the pressure profile produced by a nurse under a compression bandage be improved by providing the nurse with feedback and advice?
3) Is any improvement in bandaging technique maintained over a two week period?

Subjects

These were eighteen registered nurses who were involved in the treatment of venous leg ulcers in the community and the hospital.

Equipment

The 'Granuflex Adhesive Compression Bandage' (Convatec, Clwyd. UK) was used during the tests.
Sub-bandage pressure at three points along the lateral aspect of the leg was measured using the 'Strathclyde Pressure Monitor' developed at the University of Strathclyde.

Method

1) Nurses were asked to apply the bandage to a volunteers leg using their normal bandaging technique. For this baseline reading the digital display of the pressure monitor was covered.
2) The nurse was then provided with a bandage which had been marked at regular intervals with an oval which would attain a circular shape once the bandage had been extended according to the manufacturers instructions. No feedback from the monitor was provided until the bandager had completed this stage of the test.

3) At this stage the bandager was able to bandage while the pressure monitor showed the compression achieved, thus the bandager was receiving continuous feedback. Advice was given by EAN regarding bandage extension, overlap and desired pressures and the sub-bandage pressure was remeasured.
4) After an interval of two weeks the bandagers were asked to return for repeat testing. They had been provided with a few bandages for practise during this time

Results
For ease of analysis the pressure profile achieved was classified as being unsatisfactory, barely satisfactory or good, using the following criteria.

Unsatisfactory; Ankle pressure <18mmHg or >60mmHg,
or Calf pressure > Ankle pressure
Barely satisfactory; Ankle pressure <25 mmHg but >18 mmHg,
or Ankle pressure>52mmHg but <60mmHg,
or Calf pressure+8mmHg > Ankle pressure
Good; Ankle pressure >25 mmHg, < 52 mmHg, **and**
Calf pressure+8 < Ankle pressure.

Therefore a good profile showed adequate ankle pressure and graduation, a satisfactory profile showed insufficient or excessive pressure or poor graduation but was not an unsafe pressure, and an unsatisfactory profile had insufficient pressure or a tourniquet effect at the calf.

The pressure profiles were scored, 1= unsatisfactory, 2= barely satisfactory and 3= good and the results achieved by the nurses were as shown in fig1.

Sub-bandage pressure score

Subject	Baseline/	Using Marked Bandage/	After Training/	After 2 Weeks
1	2	2	3	3
2	2	3	3	3
3	1	3	3	3
4	1	3	2	2
5	1	2	1	1
6	1	3	3	*
7	1	1	2	*
8	1	1	3	*
9	1	1	3	*
10	1	1	1	*
11	2	1	2	2
12	1	2	3	*
13	3	2	2	3
14	1	1	3	*
15	1	1	3	2
16	2	1	2	3
17	1	2	2	3
18	1	1	2	3

* = data missing

The Wilcoxon Sign Rank Sum test was used to show that the difference between the bandaging proficiency score was significant between pre-training score and post-training score <u>and</u> that this was maintained after two weeks ($P<0.01$).

There was no difference found when using the marked bandage, ($P>0.1$).

Conclusions

Initial bandage profiles were unsatisfactory.

Training (feedback and advice) improved bandage application and this was maintained for two weeks.

It is unknown whether the use of the monitor alone would result in a similar improvement.

The longevity of the change in technique is being studied in present studies.

Phlébologie 92. Eds P. Raymond-Martimbeau, R. Prescott, M. Zummo.
John Libbey Eurotext, Paris © 1992, pp. 898-900

Algorithme de la prescription des bas de compression

Robert Stemmer, Christian Furderer

8, rue Auguste-Lamey, 67000 Strasbourg, France.

La prescription d'un bas médical de compression est une décision importante, car souvent ces bas sont à porter toute la vie pour éviter les récidives des affections veineuses et lymphatiques chroniques. Elle se base sur un raisonnement logique qui peut être résumé dans un algorithme comprotant différentes réflexions successives:

1. Un traitement compressif préalable est-il indispensable?
2. Quel traitement mettre en peuvre avant la prescription de bas médicaux de compression?
3. Eliminer d'abord les contre-indications.
4. Choisir la force de la compression.
5. Choisir le modèle de bas.
6. Prendre les mesures pour le meilleur choix.

1. TRAITEMENT PREALABLE

```
                                              oedèmes minimes
  pansements compressifs -> NON  -> varices sans oedèmes
                                              angiodysplasies simples
          OUI

                                   I.V. superficielle
  oedèmes importants       I.V. profonde
  trouble trophiques         I.V.chronique stades 1 - 3
                                   lymphoedèmes
```

2. TRAITEMENT ACTIF (préférable à une compression à vie)

```
      indication -> OUI ->chirurgie ou sclérose

          NON  ->  contre-indication temporaire ou définitive
```

3. CONTRE-INDICATIONS

MALADIES CUTANEES

NON <- derm. suintantes -> OUI -
NON <- ulcère de jambe -> OUI -
NON <- infections -> OUI -
NON <- alllergies -> OUI -

traiter jusqu'à guérison

COMPRESSION

tropforte

pouls pér. palpables -> NON ->

P < 70 mm Hg: pas de bas
70 > P < 100: - 1 classe
P > 100: = classe

OUI

trop faible

NON <- oedème -> OUI -> desinfiltrer

> 18cm cheville <18cm -> rester au pansement

NON <- hypod. aiguë -> OUI -> continuer pansement

DIFFICULTES D'ENFILAGE

toucher le gros orteil -> impossible -> aide-> NON -> pas de bas

facile — OUI

difficile -> aide mécanique
-> superposition de bas: 1 + 1 > 2
1 + 2 >> 3

4. CHOIX DE LA CLASSE DE COMPRESSION

Classe 1

troubles fonctionnels
télangiectasies
oedèmes vespéraux minimes

Classe 2

varices non compliquées
varices de la grossesse
I.V.C. stades 1 et 2
lymphoedèmes réversibles

Classe 3

I.V.C. stade 3
syndrome postthrombotique
oedème posttraumatique
lymphoedème réversible

Classe 4

oedèmes indurés
hypodermites chroniques
lymphoedèmes irréversibles

5. CHOIX DU MODELE

atteinte cuisse -> NON -> bas cuisse? -> NON -> bas jarret
OUI

collant?.-> uniquement classe 1 + 2
grossesse ?
NON

fixation -> NON -> bord adhérent
cuisse avec slip
colle
OUI

cuisse entière? -> NON -> bas mi-cuisse

OUI -> bas cuisse

6. PRISE DES MESURES

mensurations standard -> NON -> bas sur mesure

OUI

bas de série : - périmètres
- longueur

Bibliographie:

BASSI, Gl., STEMMER. R. (1983): Les traitements mécaniques fonctionnels en phlébologie, Piccin, Padova.

A comparison of class 2 and class 3 compression in the prevention of recurrence of chronic venous leg ulcers

J.R. Harper, J.J. Dale, C.V. Ruckley, B. Gibson, D. Brown, A. Nelson, M.J. Callam and R.J. Prescott

300 patients with newly healed chronic venous leg ulcers have been randomized to class 2 or class 3 knee length graduated elastic compression hosiery and followed up for up to three years. Patients were assessed by Doppler ultrasound and Duplex scanning. They were accurately fitted with hosiery and followed by four monthly visits by trained staff. Compliance was monitored and ulcer recurrence recorded. The data are currently being analysed and will be available for presentation in full.

Phlébologie 92. Eds P. Raymond-Martimbeau, R. Prescott, M. Zummo.
John Libbey Eurotext, Paris © 1992, pp. 902-903

Prevention of recurrence of chronic leg ulcer : a randomised trial of different degrees of compression

D.R. Harper, C.V. Ruckley, J.J. Dale, M.C. Callam, P. Allan, D. Brown, B. Gibson, A. Nelson, R.J. Prescott

Vascular Surgery Units, Royal Infirmaries of Edinburgh and Falkirk, Scotland, UK.

The Lothian and Forth Valley Leg Ulcer Study (1985) (Callam et al., 1985) demonstrated that of 827 ulcerated legs, 272 were in their first episode but of these 151 had not healed their ulcers over more than a year. Of the remaining 555 (67%) had had multiple episodes. Thus recurrence of leg ulceration is the predominant health care problem in this group of patients.

Compression therapy is the most important treatment option for such patients once healing has taken place especially now that high quality hosiery is widely available, national standards have been set in the U.K. (Fentem, 1986) and the physiological effects of compression therapy are better understood. For optimal haemodynamic effect the pressure should graduated, highest at the ankke and reducing towards the knee (Sigel et al., Lawrence and Kakkar,1980, Jones et al., 1980). These guidelines ensure ensure that compression therapy is regarded as effective, increasing the velocity of femoral vein flow (Lawrence and Kakkar, 1980), reducing ambulatory venous pressure (Jones et al., 1980, Horner et al.,1980) and producing symptomatic relief (Somerville et al., 1974), especially when surgery is not advised or refused. However, it is not known if the degree of pressure is important in preventing recurrence or whether any therapeutic advantage accruing to a higher compression stocking is outweighed by poor compliance or other disadvantage.

Patients and Methods

This preliminary communication describes a major ongoing trial in which patients with recently healed chronic leg ulcers were randomised to either low (approximately 20mmHg at the ankle) (Class 2) or higher pressure (approximately 30mmHg at the ankle) (Class3) graduated compression hosiery. Patients with arterial insufficiency (ankle/brachial systolic ratio <0.8), diabetes mellitus or rheumatoid arthritis were excluded. The hosiery was professionally fitted and replaced at four month intervals, being refitted if required. Compliance and ulcer recurrence were monitored.

Results

Analysis of the first 204 patients shows 106 allocated to high compression and 108 to low compression. Compliance was similar in both groups (48/106 vs 50/108). Over a 2-4 year follow up there were 16(15%) ulcer recurrences in the high compression group versus 26(24%) in the low compression group. Patient follow up in this trial and more detailed studies are continuing. At this preliminary stage we may conclude:

(i) The apparent therapeutic advantage of high compression do not appear to be jeopardised by poorer patient compliance.

(ii) Careful patient supervision in a hospital clinic and the prescription of high quality compression hose does not eliminate the problem of ulcer recurrence.

References

Callam,M.J., Ruckley,C.V., Harper,D.R., Dale,J.J. (1985). Chronic leg ulceration; the extent of the problem and the provision of care. Brit Med J. 290, 1855-6.

Fentem,P.H. (1986) Advances in elastic hosiery. Pharmacy Update 2, 200.

Jones,N.G.A., Webb,P.J., Rees,R.I., Kakkar,V.V., (1980) A physiological study of elastic compression stockings in venous disorders of the legs. Br J. Surg. 67, 569-73.

Lawrence,D. & Kakkar,V.V. (1980) Graduared, static, external compression of the lower limb; a physiological assessment. Br J. Surg. 67, 119.

Sigel,B., Edelstein,A.L., Savtch,L., Hasty,J.H., Felix,W.R., (1975) Type of compression for reducing venous stasis. A study of lower extremities during inactive recumbency. Arcg Surg 110, 38-43.

Phlébologie 92. Eds P. Raymond-Martimbeau, R. Prescott, M. Zummo.
John Libbey Eurotext, Paris © 1992, pp. 904-907

Controlling compression therapy in venous incompetence guarantees the therapeutic effect

M. Emter, K. Alexander

Medizinische Hochschule Hannover, Abteilung Angiologie, Karl-Weichert-Allee, D 3000 Hannover 61, Germany.

Compression therapy is the oldest and nevertheless in many cases the best therapy in chronic venous incompetance. To reach a decrease of venous hypertension with a consecutive lowering of edema filtration is the aim of a good therapy and minimalizes the pain of the patient.

"Bad feelings" like "hot legs", "restless legs" or pain because of swolen legs and cramps can be eliminated in a short time. Many clinicals studies did proove the positive effect of compression therapy in minimazing venous hypertension, reducing reflux and edema filtration (2, 3, 4, 6, 10, 11, 12).

But only a correct compression guarentuees the positiv effect. An adviced therapy which is not accepted by the patient will not reach the aim of preventing progress of the sickness or recurrence of venous ulcers for example. Thow the patient must be informed about the pathophysiology of the venous disturbance and consequences of the therapy. The right diagnosis and indication for compression therapy taking the personal situation of the patient in account is the basis of patients compliance. Compression always should be so "strong" and "high" as essential because overdrawn therapy will not be accepted over a long time.

Principally the length of a compreesion stocking should be identic with the hight of the venous disturbance. For prevention of a postthrombotic syndrome after a pelvic thrombosis or a thrombosis of the thigh compression panties must be used. The situation of an "uncomplicated" postthrombotic situation of the lower leg or a slight venous incompetance might be handled with a compression stocking up to knee. These advices are for the initial therapy of venous disorders. Very often by time of collateralisation it becomes possible to lower the compression class or to use a short instead of a long compression stocking. Also a persistent venous hypertension can force to a higher compression class or another size of a stocking.

The compression stockings are graded refering to the pressure they have at the ancle. The pressure should decrease continuously from distal to proximal and should have 40% of the initial pressure left at the proximal point.

By this graduation venous backflow is enforced optimal. Compression stockings class I should have an ancle pressure of 18 - 20 mmHg, class II of 25 - 32 mmHg, class III of 36 - 46 mmHg and class IV which is not used in venous disturbances very often of more than 60 mmHg.

In slight venous incompetance with the symptoms of "tired" or heavy" legs or beginning varicosity the class I compression stocking is usefull in eliminating this symptoms and preventing progress .Reffering to localisation and severity compression up to the knee can be sufficicient.

Compression class II which is in everyday usage the most adviced should be used in cases of venous incompetance because of varicosity or postthrombotic syndrome with slight edema filtration, in cases of recurrent superficial thrombophlebitis or under ideal conditions as prophylaxis after healing of a venous ulcer . After vein - stripping or extensive sclerotherapy the class II stocking gurantees a less recurrence rate if it is used for an adequate amount of time.

Chronic venous incompetance with severe edema filtration because of a postthrombotic syndrome or excessive varicosity or prophylaxis of recurrent occuring venous ulcers should be treated by class III compression stockings .

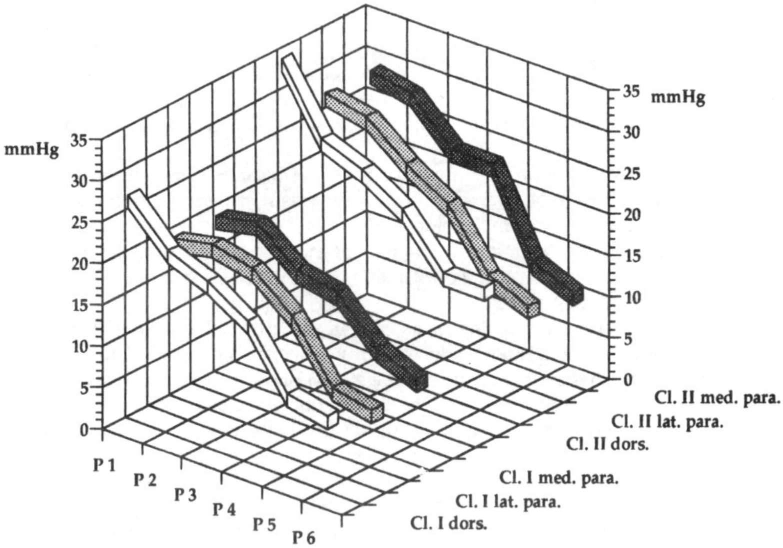

Point	P1	P2	P3	P4	P5	P6	P1	P2	P3	P4	P5	P6	P1	P2	P3	P4	P5	P6
mm Hg	20	21	17	16	11	9	20	21	20	16	9	8	28	23	21	18	11	10
SD	7	6	4	5	4	3	5	4	5	6	3	5	6	4	5	4	2	5
	medial paratibial						lateral paratibial						dorsal					

Pressure at the leg from the ancle to the thigh (P1 to P6) with compression stockings Class I (n = 50)

Point	P1	P2	P3	P4	P5	P6	P1	P2	P3	P4	P5	P6	P1	P2	P3	P4	P5	P6
mm Hg	28	27	22	22	12	10	28	27	23	20	13	11	35	27	25	22	16	16
SD	9	5	5	7	4	3	5	5	5	4	8	6	4	4	4	4	7	6
	medial paratibial						lateral paratibial						dorsal					

Pressure at the leg from the ancle to the thigh (P1 to P6) with compression stockings Class II (n = 50)

As mentioned before the class IV compression stockings are used very seldom in venous disturbances. Only in very severe postthrombotic syndromes but mainly in extense lymphatic edema which are to mobilise very difficult this class is indicated.
Contraindication are to be looked at as in every therapy. The patient should not have an arterial occlusive disease especially not combined with a diabetes or an endangiitis obliterans. In these cases must be tested very carefully wether a compression therapy would induce a decompensation of the arterial disturbance .
Cardiac insufficiency might be a contraindication of compression therapy because of mobilisation of great quantities of volume from the extremities to the heart. Excemes, dermatosis, acute ulceration and skin infection should be healed before applicating a compression stocking . As well as the direct contraindications the indirect ones should be mentioned. The patient must be able to wear the adviced compression stocking. Especially older patients or those with arthritis or arthrosis are not able to applicate stockings of higher classes by themselves.
The correct production of the material and the stockings is as well an essential as to measure which stocking is the right one for a leg. Measurement must be done at the not swolen leg, length and cicumferences at defined points should exclusively be fulfilled be exsperienced persons because fitting of the compression stocking is absolutely necessary to reach the therapeutic effect and not to loose the compliance of the patient. The positive effects of adequate compression materials was already prooved in clinical trials (1, 5, 7, 8, 9).
For a correct measurement there do exist standarized meters and tables of the producers show if a preformed stocking can be used or an individual stocking must be produced for the patient.
Controlling the adviced compression stocking at the patient should be essential to make sure that the stockings fits to the patient, thow the compliance of the patient is given and therefore the therapeutic effect is guaranteed.

In a study in 50 patients it was controlled wether the measured compression stocking* at the leg of the patient had the right pressure and the right decrease of pressure from distal to proximal (P1 at the ancle up to P6 at the thigh). With a special apparatus it is possible to measure directly at the leg the pressure of a compression stocking in every wanted level. It was measured which pressure is induced by the stocking in several places of the circumference of the legs, at the dorsal site, lateral paratibial and medial paratibial, and in several levels of the leg, six points from the ancle up to the body. Measurement was repeated five times after removal and replacement of the stockings. Data were statistically looked at with the t-test and Wilcoxon-test reffering to relation and distribution of the data. Significance level was $p<0.05$.
At the dorsal site of the leg the results showed the best reproducible data. Medial and lateral paratibial differences of data were greater. In compression stockings of class I a pressure at the ancle of 28 mmHg + 6mmHg was found at the dorsal site, medial and lateral paratibial data were 20 mmHg +5 (7)mmHg. The loss of pressure from distal to proximal was approx. 60% of the pressure at the ancle level. In compression stockings class II the results were very similar at a higher pressure, at the dorsal site 35 mmHg + 4mmHg and medial and lateral paratibial 28mm Hg + 5 (9) mmHg was measured. Also in this class the decrease of pressure was adaquate with a loss of approx. 60%.
Measurement in lying and in standing position showed differences which not were significant and the profiles of pressure over the length of the stockings did not change sigmificantly.

The studies showed that a correct measurement of the leg with the consequent choice of the adaquate compression stocking ensures the wanted effects of pressure and pressure profiles at the leg. In this trial only "high quality products" were used in which the right pressure and profile reffering to the compression class was prooved. Measurement should be done at the not swolen leg and might be done in lying position because the differences and especially the pressure profiles do not change significantly between lying and standing position. Controlling the adviced compression stocking at the patient induces an increase of compliance of the patient by ensuring that the therapautic effect causes an elimination of symptoms of venous incompetance.

* medi stockings, Bayreuth, Germany; medi stockings, USA

References

1) Bollinger, A.A. , Flußgeschwindigkeit in der Vena saphena und der Vena femoralis mit und ohne Kompressionsverbände, SWISS med 2 : 61 (1980)

2) Emter M., Pretschner D.P., Hundeshagen H., Alexander K., Determination of Changes in the Intravascular and Extravascular Compartment in the Leg -The Engymetric Double Radionuclide Method- , Nuklearmedizin (New Trends and Possibilities in Nuclear Medicine), Hrsg. H.A.E. Schmidt u. L. Czernay, Schattauer Verlag, 265 - 269 (1987)
3) Emter, M., Alexander K., Pretschner D.P., Venöse Hämodynamik und Ödembildung am postthrombotischen Bein unter Therapie, Kassenarzt 3 : 30 - 32 (1989)
4) Fischer, H. , Venenleiden (Tübinger Studie), Urban und Schwarzenberg, München (1981)
5) Fröhlich, H., Wuppermann, Th. , Verhalten der venösen Haemodynamik unter Kompressionsstrümpfen, Medita 3A : 7 (1978)
6) Haid-Fischer, F. , Haid, H. , Venenerkrankungen, Verlag Thieme, Stuttgart (1980)
7) Lofferer,O. , Mostbeck, A. , Partsch, H. , Experimentelle Untersuchungen zum Wirkungsmechanismus eines Kompressionsverbandes, in : Aktuelle Probleme der Angiologie, Band 21, Hrsg. U. Brunner, A. Bollinger, R. Stemmer, Verlag Huber, Bern, Stuttgart, Wien (1973)
8) Partsch, H. , Verbesserte Förderleistung der Wadenmuskelpumpe unter Kompressionsstrümpfen bei Varizen und venöser Insuffizienz, Phlebol. Proktol. 7 : 58 - 66 (1978)
9) Rudofsky, G. , Hämodynamische Befunde bei Gesunden und Patienten mit chronisch-venöser Insuffizienz unter Gummistrumpfkompression der Venen, in : Mikrozirkulation und Blutrheologie ; Therapie der peripheren AVK, Hrsg. H. Müller - Wiefel, Verlag G. Witzstrock, Baden-Baden (1980)
10) Schmitz, R. , Der richtige Kompressionsstrumpf, Phlebol. Proktol. 10 : 193 (1981)
11) Stemmer, R. , Die Kompressionsbehandlung der unteren Extremität, insbesondere durch Gummistrümpfe, Kassenarzt 9 : 372 (1969)
12) Wuppermann, Th. , Varizen, Ulcus cruris und Thrombose, (Begr. K. Sigg), Springer Verlag Berlin, Heidelberg, New York, Toronto, (1986)

Authors address: Dr. Michael Emter,Medizinische Hochschule Hannover, Abteilung Angiologie, Karl-Wiechert-Allee, D 3000 Hannover 61, Germany

Phlébologie 92. Eds P. Raymond-Martimbeau, R. Prescott, M. Zummo.
John Libbey Eurotext, Paris © 1992, pp. 908-910

Effets de bas de contention sur l'intolérance orthostatique au décours d'une expérience de simulation d'apesanteur

A. Güell*, M.M. Faurat*, A. Cornac*, F. Louisy**, X. Cailletaux***

** MEDES, Hôtel-Dieu, Pont-Neuf, 31052 Toulouse Cedex, France. ** CERMA, Base d'essai en vol, 91228 Bretigny-sur-Orge Cedex, France. *** Société Thuasne, 6, rue des Maronniers, BP 234, 92300 Levallois-Perret, France.*

Parmi les grands systèmes homéostasiques, la fonction cardiovasculaire du cosmonaute va être modifiée au cours, et surtout au décours du vol spatial : cela se traduira par l'apparition du Syndrome de Déconditionnement Cardiovasculaire (S.D.C.V.) qui associe au retour sur terre (Atkov *et al.*, 1987) : (1) une fréquence cardiaque de repos élevée ; (2) une baisse de la capacité à l'effort ; (3) une intolérance orthostatique pouvant aboutir à un état présyncopal voire une syncope : selon les données publiées par la NASA, 15% environ des cosmonautes présentent une hypotension artérielle soit au cours des 12 minutes qui précèdent l'atterrissage alors qu'ils sont soumis à des accélération du type +Gz, soit dans les deux heures qui suivent le retour sur terre. Plusieurs mécanismes sont impliqués dans la physiopathogénie de cette intolérance orthostatique : (1) une hypovolémie conséquence de la redistribution des liquides organiques de la moitié inférieure du corps vers les régions cardio-thoracocéphaliques (Kirsch *et al.*, 1984 ; Gauer, 1983 ; Güell *et al.*, 1982) ; (2) une atténuation de l'activité de l'arc baroréflexe (Harisson *et al.*, 1986 : Billman *et al.*, 1982) ; (3) enfin une diminution de l'activité fonctionnelle du système veineux basse pression des membres inférieurs modifiant ainsi les caractéristiques de compliance et de vidange (Louisy *et al.*, 1990 ; Güell *et al.*, 1991). L'objectif de la présente étude consiste à vérifier au cours d'une expérience de simulation d'apesanteur , si la mise en place de bas de contention élastiques VENOFLEX® au niveau des jambes peut prévenir l'intolérance orthostatique observée dans le cadre du S.D.C.V.

MATERIELS ET METHODES

• **Les sujets volontaires** : 10 sujets sains volontaires dont les caractéristiques figurent dans le tableau 1 ont participé à l'expérimentation. Chacun a donné son consentement après avoir été informé des procédures et des risques possibles inhérents à l'expérimentation. Les sujets ont été divisés en 2 groupes de 5 : chez les sujets du premier groupe, il a été placé, une heure avant le lever un système de bas de contention des jambes à un équivalent pression de 30 mmHg. Le second groupe de sujets a servi de groupe témoin.

• **La simulation d'apesanteur** : le décubitus antiorthostatique à -6° a été retenu afin de simuler la nouvelle répartition de la masse sanguine de la moitié inférieure du corps vers les régions cardiothoraco-céphalique : la durée du décubitus a été fixée à 4 jours de façon à provoquer un certain degré de déconditionnement cardiovasculaire surtout dans sa composante intolérance orthostatique.

• **L'exploration orthostatique : tilt test** : Deux explorations orthostatiques ont été éffectuées : (1) la première 24 heures avant le début du décubitus ; (2) la seconde à la fin de celui-ci. Chacune de ces explorations a été effectuée à la même heure de la journée pour chacun des sujets. L'épreuve du tilt test consistait au passage à la position +60° en 2 secondes, pendant 30 minutes, après une période en position horizontale de 15 minutes: l'épreuve était arrêtée s'il apparaissait des symptômes d'intolérance orthostatique (état présyncopal avec chute de la pression artérielle). Durant toute l'épreuve, l'E.C.G. et les pressions artérielles systolo-diastolique et moyenne étaient monitorisées.

RESULTATS

Les principaux résultats sont présentés dans le tableau 1.

• **Avant le décubitus.** Que ce soit dans le groupe témoin ou dans le groupe chez lequel les sujets ont été porteurs de bas de contention une heure avant le lever, il n'existe pas de variations significatives des pressions artérielles systolo-diastolique et moyenne entre la position horizontale et la fin du tilt test ; il est noté une augmentation de 12% en moyenne de la fréquence cardiaque. La durée totale du tilt test pour les 10 sujets a été de 30 minutes : aucun symptôme d'intolérance orthostatique n'a été noté.

• **Après le décubitus.** Chez les sujets porteurs de bas de contention la réponse des pressions artérielles au tilt test a été identique à celle observée lors de la période de référence ; la réponse de la fréquence a été également identique ; la durée totale du tilt test a été de 30 minutes et aucun symptôme d'intolérance orthostatique n'a été noté.

Chez des sujets témoins il est noté en moyenne une chute significative de la pression artérielle moyenne associée à une importante tachycardie avec apparition chez 2 sujets d'un état présyncopal ayant motivé l'arrêt du tilt test, l'un à la 5ème minute, le second à la 15ème minute : la durée moyenne du tilt test a été de 20 minutes.

Tableau 1 : Caractéristiques anthropométriques

Sujet	Age(ans)	Taille(cm)	Poids(kg)	Surface corporelle (m^2)
A	40	175	73	1.20
B	37	175	70	1.79
C	33	170	68	1.73
D	35	174	74	1.21
E	43	178	70	1.83
F	34	180	66	1.85
G	43	176	83	1.80
H	28	177	70	1.79
I	26	173	65	1.76
J	21	175	67	1.78
X	33.4	175,3	70.6	1.79
±	±	±	±	±
SE	8.2	2.75	5.2	0.3

Tableau 2 : Pression artérielle moyenne (mmHg) et fréquence cardiaque (bat/min) au cours des tilt tests avant et après décubitus chez les sujets porteurs de bas de contention (n°5, A, B, C, D, E) et chez les sujets témoins (n°5, F, G, H, I, J)

	Avant décubitus				Après décubitus			
	Horizontal		+ 60°		Horizontal		+ 60°	
Sujets	FC	PAM	FC	PAM	FC	PAM	FC	PAM
A	75	84.3	85	96.3	60	82.6	68	90.3
B	61	76.3	86	84.3	72	76	97	92.3
C	67	86	85	97.3	64	80	70	85
D	60	76.3	74	78.6	63	78.3	78	85
E	48	94.6	54	89.3	57	95	60	96.3
F	53	82	92	88	60	81	97	72
G	63	82.2	70	85	60	90	65	74
H	56	84	63	89	54	77.3	64	76
I	64	82.4	92	88.3	60	86.6	96	75.6
J	55	80.6	72	74.6	53	75.3	78	68.9

DISCUSSION

Le groupe porteur de bas de contention VENOFLEX® au niveau des jambes n'a pas présenté de chute significative des pressions artérielles lors du tilt test post décubitus : ceci serait en faveur du rôle préventif d'un tel système contre l'intolérance orthostatique.

Parmi les causes de l'intolérance orthostatique post vol spatial ou post décubitus, le rôle fonctionnel des systèmes veineux des membres inférieurs a été longtemps sous estimé. Dès les premières missions habitées de longue durée, des modifications de la compliance des membres inférieurs et par conséquent de la capacitance des veines ont été décrites ainsi qu'une baisse du tonus veineux (Moore, 1987 ; Nicogossian, 1989) : ces données ont été confirmées par les expériences de simulation de durée variable. Par ailleurs, une hypotonie de la musculature striée des jambes a également été décrite empêchant en partie aux muscles gravifiques et antigravifiques de jouer un rôle de contention favorisant ainsi une stase veineuse lors du passage de la position horizontale à la position debout. On sait que l'accumulation excessive de sang dans les jambes diminue le retour veineux du sang au cœur et grève les possibilités de régulation du débit cardiaque et de la pression artérielle. Par ailleurs les veines profondes des membres inférieurs cheminent dans le compartiment musculaire, ce dernier se comportant comme un bas élastique. Les éléments observés au cours de notre étude semblent indiquer que l'utilisation de bas de contention élastiques peut jouer un rôle non négligeable dans le maintien de l'hémodynamique veineuse.

REFERENCES

1. Atkov O., Bednenko V., Fomina G. : Ultrasound technique in space medicine. Aviat. Space Environ. Med. 1987, 58, 69-73.

2. Billman G.E., Dickey D.T., Teoh K., Stone H.L. : Effects of central venous blood volume shift on arterial baro-reflex of heart rate. Am. J. Physiol. 1981, 241, 571-575.

3. Bungo M.V., Charles J.B., Johnson P.C. : Cardiovascular deconditonning during space flight and the use of saline as a countermeasure to orthostatic intolerance. Aviat. Space Environ. Med. 1985, 56, 985-990.

4. Charles J., Bungo M. : Cardiovascular research in space : consideration for the design of the human research facility of the U.S. Space Station. Aviat. Space Environ. Med. 1980, 46, 1000-1005.

5..Echt M., Gauer O. : Changes in peripheral venous tone and central transmural venous pressure during immersion in thermo neutral bath. Pfluegers Arch. 1979, 352, 211-217.

6. Egorov A.D., Anachkin O.D., Itsexovsji O.G., Alferova Z.A., Golubtchikova Z.A., Liamin V.R., Poliakova A.P., Turtchaninova V.F., Talavrinov V.A., Turbasov V.D. : Résultats d'investigations médicales menées en 1985 lors des vols spatiaux dê longue durée. Kosm. biol. i aviokos. Med., 1988, 1, 24-29.

7. Gauer O. : Circulatory basis of fluid volume control. Physiol. Rev., 1963, 43, 423-481.

8. Güell A., Gharib Cl., Bes A., Geraud G. : Physiological effects of bedrest. Lancet, 1982, 2, 328.

9. Güell A., Braak L., Pavy Le Traon A., Gharib Cl. : Cardiovascular adaptation during simulated microgravity : Lower Body Negative Pressure to counter orthostatic hypotension. Aviat. Space Eviron. Med., 1991, 62, 331-335.

10. Gharib Cl., Maillet A., Gauquelin G., Allevard A.M., Güell A., Cartier R., Arbeille Ph. : Results of a 4 week headown tilt with and without LBNP countermeasure I volume regulating hormones. Avait. Space Environ. Med., 1992, 63, 3-8.

11. Gharib Cl., Gauquelin G., Geelen Gh., Cantin M., Gutkowskia J., Mauroux J.L., Güell A. : Volume regulating hormones in weightlessness. The Physiologist, 1985, 28, 530-534.

12. Harrison M.H., Rittenhous D., Greenleaf J.E. : Effects of posture on arterial baroreflex control of heart rate in humans. Eur. J. Appl. Physiol., 1986, 55, 367-73.

13. Jhonson R.L., Hoffler G.W., Nicogossian A.E., Bergamn S.A., Jackson M.M. : LBNP : third manned Skylab mission. In. : Biomedical Results from Skylab, Washington, 1977.

14. Kirsch K, Rocker L, Gauer O, Krause R, Leach C, Wicke MJ, Landry R. : Venous pressure in man during weightlessness. Science, 1984, 225, 218-219.

15. Louisy F., Gaudin G., Oppert J.M., Güell A., Guezennec G.Y. : Haemodynamics of the leg veins during a 30-days -6° head down bedrest with and without LBNP. Eur. J. Appl. Physiol., 1990, 61, 349-355.

16. Moore Th., Thornton W. : Inflight and postflight fluid shifts measured by leg volume changes. In : NASA TM-5820. pp. 59-65. Houston, Johnson Space Center, 1987.

17. Nicogossian A.E. : Space medicine and physiology. Washington, NASA SP-477, 1982.

Phlébologie 92. Eds P. Raymond-Martimbeau, R. Prescott, M. Zummo.
John Libbey Eurotext, Paris © 1992, pp. 911-914

Use of compression in venous disease

Lucie Beaupré

Ottawa, Ontario, Canada.

Definition

Compression is a tension at the surface of the leg (given by a tensor bandage or an elastic stocking), which works against a pathologic venous hypertension.

Indications

- *oedema of the lower extremities*
- *varicose veins and their complications*

compression is a palliative treatment only; it never cures varicose veins; it treats the symptoms not its causes.

Types of compression

Tensor bandages and stockings.

Tensor bandages

Bandage stretch	0% none	50% short	100% medium	150% long
Site of action	-deep venous system -severe oedema -varicose ulcer -deep tissues		-superficial venous system -saphenous & tributaries -light oedema	-wound protection
Duration of placement	-remains 3 to 15 days	-remains maximum of 7 days	-removable	-removable
Example	Unna boot -zincopaste -viscopaste	Elastoplaste -for use on healthy skin only	Available in pharmacies	

STOCKINGS

Compression	Extra heavy 50-60 mm Hg	Heavy 30-50 mm Hg	Medium 20-30 mm Hg	Light 10-20 mm Hg
Fabrication	custom made	serial	serial	serial
Indication	-severe lymphoedema	-post-phlebitic syndrome -moderate lymphoedema -chronic venous insufficiency	-pregnancy varicose vein -simple varicose veins with oedema -healed ulcer	-simple varicose vein -fatigue -heaviness -prevention of varicose veins
Action	deep venous system	deep venous system	superficial venous system	superficial venous system
Type	-opaque, thick and very tight -open toe	-opaque and thick -open toe	-opaque -closed toe -comfortable	-sheer -easy to wear -esthetically pleasing
% of patients	~ 1%	~ 8%	~ 12%	~ 80%

WHEN TO PRESCRIBE ELASTIC STOCKINGS?

Generally speaking, to all patients suffering from a venous pathology of the lower limbs. The stockings, by external mechanical strengths, fight against intravenous hypertension which causes varicose veins, stasis and many complications as damaging as varicose ulcers.

The absolute contraindication is arterial insufficiency grade III and IV.

WHICH STOCKINGS TO PRESCRIBE AND WHEN?

a) 50 to 60 mm Hg
Extra heavy compression stockings of 50-60 mm Hg are custom-made only. They are mainly recommended in cases of severe lymphoedema and they work at the deep venous system level. 50 to 60 mm Hg stockings are necessary to less than 1% of all venous pathologies of the lower limbs. They are very heavy, very warm, very thick and difficult to put on.

b) 30 to 50 mm Hg
Heavy compression stockings from 30 to 50 mm Hg are serial manufactured. The are especially prescribed for post-phlebitic syndrome cases. They are also recommended for chronic venous insufficiency (CVI) grade II (skin pigmentation and stasis dermatitis and grade III (varicose ulcers). They can help with cases of post-traumatic oedema and moderate lymphoedema.

30 to 50 mm Hg stockings work at deep venous system level and serve to about 8% of all venous pathologies of the lower limbs. They are opaque, heavy, non-aesthetic but still lighter than 50 to 60 mm Hg stockings.

c) 20 to 30 mm Hg
20 to 30 mm Hg stockings are serial manufactured. They are principally used for varicose veins during pregnancy, for chronic venous insufficiency Stage I, or corona phlebetatica; they are also prescribed in cases of light oedema of the lower legs or post-operatively.

20 to 30 mm Hg stockings act at the superficial venous level and help about 12% of patients suffering from venous insufficiency of the lower limbs. They are still opaque but can be completely closed and relatively comfortable to wear.

50 to 60 mm Hg, 30 to 50 mm Hg, and 20 to 30 mm Hg stockings are well-recognized in medical literature as being important in the treatment of venous diseases of the lower limbs. More contro-versial is the use of light compression stockings of 10 to 20 mm Hg.

d) 10 to 20 mm Hg

10 to 20 mm Hg stockings are largely prescribed in simple cases of varicose veins and as adjuvant to sclerotherapy. They are also efficient in relieving fatigue, heaviness, tiredness due to varicose veins or simply due to prolonged standing. After the treatment of varicose veins (surgery and sclerotherapy) has been completed, 10 to 20 mm Hg stockings are one of the best ways to prevent recurrence.

10 to 20 mm Hg stockings work exclusively on the superficial venous system and can help about 80% of all varicose patients. They are 100% sheer, elegant and easy to wear.

The following is a Canadian study made on 94 symptomatic women suffering from varicose veins, saphenous, reticulars, or telangiectasia. These patients were randomly divided and advised to wear the stockings for a week, each day from 9:00 a.m. to 5:00 p.m. The stockings used were 20 to 30 mm Hg, 10 to 20 mm Hg, and ordinary stockings of no compression.

The results show that light compression stockings relieved varicose symptoms from saphena, reticular, and telangiectasia as much as medium compression stockings of 20 to 30 mm Hg. The patients of this study considered light compression stockings more aesthetically pleasing than medium compression stockings and as attractive as no compression stockings. The patients preferred to wear light compression stockings over medium compression stockings, and further preferred wearing light compression stockings over ordinary no compression stockings.

Phlébologie 92. Eds P. Raymond-Martimbeau, R. Prescott, M. Zummo.
John Libbey Eurotext, Paris © 1992, pp. 915-917

Distensibility measurements in therapeutic elastic stockings

H.J.L. van Gerwen, A.J.M. Brakkee, J.P. Kuiper

University Hospital, department of dermatology, Postbox 9101, 6500 HB Nijmegen, The Netherlands.

Introduction

Continuous graduated compression by elastic stockings is generally considered to be a rational therapy in patients with chronic venous insufficiency because edema formation is prevented.
Another known beneficial effect of this compression is a reduction of the venous volume.
To evaluate the pressure tolerance of graded compression stockings we studied the venous distensibility in relation to the graduation of compression.

Method and Materials

Volume changes of the legs, both with and without stockings have been studied by means of strain gauge plethysmography. The patient lies in a supine position, with pneumatic cuffs around the thighs and strain gauges 5 cm above the ankle. A characteristic distensibility curve is determined by measuring the maximum volume increase Vc (%) induced by successive congestions with different cuff pressures (fig.1) and plotting Vc against the effective congestion pressure Pv. Fig.2 shows two such curves from the same ankle region of one patient, one with and and one without elastic stocking.

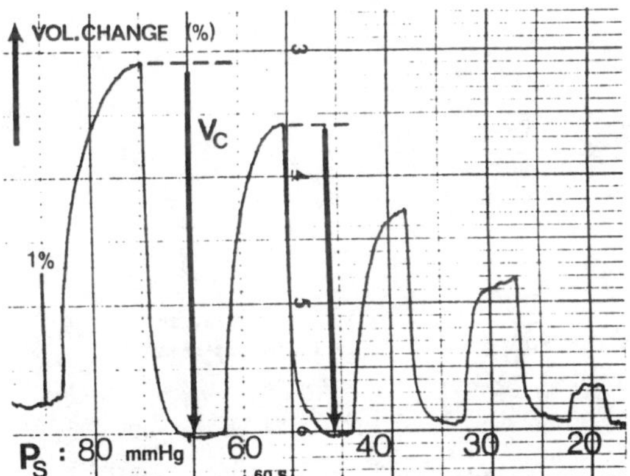

Fig.1: Registration of volume changes due to congestion with different cuff pressures (Ps).

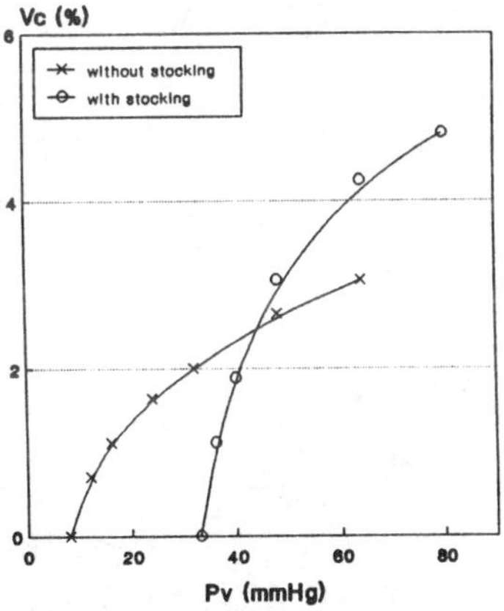

Fig.2: Distensibility curves of one patient measured at ankle region both with and without stocking.

We studied distensibility curves in 31 limbs of 20 patients known with severe chronic venous insufficiency. During four weeks those patients wore alternately during one week a made-to-measure graduated elastic stocking (**G-stocking***; G = graduated) and a special one (**A-stocking***; A = abnormal) equally made except for an area of 6-8 cm at the B1-level, where the pressure in the A-stocking was 10 mmHg lower than in the G-stocking. The stocking pressures as tested in vitro are given in fig.3.

Distensibility measurements have been carried out at the start of the test period and after each week and always in the afternoon.

At the same time limb circumferences have been measured at B, B1 and C-level using a simple measuring tape. All measurements were made both with and without elastic stockings.

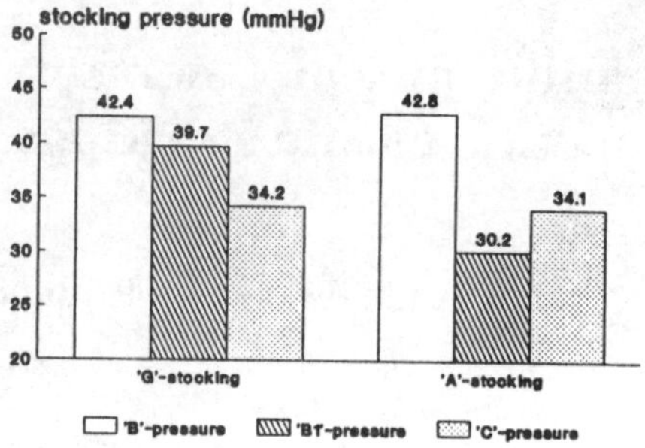

Fig.3: Mean Stocking pressure (mmHg) of 31 'G'- and 'A'-stockings measured in vitro at 3 different levels B, B1 and C.

Results

In all 31 limbs it has been found that the distensibility curves measured at the B1-level are lower with the A-stocking than with the G-stocking. In fig.4 a representative example is given. The volume reduction obtained by the A-stocking is less than by the G-stocking. This is in accordance with the results of the circumference measurements as shown in fig.5. At B and C level the effects of the elastic stockings were exactly the same and as could be expected no differences in circumference were found (fig 5a,b). At B1 level however a significant difference is found between both stockings (fig 5c).

There is also a significant difference between the circumferences at B1-level, when measured without stocking (fig.5c right).

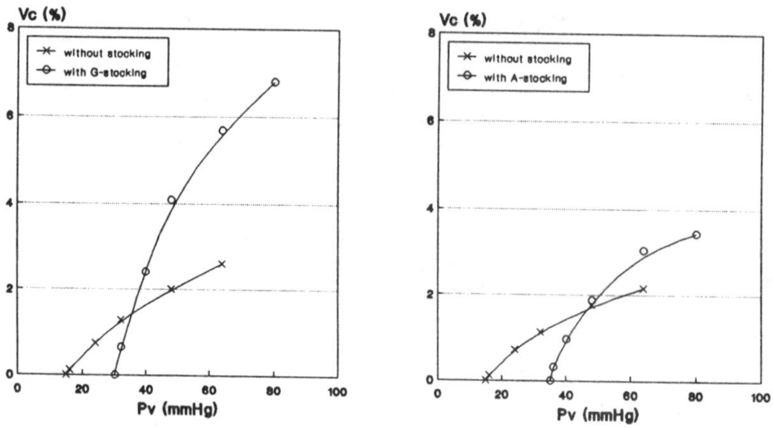

Fig.4: Representative example of distensibility measurements in one patient. The left graph shows distensibility curves measured after wearing stocking G for a one week period. The right graph shows the results after wearing stocking A for a one week period.

* Produced by **VARITEX** N.V. Haarlem, the Netherlands

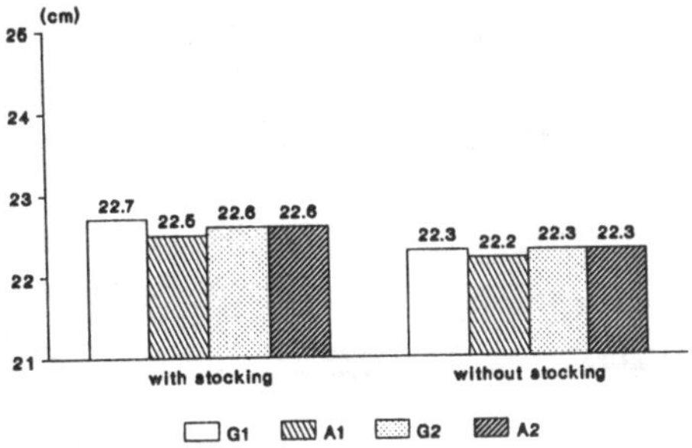

Fig.5a: Mean circumferences (cm) at B-level (n=31).

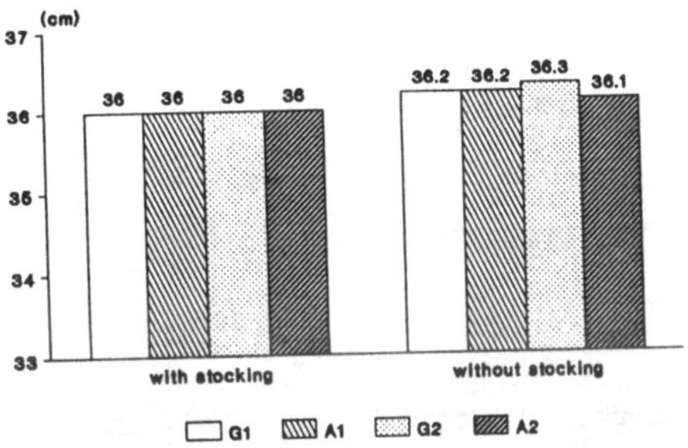

Fig.5b: Mean circumferences (cm) at C-level (n=31).

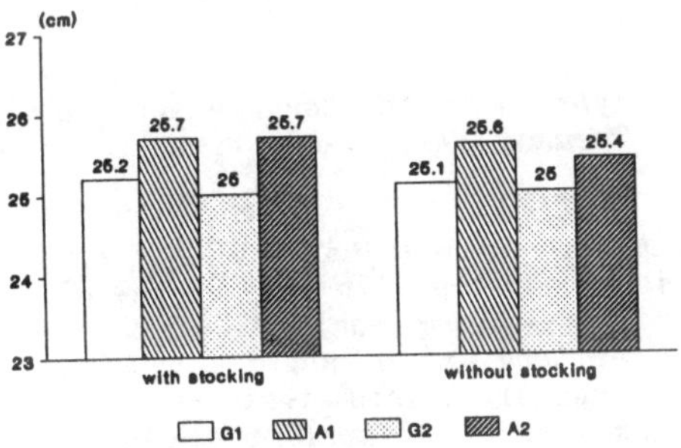

Fig.5c: Mean circumferences (cm) at B1-level (n=31).

Fig. 5a,b,c: Mean circumferences (cm) measured at 3 different levels B, B1 and C after wearing stocking 'G' and 'A' alternately for a one week period during 4 weeks.

Conclusions

All graduated elastic stockings exerting a pressure higher than the supine venous resting pressure, will in the horizontal position empty the venous system almost completely. The effect they have on the venous volume in this position is the same whether it is a pressure 1 class stocking or a class 4. In the standing position however the graduated stocking exerting the highest pressure will give the smallest venous volume. Knowing this the smaller reduction of the venous volume in the horizontal position by the A-stocking can only be explained by the fact that venous congestion was induced by a few mmHg higher compression proximally. The circumference measurements were in accordance with these findings and also revealed the formation of edema at B1 level in patients with severe chronic venous insufficiency after wearing the A-stocking.

Our final conclusion is that for patients with severe chronic venous insufficiency stockings should be made-to-measure to ensure graded compression.

Phlébologie 92. Eds P. Raymond-Martimbeau, R. Prescott, M. Zummo.
John Libbey Eurotext, Paris © 1992, pp. 918-920

A new controlled tension compression bandage

Andrew J. Carter, Mollie Davies, Andrew P. Jackson, Stephen M. Lang, Lakshman P. Nethsinghe, Kathleen M. Shawley

Smith and Nephew Research Ltd., Gilston Park, Harlow, Essex, CM20 2RQ, UK.

INTRODUCTION

The ultimate objective of compression bandage therapy is to improve the venous return of the leg (Dale, 1990). Different sub-bandage pressures are recommended for different clinical indications (Dale, 1990; Thomas, 1990), and a gradient of pressure should exist along a leg such that there are higher pressures distally than proximally (Cornwall, 1987). In practice, however, the achievement of the desired pressure and pressure gradient is not straightforward. Problems arise with accuracy and consistency (Millard et al., 1986).

The pressure under a bandage is governed by the tension in the bandage and the leg circumference according to the Laplace Law (Thomas, 1990) where Pressure = Tension/Radius.

In order to achieve a desired pressure the circumference must be known (it can easily be measured) and the required tension must be applied with some degree of accuracy. As the circumference of the leg increases from ankle to calf, a pressure gradient will automatically be created, as long as the applied tension is consistent throughout the application. The danger exists that pressure delivered to the limb may be much greater or less than the desired therapeutic pressure and that an adverse pressure gradient may be set up along the limb.

Considerable variation in extension was demonstrated by Millard et al. (1986) resulting in both ineffectively low (5mm) and dangerously high (76mm) sub-bandage pressures. Variation in bandage extension during application also resulted in the failure to achieve the required pressure gradient in 43 of 50 applications.

VERSAFLEX

The new VERSAFLEX* controlled tension compression bandage contains a unique elastomeric filament which produces a degree of tension control not found in traditional products. Once stretched beyond 30 per cent of its original length the filament exhibits minimal increase in tension for further extensions up to 150 per cent. Thus the force-extension profile of a VERSAFLEX bandage (Fig. 1) demonstrates a characteristic plateau-like region between 30 and 150 per cent extension. This is in marked contrast to the steeply increasing force produced by standard elastomers used in the production of currently available traditional compression bandages. In practice, the tension developed in a VERSAFLEX bandage

*** VERSAFLEX is a Trade Mark of T.J. Smith & Nephew Ltd.**

is less dependent on the degree to which it is extended on application. Relatively large variations in extension result in minor changes in tension (within the plateau range) and the sub-bandage pressure is thus more precisely controlled.

VOLUNTEER TRIAL

Five nurses were asked to apply either VERSAFLEX (Grade D) or DAUERBINDE K** bandages to the right leg of a healthy volunteer. Of the five, three were experienced in the application of compression bandages and two were inexperienced. Each nurse applied ten bandages of each type. The order of bandage application was randomised and the bandages were unidentified. The nurses were instructed to achieve 50 per cent bandage extension using a simple spiral wrapping technique, starting at the foot and ending just below the knee. The limb circumference was measured at five equidistant positions up the leg from ankle to calf. The extension in the bandage at each of these positions was determined by marking a 10cm length on the bandage and comparing the length of the mark after the bandage had been removed and allowed to relax for 24 hours. Interpolation of the extension readings on the force-extension profile provided tension data; sub-bandage pressures were determined through application of Laplace's Law.

Figs. 2 and 3 show the bandage extension and sub-bandage pressure results for a typical inexperienced nurse and a typical experienced nurse, respectively. The data are represented as the mean ± 2 standard deviations, as this range covers approximately 95 per cent of all results. It can be seen that the extensions achieved with VERSAFLEX are more variable than those achieved with DAUERBINDE, but despite this, the pressures produced by VERSAFLEX are more consistent than those produced by the conventional product. This is true at each measured position along the length of the limb. As expected, the inexperienced nurse achieves more variable pressures with either bandage than does the experienced nurse. However, when using VERSAFLEX, the inexperienced nurse is able to improve her pressure consistency such that it is of the same order as the experienced nurse using DAUERBINDE. In the hands of the experienced nurse the pressure consistency is improved even further.

The presence or absence of pressure gradients from ankle to gaiter, gaiter to calf, or ankle to calf has also been quantified and the results are presented in Table 1 for all 5 nurses combined. Both bandages are able to achieve a pressure fall from ankle to calf and from ankle to gaiter on most of their applications. From gaiter to calf, however, there is a significant difference between the two bandages. The new VERSAFLEX bandage achieves a positive therapeutic gradient on 94 per cent of the applications compared with only 52 per cent with the traditional bandage. Also, only 2 (i.e. 4 per cent of) applications resulted in negative (adverse) gradients with VERSAFLEX compared with 14 (i.e. 28 per cent of) with the conventional bandage.

CONCLUSION

The variability in pressures achieved in the present study with the traditional compression bandage indicates that the achievement of effective levels of compression cannot be taken for granted, even by experienced personnel. The force-extension profiles of traditional elastomers lead to bandage tensions which are very sensitive to small variations in extension. This in turn leads to a large uncertainty in the pressure generated in practice, and in the ability of the bandage to produce a therapeutic pressure gradient. In contrast, the wide plateau on the force-extension curve of the VERSAFLEX elastomer ensures the application of a consistent force to the limb over the wide range of extensions likely to be experienced in practice. As demonstrated in the present study, the bandage's ability to deliver a consistent force produces a greater number of applications in the safe and effective pressure range, and with the required therapeutic pressure gradient.

** **DAUERBINDE is a Trade Mark of Lohmann GmbH & Co. KG**

REFERENCES

Dale, J. (1990): Compression - how and why? CARE Science and Practice 8, 63-66.

Thomas, S. (1990): Bandages and bandaging: the science behind the art. CARE Science and Practice 8, 56-60.

Cornwall, J.V. et al. (1987): Graduated compression and its relation to venous refilling time. British Medical Journal 295, 1087-1090.

Millard, L.G. et al. (1986): The pressure at which nursing staff apply compression bandages when treating patients with varicose ulcers. In Phlebology '85, eds D. Negus and G. Jantet, pp. 682-685. London: John Libbey & Company.

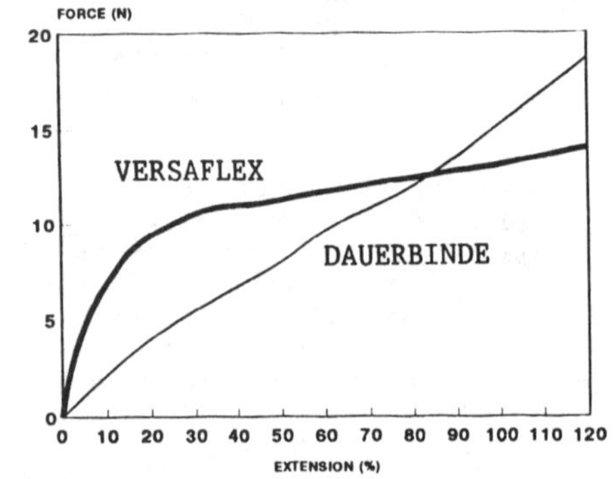

Fig. 1 Force-extension profile for VERSAFLEX and conventional compression bandage.

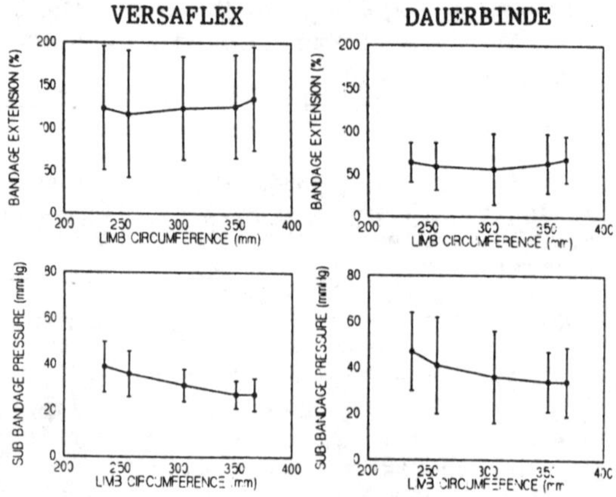

Fig. 2 Extensions and pressures obtained at different limb positions by a typical inexperienced nurse.

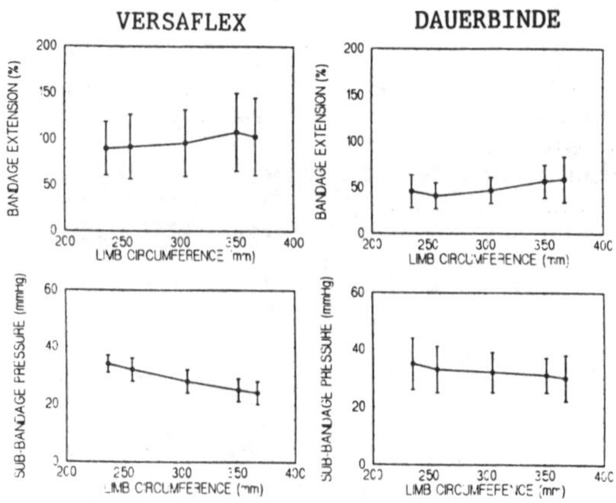

Fig. 3 Extensions and pressures obtained at different limb positions by a typical experienced nurse.

	DAUERBINDE K			VERSAFLEX		
	Positive	Zero	Negative	Positive	Zero	Negative
Ankle to calf	46 (92%)	1 (2%)	3 (6%)	48 (96%)	1 (2%)	0 (0%)
Ankle to gaiter	49 (98%)	0 (0%)	1 (2%)	49 (98%)	0 (0%)	0 (0%)
Gaiter to calf	26 (52%)	10 (20%)	14 (28%)	46 (94%)	1 (2%)	2 (4%)

Fig. 4 Pressure gradients across different parts of the leg.

Phlébologie 92. Eds P. Raymond-Martimbeau, R. Prescott, M. Zummo.
John Libbey Eurotext, Paris © 1992, pp. 921

Parvovarice : nouveau moyen compressif dans la thérapie de l'œdème veineux et lymphatique

Jean Parvulesco

Unité de Phlébologie, Clinique La Rosiaz, CH-1009 Pully-sur-Lausanne, Suisse.

La stratégie thérapeutique de l'oedème veineux et surtout lymphatique reste pour bon nombre de médecins encore obscure.

Les thérapeutiques proposés jusqu'à ce jour sont nombreuses et certaines encore sujet à discutions.

Un traitement en deux temps est unanime admis actuellement.
Il consiste en :
1.La réduction de l'oedème.
2.Le maintien du résultat obtenu.

Dans cet exposé, nos propos se limitent à décrire un nouveau modèle de bas de compression avec inclusion du gros orteil (PARVOVARICE)..

Ses qualités (compression efficace et uniforme sur la totalité de la surface du pied, bonne stabilité et bon confort) sont confirmées par une étude clinique, qui établit que ce nouveau moyen de contention constitue un réel progrès dans la thérapeutique de l'oedème veineux et lymphatique, par rapport au bas de contention classique.

Phlébologie 92. Eds P. Raymond-Martimbeau, R. Prescott, M. Zummo.
John Libbey Eurotext, Paris © 1992, pp. 922-924

Do we need custom-made elastic stockings ?

J. Heuser

Zimmermann Gmbli and Co.KO, Hauptstr. 16, D-3559 Burgwald/Eder 1, Germany.

Do We Need Custom-Made Elastic Stockings?

This is a question that has been discussed for many years now: Can the needs of all patients who require elastic stockings be adequately met by providing them with standardized articles?

In Germany, all manufacturers of compression stockings produce not only standard articles, but also custom-made stockings. This would indicate that there is a need for such special products. Is this really true, and if so, what is the percentage relation between custom-made and standard stockings?

In our attempt to answer these questions, we took the following consideration as our point of departure: There is only one therapeutic reason for wearing elastic stockings, and that is the compression that they provide: the pressure they exert on the leg. This pressure is therapeutically effective only if the stocking fits the patient's leg as well as possible.

In turn, the fit of the stocking depends upon four essential points:

1. the measurements of the patient's leg;
2. the standard stocking sizes available;
3. the elastic properties of the stocking;
4. the pressure that is medically indicated, and the decrease in pressure from distal to proximal.

Point 1:

Our study is based on a random sample of the legs of 483 patients. The measurements were made by a physician in accordance with the guidelines of the "Gütezeichengemeinschaft medizinische Gummistrümpfe" (Quality-Seal Association of German Manufacturers of Elastic Stockings). The measurements were made with a tape measure and a measuring board. We had no influence on the measuring or on the patients, since at that point of time, the physician who took the measurements did not know that we would subsequently evaluate his data.

Point 2:

As a size system, we chose the stocking sizes as defined in the guidelines of the Quality-Seal Association with reference to the body-measurement table for seamless stockings (6 sizes, Roman numeral system) and stockings with seams (11 sizes, Arabic numeral system).

Point 3:

The elastic properties of the stockings in our study correspond to the specifications of the Quality-Seal Association, which are on file with the Deutsches Institut für Gütesicherung und Kennzeichnung (German

Institute for Quality Maintenance and Designation) under the number RAL-GZ 387. This pertains especially to the properties "practical elongation", "elastic extensibility", compression classes and the pressure profile along the leg.

We chose these guide-lines of the Quality-Seal Association because they have gained world-wide acceptance, and provide the basis in this field for most countries on the world, or at least served as a model for national guide-lines, for example in England and France. Today, 20 European manufacturers are members of the Quality-Seal Association, and they are the world-wide market leaders.

Stocking properties were examined with the use of our software system DIADEM, which we used for evaluation:

On the bases of the patient's leg data, DIADEM decides whether a standard stocking will meet the patient's needs, or whether a special stocking has to be produced. The calculation is based on the properties of 10 stockings produced by Quality-Seal manufacturers and commonly available on the German market. These properties were converted into a computer program.

We developed DIADEM in 1986, in collaboration with the Institute for Informatics of the University of Marburg.

DIADEM is available to our customers and to physicians in a pocket-calculator version, and is also used in our plant as a manufacturing system for both standard and custom-made stockings.

Point 4:

We chose compression class 2, which is the one most frequently prescribed: 3.35 - 4.3 kPa. The higher the compression, the greater the likelihood that custom-made stockings will be required. For this reason, the results we obtained are all the more true for compression classes 3 an 4.

Since the data form the patients applied only to the lower leg, we restricted ourselves to below-knee stockings (AD), for which a pressure decrease of at least 30 per cent up to the knee is required.

Likewise, the longer a stocking is, the greater the likelihood that it will have to be custom-made. Again, for this reason our results are all the more true for thigh stockings or panty hose.

Here are the results of our study:

Serie / Maß

ohne Naht

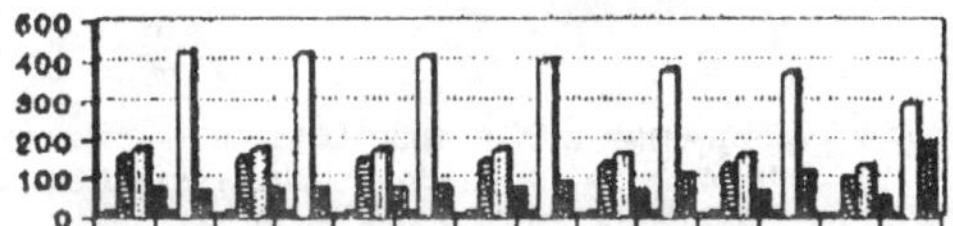

	0,29	0,47	0,57	0,65	0,82	1,00	2,00
I	11	11	9	9	10	7	2
II	156	164	148	142	134	133	101
III	176	176	173	173	161	160	133
IV	68	67	69	68	64	61	61
V	9	9	9	8	8	8	6
Serie	420	417	408	400	377	369	292
Maß	63	66	76	83	106	114	191
% Maß	13	13,7	16,6	17,2	22	23,6	39,6

Schärfe

Figure 1

Figure 1 shows the distribution of the 483 stockings among the standard sizes and the number of custom-made stockings, based on the size system for seamless stockings I - VI, with varying tolerance ranges.

The tolerance ranges are defined thus:

0,29 is equivalent to ± 17,7 %
0,47 is equivalent to ± 11,6 %
0,57 is equivalent to ± 10,0 %
0,65 is equivalent to ± 9,0 %
0,82 is equivalent to ± 7,6 %
1,00 is equivalent to ± 6,6 %
2,00 is equivalent to ± 4,4 %

This means if below-knee stockings in class 2 could be made so elastic that they would show a circumferential deviation of 17.5 per cent at every measurement site, and if we assume a correct pressure decrease of at least 30 per cent, then the proportion of custom-made stockings would amount to 13 per cent. In this extreme case, however, the technical possibilities are already exhausted.

Serie / Maß
mit Naht

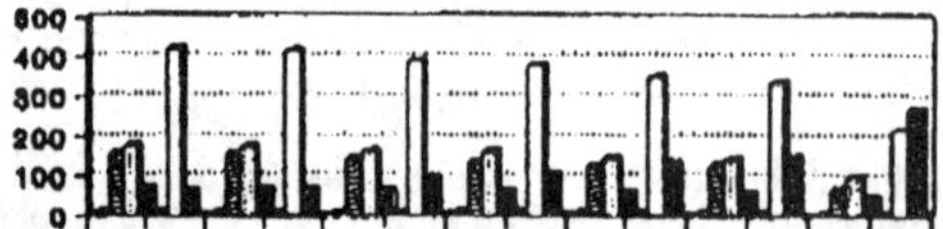

	0,29	0,47	0,57	0,65	0,82	1,00	2,00
4	11	11	9	9	8	6	2
5 / 6	166	164	143	137	128	127	67
7 / 8	176	173	163	168	147	142	99
9 /10	88	67	66	62	68	64	43
11/12	9	9	9	7	7	7	6
Serie	420	414	389	378	348	336	216
Maß	63	69	94	105	135	147	267
% Maß	13	14,3	19,5	21,7	28	30,4	55,8

Schärfe

zu "ohne Naht" - Klassen zusammengefaßt

Figure 2

Figure 2 shows the analogous evaluation for stockings with seams. Since these stockings are more sensitive to circumferential deviations, the proportion of custom-made stockings would be clearly greater than in seamless stockings, although the size system offers five additional sizes.

In the extreme case, beyond the limits of what is technically possible, the proportion of custom-made stockings also amounts to 13 per cent.

Summary:

1. If we use the Quality-Seal system with 6 sizes for seamless and 11 sizes for stockings with seams, and if we take into consideration the prescribed pressure decrease from distal to proximal, the proportion of custom-made below-knee stockings in compression class 2 amounts to at least 13 per cent of the stockings presently available.

2. Reducing the proportion of custom-made stockings by introducing size system with 'many' sizes appears to be a doubtful procedure. The great variety of leg shapes and sizes cannot be forced into a rigid size scheme.

Phlébologie 92. Eds P. Raymond-Martimbeau, R. Prescott, M. Zummo.
John Libbey Eurotext, Paris © 1992, pp. 925-926

Manufacture of graduated light compression stockings

Lucie Beaupré

Ottawa, Ontario, Canada.

That compression stockings reduce symptoms of varicose veins, such as oedema, heaviness and fatigue, is well documented in medical literature. Studies have strongly suggested that even light compression stockings (from 15 to 20 mm Hg) are efficacious in addition to being attractive. As a physician practising phlebology for many years and prescribing light compression stockings to my patients, I became interested in their manufacture when visiting a manufacturing plant. The elements of optimum combination of light compression stockings are the ideal yarns, the appropriate knitting and spandex incorporation with the degree of compression desired.

1. The ideal component yarns are one elastomeric and one non-elastomeric.

a) Spandex-lycra is preferred to rubber as the elastomeric yarns of light compression stockings.

b) The spandex must also be of low modulus, allowing a low variation of compression in a stocking in terms of the circumference of the legs. With spandex of low modulus and high elongation about 80%

Patients can wear mass produced hosiery with a relatively stable compression at a given point on the leg.

Raw nylon is chosen as the non elastomeric yarn of light compression stockings because it is stronger and more resistant than texturized or elastic nylon. The little elasticity of raw nylon avoids the solenoid effect of the yarn, therefore it does not form any ringlets.

2) The appropriate knitting of the yarns is the function of the stitches used and of the method of incorporating the Spandex.
There are two Knit Stitches:
i) Jersey Stitch - where each spandex loop is knitted to each nylon loop (used more often in knee-highs), and
ii) Float Stitch - where each spandex loop is knitted to every second nylon loop (used more often in panty-hose).

3) There are two methods of incorporating the Spandex:

- *First the knit in method - where the spandex is directly knitted to the nylon.*
- *Second the lay-in method - where the spandex is lain linearly in a given knit stitch.*

The knit-it method alone will give compression around 15 mm Hg. The knit-it method plus the lay-in allow stronger compression of 20 mm Hg and higher.

4) How to get the Degree of Compression Desired
There are two methods of determining the degree of compression; the stitches and the stretch of the spandex. The stitches, by the size of the loop, give the vertical tension: the smaller the loop, the stronger the compression. The stretch or tension applied on the Spandex, gives the lateral tension.

Remember, the compression is the function of the Law of Laplace, therefore is not uniform at the ankle.

$$\text{Compression} = \frac{\text{Tension of fabric}}{\text{Radius of the curve}}$$

The knitting machine and the tension on the elastic yarn must be set to give a degree of compression of the stocking gradually decreasing from the ankle up.

Finally, some sophisticated measurement tests following the Law of Laplace are used to control the degree of compression at different levels of the stocking. Among others, there are the Instrom test (more common in Europe) and the National Association Hosiery Manufacturers test (more common in U.S.A.).

In conclusion, efficacious light compression stockings are from 15 to 20 20 mm Hg, are made with appropriate component fibers, selective knitting, chosen degree of compression, and are controlled by scientific measuring tests.

D.
TRAITEMENT PHYSIQUE
PHYSICAL TREATMENT

Phlébologie 92. Eds P. Raymond-Martimbeau, R. Prescott, M. Zummo.
John Libbey Eurotext, Paris © 1992, pp. 929

La micro-coagulo-chirurgie selon Parvulesco : nouvelle thérapie esthétique des varicosités téléangiectasiques (microvarices)

Jean Parvulesco

Unité de Phlébologie, Clinique La Rosiaz, CH-1009 Pully-sur-Lausanne, Suisse.

Les varicosités téléangiectasiques (Microvarices) représentent une atteinte fréquente de la population féminine.

Cetains moyens thérapeutiques proposés jusqu'ici (sclérothérapie, électrocoagulation, Laser) se sont avérés peu efficaces ou même décevantes.

Préoccupés d'améliorer la gêne esthétique chez nos patients, nous avons élaboré et expérimenté pendant les 12 dernières années une nouvelle méthode de traitement.

Notre procédé est basé sur la destruction des vaisseaux téléangiectasiques par une excision micro-chirurgicale (selon notre méthode de "phlébextraction segmentaire étagée des varices") et par une micro-coagulation trans-incisionnelle.

Pour plus de précisions, voir notre livre intitulé "Microvarices (Téléangiectasies) - La nouvelle thérapie esthétique" en cours de réalisation en 1992 où notre expérience est exposée en détail.

Phlébologie 92. Eds P. Raymond-Martimbeau, R. Prescott, M. Zummo.
John Libbey Eurotext, Paris © 1992, pp. 930-932

Vascular lesions of childhood : treatment with the candela flashlamp-pumped pulsed dye laser

Mitchel P. Goldman, Richard E. Fitzpatrick, Javier Ruiz-Esparza

Dermatology Associates of San Diego County, Inc., 477 N. El Camino Real, Suite B-303, Encinitas, CA 92024, USA.

INTRODUCTION

Vascular malformations occur in childhood with notable frequency. The port-wine stain (PWS) occurs in 0.3% of births[1]. Telangiectasia (TEL) of the face in children have a reported frequency of 15%[2]. Interscapular telangiectasia occur in 39.9% of girls and 32.3% of boys between ages 6-17[3]. Capillary (or strawberry) hemangiomas (HEM) occur in 1.0-2.6% of infants[1,4]. Pyogenic granuloma (PG) is a common disorder which usually occurs after trauma, infection or under hormonal influences. It is more common in children and young adults but may appear at any age[5,6]. Even though the above-mentioned vascular lesions are not rare, their presence is oftentimes very disturbing to the child and/or parents and requires treatment.

Various treatment modalities have been used to effect resolution of vascular malformations. Unfortunately, virtually all prior modalities have been fraught with complications, especially when treatment is begun in infancy[7]. Until recently, the argon laser was the most popular therapy for PWS, HEM, TEL, and PG. However, the argon laser has a demonstrated 9-26% incidence of hypertrophic scarring[8-12] and an unknown, unspecified incidence of mild to moderate atrophic scarring. Therefore, it has been recommended that the argon laser not be used for treatment of PWS in children under the age of 17 years old.[13] In addition, the argon laser also produces scarring in HEM treated in childhood[14]. The Candela FlashLamp-Pumped Dye Laser (FLPDL) by virtue of its specific wave length and short pulse duration has been demonstrated to have a negligible risk of scarring or permanent pigmentary changes in the treatment of vascular malformations in infants and children[7,15-18]. We report our experience treating PWS, HEM, TEL, and PG in children with the FLPD laser.

One hundred and sixteen children, ages 2-1/2 weeks to 14 years with vascular malformations (port-wine stains (PWS), spider telangiectasia (TEL), capillary (or strawberry) hemangioma (HEM), and pyogenic granuloma (PG) were treated with the Candela FlashLamp-Pumped Dye Laser (FLPDL) at 585nm.
Forty-three patients with 49 separate PWS were treated with laser energies between 5.5 and 7.75 J/cm^2.

CHILDHOOD PORT WINE STAINS

TREATMENT ENERGY (J/CM^2)	# LESIONS TREATED	AVERAGE # RX	AVERAGE IMPROVEMENT	> 95% CLEAR # LESIONS	(%)	AVERAGE # RX TO CLEAR
< 6.0	5	3.8	52%	0	0%	-
6.0 - 6.75	20	3.65	74%	6	30%	5.3
7.0 - 7.75	24	3.7	69%	4	17%	3.3

Five children 4 years or younger had >95% fading with an average of 3.8 treatments with two children **0-4** having an average fading of 75% with 3.8 treatments.

Twenty-two patients, 4.5- 14 years old had an average fading of 75% with 6.5 treatments.

CHILDHOOD PORT WINE STAINS

# PATIENTS	# LESIONS	AGE RANGE	AVE AGE	AVE # RX	AVE IMPROVE-MENT	MEDIAN IMPROVE-MENT	> 95% IMPROVEMENT		
							# LESIONS	%	AVE #RX
AGE 0 - 4 YRS									
21	25	2 wk-4 yr	2.15yr	3.4	70%	75%	5	20%	3.8
AGE 4.5 - 14 YRS									
22	24	6-14 yr	10.3yr	4.0	68%	75%	3	12.5%	6.5
TOTAL 0 - 14 YRS									
43	49	2 wk-14 yr	6.2 yr	3.7	69%	75%	8	16.3%	4.8

PWS on the face, neck and torso cleared significantly better than lesions on the hand and arm.

CHILDHOOD PORT WINE STAINS

LOCATION	# LESIONS	AVE # RX	AVE IMPROVEMENT	> 95% CLEAR # LESIONS	(%)	AVE # RX
Face	33	3.5	65%	4	12%	4.0
Neck	4	5.3	90%	2	50%	4.5
Torso	6	3.0	85%	3	50%	3.0
Hand & Arm	6	3.7	63%	0	-	0

Almost all PWS lesions showed an improvement with additional treatments

CHILDHOOD PORT WINE STAINS

			IMPROVEMENT				IMPROVEMENT OF NON-CLEAR LESIONS	
# OF TREATMENTS	# LESIONS TREATED	AVE TREATMENT ENERGY	MEAN	MEDIAN	# LESIONS >95% CLEAR	(%)	MEAN	MEDIAN
1 RX	10	6.73 J	51 %	50%	1	10%	46%	40%
2 RX	12	6.96 J	70.4 %	72%	3	25%	61%	50%
3 RX	5	6.55 J	62 %	60%	0	0%	62%	60%
4 RX	4	6.86 J	70 %	70%	0	0%	70%	70%
5 RX	10	7.05 J	77.5%	80%	2	20%	72.5%	77%
6-11 RX	8	6.5 J	85 %	90%	3	37.5%	78%	80%

Twenty-three children with TEL had an average of 90% fading with 1.2 treatments at an average energy of 6.9J/cm^2.

CHILDHOOD SPIDER TELANGECTASIA

# LESIONS	# PATIENTS	AVERAGE AGE	AGE RANGE	AVERAGE # RX	AVERAGE IMPROVEMENT	TOTAL CLEARING	AVERAGE IMPROVEMENT IF NOT CLEAR
55	23	6.7 yrs	1 - 14 yr	1.2 *	90%	90%	78%

* 22% OF PATIENTS HAD A SECOND TREATMENT

Eight children with superficial HEM demonstrated 87% clearing with an average of 4.3 treatments at 7.1J/cm^2.

SUPERFICIAL CAPILLARY HEMANGIOMA

# LESIONS	DIAMETER < 1 CM	AVE AGE LESION APPEARED	AVE AGE OF RX	AVE # RX	AVE RX INTERVAL	AVE RX TIME	AVE RX ENERGY	AVE IMPROVE-MENT	TOTALLY CLEAR
8	8	3 wks	5 mos	4.3	1 mo	3.3 mo	7.1 J/cm^2	87%	3 (38%)

Ten children with PG or papular hemangiomas, had variable resolution from 0-100% with 1-2 treatments with 7 or 7.5J/cm^2.

CHILDHOOD PYOGENIC GRANULOMA OR PAPULAR HEMANGIOMA

# LESIONS	AVE AGE LESION APPEARED	AGE RANGE	AVE AGE RX	AVE # RX	AVE RX ENERGY	AVE IMPROVEMENT	TOTALLY CLEAR
10	22 mos	6 mos - 3 yr	26 mos	2.1	7.2 J/cm^2	88%	60%

There were no episodes of scarring or persistent pigmentary changes in any of the patients. The FLPDL is proven to be a safe and effective treatment modality for vascular malformations and other vascular lesions of childhood.

REFERENCES

1. Jacobs AH, Walton RG: The incidence of birthmarks in the neonate. Pediatrics 1976; 58:218-22.
2. Wenzel JE, Burgert EO. The spider nevus in infancy and children. Pediatrics 1964; 33:227-32.
3. Oster J, Nielsen A: Nuchal naevi and intrascapular telangiectases. Acta Paediat Scand 1970; 59:416-423.
4. Pratt AG: Birthmarks in infants. Arch Dermatol 1953; 67:302.
5. Lee FD: A comparative study of Kaposi's sarcoma and granuloma pyogenicum in Uganda. J Clin Pathol 1968; 21:119-28.
6. Bhaskar SN, Jacoway JR: Pyogenic granuloma: Clinical features, incidence, histology, and result of treatment: Report of 242 cases. J. Oral Surg 1966; 24:391-98.
7. Glassberg E, Lask G, Rabinowitz LG, et al: Capillary hemangiomas: Case study of a novel laser treatment and a review of therapeutic options. J Dermatol Surg Oncol 1989; 15:1214-23.
8. Afelberg DB Maser MR, Lash H, et al: The argon laser for cutaneous lesions. JAMA 1981; 245:2073-75.
9. Noe JM, Barsky SH, Geer DE, et al: Portwine stains and the response to argon laser therapy: successful treatment and the predictive role of color, age, and biopsy. Plast Reconstr Surg 1980; 65:130-36.
10. Cosman B: Experience in the argon laser therapy of port wine stains. Plast Reconstr Surg 1980; 65:119-29.
11. Apfelberg DB Kose J, Maser MR et al: Histology of port wine stains following argon laser treatment. Br J Plast Surg 1979; 32:232-37.
12. Dixon JA, Huether S, Rotering R: Hypertrophic scarring in argon laser treatment of port-wine stains. Plast Reconstr Surg 1984; 73:777.
13. Smith JD, Cook TA: Argon laser treatment of hemangiomas in children. Int J Pediatr Otorhinolaryngol 1984; 7:153.
14. Tan OT, Sherwood K, Gilchrest BA: Treatment of children with port-wine stains using the flashlamp-pulsed tunable dye laser. N Engl J Med 1989; 320:416-21.
15. Reyes BA, Geronemus R: Treatment of port-wine stains during childhood with the flashlamp-pumped pulsed dye laser. J Am Acad Dermatol 1990; 23:1142-48.
16. Sherwood KA, Tan OT: Treatment of a capillary hemangioma with the flashlamp pumped-dye laser. J Am Acad Dermatol 1990; 22:136-37.
17. Ashinoff R, Geronemus RG: Flashlamp-pumped pulsed dye laser for port-wine stains in infancy: Earlier versus later treatment. J Am Acad Dermatol 1991; 24:467-72.
18. Geronemus RG: Treatment of spider Telangiectases in children using the flashlamp-pumped pulsed dye laser. Ped Dermatol 1991; 8:61-63.

Phlébologie 92. Eds P. Raymond-Martimbeau, R. Prescott, M. Zummo.
John Libbey Eurotext, Paris © 1992, pp. 933-935

The chromatic micropuncture in the treatment of the telangiectasias

Saul Umansky, Miguel Eduardo Umansky, Pablo de Ferrari

Department of Phlebology, Clínicas Mepres. C/Rui Perez No.1.3P.Der. Avilés, 33400 Asturias, España.

SUMMARY.

The Chromatic Micro Puncture is an original technique consisting in destroying the Telangiectasias by intradermic punctures all along the vein, by mechanical destruction. We may at the same time implant some substances as Scentella Assiatica which promotes, protects and stimulates the healing of the skin, and/or a pigment which neutralise the brown colouration of haemosiderine such as those observed in the processes of Post-Flebitic Syndromes, or Pigmentations Post-Scleroterapy.

INTRODUCTION.

In this article we wish to pre-established that our experience refers to the Telangiectasia defined by Von Graf as "Pathological dilations of the most periphery of the small blood vessels".
According to dermatologists, Telangiectasias are dilations of the venous subpapilar plexi, situated within the thickness of the dermis and visible to the naked eye. They are therefore located between the epidermis and the hypodermis.
According to Tournay the majority of intradermal varices are not paiful, although sometimes they can be so, referred to as "venous sympatalgy" although in the majority of cases these play an important role in the aesthetics.
Electrocoagulation, Cryotherapy, Mesotherapy and the Laser, have only had partial succes and occasionally none, and sometimes their incorrect indications has provoked small sloughs and pigmentation which caneven be more antiaesthetic than the telangiectasia itself.
Microschlerosis, as Orbach says, "has only had partial succes", as these types of venules are too fine to be injected in most cases. It is feasible to bear in mind that the puncture and the liquid injected may produce pigmentation due to haemosiderine or the material injected as well as allergic reactions, sloughs, etc,.

MATERIAL AND METHOD: Equipment. Medicaments.

Equipment: The necessary equipment includes a Mobile Electronic Unit, a Manual Piece and a Pedal.
A Mobil Unit consists of a motor with several controls which regulates the penetration of the needle between 0.5 and 3 mms. depth, as

well as number of vibrations per second, in order to ensure the umount of medicament implanted and the force of penetration, variable according to the toughness of the skin.
The Manual Piece(sterile) has an Electromagnet inside it, which creates a pulse, which is transmited to the needle. It is similar to a pencilwhich is sharpened untill it ends in a small tube which serves as a guide for the needle and a receptacle for the material to be implanted, in which moves the needle whose purpose is to destroy the venule, as it can be replaced when bluntened and to carry out microimplants of the medicaments. The Pedal activates the Magnet Pulse.
Medicaments: Scentella Assiatica. Pigments.
Scentella Assiatica, promotes, protects and stimulates the healing of the skin: it acts regulating the incorporation of two fundamental aminoacids to the collagen of the skin, the Alanin and the Proline which stimulates the granulation tissue; in the other hand the Scentella Assiatica acts helping the correct epitelization of the skin by mens of the stimulation of the biosinthesis of the glicosaminglicanos.
Pigments are soluble materials of very small size which for our work are aproximately 6 microns in size in suspension. The transporting solvents such as Fenol Povidona with Scentella Assiatica, fill the space left by the punctures of the needle and facilitates the normal regeneration and pigmentation of the skin,

SURGERY.

This is a microsurgical procedure that may be undertaken in an out patients clinic in several sessions or in one surgical session in the operating theatre.
Anasthesia: It can be carried out without anaesthetic or with a simple Freon based spray in several sessions. It is also possible to perform the operation under general anaesthetic in one session, leaving the final retouching, if necessary, for an external consultation.
Operation: Before beginning the operation the Mobil Unit, the Manual Piece and the Pedal mus be checked. The Manula Piece is withdrawn from its sterile wrapping or from the drawer sterilised with Formaldehyde and it is connected into the Power Unit. The red button is pressed and the Mobil Power Unit is adjusted for the depth, and force of penetration and vibration rate of the needle. A team member of the surgeon presses the Pedal and controls the functioning of the needle; then the tip of the needle only is dipped in the liquid which has been previously chosen and prepaired, with or without pigment and with prior anesthetic by spray or without it, the outline of the Telangiectasia is slowly traced, taking care not to allow the needle to remain stationary on one point for more than a second.
Ideally this is done under a high power lens or microscope although it can be performed with the naked eye.
various groups of telangiectasias can be treated together depending on the patient´s tolerance or all at once leaving any final retouching for a later consultation. It is also recommended not to allow extended runs of the apparatus, I.E. not to let it run for long periods without stopping. There will be no excess of pigment in the skin if the metal tube does not touch the skin.
On the other hand, if it does, a drop of pigment will be left on the skin, which can be removed with a solution equal parts saline and alcohol/Glycerol.
The metal point must be dipped in the solution as many times as necessary remembering to mix the pigment frequently. Once surgery is finished an antibiotic cream is applied to the treated area which is then covered with a simple gause and the same treatment is recommended for several days alternating the cream with a Heparinoid gel.
After one week of combined antibiotic/heparinoid treatment, if traes

of pigment remain, alternate applications of alchol/glycerol and saline with abrasive cream can be made.
After a fortnight nearly all operative symptoms will have disappeared and long sessions may be continued fortnightly and shorter sessions weekly, if different areas are being treated.
In the inmediate postoperative period a slight oedema may arise in the area, in which case the application of cold compresses or ice bags may be made, as well as changing the antibiotic dressing for at least four days. An oral anaelgesic may also be administrated. It is recommended that the patient should not take the sun for a fornight. After a fortnight the oedema will have disappeared and most of the contusion will be resolved. The surface skin will be cure in each implantation zone and then the overall succes of the treatment may be appreciated as well as the pattients appreciation of the treatment received.

COMPLICATIONS.

Complications arising from this procedure are relatively few. Whilst some patients will show no operative inconviniences of complications, most ofthem will show some degree of contusion along the line of the treated vein or slight pigmentation, which we have to consider a slight or moderate routine disorder which may be treted as previously indicated. In some cases all the vein is not destracted at the first time, and in a second time we can retouch this vein.
The two main complications are infection and reaction to the Scentella Assiatica/Pigment.
Infection is a remote possibillity, but as the skin is allways contamined it can happen. If it does, then suitable antibiotic therapy is initiated.
Allergic reactions: As is the case with infections, Allergic reactiion is very unlikely and can be anticipated by preoperative dermatologicaltests. In the event that it occurs, treatment with cortisone cream and an orally administered antiallergic can overcome the problem.
Case Histories: Our experiences are based on 1800 cases and a follow up from one to five years.
We have found 95% of good effective results and 5% of only moderate efficacy; this latter cases resulting from a lack of experience in blending the pigments to match the patients skin colouration, and to inadequate calculations of the penetration depth of the needles.

Phlébologie 92. Eds P. Raymond-Martimbeau, R. Prescott, M. Zummo.
John Libbey Eurotext, Paris © 1992, pp. 936

La pressothérapie par bains de mercure

Michel Schadeck

École Européenne de Phlébologie, 6, rue Giordano Bruno, 75014 Paris, France.

L'utilisation de la compression dans la réduction des différents types d'oedème ou des troubles trophiques d'origine veineuse est chose courante mais se heurte régulièrement à des contraintes de confort, d'adaptation à la forme du membre et de lenteur dans les résultats obtenus.
La pressothérapie par bains de mercure est une technique également ambulatoire.
Elle consiste en l'utilisation des propriétés du mercure, fluide de haute densité (13,6) pour réaliser une compression progressive, indolore et surtout ajustée du membre supérieur ou inférieur.
Ce membre est placé verticalement dans une cuve dans laquelle le mercure va monter le long du membre puis redescendre suivant un rythme librement choisi et dépendant du contexte pathologique.
En fonction de celui-ci, des traitements d'appoints comme la compression élastique, les draînages lymphatiques manuels ou des médications veinotropes ou lymphagogues pourront être utilisés.
Les indications thérapeutiques sont donc celles des lymphoedèmes primitifs ou secondaires, les oedèmes post-thrombotiques, les troubles trophiques comme les hypodermites (lipodermatosclerosis), les ulcérations d'origine veineuse voire artérielle. En effet l'hyperhémie réactionnelle obtenue peut favoriser une meilleure perfusion de la distalité du membre.
Des essais ont également été faits sur des algodystrophies avec des résultats très encourageants.
Enfin, bien que sortant de la pathologie vasculaire pure, les oedèmes post-traumatiques du pied ou de la cheville bénéficient de façon remarquable de ce type de traitement.

En conclusion, cette méthode thérapeutique, relativement nouvelle en pratique quotidienne et donc souvent mal connue apparaît comme un moyen d'avenir dans l'approche de pathologies difficiles bien représentées par les complications vasculaires que nous fréqentons tous.

Phlébologie 92. Eds P. Raymond-Martimbeau, R. Prescott, M. Zummo.
John Libbey Eurotext, Paris © 1992, pp. 937-939

Étude de la pressothérapie par le mercure dans la récupération après effort chez le cycliste de haut niveau

F.A. Allaert*, M. Schadeck**, B. Provot***

** Department de biostatistique et information médicales CHRU Dijon, France. ** Service d'angiologie, Hôpital Notre-Dame du Bon secours, Paris, France. *** Médecine du Sport. Équipe cycliste Nationale, France.*

Lors des épreuves sportives répétées telles que les étapes des grands tours cyclistes, la qualité de la récupération après effort joue un rôle fondamental dans les performances obtenues par les coureurs.

Actuellement pour favoriser cette récupération, l'une des techniques les plus utilisées est la "récupération active". Celle-ci consiste à poursuivre un effort physique après l'arrêt de l'épreuve officielle de manière à consommer les métabolites intermédiaires produits lors de l'effort intense et dont l'accumulation est à l'origine de la gêne musculaire.

L'objectif de cette étude est d'évaluer l'intérêt d'une nouvelle méthode physique, la pressothérapie par le mercure, en complément de la récupération active après l'effort chez le cycliste de haut niveau soumis à des épreuves répétées.

MATERIEL ET METHODE

Sélection des sujets

Les sujets devaient être agés de 18 à 35 ans, être cyclistes de haut niveau, en période d'entraînement intense, répété quotidiennement sous contrôle médical. Un groupe de 11 cycliste appartenant à l'équipe National Française et devant suivre une période d'entrainement intense de 9 jours en vue d'une qualification ont accepté de participer à l'étude.

Aucun d'eux ne présentant de troubles trophiques ou cutanés au niveau des membres inférieurs, une tendance à la spasmophilie ou des troubles veineux qui correspondaient aux critère de non-inclusion, l'ensemble de ces sportifs a été retenu comme groupe d'étude.

Modalités de la pressothérapie au mercure

Le principe de cette méthode consiste en l'utilisation de deux caractéristiques essentielles du mercure: son état liquide et sa forte densité.

Lors du traitement le membre du sujet est placé dans une cuve à l'intérieur de laquelle le mercure circule.

Les vagues successives de montées et descentes permettent une compression:

- ajustée car l'état liquide du mercure assure un moulage parfait le long du membre;
- évacuatrice car grâce à sa forte densité, le mercure crée un gradiant de pression régulier et évacuateur. Lorsque le mercure est monté le long du membre, la pression au fond de la cuve est de 1 bar soit une pression identique à celle que reçoit la semelle plantaire lors de la marche, et décroit régulièrement jusqu'à la racine du membre.
- atraumatique et indolore car la technique reste dans les strictes limites physiologiques sans risque lymphatique.

Après chaque période d'entraînement de l'après midi, l'ensemble des sujets pratiquait une séance de récupération active.
Chaque jour, au terme de celle-ci , 6 d'entre eux désignés à l'avance par tirage au sort pré-établi et équilibré, bénéficiaient d'une pressothérapie au mercure.
Ce plan expérimental a été retenu de manière à garantir que chaque sportif bénéficie d'un nombre identique de séances de pressothérapie au cours des 9 journées d'entrainement et qu'aucune inégalité de traitement ne vienne ainsi entacher les résultats de l'épreuve finale de qualification.

Modalités d'évaluation des résultats
L'effet de la pressothérapie au mercure est évalué d'une part, au travers d'un critère biologique objectif, le test d'hyperhémie cutané, et d'autre part, par une série d'échelle analogiques visant à apprécier l'état musculaire subjectif du sportif.

Dans le test d'hyperhémie cutanée, le patient est allongé sur le dos en position semi-assise. On comprime l'artère fémorale du membre directement avec la sonde doppler (4 mhz), le pied étant levé à 20cm au dessus du plan de la table. La compression, aidée ou non de l'index, dure 40 secondes dans cette position et est prolongée 10 seconde sur le membre relaché. L'absence de tout flux est contrôlé directement par le doppler.
Immédiatement après relachement de la compression, on enregistre en vitesse moyenne (5mm/seconde) jusqu'au retour à la ligne à la ligne de base.
Une évaluation de l'hyperhémie cutanée est réalisée par un médecin angiologue au travers du temps de demi retour à la ligne de base pour les 6 sujets désignés chaque jour par le tirage au sort, avant et après la séance de pressothérapie au mercure.
Une diminution du temps de retour à la ligne de base, traduit une meilleure circulation sanguine , condition sine qua none à une bonne oxygénation des tissus, à laquelle vient s'opposer l'accumulation des métabolites intermédiaires produits au cours de la phase d'effort intense.

L'évaluation de l'état musculaire des sujets repose sur 12 échelles analogiques allant de 0 à 100 c'est à dire de "je ne me suis jamais senti aussi mal" à "je ne me suis jamais senti aussi bien". Six sont relatives à la Douleur et six à la sensation de Bien-être musculaire ressenties au niveau de la cuisse et du mollet.

L'ensemble de ces critères est évalué:
- pour tous les sujets, avant tout exercice physique intense, au début de leur période d'entraînement et de sélection, ;
- pour tous les sujets, d'une part,avant et après la séance de récupération active, d'autre part le matin avant tout effort physique;
- pour les 6 sujets désignés chaque jour par le tirage au sort, après la séance de pressothérapie au mercure.

Par ailleurs, bien qu'aucun effet indésirable n'ait été décrit jusqu'à présent, toute description d'une effet désagréable de la pressothérapie au mercure devait être noté par le médecin en attachant une attention particulières aux manifestations vagales.

RESULTATS

Evaluation de l'effet de la pressothérapie

Résultats des test d'hyperémie cutanée avant et après pressothérapie.
Les résultats de l'ensemble des tests d'hyperhémie cutanée avant et après la séance de pressothérapie au mercure réalisée chez les six sujets tirés au hazard chaque jour, ont été comparés par une analyse de variance sur séries appariées. Ses résultats montrent une

réduction de 2,5 secondes du temps de retour à la normale dont la signification est chiffrée à $p<0{,}001$.

Résultats des échelles d'évaluation de l'état musculaire avant et après pressothérapie.
Les résultats de chaque échelle d'autoévaluation de l'état musculaire avant et après pressothérapie ont été comparés également par des analyses de variance sur séries appariées. Quelle que soit l'échelle d'évaluation considérée, on note une évolution positive significative des résultats à $p<0{,}01$. Exprimées en pourcentage d'amélioration par rapport à la valeur initiale, ces évolutions correspondent à une diminution de 40 à 45% des 6 échelles de douleur et à une augmentation de 20 à 25% des 6 échelles de bien-être musculaire.

Tolérance
Aucune manifestation indésirable n'a été signalée par les sportifs au cours des différentes séances auxquelles ils ont été soumis.

Comparaison de la récupération avec ou sans pressothérapie
Après vérification de la comparabilité initiale, les valeurs de chacune des échelles d'évaluation de l'état musculaire obtenues immédiatement après la séance de pressothérapie ont été comparées à celles mesurées en son absence au terme d'une nuit de sommeil. Les résultats apparaissent équivalent pour l'ensemble des échelles de douleurs et significativement supérieur pour la pressothérapie pour les échelles de bien-être ($p<0{,}05$ à l'exception de la 5ème). Exprimées en terme de pourcentage d'amélioration, les résultats contrastent encore plus avec respectivement dans les groupes avec et sans pressothérapie au mercure:
- une diminution de 40 à 45% des intensités douloureuses contre de l'ordre de 25 à 35%;
- une augmentation de 20 à 25% des sensations de bien-être contre 5 à 15% au maximum.

DISCUSSION

Au terme d'une séance de pressothérapie, l'état musculaire apparaît donc similaire en matière de douleur et supérieur en matière de bien-être à ceux obtenus après une récupération d'une nuit de sommeil. Ceci constitue un élément de poids en favuer de l'utilisation de cette méthode lors des épreuves répétées.
Ces résultats laissent également espérer que cette méthode puisse suppléer aux diminutions de la récupération normale physiologique nocturne qu'entraine l'accumulation des fatigues et des stress d'épreuves successives. Pour le mettre en évidence, il aurait fallu pouvoir suivre deux groupes dont l'un aurait bénéficié quotidienement de la pressothérapie et l'autre jamais. Comme nous l'avons indiqué dans le protocole, pour des raisons d'éthique sportives liées à une compétition finale entre les sportifs du groupe d'étude , ce plan expérimental ne pouvait pas être retenu. Ce sera l'objet d'une prochaine étude, mais d'ores et déjà l'évolution des paramètres biologiques et de l'état musculaire avant et après pressothérapie et l'équivalence avec les effets physiologiques d'une nuit de sommeil laisse largement augurer de ses résultats.

CONCLUSION

Cette étude menée chez des sportifs cyclistes de haut niveau en période d'entraînement intense:
- d'une part, objective les améliorations biologiques objectives et musculaires subjectives supplémentaires obtenues par une pressothérapie au mercure alors même que les sujets viennent de bénéficier d'une récupération active bien conduite;
- d'autre part, quantifie la récupération induite par cette séance de pressothérapie comme étant équivalente à celle obtenue par une nuit entière de repos.dans un groupe témoin.

Son utilisation paraît donc pouvoir être légitimement proposée avec bénéfice en complément de la récupération active chez les sportifs soumis à des épreuves répétées

MERCURY PRESSOTHERAPY AS ANCILLARY TREATMENT FOR VENOUS ULCERS

Douglas A. Hill, M.D.

Private Practice, Calgary, Alberta, Canada

This randomized study compares the healing rate for venous leg ulcers treated with standard compression therapy (i.e. , the Unna's boot) with the healing rate of ulcers treated with the same compression therapy in combination with mercury pressotherapy. Methodology and results will be discussed.

Phlébologie 92. Eds P. Raymond-Martimbeau, R. Prescott, M. Zummo.
John Libbey Eurotext, Paris © 1992, pp. 941-942

Mercury pressotherapy in the treatment of lipodermatosclerosis

Louis Grondin, Jeannette Soriano

Circulatory Disease Center, 1504 15th Avenue S.W., 3rd Floor, Calgary, Alberta, T3C-0X9, Canada.

The importance of compression as the silent healer of veno-lymphatic disorders is presently well accepted (1). At present the international effort of standardization (2) of support garments offers to both the therapist and the researcher unsurpassed tolls in broadening the field of application of compressive therapy. Mercury pressotherapy as a new therapeutic modality (3) has offered further assistance in the management of chronic edema and lymphoedema (4).

Lipodermatosclerosis (5) has been described as an intermediate state of chronic venous insufficiency leading to further complications such as bouts of acute hypodermatitis and recurrent stasis ulcerations. Its treatment besides the daily use of compression garments has included various agents such as pentoxiphillin (6) and dapsone (7). Pentoxiphillin has the disadvantage of requiring several weeks before improvement may be observed (6), and dapsone has definite toxic side effects which limits its use and indications (7). Finally fibrinolytic agents such as stanozolol (8) and other products (9) have been found effective in reversing chronic lipodermatosclerosis and its complications.

In our experience mercury pressotherapy has demonstrated to be an excellent therapy for lipodermatosclerosis in not only reversing the underlying condition without chemotherapy, but also in preventing and reversing its complications namely, acute dermatitis and stasis ulcerations.

REFERENCES

1. Bassi, Stemmer. (1983): Traitement Mecaniques Fonctionnels En Phlebologie. *Editions Piccin.*

2. Gummistrumpfe, E.V., Schattauer. (1989). The Medical Compression Stocking. *Gutezeichengemeinschaft Medizinischer.*

3. Cartier, C.J. (1983): Traitment Des Oedemes Vascularies Des Membres Par Bain De Mercure. *Hour. Des Mal. Basc., 1983, P. 297-300.*

4. Schadech, M. (1991): Mercury-Bath Pressotherapy on Lympho-Venous Disorders. *Proceedings of The Canadian Society of Phlebology, Whistler 1991.*

5. Caille. (1985): Phlebologie en Pratique Quotidienne. *Expansion Scientifique Francaise.*

6. (1988): Haemorheologie Et Agregation Erythrocytaire. *Deuxieme Symposium International, Paris.*

7. Lack, Edward. (1989): The Use Of Dapsone In the Treatment of Lipodermatosclerosis. *Proceedings of the Phlebology Society of America.*

8. Layer, G.T. et al (1986): Stanozolol And The Treatment Of Venous Ulceration. *Phlebology, December 1986.*

9. Belcaro, G., Marelli, C. (1989): Defibritide, Elastic Compression and Lipodermatosclerosis. *Phlebology, June 1989.*

Nd-Yag laser and Argon laser for the radical and cosmetical treatment of the varicose syndrome

B. Puglisi A. Mazza F.M. San Filippo

The Authors, after an experience of 276 cases through three years describs the results and the new technique that allows to make safenotomy instead of a safenectomy by stripping.

Further the Authors underline the indications and the advantages of this new technique that's less thraumatic than stripping,doesn't give hematoma and related septic compliances and offer a best cosmetical result.

Phlébologie 92. Eds P. Raymond-Martimbeau, R. Prescott, M. Zummo.
John Libbey Eurotext, Paris © 1992, pp. 944-946

Hydrotherapy for varicose veins : a randomized, controlled trial

E. Ernst, T. Saradeth, K.L. Resch

University of Vienna, Medical School, Department of Physical Medicine and Rehabilitation, Währinger Gürtel 18-20, 1090 Vienna, Austria.

INTRODUCTION

Varicosity is both frequent and potentially dangerous. Compression stockings provide the conservative treatment of choice (1). In addition, several adjunctive measures may be considered. In particular a number of drugs have been shown to work clinically (3). Hydrotherapy has a long tradition in Europe. One of its domaines is the treatment of varicose veins (8). Yet the notion that it is effective in this condition is based purely on empiricism. The present study was designed to evaluate its usefulness in a controlled trial.

MATERIAL AND METHODS

122 out-patients gave informed consent to participate. Inclusion criteria were primary varicose veins of at least one leg as diagnosed by patients' history, symptoms, physical examination and light reflex rheography (LRR) (7). Patients were always examined by the same doctor, who was blinded to the patients' treatment. Exclusion criteria were venous insufficiency not due to primary varicosity, venous thrombosis, thromboplebitis, lymph-oedemas, congenital angiodysplasias, venous valve agenesia, venous compression syndromes, congestive heart failure, liver or kidney diseases, malignancies, acute inflammatory processes, haematologic disorders and symptomatic peripheral arterial occlusive disease.

Patients were randomized into group A and B. Group A was treated with hydrotherapy, group B was not. All concomitant therapy was left constant during the study period.

Hydrotherapy consisted of daily treatments with alternating warm and cold water (2,6,8). Treatments were administered to both legs 5 days per week. Two out of 4 different hydrotherapeutic measures (Tab. 1) were chosen intermittently, at least one and no more than three for each day.

The following variables were quantified at entry, after 12 and 24 days of therapy: foot volume by water plethysmography (4), minimal leg circumference at the ankle, venous re-fill time by

LRR (7). Subjective symptoms were quantified by visual analogue scales: frequency of cramps, stabbing pain in the calf, itching, paraesthesias, heaviness of legs, leg pain during standing or sitting, need to elevate legs during the day.

The data were evaluated as a cross-sectional comparison between A and B and expressed as means ± 1 SEM. For each group, the absolute changes relative to the respective baseline values were analysed statistically. After confirming normal distribution, the t-test was used for objective variables and the Chi-square-test was employed for subjective symptoms (after dichotomizing the analogue scales into "improvement" and "no improvement"). The null-hypothesis was rejected when p was less than 0.05.

RESULTS

At baseline, none of the variables tested yielded significant differences between group A and B. There were no drop-outs during the trial. No adverse effects were reported.
At day 12 and 24 the average foot volume in group A decreased significantly more than in group B. The circumference at the ankle decreased significantly more in group A at the end of the study. Venous re-fill time increased significantly more in group A compared to B both after 12 and 24 days of treatment (Tab. 2).
In group A subjective symptoms improved in 4 qualities: cramps, stabbing pains, itching and pain during standing or sitting.

DISCUSSION

The present results imply that hydrotherapy is effective in treating objective and subjective signs of primary varicose veins. Due to the nature of the present trial, placebo effects must be considered. These can be most impressive, particularly when evaluating subjective criteria (5). Placebo effects, however, are less likely to occur with objectively measurable variables. Therefore, we believe that the present results are (at least in part) true effects of the hydrotherapeutic interventions, unrelated to placebo. The changes in objective parameters may well be considered as small. The fact that they are statistically significant therefore indicates that they are highly uniform. The modification of LRR re-fill time, however, is more impressive. This parameter can be considered as one of the most relevant objective endpoints for evaluating primary varicosity non-invasively (6). It must be stated that no other conservative treatment of varicose veins (other than compression) is known to lead to changes which are markedly more pronounced than the ones observed in this trial.

REFERENCES

1. BROWSE, N.L., AND BURNAND, K.G., ET AL (1988) : Diseases of the veins. London: Arnold.
2. BRÜGGEMANN, W. (1986) : Kneipptherapie - ein bewährtes Naturheilverfahren. Berlin: Springer.
3. CHEATLE, T.R., AND SCURR, J.H., ET AL (1991) : Drug treatment of chronic venous insufficiency and venous ulceration: a review. *J. Roy. Soc. Med.* 84, 354–57.
4. ERNST, E., AND SARADETH, T., ET AL (1991) : A single blind randomized, controlled trial of hydrotherapy for varicose veins. *VASA* 20, 147–152.
5. ERNST, E., AND SARADETH, T., ET AL (1991) : The powerful placebo. *Lancet* 337, 611.

6. KNEIPP, S. (1898) : Gesammelte Schriften. Kempten: J. Kösel'sche Buchhandlung.
7. SHEPARD, A.D., AND MACKEY, W.C., ET AL (1984) : Correlation of venous measurements with LRR: Effect of different exercise regimes. In *Die Lichtreflexrheographie*, eds R. May and R. Stemmer. Erlangen: Perimed.
8. WINTERNITZ, W. (1877) : Hydrotherapie. Wien: Urban-Schwarzenberg.

Table 1: Daily treatments with water during the study

hydrotherapy	temperature	duration
showers of the legs *(according to Kneipp, two alternations or more, always finishing with the cold treatment)*	35–38° C 12–16° C	1–2 min 20 sec
continous cold water treatment *(according to Kneipp)*	12° C	40–80 sec
feet baths *(two alternations or more, always finishing with the cold treatment)*	35–38° C 12–16° C	5 min 15 sec
walking in cold water *(water level to the calf, leg out of the water during each step)*	10–18° C	15–50 sec

(before treatments both legs had to be agreeably warm)

Table 2: Objective variables in group A and B (means ± 1 SEM)

Parameter [units]	Group	baseline	day 12	day 24
foot volume (ml)	A	3154 ± 35	3104 ± 34 *	3110 ± 35 *
	B	3081 ± 32	3059 ± 32	3081 ± 33
minimal circum–ference (cm)	A	22.09 ± 0.17	21.96 ± 0.16	21.90 ± 0.16 *
	B	21.85 ± 0.13	21.82 ± 0.13	21.91 ± 0.13
venous re-fill time (sec)	A	27.1 ± 1.8	32.2 ± 2.0 *	31.0 ± 2.1 *
	B	27.6 ± 1.7	25.2 ± 1.6	28.2 ± 1.8

* = significant inter-group difference of absolute changes ($p < 0.05$)

PHYSICAL EXERCISE TRAINING AS THERAPY FOR PATIENTS WITH CHRONIC VENOUS INCOMPETENCE (CVI)

Jünger M, Jünger I, Rahmel B, Rassner G

Dep. of Dermatology, Univ. Hospital, 74 Tübingen, Germany

A special physical exercise training was developed for patients with CVI in order to improve function of calf muscle pump. Patients have been performing this training regularly between 2 to 4 times a week, meanwhile for up to 12 months. Before and during training movement of upper ankle joint and ulcer size have been measured, patients' complaints like pain and swelling have been quantitated by means of a scale from 0 (no complaints) to 10 (maximal complaints). Calf muscle pump function has been measured by phlebodynamometry, venous drainage by plethysmography and skin microcirculation by transcutaneous oxygen tension ($tcPO_2$) measurement at distal medial lower limb. 39 patients, 19 women and 20 men, with mean age of 56 ± 9 years have been taking part into the training. At the beginning 12 patients suffered from venous ulcers, 27 from swelling, hypodermitis or dermatoliposclerosis. Before therapy the following mean values were measured: swelling 4,7 ± 2,8 AU; pain 4,7 ± 3 AU; dorsal movement of upper ankle joint 9 ± 11°; plantar movement 32 ± 12°; phlebodynamometry 30 ± 27 mmHg; venous drainage 61 ± 27 ml/100ml/min; $tcPO_2$ 28 ± 19 mmHg. All these values indicate an impaired venous macro- and microcirculatory drainage which caused reduced movement of ankle joint. Physical training lead to improvement of both the clinical situation and the measured parameters on average. Therefore regular physical training should be part of a therapy regimen in CVI.

Effect of dressings on ultrasound transmission

Callam MJ, Marshall I, and Lothian & Forth Valley Leg Ulcer Group

Department of Vascular Surgery, Bedford Hospital, Bedford

Department of Vascular Surgery, Royal Infirmary, Edinburgh

Ultrasound has been shown to have a beneficial effect on tissue healing if given at an appropriate frequency and intensity. A controlled trial in the treatment of chronic leg ulceration showed a significant improvement in the group treated with ultrasound compared to the control group. However the benefit of ultrasound was limited as the probe could only be placed on the area around the ulcer, rather than on the ulcer base itself, as direct application was too painful. A further disadvantage was that the ulcer area had to be exposed for each treatment. A study has been carried out to assess the ultrasonic transmission properties of dressings which would allow regular treatments without disturbance of the wound contact layer and direct insonnation of the ulcer base.

Five dressings of each type were assessed using ultrasound at 0.25 Watts and 1.5MHz; a frequency and power ratio shown to be effective.

Transmission of Ultrasound through Dressings

Dressing	Mean Voltage meas'd	%decrease in intensity	Dressing	Mean Voltage meas'd	%decrease in intensity
None	13.06	-	Granuflex	0.00	100
Coloplast	9.73	44.5	Geliperm	12.47	8.8
Intrasite	3.48	92.9	Silastic Gel	12.49	8.5
Biotrol	0.00	100			

Intensity is proportional to $Voltage^2$

This study shows that either Geliperm or Silastic Gel would be an appropriate dressing during ultrasound treatment

Phlébologie 92. Eds P. Raymond-Martimbeau, R. Prescott, M. Zummo.
John Libbey Eurotext, Paris © 1992, pp. 948-951

Le drainage veineux manuel (méthode C. Garde, Quiberon)

Claude Garde

93, avenue du Bac, 94210 La Varenne Saint-Hilaire, France.

RAPPEL PHYSIOLOGIQUE ET CONCEPT GENERAL.

Le système veineux a plusieurs propriétés et plusieurs fonctions.

C'est un système capacitif réservoir, à basse pression, ayant de larges capacités de soutien et d'adaptabilité.

Il est chargé du drainage et de l'épuration des tissus inondés par le catabolisme cellulaire, de la thermorégulation et de la volémie

Le système capillaire, qui le précède, est lui chargé des échanges sang -> tissu mais aussi tissu -> sang. Les mécanismes de ces échanges sont liés aux lois classiques de l'osmolarité, de la pression oncotique des protéines, des différences de pression capillaro-tissulaire, mais aussi à des phénomènes actifs de résorption (pinocytose).

L'espace interstitiel est le lieu des échanges cellulaires et le berceau de la trophicité cutanée. Faisant office d'éponge, il peut capter l'eau en surchage (non réabsorbée par le système capillaro-veinulaire) et les macromolécules non réabsorbées par le système lymphatique.

Le système lymphatique : adjoint fondamental de l'épuration interstitielle, réabsorbe lui aussi l'eau tissulaire, mais aussi les macromolécules responsables de la pression oncotique et donc de l'oedème inflammatoire. Il existe un lien entre tous ces milieux (veineux, capillaire, interstitiel et lymphatique), c'est le sens circulatoire des liquides (sang, lymphe, eau interstitielle). La pression y joue un rôle prépondérant aidée en cela par les mécanismes précités.

• Que se passe-t-il au nouveau des territoires de drainage ?

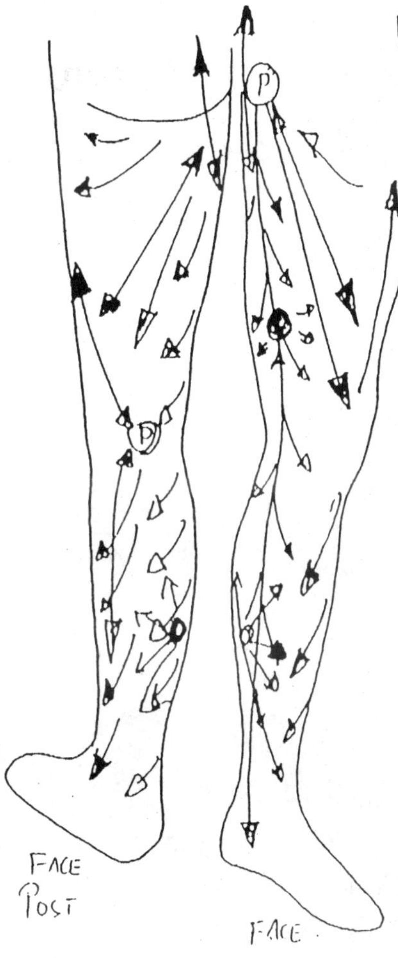

Par les siphons (P) le réseau superficiel est mis en pression, et se dilate suivant les lois de la gravité, mais aussi de la proximité de l'onde de pression.

Si un siphon demeure continent, il agit comme un aspirateur de surface et, finalement minimise la surcharge de pression superficielle en réinjectant le sang à l'intérieur.

Globalement, les veines circulent à contre-sens se remplissant alternativement à chaque contraction musculaire, ou lors de la position immobile prolongée. C'est au niveau des siphons (P) qu'elles sont les plus grosses puis se divisent comme un fleuve et ses affluents mais aussi en boucle de raccordement (schéma 2) (réseau maille). Ceci explique certains échecs thérapeutiques. Cette contre-pression est répercutée au niveau des capillaires du réseau sous-papillaire, de là, naitra l'oedème sus aponévrotique déclive.

PRINÇIPE DE DRAINAGE VEINEUX MANUEL

Le drainage veineux manuel se propose de restaurer un gradient de pression interstitiel, capillaire, veine superficielle, veine profonde de telle façon que, la pression interstitielle soit supérieure à la pression capillaire, supérieure à la pression de la veine superficielle, supérieure à la pression de la veine profonde et que par conséquent les tissus soient épongés de leur masse liquidienne de stase (amélioration du drainage et de l'épuration tissulaire).

Il s'agit donc d'évacuer toute la surface vers la profondeur.

• ***Conditions de faisabilité :***

1) que le pression des veines profondes soit égale ou inférieure à la pression des veines superficielles. Pour cela le patient sera en position allongée, membre en complète relaxation musculaire éventuellement en léger tredelenburg. Dans ce cas PVS = PVP. On demandera au patient de pratiquer une respiration abdominale en faisant simplement fonctionner le diaphragme, afin de créer une pression intrathoracique négative.

2) que la pression des branches et micro-branches soit supérieure à la pression des siphons.

3) que la pression capillaire soit supérieure à la pression des veinules.

Les territoires seront drainés les uns après les autres.

D'abord un massage lymphatique rapide. On commencera par les territoires les plus importants et les plus étendus.

DOS
(Semelle de LEJARS ---> Crosse saphène interne
(Les perforantes COCKET la BOYD la HUNTER
(les périnéales
(La saphène antérieure
(La saphène externe
(La saphène postérieure.

puis : profils (droits = gauche

- drainage du réseau saphène externe de facon confluente (descendant sur la cuisse vers le pli poplité - montant du pied sur la face externe du mollet jusqu'au pli poplité).

puis :

	(La saphène interne ...LEJARS
VENTRE	(Le mollet, la saphène externe (la cuisse).
	(Le GIACOMINI les veines pudendales
	(Les veines de COCKETT

Forme du massage :

Confluant sur le siphon
Confluant par rapport à l'axe veineux.

EXPLICATION SUR LE TERRITOIRE VEINEUX

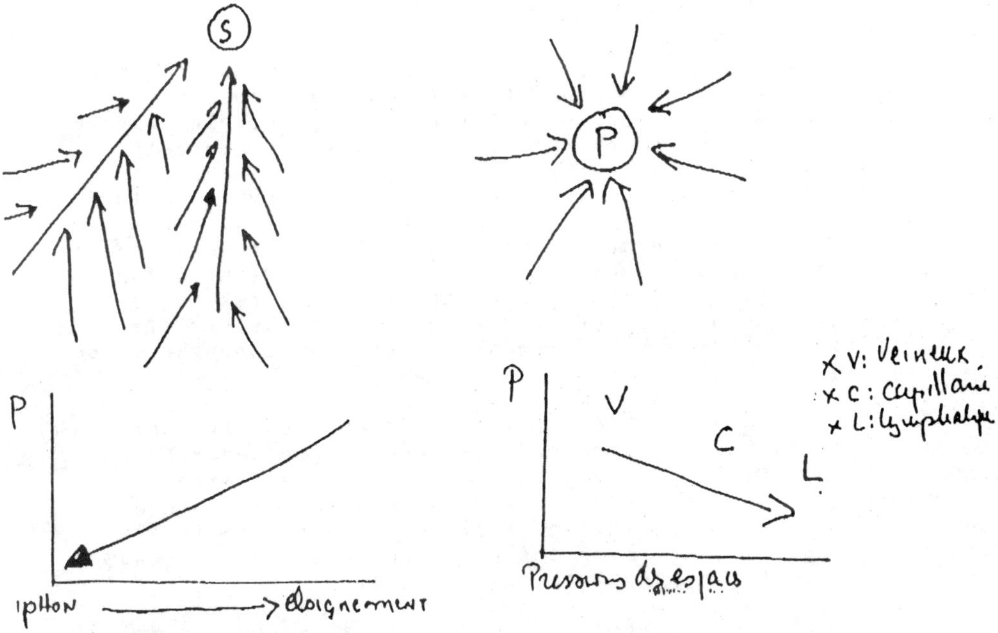

On adjoindra une substance levant le spasme capillaire à titre de produit de massage.

Phlébologie 92. Eds P. Raymond-Martimbeau, R. Prescott, M. Zummo.
John Libbey Eurotext, Paris © 1992, pp. 952-954

Interest of holo-energetic methodology in chronic leg pain

Jean Ratte

Centre Médical Rouleau, 161, avenue Rouleau, 305, Rimouski, G5L 5T3, Québec, Canada.

In a well-equipped metropolitan university center with many specialists, there is a lot of screening before the vascular surgeon sees a patient with chronic leg pain. In private practice since 1973 in a peripheral rural area, we see more leg problems not explained by classical vascular medicine. These complaints, despite normal Doppler and plethysmography since 1975, led us study acupuncture in 1977 and osteopathy in 1984. Persistent leg pain, despite these therapeutic approaches and normal vascular, orthopedic and neurological work-up, prompted us to study holo-energetic methodology which is based on the vascular resonance of the wrist's arteries when different frequencies of the visible electromagnetic spectrum (Wratten-Kodak filters) are brought close to the body.

Each artery, cubital, radial and its first branch in the snuffing-box, has a different resonance's frequency to the photons of the specific filters. Each artery is tuned with a different"program" of the nervous system's computer. Interference between programs produces a longitudinal non linear wave in the wall of the arteries, that is perceived by the examinator's thumb, lying flat on specific spots of the wrist. (1).

These longitudinal intraparietal waves, so called waves of Lamb, are different from the pressure wave and from the velocity waves detected by Doppler. (2,3,4).

A systematic study of this vascular resonance phenomenon between electromagnetic waves and the vascular system allowed Claude Piro and André Secondy from Montpellier (France) to correlate different complaints with the different resonance frequencies. They have been able to devise an organigram systhesizing a vibratory semeiology that is often perturbed in patients with unexplained leg problems.

Although it is not a medical technology, this methodology points out some subtle problems in relation to gravitational waves from the environment, not amenable to classical medicine, and allows their solution.

The understanding of this vascular resonance requires an overview of modern physics. Einstein described the particle-like aspect of the electromagnetic wave (photon) in the photo-electric effect (1905). De Broglie (1924) described the wave like aspect of matter that gave rise to the electron microscope, semi-conductors and informatic. Quantic physics is based on this wave-particle complementarity. The vibratory nature of atoms is used in atomic clocks. The magnetic resonance demonstrates this oscillatory nature of nucleus and electrons which are able to react to and emit radio frequencies detectable outside of the body. (5).

The physics of condensed matter reveals the production of acoustic waves or phonons under the excitation of photons. (6). The supraconductivity of matter and the superfluidity are another index of the wave-like behavior of solid states.

The particle-like behavior of waves of the different fields gives us, besides the well-known photon, the graviton, the gluon and the intermediary or weak vector boson, all quantized aspects of radiative energy.

Previous work in Chronobiology has shown a more complex but similar behavior in living matter at the level of cells, organs, systems and organisms. (7). The surface of all membranes of the body has been estimated to 840 square acres, the surface of Central Park. (8). The length of the whole vascular system has been evaluated to 60,000 miles, two times the circumference of the Earth at the equator. (9). The body acts as a resonant cavity and the arteries act as Fabry-Perot interferometers which amplify the resonance and act also as waves-guides which select the frequencies.

The fractal geometry shows the self-similarity of the vascular system. (10). Already 50 years ago, Leriche said that each segment of artery and vein, in their common sheath, was a miniature heart. This same fractal geometry shows that the area of the whole vascular system is infinite in a finite volume. These geometric considerations explain the possibilities of the vascular system as a resonator and amplifier able of detecting and emitting gravitational interactions that are 10^{38} less intense than electromagnetic interactions. It is our hypothesis that the human body, owing to the vascular system, is able of realising the unification of the four fondamental interactions, looked for by physicists. This work is a forerunner of phlebology of the third millenarium.

References:

1- Claude Piro. Methodologie holo-énergétique. Socapress ed. Perpignan 1991.

2- Robert Lemaire. L'écoulement du sang dans les artères athéromateuses. Essai de biomécanique médicale. Laboratoire L. Lafon ed.

3- R.Comolet. Mécanique expérimentale des fluides. Masson ed. Paris 1969.

4- H.Lamb. Hydrodynamics. 1932. (Reprinted in Dover Publications New-York).

5- David D.Stark, W.G. Bradley Jr. Megnetic resonance imaging. Mosby 1988.

6- C.Kittel. Introduction to solid state physics. 4th ed. Wiley. New-York 1971.

7- J.Ratte, F.Halberg et al. Circadian variation in the rejection of rat kidney allografts. Surgery vol.73, Jan.73.

8- W.Drost-Hansen et al. Liquid Asset. The Sciences. Oct.1989.

9- Steven Vogel. Vital Circuits. Oxford University Press. 1991.

10- B.Mandelbrot. Les objets fractals. 3ième ed. N.B.S. Flammarion 1989.

XIV.
TRAITEMENT CHIRURGICAL
SURGICAL TREATMENT

A.
TECHNIQUES CHIRURGICALES
SURGICAL TECHNIQUES

Phlébologie 92. Eds P. Raymond-Martimbeau, R. Prescott, M. Zummo.
John Libbey Eurotext, Paris © 1992, pp. 959-961

Chirurgie ambulatoire des varices

Jacques Dortu

Société Française de Phlébectomie Ambulatoire, 2, rue des Glières, 74000 Annecy, France.

Les explorations modernes ont fait exploser les conceptions " monolithiques " de l'insuffisance veineuse, trop souvent reduites aux seules saphenes.

Ces explorations ont permis de demembrer la maladie variqueuse, d'en reconnaitre le caractere multiforme et d'en decrire, avec une vision renouvellee, de tres nombreuses variantes anatomiques ou physiopathologiques.

Ces situations , si diverses , reclament des traitements adaptes , personnalises , eclectiques. Les nouvelles techniques d'eveinage ambulatoire apportent une reponse selective et meme superselective a de telles situations.

Enfin, certaines exigences liees a la demande de nos patients, a l'ethique des medecins et aux contraintes sociales obligent:

- A limiter le traumatisme tissulaire lie a nos traitements
- A reduire l'incapacite qui en resulte
- A preserver l'image corporelle de nos patients par une une recherche esthetique attentive.
- A ameliorer nos resultats a long terme

LIMITER LE TRAUMATISME THERAPEUTIQUE

Il convient d'observer quelques regles: instrumentation adaptee, main super-legere, minutie, permettront de menager les divers plans epidermiques, hypodermiques, aponevrotiques et profonds, lors de l'acces aux axes variqueux; Ligatures et bandages enfin, meritent une attention particuliere.

1- Au plan epidermique: les mini-incisions (1-2 cms) seront fermees par sutures allegees. On leur preferera les micro-incisions (1-2 millimetres) qui seront closes par simple rapprochement de leurs levres a l'aide de steristrip.

2- Au plan hypodermique, un bon reperage pre-operatoire permet un abord immediat des varices, une reduction sensible de la dissection perivariqueuse et en consequence, une epargne des tissus adjacents conjonctifs, nerveux ou lymphatiques.

3- Aux plans aponevrotiques et profonds, les memes regles seront observees.

4- L'extraction des varices, troncs et perforantes devra s'accompagner du minimum de delabrement tissulaire .

5- Les ligatures hemostatiques seront reservees aux crosses et emergences des varices suprameliques en racine de cuisse. A ces divers niveaux, en effet, le bandage elastocompressif n'est pas a meme d'assurer une hemostase sure.

Partout ailleurs, par contre, les ligatures hemostatiques seront inutiles, l'hemostase etant parfaitement controlee par le bandage elastocompressif.

6- L'utilisation des methodes de contention se generalisent. Elles sont plus ou moins lourdes et donc plus ou moins contraignantes a mettre en place par le medecin ou a supporter par le malade.

Le bandage elastocompressif de type phlebologique comporte le maximum d'avantages:

- Antalgique par maintien ferme des tissus traumatises
- Anti-inflamatoire par reduction des exsudations sero-hematiques et des ecchymoses, par resorption acceleree des debris cellulo-graisseux.
- Hemodynamique enfin par acceleration importante des flux profonds.

Le bandage elastocompressif superposera successivement:

- une compression selective du lit variqueux
- une compression inextensible (composante hemostatique)
- une compression elastique (composante hemodynamique)

Il resulte de ces regles une reduction considerable des nuisances therapeutiques.

REDUIRE L'INCAPACITE

En cette matiere, la demande de nos patients est de plus en plus claire. Un certain nombre de gestes devront etre mis en oeuvre pour permettre une ambulation immediate, une reprise d'activite professionnelle sous 24 heures et une reprise sportive sous 15 jours.

1- L'anesthesie locale, a la lidocaine avec ou sans epinephrine, **permet seule la mobilisation immediate du patient des la fin de l'intervention.**

Les autres anesthesies, locoregionales, tronculaires, epidurales, provoquent une anesthesie motrice de 3 a 5 heures.

La neuroleptanalgesie ou l'anesthesie generale comportent des contraintes plus lourdes et prolongees.

2- L'allegement du geste therapeutique et le bandage elastocompressif, nous l'avons vu, vont aussi concourir a la reduction de l'incapacite par leurs vertus antalgiques.

PRESERVER L'IMAGE CORPORELLE

Les exigences esthetiques sont maintenant ouvertement formulees par nos patientes (et nos patients). Pour eux, la correction du prejudice esthetique l'emporte souvent sur le souci de rehabilitation fonctionnelle.

Les preoccupations des praticiens et l'evolution technique permettent de concilier esthetique et obligation de resultat et apportent une reponse:

- En cernant avec precision l'espace therapeutique
- En controlant les conditions de cicatrisation epidermique et conjonctives.

En prevenant les reactions disgracieuses secondaires telles que pigmentation ou telangiectasies .

Micro-incisions, main legere, contention efficace, anti-inflammatoires, en reduisant ces risques immediats, allegent les retouches esthetiques ulterieures.

AMELIORER LE RESULTAT A LONG TERME

Apres chirurgie conventionnelle ou sclerose, l'instabilite de certains resultats a moyen ou long terme contraignent a un suivi therapeutique lourd et non denue d'inconvenients:

- Les reinterventions sont sources de stigmates cicatriciels et les scleroses iteratives sources de pigmentations residuelles.
- Elles peuvent favoriser le developpement de telangiectasies diffuses ou l'extension variqueuse a d'autres territoires.

Dans tous ces cas , la responsabilite de telles evolutions incombe a l'inadequation qui s'exprime entre les therapeutiques mises en oeuvre et les caracteristiques de l'insuffisance veineuse a traiter.

Les therapeutiques au protocole trop rigide s'averent , des lors, incapables de s'adapter a l'extreme diversite des situations rencontrees.

Les criteres fondamentaux qui permettent de maitriser de telles situations sont triples :

1- <u>L'analyse exhaustive de l'insuffisance veineuse,</u> clinique, Doppler, echoDoppler, varicographique,fournira les donnees les plus fines sur les conditions anatomiques, morphologiques, hemodynamiques, trophiques de l'insuffisance veineuse.

2- <u>La cartographie variqueuse</u>, document evolutif, permet l'autocritique, par confrontation avec les donnees fournies par un nouvel examen ou par les controles operatoires et post- operatoires.

3- <u>Le bon choix therapeutique</u> enfin, car l'extreme diversite de la maladie variqueuse necessite une demarche therapeutique souple et adaptative et une selection technique avisee .

LES TECHNIQUES D'EVEINAGE AMBULATOIRE

Elles apportent des reponses selectives et meme superselectives a ces diverses situations.

Stripping par invagination, cryochirurgie, phlebectomie ambulatoire, chiva, techniques en evaluation ont en commun d'etre ambulatoires " en temps reel".

Encore faut-il faire le bon choix, encore faut-il aussi maitriser les techniques afin d'en retirer le meilleur profit pour nos malades.

<u>Mais il convient aussi de se rappeler qu'aucune de ces methodes ne peut se pretendre universelle.</u>

Quelques experts dans les techniques d'eveinage ambulatoire vont nous faire profiter de leur grande experience.

Nous avons reserve le maximum de temps pour la discussion .

N'hesitez pas a poser vos questions ; Bien souvent les questions les plus simples sont l'expression de l'interet general .

Phlébologie 92. Eds P. Raymond-Martimbeau, R. Prescott, M. Zummo.
John Libbey Eurotext, Paris © 1992, pp. 962

Place et évolution du traitement des varices par la chirurgie ambulatoire en Suisse

Michel Gross

Avenue de la Gare, 10, 1003 Lausanne, Suisse.

RESUME

Dans l'antiquité gréco-romaine, la chirurgie des varices se pratiquait ambulatoirement.

Au début du XXe siècle, les opérés des varices étaient immobilisés et alités, ce qui favorisa la maladie thrombo-embolique et ses conséquences parfois mortelles.

Pour pallier cet inconvénient, les docteurs Fred BLANCHOD de Lausanne et Karl SIGG de Bâle préconisèrent le traitement sclérosant effectué, évidemment, ambulatoirement.

Actuellement, la chirurgie classique (crossectomie, stripping et incisions étagées) effectuée sous anesthésie générale ou loco-régionale, avec hospitalisation de plusieurs jours, coexiste avec la sclérothérapie, alors que la phlébectomie ambulatoire, sous l'impulsion du Dr Robert MULLER de Neuchâtel, fait de plus en plus d'adeptes dans notre pays.

Des équipes mixtes de chirurgiens, de phlébologues et de dermatologues développent les principes mis en pratique par le Dr Robert MULLER en favorisant de plus en plus le traitement chirurgical ambulatoire des variqueux.

Phlébologie 92. Eds P. Raymond-Martimbeau, R. Prescott, M. Zummo.
John Libbey Eurotext, Paris © 1992, pp. 963

Pins maritimes. Varicosités et veines de drainage

Robert Muller

9, rue du Seyon, CH-2000 Neuchatel, Suisse.

Le sang circule des artérioles dans les capillaires, puis dans les postcapillaires et enfin dans les veines de drainage. S'il y a hypertension dans le réseau veineux, par voie rétrograde, elle dilate les postcapillaires. Leur paroi, réduite à une couche, l'intima, est fragile, sensible à l'équilibre hormonal et aux traumatismes. Ces varices postcapillaires s'appellent en allemand des Besenreiser et en français des varicosités en brindilles de genêt.

L'association des varicosités et des veines de drainage forme le syndrome du pin maritime: Un tronc, des branches, des branchioles, des rameaux dessinés par les veines de drainage et la frondaison des varicosités. De nombreuses mini-perforantes s'étagent de la racine aux rameaux. Il n'y a aucun traitement efficace (durable) des varicosités si on n'élimine pas les veines de drainage, surtout les mini-perforantes.

Parfois, la veine de drainage n'est pas visible, car la perforante arrive de la profondeur au milieu d'une tache de varicosités.

Ces "pins maritimes" sont fréquents. C'est le "pain" quotidien du phlébologue. Il faut surtout éviter tout traitement thermique ou électrique qui fait des cicatrices punctiformes cumulatives. Le pire de tous est le laser.

Dans une séance, on marque les veines de drainage, on les anesthésie, on microsclérose toutes les varicosités par Sclérémo 5 ml + 1 ml Lidocaïne 1% adrénalinée, on élimine par phlébectomie ambulatoire toutes les veines de drainage et on termine le pansement par une forte compression qu'on peut exercer dès le 2ème jour déjà par un bas compressif **VARISMA** classe de compression 3, pendant environ 3 semaines.

Résultats lointains

Si on a exceptionnellement réussi à éradiquer toutes les mini-perforantes, on n'observe pas de rechute, même après des années.

En général, il faut reprendre par microsclérose les varicosités disséminées tous les 1 à 3 ans.

The superficial varices clinical surgery in Italy

Pier Antonio Bacci

Centro di Flebologia - Universita di Siena Italy

The superficial varices of the lower limbs are the expression of various causes; a particular importance have the overweight, the intestinal diseases, the foot, the heredity, the constitutionality, the childbirth and the cutaneous system tone.

And more, over these reasons there can also be some infective, immunity, mechanical or degenerative problems that may damage the walls and the valves causing the varicose disease.

Nowadays in Italy we strongly tend to make a right prophylactic diagnosis to establish if the saphena-femoral crosse is inadequate or imbalanced.

In the first case we can adopt a therapeutical method such as the external anaplasty valve (in various ways) or the perivenous sclerotherapy.

In the second case we should apply a radical crossectomy, the antireflux ligature or the clips, which are all technics used to avoid the saphena-femoral reflux.

The remaining saphenical trunk can be treated both with a wrecker therapy (such as stripping, phlebectomy or cryosurgery) both with a conservative method (such as aimed ligatures, partial phlebectomy, or the two times surgery).

There are some basical lines that always wants the local anaesthesia, early ambulation, complete pre-surgical diagnosis and a therapeutical strategy that's execute for the most part by:

1. The saphena-femoral crosse correction by crossectomy or anaplasty valve or clips.
2. Aimed ligature of the piercings and imbalanced trunks phlebectomy.
3. In the second time correction of a possible damage in the external saphena with micro-phlebectomy and finishing of the small remaining piercings, integrated by sclerotherapy.

Concluding: a perfect diagnosis using bloodless methods and aimed and functional surgical therapies.

Ambulatory surgery in United States

Anton Butic, John J. Bergan

Private Practice

This history and the current use of ambulatory surgery in the treatment of primary varicose veins is outlined. The information is based on personal experience and a survey of physicians of the North American Society of Phlebology and of the Venous Forum.

Day care varicose vein surgery - Audit, logistics and results of a 4-years pilot study

H.J. Schubert

Chirurgische Tagesklinik Traunreut (CTT)

The POSTER shows features of the unit (floor plan, recovery and OP-area, monitoring equipment, staff, etc.) and statistical data (operative spectrum of radical varicose vein surgery, complication and infection rate, hospital transfer and overnight stay rate). Operative techniques as well as the preferable gentle local/i.v. combination sedoanalgesia and perioperative regimen are clearly demonstrated.

Case reports (typical day care examples and follow-ups, photodocumentation of preoperative and intraoperative findings and postoperative results) complete the demonstration.

The poster documentation gives an impressive survey on surgical audit, logistics, preferable methods and results in ambulatory varicose vein surgery based upon a 4-years experience in a pilot freestanding surgicenter project for polyvalent day surgery of an average southern German town of 21,000 inhabitants nearby Munic.

The management of ambulatory varicose vein surgery

H.J. Schubert

Chirurgische Tagesklinik Traunreut (CTT), D-8225 Traunreut, FRG

The VIDEO (VHS) presents the typical day care management of radical elective varicose vein surgery in a freestanding German surgicenter nearby Munic.

The patient is followed from entering the unit, during the pre- and postoperative periods, until leaving the day clinic some hours after the intervention.

Operation technique and the preferable gentle method of combined local/i.v. sedoanalgesta and its positive influence on the patient in the course of the procedure as well as on the postoperative early mobilisation phase are impressively shown.

Phlébologie 92. Eds P. Raymond-Martimbeau, R. Prescott, M. Zummo.
John Libbey Eurotext, Paris © 1992, pp. 966-968

L'esthétisme en phlébectomie ambulatoire (méthode de Muller)

Isabelle Constancias-Dortu, Jacques-Antoine Dortu

2, rue des Glières, 74000 Annecy, France.

* <u>LA PERFORMANCE ESTHETIQUE</u> , par principe , **n'est qu'un sous-produit du geste thérapeutique au cours des Phlébectomies Ambulatoires (P.A.)** .
* **Mais la préocupation esthétique de nos malades n'est pas rare** , même si elle reste informulée (4,5) . **Elle mérite une écoute attentive** et recoit une réponse qui passe par :

  - Le trés normal respect de leur intégrité corporelle
  - Le souçi de minimiser le traumatisme thérapeutique
  - Des artifices techniques
  - L'utilisation de méthodes de contention efficaçes

* Cette réponse est différente selon qu'on pratiquera une P.A. conventionnelle ou une P.A. à visées esthétiques :

DANS LE CAS D'UNE <u>P.A. CONVENTIONNELLE le projet essentiel reste la correction immédiate du trouble hémo-dynamique et la suppression totale du tissu veineux altéré</u> .

DANS LE CAS D'UNE <u>P.A.à VISEES ESTHETIQUES</u> , <u>on s'adresse aux anomalies veineuses ou veinulaires dont les incidences pathologiques ou l'évolutivité sont modestes</u> , <u>voire nulles</u> .

* **Cadre général de la Phlébectomie ambulatoire** (6) :
  - <u>La P.A. a pour objet le traitement des anomalies</u> veineuses superficielles <u>pathologiques</u> .
    Elle devra s'arrêter en territoire sain .
  - <u>Son champ d'action est strictement supra-fascial</u> .
    <u>L'abord des zones sous-aponévrotiques ne concerne pas la P.A.</u> :
    . Jonction saphéno-fémorale
    . jonctions saphéno-poplitées complexes
    . Ligatures sous-aponévrotiques (perforantes)

* **Limites de la P.A. à visées esthétiques :**
  - <u>Parfois</u> , on sera <u>tenté de</u> corriger certaines disgraces physiologiques telles que :

. les veines " apparentes " à travers des épidermes minces . pales . ou chez les sujets maigres .
. Les veines hypertrophiées des manuels . des athlétes des danseurs ...
. Les dilatations veineuses généralisées qui sont le fait des grandes atonies veineuses .

* **La mise en oeuvre de La P.A. à visées esthétiques interviendra :**
  - <u>aprés analyse de la motivation du patient</u>
    . demande expresse
    . rejet de toute autre thérapeutique
    . référence à un résultat connu
  - <u>aprés analyse des facteurs de risque esthétique</u> :
    . qualité de la peau (carnation . texture)
    . anomalies de la pigmentation
    . troubles trophiques
    . anomalies capillaires associées
    . anomalies cicatricielles (chéloîdes,migrations pigmentaires . élargissements cicatriciels)
    . stigmates inesthétiques des traitements antérieurs chirurgicaux ou phlébologiques .
  - <u>aprés analyse du terrain psychologique</u> du patient ?!

* **Caractéres particuliers à la réalisation de la P.A. à visées esthétiques :**

Un certain nombre d'artifices techniques seront exploités :
  - <u>Le marquage</u> sera minutieux : trait ténu et précis
  - <u>L'usage du DOPPLER permettra repérage et marquage des perforantes</u> d'alimentation . Leur tronc et leurs racines devront être emportés .
  - <u>La pénétration trans-épidermique fera appel à des micro-incisions ou à des micro-ponctions</u> :
    . Les micro-incisions seront minimes (1 mm) .
    . les micro-incisions seront toujours sagittales
    . Les micro-ponctions (Aiguille de 11/10°) seront perpendiculaires au plan cutané .
    . Leurs cicatrisations sont comparables .
  - <u>On utilisera les crochets acérés de petites tailles</u> N°1 ou N°2 ;
    La prise de varice restera trés superficielle .
  - <u>On éliminera les debris cellulo-fibreux</u> qui pourraient gêner l'affrontement des lévres de l'incision
  - <u>Le bandage élasto-compressif</u> sera renouvellé lors du 1° pansement et porté quelques jours de plus , si les réactions tissulaires ont paru notables .

* **Les indications de la P.A. à visées esthétiques** porteront principalement (1) :
  - <u>Aux membres inférieurs</u> (3)
    . **Sur les axes d'épuisement capillaro-veinulaires** et en particulier sur leur veinule **" de drainage "** .
    . **Sur les varicoses " pariétales pures "** .
    . **Sur les perforantes insuffisantes alimentant** directement **les formes " télangiectasiques pures "**
    . **Sur les varices à incidence hémodynamique faible .**

. **Sur les varices résiduelles ou ré-évoluées aprés chirurgie** (classique ou autre)

- Aux membres supérieurs et à l'abdomen
  . Le plus souvent sur des varices aprés phlébite superficielle ou profonde
  . Ces indications méritent réflexion , en raison des faibles conséquences hémodynamiques et évolutives de ces varicoses .
- Au visage
  . Sur les réseaux peri-orbitaires ou temporaux

INCIDENTS

* **Les incidents notables sont rares** : Ce sont ceux de la P.A.
* **Mais quelques incidents sont plus regrettables au cours des P.A. à visées esthétiques** ; Ce sont plus particuliérement :
  - Les poussées de télangiectasies , qui sont le fait des terrains peu favorables (érythro-cyanose , capillaroses pré-existantes , cellulite) .
  - Les élargissement cicatriciels chez les sujets présentant une surcharge pondérale , une cellulite .
  - Les migrations pigmentaires peri-cicatricielles .

Ils seront évités (ou limités) en réduisant le traumatisme tissulaire (micro-incisions minimes . main légére) , en prêtant la meilleure attention à la contention (2) et en prescrivant veinotoniques voire anti-inflammatoires .

Ils peuvent être corrigés par des traitements spécifiques.

CONCLUSIONS

La demande esthétique en thérapeutique phlébologique s'affirme de plus en plus . La P.A. (méthode de MULLER) est parfaitement adaptée à satisfaire cette demande .

L'affinement du matériel , du protocole et du geste technique ont permis d'élargir les indications de la méthode au domaine de l'esthétique avancée avec (photo 7) :

* des contraintes particuliérement allégées
* des résultats encourageants pour le praticien
* des résultats satisfaisants pour le patient .

BIBLIOGRAPHIE

1 - CONSTANCIAS-DORTU I. , DORTU J-A.
Indications de la P.A.
Phlébologie , 1987 : 44 (n°4) : p. 671-681

2 - DORTU J. (1987) : Il bandagio elasto-compressivo . In La la flebectomia ambulatoriale . ed. Salus internazionale , p.52-55 . Roma .

3 - DORTU J. (1987) : P.A. ; Approches anatomo-cliniques . Phlébologie 89 , Ed. A.DAVY . R. STEMMER , John Libbey Eurotext ; p.1076-1079 . London .

4 - GUILLEROT E. (1985) : La demande esthétique en phlébologie . Phlébologie . 38 (n°4) : p. 647-651 .

5 - MULLER R. (1985) : L'esthétique en phlébologie . Phlébologie . 38 (n°4) : p. 673-676 .

6 - MULLER R. . BACCI P.A. (1987) : La flebectomia ambulatoriale . ed. Salus internazionale . Roma .

Phlébologie 92. Eds P. Raymond-Martimbeau, R. Prescott, M. Zummo.
John Libbey Eurotext, Paris © 1992, pp. 969-971

Indications de la phlébectomie ambulatoire

Jacques-Antoine Dortu, Isabelle Constancias-Dortu

2, rue des Glières, 74000 Annecy, France.

BREF RAPPEL sur la Phlébectomie Ambulatoire (P.A.) (3 , 8) :

*** La phlébectomie ne retire que des veines pathologiques :**
Elle s'arretera donc en territoire sain .
*** La phlebectomie reste toujours supra-fasciale :**
Elle ne franchira pas le fascia superficialis .

* Anatomie et physio-pathologie des varices ont considerablement progressé graçe aux acquits de la P.A. ;
Ses indications en sont devenues plus préçises .

LES INDICATIONS ANATOMIQUES AU MEMBRE INFERIEUR (2, 3)

1) - Les indications à la cuisse porteront :

Sur les axes longitudinaux (1) Fig. 1
- Récidives tronculaires saphéniennes aprés chirurgie .
- Saphénes accessoires antérieures ou postérieures échappées au stripping ou autonomes , alimentées par des perforantes insuffisantes (grand adducteur ou Dodd) ou une varicose honteuse externe .
- Saphénes internes sans insuffisance ostiale alimentées par une perforante pathologique sous-jacente à la crosse
- Veines crurales externes .

Sur les axes collatéraux (4, 2) Fig. 2
- Veine oblique antero-latérale de cuisse
- Veine de Cruveilhier
- Veine de Giacomini
- Veines crurales postérieures

Sur les reflux de racine de cuisse (4, 6) Fig. 5
- **Varicoses " supra-mêliques "** tributaires de veines inguinales , honteuses externes , hémorroïdaires ou fessiéres

2) - Les indications à la jambe porteront :
Sur les axes longitudinaux Fig. 1
* Saphéne interne * Veine de Leonard (5) * Saphéne tibiale
Ces 3 réseaux (Trépied saphénien) pouvant avoir évolué :

> de manière autonome . à partir de perforantes insuffisantes primitives (Boyd , antérieure du jumeau interne , Cockett par voie antigravitationnelle)
> ou aprés chirurgie (stripping court ou long) à partir des mêmes perforantes insuffisantes laissées en plaçe .

* Varices peroniéres superficielles
* Saphéne externe à crosse simple

Sur les axes collatéraux (4)

* Veine oblique antero-externe de jambe (5)
* Anastomotiques gémellaires externes et internes (supérieures ou inférieures) .
* Reticulum antéro-externe de jambe ou reticulum du mollet

Sur les reflux de creux poplité (4)

* Varices " **fosse poplitée** " internes et externes (supérieures ou inférieures) .

3) - Les indications au genou et au pied porteront sur :

* le cercle peri-rotulien et les varices pré-rotuliennes
* les réseaux infra-malléolaires et dorsaux du pied .

4) - Les indications physio-pathologiques porteront sur les varices compliquées de troubles trophiques :

* Ulcéres (de préference aprés cicatrisation)
* Hypodermites scléreuses (aprés réduction par botte)

INDICATIONS AUX MEMBRES SUPERIEURS . Elles porteront :

- Sur des réseaux variqueux aprés phlébite superficielle ou profonde .
- Indications rares et à discuter , compte tenu des faibles , sinon inexistantes , conséquences hémodynamiques de ces varicoses et de leur évolutivité quasi-nulle .

INDICATIONS SUR LES TERRAINS POST-PHLEBITIQUES

- La P.A. sera mise en oeuvre sur les varices post-phlébitiques aprés exploration minutieuse des réseaux profonds et superficiels par Doppler . echographie , plethysmographie .
  * Les varices et leurs perforantes insuffisantes , dont l'exclusion au cours des épreuves fonctionnelles aura démontré la nocivité , pourront être phlébectomisées .
  * Les axes superficiels vicariants seront respectés .
  * Des précautions devront être prises (Bilan biologique . compression prolongée , héparines bas poids moléculaire)

INDICATIONS SUR LES PHLEBITES SUPERFICIELLES (8)

- Les thromboses post-sclérothérapiques et hémorroïdaire externe sont une bonne indication de P.A. : La sédation des troubles inflammatoires est spectaculaire et immédiate .

INDICATIONS ESTHETIQUES (7)

- **Les indications esthétiques enfin** concerneront les P.A. portant sur les anomalies veineuses ou veinulaires dont les incidences pathologiques ou l'évolutivité sont modestes , voire nulles , et porteront principalement :

* Au membre inférieur
  . sur les axes d'épuisement télangiectasiques , et en particulier sur leurs veines dites " de drainage " .
  . sur les varicoses " pariétales pures "
  . sur les perforantes insuffisantes alimentant directement les formes " télangiectasiques pures "
* Au membre supérieur et à l'abdomen
  . le plus souvent sur des varices secondaires
* Au visage
  . le plus souvent sur les réseaux peri-orbitaires ou temporaux

- La décision sera prise sur un certain nombre de critéres :

*** - consentement " eclairé " du patient**
*** - appréciation des " facteurs de risque généraux "**
*** - appréciation des " facteurs de risque esthétique "**
*** - et sur le terrain psychologique du patient .**

CONCLUSIONS

Les évolutions techniques ,l'exploitation systématique des moyens d'exploration fonctionnelle et une expérience de plusieurs décennies , ont permis :

* de reconnaitre l'extrême diversité des indications de la P.A.
* d'en préciser la place au sein de l'arsenal thérapeutique de l'insuffisance veineuse .

BIBLIOGRAPHIE

1 - CONSTANCIAS-DORTU I. , DORTU J.A.
Indications de la Phlébectomie Ambulatoire .
Phlébologie , 1991 : 44 , n°3. : 671-681 .

2 - DAVY A. , OUVRY P. , GUENNEGUEZ H.
A propos des saphénes antérieures de cuisse
Phlébologie , 1985 . 38 : 279-292

3 - DORTU J. : La phlébectomie ambulatoire .
Impact Médecin , 1990 . 64 , XII-XV

4 - DORTU J. : Anatomie clinique des collatérales variqueuses
Phlébologie , 1989 ; 42 (n°4) : 553-566

5 - DORTU J. : Anatomie clinique de la veine de LEONARD ;
Communication à la II° journée de l'Union Internationale de Phlebectomie Ambulatoire 28/30-10-1989 (Arezzo) .

6 - DORTU J. , DORTU J.A.
Les veines honteuses externes : Etude anatomo-clinique .
Phlébologie , 1990 ; 43 (n°2) : 329-355

7 - GUILLEROT E. : La demande esthétique en phlébologie .
Phlébologie , 1985 ; 38 : 647-651 .

8 - MULLER R. BACCI P.A. : La flebectomia ambulatoriale .
Salus édit. , Roma , 1987 .

Phlébologie 92. Eds P. Raymond-Martimbeau, R. Prescott, M. Zummo.
John Libbey Eurotext, Paris © 1992, pp. 972-974

La phlébectomie ambulatoire (méthode de Muller) : ses raisons, sa place dans le traitement des varices

Jacques Dortu

Société Française de Phlébectomie Ambulatoire, 2, rue des Glières, 74000 Annecy, France.

Depuis MAYO (1905) Et BABCOCK (1906), depuis SICARD (1926) et TOURNAY (1929) , chirurgie et sclerose representent les methodes de reference dans le traitement des varices .

Protocoles precis , pratique scrupuleuse , mise en oeuvre par des specialistes avertis , debouchent sur des resultats de qualite .

Dans un tel contexte, pourquoi recourir a la Phlebectomie Ambulatoire (P.A.) ?

- L'analyse sincere de certains resultats peu satisfaisants (varicoses residuelles, evolutions ulterieures, repermeations, stigmates cicatriciels regrettables, pigmentations inesthetiques etc...) montre les limites de la chirurgie et de la sclerose .
- Les progres de l'analyse de l'insuffisance veineuse superficielle permettent de mieux apprecier les frontieres de la chirurgie conventionnelle ou de la sclerose et permettent une approche de plus en plus selective des varices qui offre une place naturelle a la P.A. .
- Les preoccupations des malades desireux d'eviter une anesthesie generale ou une reduction de leur activite professionnelle, leurs exigences esthetiques, meritent une ecoute attentive et une reponse qui passe par l'utilisation de l'anesthesie locale, la limitation du traumatisme therapeutique, une contention methodique (aux vertus hemostatique, antalgique, hemodynamique), le respect de leur integrite corporelle et enfin une ambulation immediate .

La P.A. s'integre d'une maniere correcte dans un tel cadre .

GESTE TECHNIQUE SIMPLE, LA P.A. OBEIT A UN PRINCIPE SIMPLE :

- Sous anesthesie locale, la P.A. doit emporter les trajets variqueux, les perforantes insuffisantes et les autres sources de reflux qui les alimentent .
- L'eradication du tissu veineux malade doit etre totale .

Cette notion d'eradication totale est d'une grande importance; La negliger expose d'emblee a la persistance d'ectasies variqueuses et, a terme, a la re-evolution quasi constante des reseaux variqueux laisses en place, meme si un affaissement spectaculaire avait pu etre note d'emblee .

Ces re-evolutions sont en relation avec l'ouverture de nouvelles perforantes insuffisantes sur les axes variqueux negliges, parfois rapidement (2-3 jours) ou dans les mois suivants .

Il convient d'epargner les reseaux veineux sains ; Mais en ce qui concerne les saphenes variqueuses, on preservera seulement les saphenes stheniques " a parois musclees " (les saphenes astheniques "a parois delabrees" devront etre eradiquees en totalite, leur capacite de recuperation, et donc leur utilisation, etant illusoire) .

Geste simple la P.A. permet d'echapper aux lourdes contraintes de l'hospitalisation ; Mais en contre-partie, une parfaite connaissance de l'anatomie moderne des veines superficielles, un usage rigoureux des methodes d'exploration, et l'acquisition d'une solide maitrise technique seront indispensables pour faire face a l'extreme diversite des situations que l'on rencontrera.

BILAN PRE-DECISIONNEL DE LA P.A.

L'analyse clinique apportera des arguments precieux a la mise en oeuvre de la strategie therapeutique.

Les analyses para-cliniques sont incontournables .

- L'analyse Doppler etablira un trace fidele des reflux tronculaires et localisera les perforantes insuffisantes axiales ou extra-axiales .
- L'analyse Echo-Doppler appreciera la morphologie des perforantes et explorera les secteurs delicats inguinaux et poplites .
- La varicographie explorera les situations complexes au niveau supra-melique, inguinal ou poplite .

TECHNIQUE : L'INSTRUMENTATION

Elle sera simple, mais un peu de sophistication ne nuit pas :

- Lame de bistouri No 11 ou aiguille de 22 g 1/2
- Crochets aceres de MULLER-DORTU No 1, 2 et 3 a manches ergonomiques
- Crochets mousses de DORTU-RAYMOND MARTIMBEAU de 2 mms et 2,5 mms
- Mini-stripper externe de DORTU, en tire-bouchon
- Mini-stripper interne de DORTU, a double olive, permettant des Mini-VAN DER STRICHT.
- Quelques pinces , LERICHE, SEMKIN, Micro-mosquito

TECHNIQUE : LE PROTOCOLE OPERATOIRE sera strict et comprend :

- Marquage cutane des varices, reperees manuellement, visuellement et au Doppler
- Aseptie chirurgicale
- Anesthesie locale a la lidocaine 1% epinephrine ; On controlera, par aspiration, que l'injection poussee le long du trajet variqueux, n'est pas intra-vasculaire .
- La penetration cutanee se fera par micro-incisions de 1 a 2 mms ou par micro-ponctions a l'aiguille .
- A l'aide des crochets, les troncs variqueux seront extraits en totalite, ainsi que les perforantes qui les alimentent.

- La fermeture cutanee se fera par simple rapprochement des levres des micro-incisions a l'aide de micropore .
- Le bandage elasto-compressif superposera
  * une compression selective du lit variqueux
  * une compression inextensible , inamovible
  * et une compression par bande bi-elastique qui sera portee du lever au coucher .

SUITES ET SURVEILLANCE comportent :
- Lever et marche immediats
- Reprise de l'activite le jour meme ou le lendemain
- Reprise sportive le 14eme jour

- On supprimera les compressions selectives et inextensibles le lendemain, les micropores le 7eme jour et la compression elastique le 14eme jour

- Antalgiques et anti-inflammatoires seront prescrits a la demande; Les heparines bas poids moleculaire seront prescrites en cas de facteur de risque .

LES INCIDENTS NOTABLES sont rares :
- Hematomes tres localises
- Reactions cellulitiques apres resections difficiles
- Varicosites reactionnellles sur les terrains defavorables
- Dysesthesies des regions malleolaires ou pedieuses

LES INDICATIONS DE LA P.A. portent essentiellement sur les varicoses ne dependant pas d'une insuffisance ostiale ou d'un reflux mineur :

*** Varicoses des axes longs :** recidives sapheniennes tronculaires apres chirurgie, varices des veines saphenes accessoires et crurale externes, de la saphene tibiale, de la veine de Leonard, de la peroniere superficielle , de la saphene externe .

*** Varicoses des axes collateraux :** varices obliques antero-externes de cuisse et de jambe, des veines de Cruveilhier ou de Giacomini ou varices gemellaires .

*** Localisations particulieres :** reflux de racine de cuisse non sapheniens (inguinaux, honteux externes, hemorroidaires ou fessiers), varices "fosse poplitee", varices du genou , de la cheville , du pied .

*** Indications de caractere particulier (indications mesurees)** varices avec troubles trophiques (hypodermites, ulceres), varices post-phlebitiques (apres analyse precise), indications esthetiques (decision mesuree) des membres, des bras, du visage .

EN CONCLUSION, la <u>bonne analyse</u> de l'insuffisance veineuse debouche sur les <u>bonnes indications</u> .
<u>Les bonnes indications font les bons resultats</u> :

- **bons resultats anatomiques**
- **bons resultats fonctionnels**
- **bons resultats esthetiques**
- **et stabilite a long terme** ou sous l'influence des facteurs d'evolution (grossesses) n'excluant cependant pas une surveillance reguliere ou la sclerose reprend ses droits, ne necessitant que peu de sceances, a faible concentration .

Phlébologie 92. Eds P. Raymond-Martimbeau, R. Prescott, M. Zummo.
John Libbey Eurotext, Paris © 1992, pp. 975

Microsurgical phlebectomy for the treatment of varicose veins

H.A.M. Neumann

Department of Dermatology, University Hospital Maastricht, P.O. Box 5800, 6202 AZ Maastricht, The Netherlands.

Sclerotherapy is nowadays widely used for the treatment of varicose veins, specially reticular and sidebranch types.

However some anatomic sides as the foot, the ankle and the popliteal fossa are rather difficult and sometimes even dangerous to treat by sclerotherapy.

Robert Müller, a Swiss dermatologist, developed in the fifties a technique by which it is possible to remove varicose veins through multiple micro incisions. This technique is time consuming but leads to excellent cosmetic results.

From the mid seventies Müller introduced his technique also for the treatment of varicose veins of the foot and other difficult areas.

In the last years we build up our own experience with this technique on patients with varicose veins in these areas. We find this technique extremely helpful for the treatment of this type of varicoses. Optimal results for patients with varicose veins can be obtained by using a good combination of: high selective surgery to eliminate major reflux, sclero-compression therapy and percutaneous microsurgical phlebectomy. The choise of treatment is based on good clinical investigation as well as non-invasive instrumental diagnostics like light reflection rheography and Doppler ultrasound.

Treatment starts with elimination of the major points of reflux, as the femoral saphenous and popliteal saphenous junction. The next step will be sclerotherapy and/or microsurgical phlebectomy of saphenous veins and sidebranches. Finally we treat the reticular varicosis and venectasien by sclerotherapy.

AMBULATORY PHLEBECTOMY WITH MULLER TECHNIQUE.

F. Pollice.

Cardiovascular Surgery, University of Bari.

The management of uncomplicated varicose veins(V V)continues to be controversial.Cosmesis, short recovery time,early return to work,cost and recurrence rate are critical determinants. Classic radical stripping procedures are associated with long convalescence,occassionally unacceptable scarring and 10-15% recurrence.Compressive sclerotherapy with high ligation, has at best a 25% recurrence.This preliminary report describes the technique of stab evulsion phlebectomy originally described in 1975,but now resurrected and performed in an ambulatory outpatient setting.In an office setting and under 0.50% Xylocaine local anesthesia and following meticulous marking of all V V,a high ligation of the source of reflux is done.All V V are evulsed with the Müller hooks through multiple(25-40)mini stab incisions(11 blade)2-3mm long,which are closed with steristrips.In the period 1981-1990,574 patients have been operated on.Post operative pain was minimal and easily controlled by NSAID.All immediately resumed normal daily activities.Cosmesis was excellent in all cases.This technique effectively and completely removes all varicosities,eliminates the proximal source of reflux previously mapped with Doppler ultrasound,disconnects the distal perforants,yet leaves in situ the undamaged trunk veins,which can be used as future vein grafts.Recovery is immediately,cosmesis and patient acceptance excellent and expected recurrence,less than 10%.This manuscript will illustrate the technical details of the ambulatory stab evulsion phlebectomy.

Phlébologie 92. Eds P. Raymond-Martimbeau, R. Prescott, M. Zummo.
John Libbey Eurotext, Paris © 1992, pp. 977

D'autres armes thérapeutiques dans le traitement chirurgical de la maladie variqueuse essentielle. La phlébectomie ambulatoire

Gérard Lange

Tours, France.

Cette technique de stripping par invagination sur fil, décrite et réalisée depuis plus de vingt ans par le Professeur Jean VAN DER STRICHT (Belgique) est ici traitée de façon à reconnaitre à la fois les sites d'injection de l'anesthésie qui est soit purement locale, soit locale associée à une neuroleptanalgésie.

La crossectomie qui est réalisée de manière tout à fait conventionnelle comme dans tous les autres cas de stripping, est décrite succinctement, et la technique de guidage du fil puis de stripping par invagination y est montrée de manière précise sans omettre les difficultés qui peuvent être rencontrées, de rupture ou de téléscopage anormal de la veine.

Les résultats immédiats et à moyen terme sont également recueillis de façon à ne pas avoir une approche trop précaire de la technique.

Rappelons ici, qu'il s'agit d'un stripping et bien que la technique soit réalisée sous anesthésie locale, elle nécessite un arrêt de travail qui peut être racourci ,mais qui reste néanmoins constamment supérieur ou égal à un semaine.

VARICOSE VEIN AVULSION AS OUTPATIENT SURGERY

Germano Lucertini and Attilio Misuri

Cattedra di Chirurgia Vascolare - Università degli Studi di Genova (Italia)

Value of saphenous collaterals avulsion through short skin incisions is well proved. This technique, described in Europe firstly by Muller, is currently used as complementary procedure of saphenous vein stripping. It can be performed as alone technique for outpatients. Avulsion of saphenous collaterals was performed in 96 outpatients (10 males and 86 females, aged 18 to 64 years). This technique usually requires local anaesthesia, rarely general anaesthesia. After avulsion of varicose veins the skin incisions were not sutured and were dressed in sterile fashion. An elastic bandage was applied. All patients can walk immediately after the treatment. The technique has indications for isolated varicose veins, also dependent from one incompetent communicating vein, and for residual varicose veins after saphenous vein stripping. The procedure was well tolerated and can be complicated in some cases by small haemorrhages, spontaneously solved. The results were satisfactory as functionally as well cosmetically in each case. Based on our experience, varicose vein avulsion for described indications is considered by us as preferential treatment, alternative to sclerotherapy and ligation and division of venous collaterals.

Phlébologie 92. Eds P. Raymond-Martimbeau, R. Prescott, M. Zummo.
John Libbey Eurotext, Paris © 1992, pp. 979-981

Modern surgery of varicose veins : removal of branches by crochet hook

Tamás Sándor, Imre Jakab, Gábor Turcsányi

Department of Surgery, Teaching Hospital, Semmelweis Medical University H-1125, Budapest, Kútvölgyi út 4., Hungary.

SUMMARY

Basic principles of modern surgery of varicose veins - crossectomy, stripping and deep ligation of the incompetent perforating veins - are well established. However, the removal of the secondary branches can be carried out in different ways. A crochet hook was used for this purpose. A minute stab incision of 3-5 mm was made over the tensed vein with a fine pointed scalpel and the branch was pulled out by a sterile crochet hook. The varicose channel was caught, dissected and spun out. The vein can be followed by its traction till a new mini incision is required. 501 operations were performed with this technique. Minimizing the size of the incisions not only reduced the postoperative pain and the recovering time but provided an excellent cosmetic result as well.

INTRODUCTION

In Hungary the varicose veins of the lower limbs have been operated with the old Trendelenburg-Madelung method by generations of surgeons resulting a 56-65 % recurrence rate. New trends in varicosity surgery started only in the late seventies.

Nowadays the basic principles of the operation are well established. These are: crossectomy, stripping and ligation of the incompetent perforating veins. However, the removal of the secondary branches can be carried out in different ways including the simple thorough excision, the use of the Klapp's, or the Smetana's knives and the application of the different phlebo-extractors and phleboaspirators as well. We applied a simple crochet hook for this purpose.

MATERIAL AND METHODS

From September 1987 till October 1991 501 patients, 175 men and 326 women were operated. Age ranges from 22 to 76 years: mean 43 years.

Operative technique

1. Crossectomy

Skin incision was made in the groin fold. The great saphenous vein was tied flush at the femoral vein and dissected with ligation and division all the groin tributaries.

2. Stripping

The Nabatoff stripper was introduced in the great saphenous vein at the medial side of the internal malleolus. The trunk vein was stripped always from above downwards.

3. Ligation of the incompetent perforating veins

At the ankle region in the Linton line the incompetent Cockett's perforators and the other incompetent perforating veins were exposed by a skin incision of 10 mm and ligated subfascially.

4. Removal of side branches by crochet hook

A minute stab incision of 3-5 mm was made over the tensed vein with a fine pointed scalpel. A sterile crochet hook was introduced trough the stab into the subcutaneous tissue and the branch was pulled out. With the help of fingertip the vein can be felt and found more easily. Then the venous channel was caught with two mosquito forceps, dissected and the vein stumps were spun out and extracted in both directions. The vein can be followed by its traction till a new mini incision is required. This way long tortuous veins could be removed. A single fine stich was enough for skin closure.

RESULTS

Compared to the Trendelenburg-Madelung operation and other traditional techniques a significant reduction of postoperative pain was observed. The majority of the patients did not need any analgesic therapy. With compression bandages the patients were mobilized at the evening of surgery or, if peridural or spinal anaesthesia was used, the following day. Later the mini stab incisions became practically invisible. Haematomas and small local infections were seen in 10 cases. 2 cases of calf thrombosis were cured by anticoagulant therapy. Small recidives in 11 cases (2,1%) could have been treated easily either by sclerotherapy or by using again the crochet hook.

DISCUSSION

Hook technique for varicosity operations has been used in Switzerland from the middle of the eighties (Oesch and Fischer, 1987). Várady reported excellent cosmetic results with fine phleboextractors (Várady, 1988). Radisic (1987), Fratila and Rate (1989) and Scuderi (1990) applied also mini-, or micro-interrupted incisions to removal of varicose veins. Acsády (1986) recommended the crochet for side branch, reticular and spider web varicosity and also for local recidives. Especially when female patients are operated, apart from the functional result the cosmetic success is also of great importance. With the interrupted micro stab incisions using a simple crochet hook, the rough operative scars can be avoided.

CONCLUSION

The removal of the varicose veins by crochet hook not only improves the cosmetic result but reduces the postoperative pain and the recovering time as well.

REFERENCES

Acsády, Gy. (1986): Exhairesis of the varicose veins by crochet hook. In The diseases of the veins and their treatment, ed. A.Nemes, p.96. Budapest: Medicina (In Hungarian)

Fratila, A. - Rate, E. (1989): La phlebectomie moderne. In Phlebologie'89, eds. A.Davy, R.Stemmer, pp.1063-1065. London, Paris: John Libbey and Co.

Oesch, A. - Fischer, C. (1987): The removal of varicose veins by mini stab incisions: a promising new surgical method. In Abstr. of IV. European-American Symposium on Venous Diseases, p.10.1., Washington, D.C., U.S.A.

Radisic, J. (1987): Perkutane Varizenexhairese - ein neues chirurgisches Verfahren der Beinvarikose. Phlebol. u. Proktol. 16: 115-119.

Scuderi, A. (1990): Surgery of the varicose veins by mini- or micro-interrupted incisions and pst-surgical bandages with elastic stockings, In Abstr. of V. European-American Symposium on Venous Diseases, p 4D6, Vienna, Austria.

Várady, Z. (1988): Microchirurgischen Phlebextraktion nach Várady in der Varizenchirurgie. Phlebo. Internationales Diskussionsblatt.1:8-9.

Phlébologie 92. Eds P. Raymond-Martimbeau, R. Prescott, M. Zummo.
John Libbey Eurotext, Paris © 1992, pp. 982

The treatment of the varicous syndrome by an aesthetical surgery

Angelo Scuderi, Helio Nigri

« Inspecmoc », Inst. Soroc. de Pesq. de Molestias Circulatorias, Caixa Postal 493, Sorocaba 18001 SP, Brasil.

The authors show in this video the technique of varicous surgery that they use normally in their clinic with local anaesthesia and interrupted mini incisions with mini hooks or crochet needles. This technique is used also with epidural anaesthesia when the "stripper" of the saphena vein is required. Just after the surgery they don´t use the traditional bandages anymore. They uses directly above the skin the elastic stockings. With this bandaging technique they have advantages over the traditional technique in the physiological and aesthetical topics. The time of recovery was shortened. The technique of bandage doesn´t require special handcraft -anyone can do it-. The healing of the small incisions are easier and better. The post-surgical oedema is avoided. The conclusion is that with this technique of surgery and bandage the authors had better results than the traditional method.

Phlébologie 92. Eds P. Raymond-Martimbeau, R. Prescott, M. Zummo.
John Libbey Eurotext, Paris © 1992, pp. 983-985

Un « crochet » phlébodisséqueur dans la chirurgie des varices

R. Bisacci, A. Colasanti, G. Genovese

Istituto di Clinica Chirurgica Generale, Università degli Studi di Perugia, Italia.

La chirurgie traditionnelle des varices s'est récemment enrichie de techniques complémentaires qui en réduisent la difficulté et qui en facilitent l'exécution. La demande incessante de traitements avec des buts esthétiques a fait répandre la technique de la phlébectomie par des mini-incisions, soit dans le cabinet de consultation (phlébectomie selon Muller) soit comme un moment complémentaire aux interventions de stripping (phlébectomie par des mini-incisions ou phlébectomie esthétique). La phlébectomie par des mini-incisions permet l'ablation des veines variqueuses et des perforantes incontinentes (à l'exception de la crosse, de la spahène au niveau de la cuisse et des grosses perforantes incontinentes), sans devoir recourir aux points de suture, cela représente una valable alternative à la saphénectomie "plurisegmentaire", où l'on recourt à plusieurs incisions cutanées qui parfois aboutissent à des cicatrices inesthétiques.
Pour améliorer cette technique, nous avons réalisé un nouvel instrument qui réunit les caractéristiques du crochet de Muller et du phlébodisséqueur, et qui permet, à travers la mini-incision, de s'accrocher et donc d'isoler du tissu sous-cutané des segments de veines, en réduisant radicalement le nombre de mini-incisions que l'on doit effectuer sur la peau.

MATERIELS ET METHODES

Notre crochet phlébodisséqueur est composé d'une tige en acier trempé de 15 cm de longueur et de 1,5 mm de diamètre qui s'emboîte dans un manche où elle est introduite de façon que la partie de l'instrument utilisable soit réglée par l'opérateur.
A son extrémité la tige se termine par deux spirales, une plus ample que l'autre qui donne à cette extrémité la forme d'un anneau ouvert, la partie terminale de l'anneau ouvert est à forme de crochet. Les spirales de l'instrument sont aplaties et émoussées le long du bord supérieur pour faciliter la dissection.
Le diamètre de l'anneau ouvert qui résulte de la succession des spirales a été réalisé avec des mesures de différents calibres (2,5 - 3 - 3,5, 4 mm) (Fig.1).
Après la mini-incision cutanée l'instrument est utilisé comme crochet pour repérer la veine qui est ensuite repérée avec la

pince Mosquito (Fig.1) et puis tendue et amenée à l'extérieur selon la technique décrite par Muller. Le crochet est ensuite introduit dans la mini-incision pour encercler la veine avec una manoeuvre de vissage et puis l'extrémité en forme d'anneau est poussée sous la peau pour isoler le vaisseau repéré. Pour cela le bord émoussé du crochet est très utile.
L'opérateur règlera la longueur de la tige selon la longueur de la veine à isoler (Fig.2, 3).

DISCUSSION

La nécessité de faciliter l'ablation de longs segments de varices et de réduire le nombre de mini-incisions a poussé à la réalisation de cet instrument.
La technique classique de la phlébectomie selon Muller prévoit l'ablation des veines repérées avec une manoeuvre de tension avec la pince Mosquito, aussi bien directement qu'avec une manoeuvre d'enroulement sur la pince. Cette technique peut être aisée dans certains endroits (intérieur de la cuisse) ou difficile dans d'autres (genoux), en outre elle est peut être compliquée aussi bien à cause de la fragilité de la paroi veineuse qu'en présence de varices déjà soignées avec une thérapie sclérosante.
Le nouveau crochet phlébodisséqueur permet de repérer et d'accrocher de façon adéquate la veine à soigner, en position pour l'entourer en pénétrant à travers la mini-incision; grâce à sa forme en spirale notre instrument permet de disséquer de longs segments de veines. L'action phlébodisséquant est semblable à celle réalisée avec d'autres instruments (anneau de Mayo, phlébodisséqueur de Corcos, etc.) mais elle se distingue de ceux-ci par la possibilité d'être utilisée comme crochet et par le fait de pouvoir pénétrer à travers les mini-incisions pour isoler les veines repérées.

FIG.1

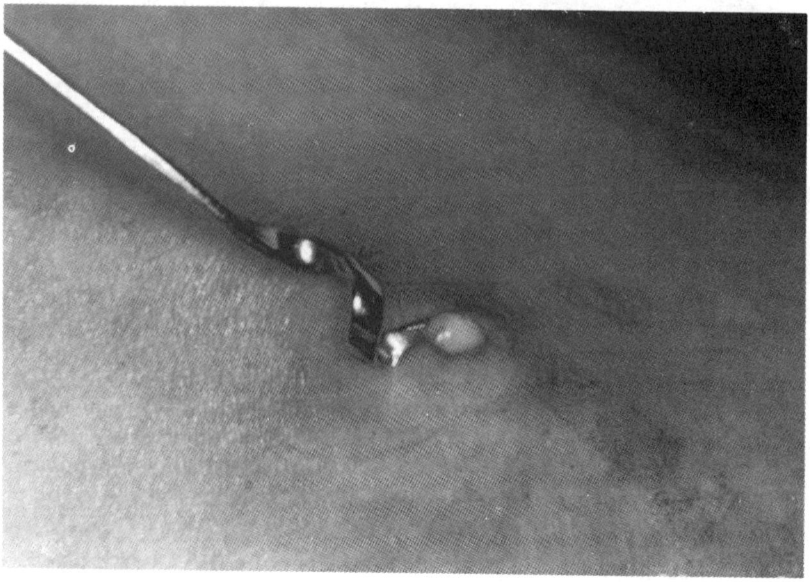

FIG.2

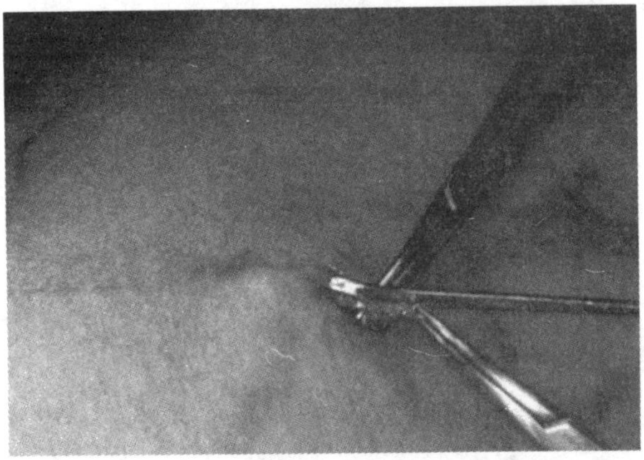

FIG.3

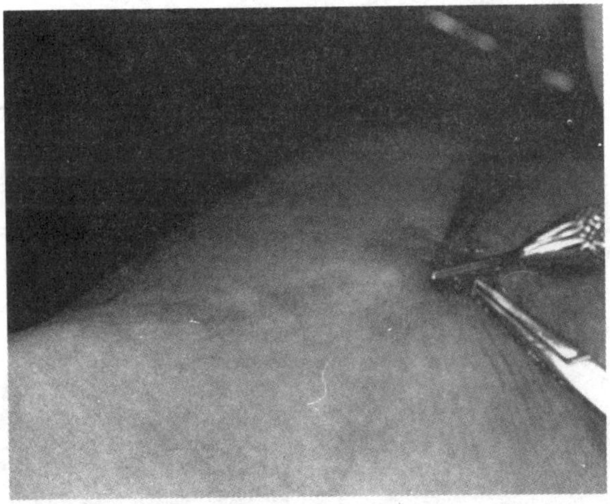

BIBLIOGRAPHIE

1) BACCI P.A.: *L[illegible] ambulatoriale (secondo Muller).* Atti Congresso Internazionale Terapia Chirugica e Sclerosante. Cortona 16 - 19 aprile 1986.

2) BRACALE G.C., BERNARDO R., SELVETELLA L., PORCELLINI M., SCAGLIONE E.: *Terapia chirurgica complementare, Corso di aggiornamento varici degli arti inferiori e sindrome post-flebitica.* 90 Congresso SIC Roma 1988.

3) CORCOS L., PERUZZI G.P. et al.: *Radical cosmetic surgery of varicose veins of lower limbs.* Actes X Congrès Mondial Union Internationale de Phlébologie, Strasbourg 25-29 settembre 1989.

4) DEI SANTI V., BOSELLI C., et al.: *Nuovi orientamenti in tema di chirurgia delle varici. Flebectomia ambulatoriale secondo Muller.* Flebectomia estetica. Act chir. italica 44, fasc. 5., 1988. varici reticolari. *Act. chir. italica 44, fasc.5, 1988.*

5) *FRATILA A., RABE E.:* La phlébectomie moderne. *Actes X Congrès Mondial Union Internationale de Phlébologie, 1063-1065. Strasbourg 1989.*

6) *MULLER R.* : Traitement des varices par la phlébectomie ambulatoire. *Med. et Hyg., 28n, 1424, 1970.*

Phlébologie 92. Eds P. Raymond-Martimbeau, R. Prescott, M. Zummo.
John Libbey Eurotext, Paris © 1992, pp. 986-988

Un artifice de guidage des strippers rigides. Application à la phlébectomie ambulatoire de la saphène interne

N. Fays, J. Fays

40 avenue Foch, 54000 Nancy, France.

Il est admis couramment que la phlébectomie de la saphène interne est "réservée" au Chirurgien (MULLER)(2)). Cependant quelques auteurs (DORTU (1), TRAUCHESSEC (3), VERGEREAU (4))ont démontré que le stripping de cette veine pouvait être réalisé selon les principes de la phlébectomie ambulatoire. Dans cette optique, nous avons mis au point un artifice de "pilotage" des classiques strippers rigides à boule au moyen d'un guide d'angiographie. Ce matériel va permettre de pousser facilement le stripper, en toute sécurité et sans risque de fausse-route, et de minimiser les incisions cutanées.

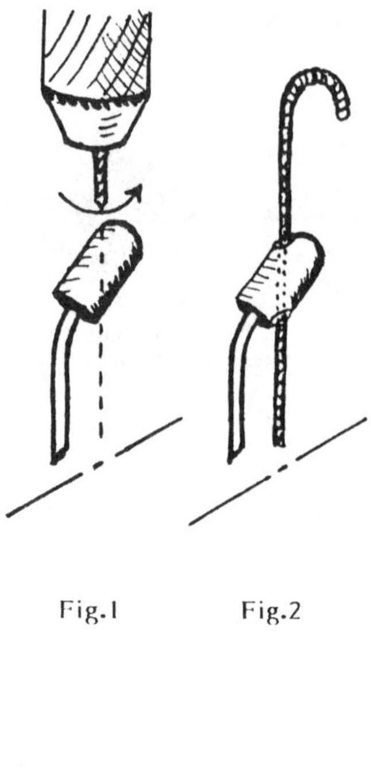

Fig.1 Fig.2

I . MATERIEL ET METHODE

L'instrumentation, en dehors de celle couramment utilisée en phlébectomie ambulatoire, comporte deux éléments fondamentaux :

- un stripper rigide aux extrémités garnies d'un embout cylindrosphérique, enbout dans le grand axe duquel nous avons foré une lumière longitudinale de 1mm. de diamètre (Fig.1);
- un guide à ressort en "J" de cathétérisme vasculaire que l'on enfile dans la lumière de l'embout pour servir de tuteur au stripper (Fig2.) lorsqu'on l'introduit et le propulse dans la saphène.

La préparation du patient est identique à celle d'une phlébectomie ambulatoire : désinfection de tout le membre inférieur, marquage cutané du trajet saphénien, le long duquel est effectuée une anesthésie locale à la xylocaïne bicarbonatée.

Le protocole opératoire se divise schématiquement en trois temps:

1. Introduction du stripper

La veine saphène interne est abordée à la face supéro-interne de la jambe. Par une micro-poncture, le vaisseau est extrait au moyen du crochet de Muller sur lequel on pratique au bistouri une veinotomie. Par cet orifice le guide d'angiographie est introduit et on le pousse jusqu'à sa palpation au dessus du pli de l'aine. Le guide, en raison de sa conformation en "J" et de sa souplesse, glisse dans les sinuosités veineuses et n'a aucun tendance à s'introduire fortuitement dans les veines afférentes. L'extrémité libre du guide est ensuite enfilée dans la lumière de l'embout perforé du stripper et on pousse la tige de cet instrument jusqu'à ce qu'on palpe son extrémité au niveau de la crosse de la saphène.

2. L'abord de la crosse

Grâce à l'embout du stripper, palpé facilement au triangle de Scarpa, on détermine avec précision la projection cutanée de la crosse de la saphène sur laquelle on réalise au bistouri une ouverture cutanée de 6mm. de long environ; cette voie d'abord très limitée est généralement suffisante pour réaliser la crossectomie. Par cet orifice on introduit un petit dissecteur vasculaire qui, manipulé comme un crochet de Muller,(2) permet d'extraire la veine. On recherchera également toutes les collatérales qui s'abouchent à ce niveau. Par une petite veinotomie sur le guide, bien visible grâce à la transparence de la paroi veineuse, on retire l'extrémité distale du guide à la pince à disséquer. En poussant sur le manche du stripper, l'embout s'extériorise sans problème par la petite ouverture cutanée, alors que, sans l'artifice du guide, l'extraction au doigt d'un stripper rigide impose une incision cutanée plus étendue et un geste plus laborieux. On réalise ensuite une triple ligature transfixiante de la saphène, le plus loin possible en aval, ainsi qu'une ligature-section de toutes les collatérales accessibles.

3. L'extraction de la saphène

Après avoir fixé par une double ligature la saphène au stripper, on sectionne cette veine au ras de l'embout. Il suffit alors de tirer sur la tige de cet instrument pour extraire la veine par invagination.
Le suites opératoires sont des plus simples. Après avoir posé un point de suture cutané sur la contre-incision de l'aine, on installe un pansement compressif hémostatique.
Le patient est autorisé à quitter le cabinet médical, 20 minutes après la fin de l'intervention. Soulignons que, comme toute phlébectomie ambulatoire, ce geste n'implique pas d'arrêt de travail.

II . RESULTATS

Nous n'avons réalisé jusqu'à ce jour que 25 phlébectomies de la saphène interne par cette méthode avec un recul de 3 mois à 4 ans. Ce sccore est sans doute très faible mais nous sommes très économes de saphènectomies dont les indications sont pour nous les suivantes :

-Varicose marquée avec stase veineuse importante de ce territoire

-Reflux saphénien massif prouvé par échodoppler, voire phlébographie dynamique.

Nous n'aons jamais constaté d'échecs ou d'incidents, en particulier pas d'hémorragie importante ni de troubles sensitifs. Les cicatrices cutanées sont pratiquement invisibles quelques semaines après l'intervention.

On peut reprocher à ce procédé d'oublier parfois de ligaturer certaines collatérales de la crosse, surtout s'il existe des afférentes sous-aponévrotiques. En fait la ligature de tous ces vaisseaux, établie classiquement comme un dogme, est-elle justifiée. Le récente communication de DORTU (1) est loin de confirmer cette théorie.

EN CONCLUSION ce procédé d'éveinage de la saphène interne est moins lourd que les autres techniques de stripping. Les risques de fausses-routes ou d'échecs sont peu probables. Il apparait qu'il peut être réalisé par tout praticien fervent de la phlébectomie ambulatoire.

BIBLIOGRAPHIE

(1) .DORTU J. (1992).Phlébectomie ambulatoire de la crosse de la saphène interne. La "crossectomie sus-faciale". *Réunion de la Société Française de Phlébectomie Ambulatoire du 20 mars 1992 à Paris*. A paraître.

(2) .MULLER R. . (1987). La phlébectomie ambulatoire. *Helv. chir. Acta* . 54, 555-558

(3) .TRAUCHESSEC J.M.VERGEREAU R.(1992). La "Gévaudanaise". *Réalités thérapeutiques en Dermato-Vénéréologie*.16, 20-27

(4) .VERGEREAU R, TRAUCHESSEC J.M. .(1990). Eveinages sur tige. *J. Méd. Esth. et Chir. Derm.* 17, 125-131

Phlébologie 92. Eds P. Raymond-Martimbeau, R. Prescott, M. Zummo.
John Libbey Eurotext, Paris © 1992, pp. 989-991

Phlébectomie esthétique de la saphène externe

Robert Vergereau*, Jean-Marc Trauchessec**

** Centre Médical Ambulatoire « Les Champs Élysées », 12, avenue de la Gare, 63130 Chamalières-Royat. ** 25, rue de la Faisanderie, 75116 Paris, France.*

La phlébectomie esthétique de la saphène externe variqueuse est présentée selon deux méthodes : endo-éveinage et exo-éveinage.
La phlébectomie de la saphène externe pose le problème technique (1) de son éveinage et celui esthétique de la diminution de la cicatrice du creux poplité.
Nous pratiquons les phlébectomies de la saphène externe (5) sous anesthésie locale (3) qui offre deux avantages :

- perception des sensibilités proprioceptives profondes que le patient peut, et doit, signaler,
- déambulation immédiate au sortir du bloc diminuant le risque thrombogène post-opératoire.

L'endosaphénectomie utilise un éveineur semi rigide, tige métallique de longueur variable jusqu'à 50 cm, terminé à chaque extrémité par une ogive variant de 2,5 mm à 4,5 mm de diamètre (6). Chaque ogive est angulée à 135° par rapport à la tige, opposée symétriquement l'une par rapport à l'autre.

L'exosaphénectomie utilise des crochets dits de MULLER (4) tels qu'ils ont été améliorés selon VERGEREAU.

TECHNIQUE DE L'ENDOSAPHENECTOMIE

La saphène externe est isolée en arrière de la malléole externe. La tige est introduite dans la lumière variqueuse puis délicatement poussée jusqu'au creux poplité où elle est extériorisée à la peau. Une ligature à la base de l'ogive permet l'endo-éveinage par invagination ou par pliage pariétal en accordéon.

En cas de rupture variqueuse en milieu de mollet, une troisième incision courte retrouve la tige et utilise l'autre ogive vacante pour l'éveinage du trajet restant.

TECHNIQUE DE L'EXO-SAPHENECTOMIE

La saphène externe est isolée le long de son tronc. Par une courte incision de deux millimètres, le crochet charge les tissus fibreux sous cutanés qui sont sectionnés dans et sur le coude du crochet. Au niveau de l'aponévrose, le crochet effectue l'opération identique pour la perforer. A travers la solution de continuité, le crochet charge la varice saphène externe. Si le nerf saphène externe est stimulé, le crochet modifie l'orientation de son incidence pour agripper le tronc veineux. L'exosaphénectomie peut ainsi éveiner les dédoublements saphéniens externes (2), les récidives variqueuses ampullaires après crossectomie (8).

La jonction saphénopoplitée est interrompue au ras de la veine poplitée par une torsion circulaire sans ligature ni une seule goutte de sang évacuée.

Les suites opératoires sont relativement simples (7). Les complications limitées à des dysesthésies peu fréquentes spontanément résolutives. La cicatrice dans le creux poplité mesure 1 cm en cas d'endo-éveinage et 2 à 3 millimètres, en cas d'exo-éveinage, garantissant le résultat esthétique de l'intervention;

Références :

1. FURDERER C.R. et al. (1986) :
"Les crosses saphéniennes : Anatomie et concepts thérapeutiques";
Phlébologie ; 39 ; (1) ; 3 - 14.

2. GILLOT C. (1987) :
"Anatomie chirurgicale des perforantes de la jambe";
Phlébologie ; 40 ; (3) ; 563 - 574.

3. LAREDO J.C. (1988) :
"Alternatives thérapeutiques en phlébologie";
La vie médicale ; N. 4 ; 182 - 183.

4. MULLER R. (1970) :
"Traitement des varices par la phlébectomie ambulatoire";
Médecine et Hygiène ; 28 ; p. 1424.

5. MULLER R. (1966) :
"Traitement des varices par phlébectomie ambulatoire";
Phlébologie ; 19 ; (4) ; 277 - 279.

6. VERGEREAU R. & TRAUCHESSEC J.M. (1990) :
"Eveinages sur tige";
J. Méd. Esth. et Chir. Derm.;
Vol; XVII ; N° 66 ; 125 - 129.

7. VERGEREAU R. & TRAUCHESSEC J.M. (1990) :
Lettre à la rédaction "Nouvelles techniques d'éveinage";
Phlébologie ; 43 ; N° 2 ; 357-359.

8. VERGEREAU R. & TRAUCHESSEC J.M. (1992) :
"Eveinage ambulatoire : pièges anatomiques" ;
Réalités thérapeutiques en dermatovénérologie ;
N° 16 ; 28 - 35 (1ère partie).

Phlébologie 92. Eds P. Raymond-Martimbeau, R. Prescott, M. Zummo.
John Libbey Eurotext, Paris © 1992, pp. 992-993

Phlébectomie du pied

Robert Vergereau*, Jean-Marc Trauchessec**

** Centre Médical Ambulatoire « Les Champs Élysées », 12, avenue de la Gare, 63130 Chamalières-Royat. ** 25, rue de la Faisanderie, 75116 Paris, France.*

La phlébectomie du pied par exo-éveinage présente des caractéristiques particulières liées à l'anatomie topographique et à la compression sélective du pansement. Sans en être une indication particulière (1), les veines du pied bénéficient des avantages de la phlébectomie (5).

Au pied, l'on préfère parler de veines dilatées que de varices, les valvules étant anatomiquement réduites et non fonctionnelles.
De nombreuses perforantes relient le système veineux superficiel à l'abondant système veineux profond. La perforante la plus volumineuse se situe souvent dans le premier espace interosseux.
La perforante sous malléolaire interne émerge à l'aplomb du paquet vasculonérveux tibial postérieur, présente des circonvolutions multiples allongeant considérablement son trajet. Les veines malléolaires externes sont accompagnées des filets nerveux sensitifs du nerf saphène externe responsable de dysesthésies le long du bord externe du pied.

Sur le coup de pied, les filets nerveux sensitifs cheminent en position sus aponévrotique, immédiatement au contact et en dessous des veines à exo-éveiner.

La technique d'exo-éveinage (2) est celle de la phlébectomie ambulatoire décrite par MULLER (3), pratiquée avec la sécurité de l'anesthésie locale (8).
L'agrippage, à travers la solution de continuité, doit parfois être relativement profond, proche d'éléments nobles.
La laxité cutanée favorise, par glissement de la peau, la dissection des veines sur des trajets allongés évitant la multiplicité des solutions de continuité.

La compression sélective du pansement atteint les plus hautes pressions (6). Le bandage comporte deux étages compressifs dont le deuxième, maximum la première journée, sera diminué ensuite pour éviter les phénomènes de névrite.

L'oedème résiduel dure plus longtemps que dans les phlébectomies d'autres topographies (4). Le recours à une compression prolongée et à des drainages lymphatiques sera poursuivi jusqu'à restitution ad integrum.

L'observance des nécessités intrinsèques de la phlébectomie podale garantit un résultat fonctionnel et esthétique gratifiant pour les patients (7).

Références :

1. CONSTANCIAS-DORTU I. (1987) :
"Indications thérapeutiques de la phlébectomie ambulatoire".
Phlébologie ; 40 ; (4) ; 853 - 858.

2. MAULER T. (1983) :
"Phlébectomie ambulatoire";
Thèse Lausanne - Suisse.

3. MULLER R. (1978) :
"La phlébectomie ambulatoire";
Phlébologie ; 31 ; (3) ; 273 - 278.

4. TRAUCHESSEC J.M. & VERGEREAU R. (1987) :
"Suites opératoires après phlébectomie ambulatoire";
J. Méd. Esth. et Chir. Derm. ; Vo. XIV ; N. 56 ; 337 - 343.

5. TRAUCHESSEC J.M. & VERGEREAU R. (1991) :
"La phlébectomie" - Tempo Médical ; N. 426 ; 25 - 29.

6. VERGEREAU R. (1985)
"Phlébectomie ambulatoire";
J. Méd. Esth. et Chir. Derm.; Vol. XII ; 46 ; 109 - 113.

7. VERGEREAU R. & TRAUCHESSEC J.M. (1987) :
"Varices : Intervention en ambulatoire";
Le Généraliste ;N. 909 ; 8 - 12.

8. VIDAL-MICHEL J.P et Al. (1989) :
"L'anesthésie locale au cours de la phlébectomie ambulatoire : appréciation du risque par dosage de la lidocaïnémie";
Congrès Mondial de Phlébologie ;
Editions John Libbey Eurotext Ltd ; N. 403 ; p. 1118.

Les varices du pied

Dr. méd. Jean Parvulesco

Clinique La Rosiaz, CH-1009 Pully/Lausanne

L'atteinte du pied par la maladie variqueuse est fréquent et invalidante tant sur le plan de la gêne fonctionnelle que sur celui de la gêne esthétique.

Les rares moyens thérapeutiques proposés jusqu'ici pour les varices du pied sont apparus comme inefficaces ou dangereux.

C'est la raison qui nous a déterminés à faire une analyse approfondie sur ce sujet ignoré par tous les traités de phlébologie et d'apporter notre technique chirurgicale («La phlébextraction segmentaire étagée des varices») à l'aide de patients porteurs de varices du pied.

Pour plus de précision, voir notre livre intitulé «Les varices du pied de la chirurgie à l'esthétique», Édition Arnette, Paris, 1991, où notre expérience est exposée en détail.

Phlébologie 92. Eds P. Raymond-Martimbeau, R. Prescott, M. Zummo.
John Libbey Eurotext, Paris © 1992, pp. 995-997

Exo-éveinage esthétique des veines du visage

Jean-Marc Trauchessec*, Robert Vergereau**

** 25, rue de la Faisanderie, 75116 Paris. ** Centre Médical Ambulatoire « Les Champs Élysées », 12, avenue de la Gare, 63130 Chamalières-Royat, France.*

L'exo-éveinage esthétique des veines du visage devient un nouveau champ thérapeutique de la phlébologie et, en particulier, de la phlébectomie (3).
Nous devons à Robert MULLER (2) de nous avoir montré pour la première fois le résultat d'un exo-éveinage esthétique d'une veine de la paupière inférieure.
La demande esthétique apparaît, nous devons apporter des solutions (5).

La pratique des exo-éveinages au visage (6) nécessite une connaissance précise de l'anatomie dermatologique veineuse et nerveuse.

Les veines cutanées du visage se drainent :

- dans la veine temporale superficielle pour les veines de la région temporo-frontale ;
- dans la veine ophtalmique supérieure pour les régions centro-frontales et de la racine du nez via les veines sustrochléaires et angulaires ;
- dans la veine ophtalmique inférieure pour les veines de la paupière inférieure ;
- dans la veine faciale pour les territoires jugaux ;

Les veines ophtalmiques supérieures et inférieures sont en rapport avec le sinus caverneux et le sinus ptérygoïdien.

Les veines dermiques du visage sont en rapport avec des trajets nerveux sensitifs et moteurs.
Les nerfs sensitifs couvrent la région périorbitaire :

- Nerf ophtalmique V3 pour le front et les paupières supérieures,
- Nerf maxillaire supérieur V2 pour les paupières inférieures.

Les nombreuses anastomoses entre ces deux territoires palient à d'éventuelles sections de filets sensitifs.
Les nerfs moteurs dépendent de la branche temporofaciale du VII. Le rameau frontal sous croise constamment les veines verticales de la queue du sourcil. Les rameaux palpébraux sous croisent les veines cutanées obliques de la région palpébrale inféro-externe.

La section de ces rameaux et de l'anastomose palpébrofrontale peut laisser une parésie sans suppléance.

La technique opératoire (1) se déroule en phases codifiées :
- Repérage permanganaté des trajets veineux.
- Anesthésie locale ou tronculaire.
- Solution de continuité sans bistouri (4).
- Agrippage de la veine au moyen d'un crochet fin, sous grossissement optique de 3.
- Extraction veineuse par exo-éveinage à la pince fine (7).
- Pansement compressif le long des trajets exo-éveinés. Aucune ligature ni coagulation n'est nécessaire.

Nous n'avons eu aucune complication dans notre série inaugurale de 34 patients.

Ainsi pratiqué, l'exo-éveinage esthétique des veines du visage ne laisse aucune trace visible, à la grande satisfaction des patients.

Références :

1. GUILLEROT F. & DAVY A. (1987) :
"Technique de la phlébectomie ambulatoire"
Phlébologie ; 40 ; (4) ; 859 - 863.

2. MULLER R. (1989) :
"L'esthétique en phlébectomie ambulatoire"
J. Méd. Esth. et Chir. Derm.
Vol XVII ; N. 62 ; 155 - 158.

3. TRAUCHESSEC J.M. et al. (1988) :
"Les phlébectomies ambulatoires";
Bulletin d'esthétique dermatologique et de cosmétologie - N° 42 - p. 55 à 60.

4. TRAUCHESSEC J.M. & CHOUKROUN P.L. (1989) :
"Phlébectomie ambulatoire";
Congrès Mondial de Phlébologie ;
Editions John Libbey Eurotext Ltd ; N. 389 ; p. 1081 . 1082.

5. TRAUCHESSEC J.M. & VERGEREAU R. (1990) :
"Aesthetic Phlebectomy";
Communication au XIth Congress of the International Society for Dermatologic Surgery.
Florence ; 103.

6 TRAUCHESSEC J.M. (1991) :
"Eveinage Esthétique du visage";
Réalités thérapeutiques en Dermato-Vénérologie ;
N. 7 ; 70.

7. TRAUCHESSEC J.M. (1991) :
"Phlébectomie des veines esthétiques du visage";
Abstract Dermato ; N° 129 ; 32.

Phlébologie 92. Eds P. Raymond-Martimbeau, R. Prescott, M. Zummo.
John Libbey Eurotext, Paris © 1992, pp. 998-1001

Cryosurgery of varicose veins

Claude Garde

93, avenue du Bac, 94210 La Varenne Saint-Hilaire, France.

Cryosurgery of varicose veins has been performed since 10 years [1,2], been a relatively new technique. It presents some advantages when compared to classical therapeutic regimens for varicose veins:

- it is easily applied and well tolerated by the patient,
- it is a safe technique,
- it exhibits good cosmetic results.

Materials and methods

In a period of 6 years more than 800 patients with insufficient long, short and in some cases anterior saphenous veins have been treated by cryosurgery [3]. Sixty per cent of the patients have been followed up for detecting long-lasting results. A fine 50 cm-long closed metallic tube adequate to be inserted in the vessels has been used as a cryoprobe. Circulation of nitrous oxide, used as refrigerant, in the probe is switched on by a trigger (fig. 1). The probe contacts tissue at a temperature of -80°C. Before inserting the cryoprobe the sapheno-femoral and the sapheno-popliteal junctions as well as all tributaries have to be classically ligated and interrupted under local or regional anaesthesia and aseptic conditions (figs. 1,2). The lower part of the vein remains open with two forceps and the cryoprobe is inserted in the lumen of the vein after a freeze-test at its visible part.

Results

By inserting the cryoprobe from the groin up to the knee and from the knee up to the ankle the vein valves were destroyed.

Cryostripping was applied by a single incision of the saphenous vein at the groin or at the popliteal fossea, inserting the cryoprobe in the vein lumen and freezing it at the lower part of the vein [4,5]. The vessel wall became weak at this level and broke. This result could be sometimes better obtained by a 2 mm-large incision and cutting the vein on the probe edge. A strong attachment of the probe on the vessel wall was achieved and the vein was returned inside-out by slow removing of the cryoprobe upwards.

Cryosclerosis was performed by a 10 seconds-freeze time every 2 cm of the vein [4]. The cryoprobe was slowly removed out after each freezing session.

The results of cryosurgery of varicose veins were generally comparable to those obtained by classical sclerotherapy or ambulatory phlebectomy. About 4% of the patients treated by cryostripping recurred due to a perforating vein or a new sapheno-femoral junction [6,7]. On the other hand, more than 20% of the patients with cryosclerosis presented recurrences because of recanalisation of the long saphenous vein. In all these cases the diameter of the vessel was >7 mm before operation. The recurrent patients were successfully treated by local sclerotherapy (thrombovar 1%) or ambula tory phlebectomy.

Immediate complications of cryostripping consisted of haematomas along the internal part of the leg in about 30% of the patients usually disappearing into one month, pigmentation and induration under the knee especially when the vein was broken without ligation and surgical division, and rare disorders of the local nerves after long freezing under the knee. On the other hand, the complications of cryosclerosis were haematomas along the internal part of the thigh with pigmentation in less than 5% of the patients disappearing usually into a period of 6 months and rare disorders of the local nerves with resisting pain in 3 patients, which eased in 1-2 years. Local necrosis was observed in one patient [3].

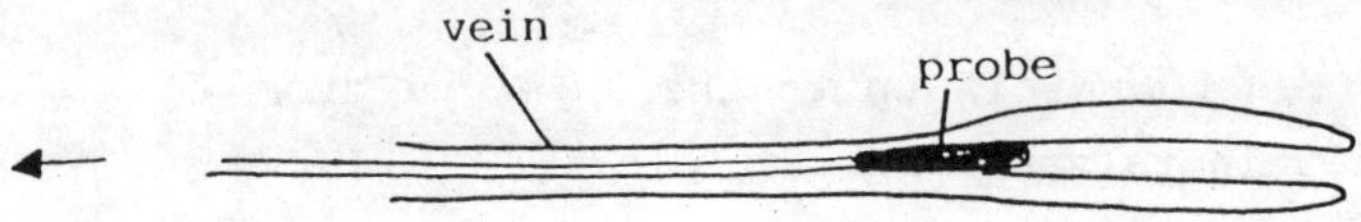

CRYOSTRIPPING

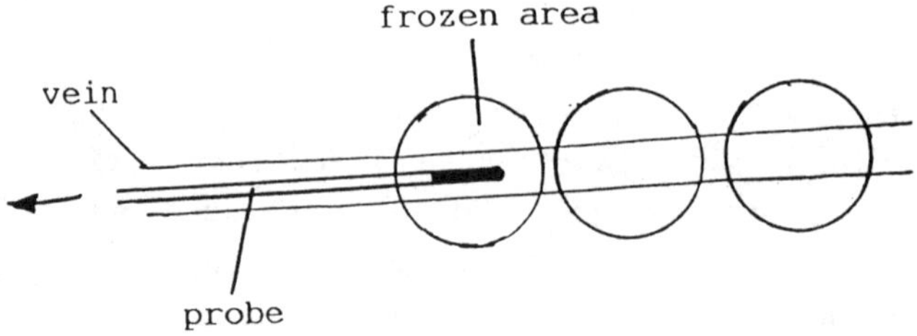

CRYOSCLEROSIS

Legends to the figures

Figure 1. The cryoprobe is introduced as far as possible in the lumen of the long saphenous vein.

Figure 2. The cryoprobe is slowly removed in order to froze or to strip the vessel.

Discussion

Treatment of varicose veins aims to stop blood circulation in the vessel. For this purpose mechanical techniques e.g. removing veins by stripping or interrupting the sapheno-femoral and sapheno-popliteal junctions by phlebectomy, and chemical methods e.g. occlusion of vessels by sclerotherapy have been mostly used. Alternative regimens such as electrocoagulation and cryotherapy are based on the effects of temperature on the tissues and represent the physical technique. By electrocoagulation the veins are occluded, by cryosurgery two effects can be produced: vein occlusion after denaturation of the endothelial cells of the vessel wall after intracellular cristallisation because of quick freezing, or vein stripping after strong attachment of the cryoprobe to the vessel [1,2].

Cryostripping presents some advantages when compared to surgical short stripping. A single upper incision is needed and only few haematomas are observed, resulting in continous work without intermissions for compression.

Indications for cryosurgery of the varicose veins can be:

- insufficient long saphenous with a diameter <6mm with or without varicose tributaries,
- old or adipose patients or patients under coumarine treatment [4,5],
- patients not willing to get general anaesthesia.

In conclusion, cryosurgery is a fast and safe method for the treatment of selected varicose disorders exhibiting good cosmetic results [6,7].

BIBLIOGRAPHIE

1- LE PIVERT P et al. Cryochirurgie à l'aide de sondes souples semi-rigides originales : rapport préliminaire. Lyon Medical 1981;245:207-211.

2- LE PIVERT P. Basic considerations of the cryolesion. in ABLIN JA ed. Handbook of cryosurgery, New York, Marcel Dekker inc.1980.

3- GARDE C, JANNEAU D. La cryochirurgie des varices. Artères et veines 1988;1:26-34.

4- GARDE C. Cryosurgery of varicose veins. Proceeding of the national conference of the Canadian Society of Phlebology. Banff, Alberta, 1988(abstract).

5- GARDE C. New methods in phlebology. First meeting of International Academy of Phlebology. Montreal 1990(course).

6- GARDE C. New methods in phlebology. Proceeding of the I.A.P. Second meeting, Houston 1991;course in phlebologia:417-419.

Phlébologie 92. Eds P. Raymond-Martimbeau, R. Prescott, M. Zummo.
John Libbey Eurotext, Paris © 1992, pp. 1002-1004

Intérêt de la cryochirurgie dans le traitement des varices des membres inférieurs

J.M. Coget - J.P. Millen

- historique,
- but de la méthode :
  - dans la chirurgie,
  - dans la sclérose.
- matériel,
- technique,
- discussion :
  - avantages,
  - inconvénients.
- intérêt régional,

comparatif :
  - chirurgie par stripping normal,
  - chirurgie sur fil,
  - chirurgie par phlébectomie.

Aprés une phase d'engouement, nettement médiatisée, voici quelques années, la technique de cryochirurgie et de cryosclérose des varices semble subir comme toute technique nouvelle, une certaine éclipse, et ceci malgré les publications volontiers optimistes des adeptes de cette méthode.
Nombreux sont les chirurgiens, qui ont taté de cette technique, mais sans s'y attarder et ont rapidement abandonné devant les servitudes qu'elle pouvait entraîner, restant alors à leurs techniques premières, plus faciles, moins astreignantes que la cryochirurgie inovante, donc rompant avec leurs habitudes - reste aussi que cette technique n'a été qu'une modification de la technique classique d'éveinage, la cryosclérose étant rapidement abandonnée car l'irritation induite au niveau de l'endothélium n'était que temporaire et n'engendrait pas de scléroses comme celles provoquées par les produits chimiques, mais une inflammation rapidement réversible, rendant ainsi le résultat final aléatoire dans les quelques mois suivant l'application.
Les techniques d'éveinage se sont depuis quelques années modifiées. La durée d'hospitalisation d'une part, s'est particulièrement réduite, pour aboutir à des séjours monojournaliers en Hôpital de jour, les anesthésies d'autre part, fonction bien entendu des techniques et surtout des anesthésistes eux-mêmes, qu'il s'agisse de l'anesthésie générale ou régionale, telle que la péri-durale, cédent le pas à l'anesthésie locale. Toutes ces évolutions nécessitent alors une moindre agressivité sur la veine et les tissus périveineux. Le ramonage par cathéter métallique, muni d'une grosse boule aux bords tranchants a vécu, aux dépends de l'invagination sur fil, pronée par VANDERSTRICHT depuis plus de trente ans. La cryochirurgie rentre dans ce cadre particulièrement élègant d'éveinage, pour qui sait l'utiliser dans ce sens.
Nous pensons toutefois que la bonne manipulation des cryodes, donne des possibilités que ne permettent pas les techniques classiques.
Quel est le matériel utilisé ?
Nous employons un matériel simple, commercialisé par les Etablissements.
Les sondes sont reliées à un détendeur, le produit de congélation est le PROTOXYDE D'AZOTE.
Les sondes sont de plusieurs types :

- les unes sont à bout émoussé, rond, de 2 1/2 mm d'épaisseur, longues de 80 cms. La congélation s'opére sur les trois derniers centimétres uniquement. La température atteinte en 3 secondes est de l'ordre de - 50°. Cette sonde permet de cathétériser la saphéne interne sur les deux tiers de son tiers, parfois complétement chez les sujets de petite taille. Nous utilisons aussi la sonde à bout pointu, plus fine, elle est plus petite, mais présente les mêmes caractéristiques de congélation que la précédente. Elle peut plus facilement transperçer la veine, mais surtout son diamétre inférieur permet de cathétériser des veines plus fines et parfois tortueuses.

Technique :

- le cathétérisme avec la sonde à bout émoussé est relativement facile sur toute la longueur de la veine, surtout lorsqu'elle est rectiligne.

Deux possibilités s'offrent alors au chirurgien :

- soit arracher le segment inférieur sans faire d'incision,
- soit faire une ligature du segment distal de la veine avant de réaliser l'éveinage.

Cette seconde alternative à notre faveur, car elle permet de :

- mieux contrôler l'hémostase du segment distal,
- de faciliter l'extraction de la veine avec un temps de latence de congélation normale permettant un éveinage par invagination et respectant les tissus périveineux,
- de réaliser l'extraction des hématômes avant la compression.

La sonde biseautée, plus fine, de par sa forme, favorise le cathétérisme de veines plus étroites. Elle permet, en cas de veine trés tortueuse, de la transpercer, pour la reprendre ensuite et ainsi d'arracher des zônes d'accés difficiles, voire impossibles sans de nombreuses cicatrices, même minimes, comme le réclame la technique de phlébectomie ambulatoire.

Ainsi, l'on pourra trés facilement, cathétériser les collatérales sur leur trajet de 40 cms environ, que l'on arrachera ensuite sans aucune cicatrice intermédiaire.

Avantages :

Ils sont assez faciles à mettre en exergue pour qui sait manipuler cette technique. Elle permet un éveinage par invagination, donc peu traumatisante pour les tissus péri-veineux.

Elle permet d'aller chercher des collatérales importantes, tant au mollet qu'à la cuisse sans opérer de cicatrices inesthétiques, sachant que le souci esthétique est revendiqué à juste titre, tant par les femmes que par les hommes.

Les hématômes sont toujours assez nets, d'autant que le froid en général inhibe la coagulation.

Il semble s'agir du seul inconvénient majeur, qui requiert alors rapidité, dextérité, pour une utilisation rapide du froid.

Le second inconvénient pourrait être l'utilisation d'un gaz, d'un coût assez élevé, à la charge de la clinique mais en général une bouteille permet environ 60 à 80 manipulations.

Les résultats :

Ils permettent une meilleure extraction des paquets variqueux. Une fois repérée et marquée, la varice ectopique peut être attaquée par une incision minime, les gros paquets variqueux peuvent être abordés par une seule incision. L'hématôme résiduel est souvent facile à exprimer.

Cet abord de la collatéralité, nous paraît particulièrement important car permet de réduire le nombre de séances de sclérose post-opératoire.

Existe-t-il des réactions importantes ? Il est évident que des phénomènes inflammatoires peuvent apparaître. Ils sont transitoires et obéissent parfaitement à la prescription d'A.I.N.S..

Les hématômes se résorbent et dans aucun cas nous avons observé de troubles cutanés secondaires à une congélation trop intense.

De même, les suites lointaines ne sont pas aggravées de plus de troubles nerveux. Les douleurs sur les trajets variqueux nous paraissent en moyenne moins importantes permettant une déambulation immédiate, fonction bien entendu de l'anesthésie.

Sur plus de 500 cas réalisés, nous n'avons jamais eu de complications particulières en rapport direct avec le froid.

Les complications sont toujours celles que l'on trouve au cours des stripping, quelque soit la technique utilisée.

Comparativement au stripping :

- nous n'utiliseront plus de strippeur métallique qui obligeait de prendre une tête relativement grosse, donc le délabrement péri-veineux était toujours important. Nous faisons bénéficier nos patients de stripping sur fil, selon la technique de VAN DER STRICHT, que nous utilisons depuis 1968.

Technique simple, peu traumatique, elle ne peut intéresser que le tronc principal. Elle a pour elle, élégance et innocuité, ce qui en fait est une technique de choix.

La phlébectomie par mini-incision est une technique facile, mais qui nécessite de multiples incisions, parfois inesthétiques, dans de trop nombreuses mains inexpérimentées. D'autre part, elle ne peut intéresser que

les collatérales, les reflux principaux devant subir un éveinage.
Nous pensons donc que la cryochirurgie en dehors de toute cryosclérose, représente lorsque les collatérales sont nombreuses, mal systématisées, donc difficile d'accés, une technique de choix aprés un marquage correct, qui permet un maximum d'ablation sans cicatrices importantes.
Elle permet donc un maximum chirurgical, esthétique, sans réaction importante des tissus sous cutanés, laissant alors un moindre travail de sclérose.
Méthode que l'on peut réaliser soit sous anesthésie générale, régionale ou locale, l'utilisation d'une cryosonde permet de cathétériser plus facilement les troncs un peu tortueux ou voire anévrismaux. Nous lui reconnaissons une supériorité dans le traitement des saphénes antérieures, des saphénes postérieures et des collatérales permettant l'ablation des paquets variqueux souvent inaccessibles aux techniques classiques.
Disons que cette méthode permet une chirurgie esthétique, plus complète, mais ne représente qu'un moyen d'approche de la chirurgie des varices. Libre à chacun de l'appliquer.

Références :

Milleret R - Mon expérience de la cryochirurgie des varices
Phlébologie 1989, 42, 573
Van Der Strich - saphénectomie par invagination sur fil
P.M. Paris 1963, 21, 1081
Van Der Stricht - nouvelles statistiques dans le traitement des varices
Phlébologie 43, 4 - 521 - 526
Le Pivert . P - Cryochirurgie contrôlée des varices des membres intérieurs. Une approche thérapeutique nouvelle. A propos de 350 cas
123 - 148
Le Pivert . P - La cryochirurgie des varices
Journal Med esthétique et chirurgie derma.
Vol. 19, 73 - Mars 92, 31-33

La ligature simple de la crosse de saphène interne a-t-elle des indications en pathologie variqueuse ?

M. Lefebvre-Vilardebo, C. Daniel

Clinique Albert 1er 92500 Rueil-Malmaison France

Quelle conduite tenir devant une volumineuse saphène antérieure (SA) de cuisse alimentée par une crosse de saphène interne (SI) incontinente alors que le tronc est sain ? Que faire devant un reflux permanent de la crosse de SI bloqué à 10-15 cm sur un tronc peu dilaté ? Un éveinage, voire une crossectomie SI semblant disproportionnés, nous avons proposé une ligature simple de la crosse avec respect de ses collatérales, conservation complète du tronc et éventuelle exérèse de la SA. 36 patients (soit 41 SI) ont été opérés (34 femmes et 2 hommes) sous anesthésie locale. 85% patients ont pu être suivis cliniquement et en écho-doppler La médiane de recul est 21,5 mois(3 mois à 47 mois). Une sclérothérapie a été entreprise 27 fois sur le membre. Les suites opératoires ont été marquées par 2 thromboses segmentaires de la SI totalement recanalisées sans sequelles sous anticoagulant. La symptomatologie pré-opératoire, pricipalement lourdeur, a toujours notablement diminué. Les patientes ayant subi un éveinage controlatéral semblent avoir une évolutivité moindre de la maladie variqueuse du côté de la ligature. Ce contraste a été notamment mis en évidence chez une patiente à l'occasion d'une maternité. Dans tous les cas, le doppler a confirmé le retour, puis le maintien d'un flux de sens physiologique dans le tronc SI, le sang se draînant (en flux inversé) par les collatérales superficielles de la crosse. Dans tous les cas, le calibre du tronc SI a diminué entre le pré-opératoire (en moyenne 6 mm à mi-cuisse, 4 mm au condyle et 3,5 mm au 1/3 supérieur de jambe) et le 6° mois post-opératoire (4 mm, 3 mm et 3 mm). Le calibre minimum semble devoir être atteint au 6° mois post-opératoire. En conclusion, chez des patients bien sélectionnés dont le tronc de SI apparaît encore sain en dessous d'une crosse nettement1 incontinente, il peut être logique de proposer une ligature simple de la crosse. Le suivi à plus de 5 ans de ces patientes est indispensable pour confirmer ces résultats.

Phlébologie 92. Eds P. Raymond-Martimbeau, R. Prescott, M. Zummo.
John Libbey Eurotext, Paris © 1992, pp. 1006-1008

Intérêt d'une chirurgie extensive d'exérèse des varices. À propos de 380 eveinages saphènes internes

M. Lefebvre-Vilardebo, C. Daniel*

*Centre de Chirurgie Esthétique des Varices, 66, avenue Victor Hugo, 75116 Paris, France. * 2, rue de la Réunion, 92500 Rueil-Malmaison, France.*

Les méthodes de destruction des varices sont la sclérothérapie et la chirurgie d'exérèse. Chacune a ses partisans, mais aussi son taux d'échecs et de récidives. Ce taux est étroitement lié à l'utilisation exclusive d'une méthode. L'association des deux donne probablement une plus grande fiabilité de résultats. Mais reste à déterminer la part de chacune dans la stratégie thérapeutique de chaque patient. Un consensus s'est peu à peu dégagé sur le rôle dévolu à la chirurgie en cas de reflux majeurs : crossectomie avec ou sans éveinage, ligature ou arrachage des perforantes incontinentes. La sclérothérapie complémentaire post-opératoire traite alors toutes les varices laissées en place. Mais cette sclérothérapie, sur des varices de gros calibre ou à faible réactivité aux produits sclérosants, peut être longue et difficile, voire totalement inefficace. Que l'échec soit avoué ou non, le risque est grand de voir le patient lassé abandonner son traitement et entraîner ultérieurement d'autres patients potentiels vers le refus d'un traitement. La mise en confiance par des résultats rapides nous paraît primordiale.

METHODES

Notre stratégie actuelle comprend donc, dans le territoire de la saphène interne (SI) avec reflux ostial, une crossectomie élargie (1), l'éveinage SI court ou long selon le bilan opératoire et l'exérèse de tous les troncs stratégiques (saphène antérieure, SI accessoires) et des branches variqueuses maîtresses. La sclérothérapie post-opératoire traite alors aisément les petites varices résiduelles. Une cartographie variqueuse dynamique quantifiée, résultat du bilan pré-opératoire clinique, ultrasonique et éventuellement varicographique, apparaît la clé de décision du protocole thérapeutique propre à chaque patient.

Le traitement chirurgical est réalisé sous anesthésie loco-régionale, par anesthésie du nerf crural à l'aine, avec hospitalisation de 48 h, membre par membre en raison de la contrainte limitative de durée d'intervention liée au type d'anesthésie. L'anesthésie locale, par l'absence de vasodilatation qui l'accompagne, aidée par la technique d'éveinage par invagination, permet de réduire considérablement les hématomes et donc de simplifier les suites opératoires et d'améliorer la qualité de la convalescence. L'intervention est précédée la veille au soir d'un marquage variqueux cutané clinique et/ou échographique. Le pansement est refait le lendemain de l'intervention, avant le retour au domicile.

MATERIEL ET RESULTATS

De juillet 1989 à juillet 1991, 285 patients ont été opérés pour réaliser 380 crossectomies avec éveinages SI par invagination (3) (37,9 % jusqu'à la jarretière et 62,1 % jusqu'au cou de pied). Ces éveinages ont été associés dans 85,5 % des cas à des varicectomies par micro-incisions esthétiques étagées, selon la technique de Müller (2). En fonction de la bilatéralité des lésions et d'une éventuelle intervention sur les saphènes externes, 110 patients ont été opérés 2 fois et 5 opérés 3 fois. Les seuls incidents liés à l'anesthésie sont des petits hématomes inguinaux localisés autour du point de ponction, par embrochage de l'artère circonflexe iliaque superficielle, sensibles à la marche pendant quelques jours. La marche précoce, en moyenne 2 heures après l'intervention, et la reprise d'une activité personnelle subnormale dès le lendemain sont les meilleurs atouts de l'acceptation de cette stratégie multi-séquentielle. Le délai de reprise de l'activité professionnelle varie de 4 à 15 jours et dépend moins de l'intervention que du type de profession et du risque de stase veineuse prolongée. Aucune complication hémorragique ou infectieuse n'a été notée, mais 2 anesthésies partielles du territoire saphène interne jambier, sans paresthésies, apparaissent définitives (0,52 %). Ces troubles sensitifs sont séquellaires d'un traumatisme du nerf, "cravaté" par une branche veineuse résistant à la traction lors de l'invagination. Les complications mineures comprennent 18,6 % d'indurations sur les trajets d'éveinage ou de varicectomies et 6,2 % d'anesthésies cutanées suspendues sur quelques centimètres par "lésions par crochets" d'un rameau sensitif cutané, toutes complications complètement résolutives en moins de 6 mois.

L'impact psychologique post-chirurgical est majeur pour le patient par disparition de toutes les grosses varices initiales. Le taux de satisfaction du chirurgien est de 85 % sur le plan variqueux au 30ème jour post-opératoire, l'insatisfaction provenant de la persistance de varices insuffisamment déconnectées et susceptibles de résister aux scléroses. Neuf mois après chirurgie, le résultat esthétique est jugé bon dans 90 % des cas avec invisibilité presque totale de toutes les "traces chirurgicales", les 10 % restants concernant la persistance de pigmentations sur les trajets d'exérèse. La sclérothérapie est idéalement, et habituellement, entreprise entre le 45ème et le 60ème jour post-opératoire. Le délai est parfois plus long, jusqu'à 3 mois, voire 6 mois, en cas d'indocilité des patients. Les scléroses sont en règle générale faciles car s'attaquant à des varices de calibre modéré et peu alimentées. Pour preuve, le nombre de séances de sclérothérapie post-opératoire par patient pour obtenir l'éradication des varices a diminué en moyenne de 13 à 6 depuis la mise en route de cette stratégie chirurgicale plus extensive. Cette rapidité de résultats permet de réaliser plus de scléroses esthétiques, d'établir un meilleur contrat de confiance avec les patients et d'améliorer la fidélité dans le suivi à long terme.

CONCLUSION

Si l'on considère le traitement d'un patient variqueux comme devant être rapide, peu agressif, esthétique et fiable, la politique d'une chirurgie extensive d'exérèse, réalisée selon des normes esthétiques, apparaît être une solution séduisante. Certes, elle allonge la durée des interventions (de 30 à 60 minutes), mais elle diminue la période de sclérothérapie (de 3 à 4 mois environ). Et cette réduction de traitement par le phlébologue pour chaque patient est largement compensée par l'accroissement de clientèle né de la satisfaction des patients...

REFERENCES

1. Lefebvre-Vilardebo M. - Carrefour saphéno-fémoral : étude anatomique et concepts de prévention des récidives variqueuses. - J. Mal. Vasc., 1991, 16, 355-358

2. Müller R.- La phlébectomie ambulatoire. Phlébologie, 1978, 3, 273-278.

3. Van der Stricht J. - Saphénectomie par invagination sur fil. Phlébologie 1963, 16, 21-24.

Phlébologie 92. Eds P. Raymond-Martimbeau, R. Prescott, M. Zummo.
John Libbey Eurotext, Paris © 1992, pp. 1009-1011

Chirurgie variqueuse et anesthésie locale

M. Lefebvre-Vilardebo

Centre de Chirurgie Esthétique des Varices, 66, avenue Victor Hugo, 75116 Paris, France.

Il est évident que la chirurgie des varices ne nécessite aucun relâchement musculaire. La conservation de la motricité per-opératoire (au moins partielle) et le lever très précoce sont même les meilleurs moyens de lutte anti-phlébite. Par ailleurs, l'absence de vasodilatation per-opératoire, voire la vasoconstriction "d'éveil" permettent de réduire au minimum les hématomes, aidées, il est vrai, par des techniques chirurgicales peu traumatiques telles que l'éveinage par invagination. Alors pourquoi continuer à opérer sous anesthésie générale ou même sous péridurale, alors que l'anesthésie locale (AL) permet la même qualité d'intervention ? Les habitudes commencent à changer, notamment pour l'exérèse de la saphène interne (SI). Mais en fait, deux types d'AL, tronculaire et directe, seules ou en association, permettent de mener à bien toute la chirurgie variqueuse, quel qu'en soit le territoire et qu'elle soit de première intention ou pour récidive.

METHODES

L'AL directe, par infiltration sous-cutanée sur le trajet des varices, est la plus simple à réaliser, mais elle devient contraignante pour l'opérateur et pénible pour le patient lorsque le réseau variqueux est étendu. Isolée, elle est surtout indiquée pour des exérèses restreintes ou dans des territoires non systématisés. Pour une chirurgie extensive, il est préférable d'utiliser une anesthésie tronculaire (1). Le territoire sensitif du nerf crural correspond au trajet de la SI et de la grande majorité de ses collatérales. Réalisée juste en dessous du ligament inguinal et associée à une AL directe du pli inguinal, l'infiltration péri-nerveuse permet une crossectomie élargie et un éveinage jusqu'au pied. L'anesthésie du nerf grand sciatique à la face postérieure du tiers supérieur de cuisse, sur le patient en decubitus ventral, associée à une anesthésie de surface permet une bonne chirurgie du creux poplité et un éveinage saphène externe. Une AL directe complémentaire sur leur trajet permet l'exérèse des branches variqueuses au-delà des territoires tronculaires insensibilisés.

Ces méthodes d'anesthésie nécessitent une bonne connaissance de l'anatomie et la qualité de leur résultat dépend beaucoup de l'expérience de l'opérateur. Les techniques opératoires doivent être adaptées à l'AL : traction douce avec les écarteurs, éveinages par invagination, utilisation d'électrocoagulation bipolaire en chirurgie poplitée. Et la réalisation de l'AL doit être adaptée au programme chirurgical de chaque patient, fonction de la topographie de son arbre variqueux. Cette interdépendance de l'anesthésie et de la chirurgie impose une étroite collaboration dans l'équipe opératoire.

MATERIEL

De juillet 1989 à octobre 1991, la totalité des actes de chirurgie veineuse (soit 668 interventions) a été réalisée sous AL : 412 crossectomies élargies avec éveinages SI (256 longs et 156 courts), 112 crossectomies avec éveinage SE ou exérèses de perforante poplitée, 59 reprises inguinales et 12 reprises poplitées pour récidives, 33 ligatures de crosses SI, 10 thromboses veineuses fémorales, 30 varicectomies isolées. Des varicectomies par micro-incisons étagées ont été associées dans 79 % des cas. Une durée d'intervention supérieure à 90 minutes étant une contrainte limitative pour le confort du patient, le nombre d'axes saphéniens à traiter peut conditionner le nombre d'interventions pour chaque patient (147 patients ont subi 2 interventions, et 20 patients 3 interventions). Chaque territoire SI est en effet opéré séparément, les 2 SE pouvant être traitées en un seul temps.

RESULTATS

Une prémédication par Flunitrazépam 2 mg absorbée une demie heure avant le début de l'AL et un environnement musical per-opératoire ont suffi dans 86 % des cas pour rendre l'intervention très confortable. Un complément de neurolept-analgésie légère a été nécessaire pour les autres patients plus anxieux ou émotifs et pusillanimes. Les AL tronculaires sont facilitées par le repérage du nerf à l'aide d'un stimulateur électrique. La stimulation des fibres motrices engendrant des contractions musculaires permet de guider l'approche de la pointe de l'aiguille au contact du nerf et de rechercher sélectivement les différentes branches de division, notamment au niveau du nerf crural. L'aide du stimulateur est devenue indispensable dans notre expérience pour une fiabilité totale des anesthésies tronculaires. La durée de réalisation du protocole anesthésique, dépendante de l'expérience de l'opérateur, est de 20 minutes en moyenne. L'anesthésique utilisé est la lidocaïne 1 %, l'adrénaline n'étant associée d'un côté que dans les rares cas d'intervention longue bilatérale. La dose utilisée pour chaque intervention varie de 200 à 900 mg avec une moyenne de 500 mg. Aucune complication liée à un possible surdosage n'a été observée. Cette absence de risques a déjà été démontrée par Vidal-Michel (1990) (2).

Contrairement aux données classiques, nous n'avons observé aucun délai d'action, que l'anesthésie soit directe ou tronculaire. La marche a pu être reprise 1 à 3 heures après la fin de l'intervention, ce qui représente environ 4 heures d'anesthésie crurale. Le "bloc moteur" sciatique est rare et gêne peu la marche. Les seuls incidents possibles liés à la technique sont des hématomes infiltrants localisés de la région inguinale par embrochage de l'artère fémorale ou surtout de l'artère circonflexe iliaque superficielle, entraînant pendant quelques jours une petite gêne à la marche. Les quelques névrites crurales transitoires, secondaires à la recherche de paresthésies de repérage, ont disparu depuis l'utilisation du stimulateur.

Le taux de satisfaction des patients est évalué à 92 %. Les mécontents se situent dans la partie initiale de notre série, essentiellement par insuffisance d'étendue du territoire crural anesthésié. L'expérience de la technique et l'aide du stimulateur sont un gage de satisfaction. La simplicité des suites opératoires et la qualité de la convalescence par diminution des hématomes et l'impression d'une moindre agressivité chirurgicale compensent largement les désagréments des infiltrations.

REFERENCES

1. Straja A. - Anesthésie loco-régionale du membre inférieur. In Précis d'anesthésie loco-régionale. Gauthier - Lafaye P. p. 135-153. Ed. Masson, Paris. 1988.

2. Vidal-Michel J.P., Arditti J., Bourbon J.H., Bonerandi J.J. - L'anesthésie locale au cours de la phlébectomie ambulatoire selon la méthode de R. Müller - appréciation du risque par dosage de la lidocaïnémie.

Phlébologie 92. Eds P. Raymond-Martimbeau, R. Prescott, M. Zummo.
John Libbey Eurotext, Paris © 1992, pp. 1012-1014

Major venous surgery in an ambulatory setting

Enrique G. Bertranou, Marcelo O. Montanelli, Hugo L. Fausti, Esteban H. Elena

Sección Flebología, Hospital Privado de Comunidad, Calle Córdoba 4545, 7600 Mar del Plata, Argentina.

SUMMARY:
The ambulatory surgery goal is to provide an effective, complication-free and expeditious treatment. Preliminary results of ambulatory major venous surgery (long saphenous stripping and perforating veins ligation) are presented. Patients between 40 to 60 years old with normal pre-operative clinical check-up and convenient family support are admitted in the hospital at 6:00 a.m. and varicose veins and perforating veins are carefully marked. Peridural anesthesia at 6:30 a.m. and surgical procedure between 7:00 to 8:45 a.m. are performed. The patient with tight elastic bandage is controlled in a day case unit up to dismissal around 6:00 p.m. Thirty seven patients were evaluated:
25 women (mean age 45.5±10 years) and 12 men (mean age 52.2±13 years) presenting mainly pain, sensation of heaviness, edema and itching were operated upon in a 22 months period. Surgical procedures: isolated long saphenous vein stripping, 23; long saphenous vein stripping + perforating vein ligation, 10; isolated perforating vein ligation (Cockett-Sherman)), 4. Complications: small groin hematoma in 2 patients. Outpatient visits since diagnosis up to the final dismissal: 4. All patients returned uneventful to their regular activities on the 8th postoperative day. The conclusions of this preliminary study are: 1) Major venous surgery may be performed in an ambulatory setting with excellent patient compliance. 2) The procedure resulted efficient, major complication-free, and expeditious. 3) The prosecution of the program will permit a long-term evaluation in a greater number of patients.

INTRODUCTION:
As part of the reorganization of the phlebology in a 230 bed community hospital, it was necessary to implement an ambulatory setting for major venous surgery, which has been proved to be feasible, effective and with low complication prevalence by Bishop et al (1986). The first step was to define the pathology amendable to surgery and to determine clear cut indications. The classification followed is: 1) Minor venous surgery: local anesthesia, no intervention on saphenous femoral junction, no intervention on femoral and/or iliac veins. 2) Major venous surgery:

local, peridural or general anesthesia, long saphenous stripping, perforating veins ligations (Cockett, Sherman), no intervention on femoral and/or iliac veins, no anticoagulants. 3) Great vein vessels surgery: general anesthesia, with femoral and/or iliac surgery, with anticoagulants and/or A-V fistula. Concerning indication for major surgery, the inclusion criteria are: 1) age: between 40-60 years; 2) normal preoperative clinical checkup; 3) convenient patient and family understanding of the pathology and treatment. These conditions, regarding ambulatory surgery, have been extensively analyzed by Ferraina (1991). With the goal of providing an effective, complication-free and expeditious treatment, major venous surgery in an ambulatory setting was established. The purpose of the present work is to analyze the results of the first 22 months.

PATIENTS AND METHODS:
Thirty seven patients were operated upon under the ambulatory setting, being 25 women (mean age 48.5±10 years) and 12 men (mean age 52.2±13 years). Twenty three patients presented varicose veins with saphenous-femoral junction incompetence, 10 patients saphenous-femoral junction incompetence + perforating veins incompetence, and 4 patients presented isolated perforanting veins incompetence. The personal history and clinical features of the patients are shown in tables I and II.

Personal History	
Sedentarism	76%
Up-right posture	49%
Mother's varicose veins	49%
Father's varicose veins	37%
Sibling's varicose veins	54%

Clinical Features	
Heaviness	73%
Pain	62%
Edema	51%
Itching	51%

The body mass index (BMI) was normal in 30 patients and obesity was present in 7 patients.
Surgery performed: long saphenous vein stripping + stab evulsion phlebectomy 23 patients; long saphenectomy vein stripping + perforating veins ligations 10 patients; isolated perforating veins ligations (Cockett) 4 patients.
Patient is admitted in the hospital at 6.00 a.m. and varicose veins and perforating veins are carefully marked. Peridural anesthesia at 6.30 a.m. and surgical procedure between 7.00 to 8.45 a.m. are performed. The patient with tight elastic bandage is controlled in a day case unit up to dismissal around 6.00 p.m. A brochure is given to patients and family, explaining the indication to be followed during the next 7 days, including management of Trendelengurg position, bed rest, activities, elastic bandages and platelet antiagregant drug. Telephone calls are made after surgery to ensure the uneventful postoperative period. The total number of outpatient visit since diagnosis up to final dismissal is four.

RESULTS:
All patients returned uneventful to their regular activities on the 8th postoperative day. Mid term follow up was good, without varicose vein recurrence and with improvement of hyperpigmentation and lipodermosclerosis in cases of incompetent perforating veins ligation. Two small groin hematomas were found at the first postoperative outpatient visit (8th postoperative day). No wound infection was detected.

DISCUSSION:
It is necessary to explain the age as the inclusion criteria in the major venous surgery. In patients younger than 40 years old the

preservation of the proximal end of the long saphenous vein for eventual coronary bypass, even in presence of saphenous-femoral junction incompetence, is advisable. In these cases the low long saphenous ligation (knee level) is easily performed, accompanied with stab evulsion saphenectomy. In cases older than 60 years the same surgical procedure is carried out, not to preserve the proximal long saphenous veins, but to minimize surgery and avoid the saphenous-femoral junction approach. Bishop et al (1986) reported a good result of surgical treatment of varicose veins in an ambulatory setting with local anesthesia and a low incidence of wound infection. The present work performed with peridural anesthesia shows also good results without wound infection. Local anesthesia is utilized for stab evulsion phlebectomy (Goren et al 1991) named also ambulatory phlebectomy by Muller (1978) which has been performed in a large number of cases (246 patients) in the first 22 months of work.

CONCLUSIONS:

1) Major venous surgery may be performed in an ambulatory setting with excellent patient compliance. 2) The procedure resulted efficient, major complication-free, and expeditious. 3) The prosecution of the program will permit a long-term evaluation in a greater number of patients.

REFERENCES:

Bishop C.C.R., Jarrett P.E.M. (1986): Outpatient varicose vein surgery under local anaesthesia. Br.J.Surg. 73, 821-822.

Ferraina P.A. (1991): Cirugía ambulatoria. Rev.Arg.Cir. Nº Extraordinario, Relatos 1991, 1-61.

Goren G., Yellin A.E. (1991): Ambulatory stab evulsion phlebectomy for truncal varicose veins.

Muller R. (1978): La phlebectomie ambulatoire. Phlebologie 31, 273-278.

Phlébologie 92. Eds P. Raymond-Martimbeau, R. Prescott, M. Zummo.
John Libbey Eurotext, Paris © 1992, pp. 1015-1017

La gévaudanaise

Jean-Marc Trauchessec*, Robert Vergereau**

** 25, rue de la Faisanderie, 75116 Paris. ** Centre Médical Ambulatoire « Les Champs Élysées », 12, avenue de la Gare, 63130 Chamalières-Royat, France.*

La Gévaudanaise est une exosaphénectomie esthétique de la saphène interne variqueuse sans contre-incision le long du membre inférieur.
Son nom provient d'une ancienne province française, le Gévaudan, où cette intervention chirurgicale a été réalisée pour la première fois en 1986 (3).

Le matériel utilisé correspond à celui de la crossectomie et celui de l'exo-saphénectomie esthétique.
Le matériel de crossectomie est classique : bistouri, écarteurs, pinces, ciseaux, sutures.
Le matériel de l'exo-saphénectomie sans contre-incision, consiste en un dissecteur éveineur breveté, le D.E.T.(Dissecteur Eveineur de Trauchessec). L'instrument se compose d'une tige rigide, longue de 60 cm, munie à l'extrémité proximale d'une poignée ou d'un système de préhension.
L'extrémité distale possède un anneau semi-tranchant ou tranchant.
L'anneau semi-tranchant inclut dans sa gorge un filin d'acier commandé par les poignées proximales dont le rapprochement resserre le fil d'acier autour de la saphène interne (6).
L'anneau tranchant, évolution technique du dissecteur éveineur, évite le fil d'acier.
Le tranchant sectionne la saphène interne par mouvement de pulsion rotation imprimé à la portion proximale du dissecteur éveineur.

La Gévaudanaise se déroule sous anesthésie locale, en ambulatoire, dans sa version princeps (1).
La région inguinale et le tronc saphénien sont infiltrés de lidocaïne à 0,5% adrénalinée.
La crossectomie de la saphène interne débute par une incision de 4 à 5 cm, parallèle au pli de l'aine, un centimètre au dessus de celui-ci. Dissection de la crosse et des afférences qui sont sectionnées.
Une ligature est posée au ras de la veine fémorale (8).

La portion proximale du tronc saphénien est passée à l'intérieur de l'anneau du dissecteur puis tendue par une pince. L'anneau est progressivement poussé vers la région dis-

tale du membre, il effectue l'exo-saphénectomie ou dissection périsaphénienne (7).
A l'étage sural, la saphène interne est sectionnée sans aucune incision cutanée :
soit par effet de lasso dû à la traction du filin d'acier (4),
soit par le tranchant de l'anneau du dissecteur éveineur sans fil.
La saphène interne désolidarisée est retirée sans traction par l'unique orifice inguinal.

Suture de l'orifice inguinal, pansement compressif du membre inférieur, le patient opéré sort du bloc opératoire en marchant.

Une expérience de 600 cas ne nous a apporté aucune complication grave. L'analyse des résultats montre des suites plus simples comparées à d'autres techniques.
Les avantages de la Gévaudanaise se résument en une trilogie (9) :

- Efficacité phlébologique de l'exo-éveinage (2) :
  . Ablation constante des trois tuniques pariétales,
  . Eveinage des dédoublements ou trifurcations saphéniens,
  . Eveinage sans risque des saphènes internes thrombosées.

- Sécurité de l'anesthésie locale :
  . réduit le saignement per-opératoire par conservation du tonus veino-constricteur,
  . prévient les risques de thrombose par la déambulation immédiate.

- Résultat esthétique :
  Aucune trace le long du membre inférieur car aucune incision cutanée (5).

La Gévaudanaise apporte une solution éclairée, ergonomique, dans le traitement esthétique des saphènes internes variqueuses.

Références :

1. CARBILLET F. (1987) :
"Phlébectomie ambulatoire, indications et résultats esthétiques au niveau des membres inférieurs";
J. Méd. Esth. et Chir. Derm ; 14 ; 56 ; 331 - 335.

2. MAYO C.H. (1906) :
"Treatment of Varicose Veins";
Surgery Gynecology and Obstetrics ; 2 ; 385 - 388.

3. TRAUCHESSEC J.M. (1986) :
"La Gévaudanaise" ; Association en chirurgie phlébologique ambulatoire d'une crossectomie et d'une saphénectomie sans contre incision.
J. Méd. Esth. et Chir. Derm. ; Vol XIII ; N° 51 ; 227 - 231.

4. TRAUCHESSEC J.M. (1987) :
Technique chirurgicale : "La Gévaudanaise" ;

La Lettre de l'angiologie ; n° 23 ; 5 - 7.

5. TRAUCHESSEC J.M. (1987) :
Pour une saphénectomie esthétique ;
Phlébologie ; 40 ; (2) ; 409 - 422.

6. TRAUCHESSEC J.M. (1987) :
Comment se servir du DET (Dissecteur Eveineur de Trauchessec) ;
Les nouvelles dermatologiques ; Volume 6 ; n° 4 ; 352 - 353.

7. TRAUCHESSEC J.M. & VERGEREAU R. (1989) :
"Le stripping court sans contre-incision";
Giornate Flebologiche Algheresi ;
I Incontro Sardo-Catalano di Flébologia - p. 645 - 650.

8. TRAUCHESSEC J.M. & VERGEREAU R. (1992) :
"La Gévaudanaise" ; Réalités thérapeutiques en dermatovénérologie ; n° 16 ; 20 - 27.

9. VERGEREAU R. & TRAUCHESSEC J.M. (1991) :
"La Gévaudanaise : analyse de 500 cas";
Act. Méd. Int. - Angiologie (8) ; n° 128 ; 1555 - 1560.

Phlébologie 92. Eds P. Raymond-Martimbeau, R. Prescott, M. Zummo.
John Libbey Eurotext, Paris © 1992, pp. 1018-1020

Eradication ambulatoire des varices : méthode CARSENA

Jean-Louis Masson

Centre de Chirurgie Ambulatoire, 3, rue d'Angleterre, 06000 Nice, France.

La méthode CARSENA, ou Chirurgie Ambulatoire Réticulaire et Saphéniene des Ectasies variqueuses par une Nouvelle Association thérapeutique, tire son nom d'Aloïs Carsena chirurgien niçois, auquel Ambroise Paré attribue l'introduction, en Europe en 1543, du principe de la ligature vasculaire qu'il ramena de sa captivité chez les barbaresques, et qui remplaça définitivement la cautérisation.
Cette méthode est essentiellement constituée par l'association de trois techniques sûres efficaces, non invasives et esthétiques, pouvant être utilisées séparément, mais le plus souvent en association synergique, selon une stratégie globale très efficace donnant d'excellents résultats à cours terme et à long terme:
-LA PHLEBECTOMIE AMBULATOIRE SELON LA TECHNIQUE DE R. MULLER qui a actuellement trente ans de recul, avec plus de 35 000 interventions
-LA CROSSECTOMIE + STRIPPING COURT AMBULATOIRES de la saphène interne à l'"AZURSTRIP"[1], dont les principes imaginés par Mayo en 1907 sont bien au point, mais dont la réalisation a été révolutionnée par l'"AZURSTRIP" qui permet, après la crossectomie, un stripping exosaphénien, cruro-jambien, par une seule incision inguinale de 1,5 cm.
-LA PHOTOCOAGULATION LASER + microangiosclérose, enfin, qui permet depuis 1982 grâce aux Lasers Co2 et Argon de venir enfin à bout des télangiectasies que la microsclérose classique ne peut traiter.
Il évident que ce traitement qui se veut éradicateur, donc définitif, au moins en ce qui concerne l'évolution de la maladie variqueuse, est basé sur des notions précises:
- Concernant l'évolution de la varicose: critique constructive avec analyse des mauvais résultats des autres méthodes (purement médicales: créno et physiothérapie, médications veinotropes, contention; méthodes phlébologiques: sclérothérapie, cryothérapie, CHIVA; méthode chirurgicale: le grand stripping classique).
- L'avènement de la chirurgie ambulatoire avec ses critères précis, ses techniques non invasives (microchirurgie, Laser chirurgie, chirurgie à distance par vidéoendoscopie), ses corrélations médicales liées à la biochimie médicale, aux médecines physiques et esthétiques et surtout à l'analgo-anesthésie.
- Enfin, l'exploration cartographique de l'hémodynamique veineuse par imagerie traitée (en particulier l'écho-Döppler).

1/ La phlébectomie ambulatoire selon R. Muller est réalisée de manière classique, grâce aux crochets de Muller à triple contre-condure, qui permettent d'extraire les veines pathologiques par des incisions de l'ordre du millimétre qui

[1]"AZURSTRIP", mis au point en 1988 par le Dr. J.L.Masson

disparaîtront totalement, le tout sous anesthésie locale stricte. L'extirpation est systématique sur les varices tronculaires de jambes, réticulaires, perforantes, saphènes externes et veines de drainage des télangiectasies; elle est courante dans les diverses écharpes veineuse latérales, les pré tibiales, varices des genoux et des pieds; plus rare mais très possible dans les varices postérieures de cuisse (communicantes "type Giacomini"), les varices paravulvaires et de la fesse; enfin on peut opérer hors des membres inférieurs (visage, main, bras.). Les résultats sont excellents à 95% et les incidents et complications mineurs.

2/ **La crossectomie + stripping court ambulatoires**, concernant l'éradication des reflux saphéniens internes, est réalisée par une petite incision inguinale unique de 1,5 cm, permettant, après crossectomie radicale classique, le stripping externe ou exosaphénien grâce à l'"AZURSTRIP", (strippeur tubulaire tranchant à une extrémité et muni d'un manche semi-rigide à poignée à l'autre extrémité), qui descendra jusqu'à l'origine de la saphéne jambière au dessous du condyle interne du genou ou bien souvent jusqu'à la zone de phlébectomie, si une phlébectomie tronculaire a été pratiquée à la jambe au genou ou au bas de la cuisse. Cette intervention, nécessaire dans plus de 80% des cas, et bilatérale dans plus de 70% des cas, doit tenir compte des anomalies que l'on peut rencontrer tant au niveau de la crosse (variations d'implantation et des collatérales), qu'au niveau du tronc saphénien (saphénes accessoires internes ou externes, double tronc superposé, drainage fémoral direct). Les résultats de cette intervention sont constamment simples, en dehors de quelques hématomes spontanément résorbables et de rares tromboses superficielles sur un tronc saphénien laissé en place après crossectomie simple.

3/ **La photocoagulation LASER + microangiosclérose**, permet le traitement esthétique des télangiectasies et varicosités. La sclérose fine classique est en effet limitée par le diamètre des vaisseaux inférieurs à 0,5mm, et la phébectomie, elle, ne commence guère à être réalisable qu'à partir d'un diamètre de 1mm. Les LASERS CO2 (utilisé en pulses à des puissances de 3 à 6 watts) ou Argon (utilisé en continu et en large défocalisation) permettent de réaliser l'éradication progressive (en trois à six séances, espacées d'environ 3 semaines chacune) des varicosités fines et des télangiectasies pseudo-angiomateuses, surtout dans les localisations réputées dangereuses à la sclérose (tibias, malléoles et pieds). Les résultats sont excellents quand le traitement peut être mené à son terme.

L'intérêt de la méthode CARSENA consiste en l'obtention d'excellents résultats par une stratégie évolutive de l'association des trois techniques, basée sur l'éradication des ectasies veineuses, des perforantes et des reflux saphéniens visualisés cliniquement et cartographiquement à l'aide du Döppler. La pratique globale habituelle consiste à effectuer à quelques heures ou jours d'intervalle les phlébectomies nécessaires + les crossectomies plus stripping court si besoin uni ou bilatéraux et enfin les séances de Laser qui seront étalées sur quelques mois. Il est cependant possible dans certains cas de pratiquer une crossectomie première, des phlébectomies préalables ou des actes isolés, mais ces actes ne sont valables que dans des cas particuliers et bénins et l'on sort alors du principe de la méthode. La méthode est également très intéressante dans les varices résiduelles ou récidivées après sclérose ou stripping classique, dans les ulcères et la dermatopathologie variqueuse en général, dans les thrombophlébites superficielles enfin qui constituent à nos yeux une urgence chirurgicale phlébologique. Reste le cas problématique des grosses jambes à trois facteurs (insuffisance veineuse, lymphoedème, cellulite), où la méthode, certes très efficace sur le facteur veineux doit être étayée par les techniques physiques type drainage lymphatique et pressothérapie pendant plusieurs années et éventuellement lipoaspiration.

Il s'agit donc d'une méthode simple, utilisable dans la majorité des varicoses, qui grâce à la synergie de trois techniques ambulatoires utilisées selon une stratégie bien déterminée, permet d'obtenir 95% d'excellents résultats, durables, même à très long terme, avec un confort et un bien-être pré, per et post opératoire optimum et, une satisfaction esthétique supérieure à tout ce qui avait été proposé jusque là.

Références

-Franceschi, C. (1988), *Théorie et pratique de la cure conservatrice et hémodynamique de l'insuffisance veineuse en ambulatoire (CHIVA)*, Editions de L'Armançon.
-Masson, J.L. , Serres, P., Noël de la Paquerie, P. M. , (1989), Insuffisance veineuse des membres inférieurs. in Les cahiers de médecine esthétique, n° 6, éd. Solal.
-Masson, J. L., (1991), *Méthode CARSENA - Eradication ambulatoire des varices*, éd. Solal.
-Muller, R., (1984), "La phlébectomie ambulatoire", Nouv. dermatol. n°3, pp.55-57.
-Muller, R. (1966), "Traitement des varices par la phlébectomie ambulatoire". Bull. Soc. Fr. Phleb., n° 19, pp.277-279.
-Ramelet, A. A., Montini, M.,(1988) : *Phlébologie*, éd. Masson

Phlébologie 92. Eds P. Raymond-Martimbeau, R. Prescott, M. Zummo.
John Libbey Eurotext, Paris © 1992, pp. 1021-1022

Faut-il conserver l'axe saphénien dans la chirurgie ambulatoire des varices ?

Ph. Blanchemaison, Ph. Gorny

Centre de Phlébologie Ambulatoire (CPA), Paris, France.

Le réseau veineux superficiel des membres inférieurs est un réseau maillé de veinules d'un calibre croissant multiramifié entre elle, aboutissant aux veines de drainage ou plutôt veines collectrices dont les plus importantes sont les saphènes. Deux arguments conduisent les thérapeutes de la veine à l'idée de diminuer la pression intraveineuse responsable des varices tout en conservant l'axe saphénien :

1) La notion de veine saphène de drainage, ou collectrice, qui explique que son ablation peut entrainer en dehors de toute malfaçon chirurgicale, une mise de surcharge des territoires cutanés, responsable de varicosités post-éveinage (qui n'apparaissent que si l'axe saphènien est unique ; mais le plus souvent, l'éveinage concerne un dédoublement sus-aponévrotique du tronc saphènien alors que la vrai saphène, hypoplasique, reste en place dans son dédoublement d'aponévrose, continuant à offrir une possibilité de drainage).
Les proposition de techniques conservatrices par les thérapeutes de la veine ont été multiples, depuis des scléroses de crosse, les crossectomies, isolées avec phlébectomies, les éveinages courts ou partiels, jusqu'à la conservation totale avec la CHIVA.
Les études publiées dans les années 60, comparant crossectomies et éveinages, concluaient à la supériorité de l'éveinage. De nouvelles études sont en cours de publication, aboutissant à des résultats inverses, notamment graâce à l'apport des examens ultrasonores.

2) Le développement des pontages saphèniens.
S'ils restent encore peu employés au dessus du genou, ils sont par contre amenés à se développer en distalité et surtout au niveau coronaire. Les

cardiologues seront donc amenés à demander aux phlébologues des critères d'exploration pour définir les troncs saphèniens utilisables pour les pontages coronariens. A partir de quand une veine saphène n'est elle plus utilisable pour faire un greffon veineux ? Il faudra également tenir compte de l'étonnante capacité de récupération d'une veine ectasique en fonction des conditions de pression, d'oxygénation et de nutrition de la cellule endothéliale.
Il sera en 1992 de plus en plus difficile de retirer systématiquement les axes saphéniens sans définir de véritables critères de lésions irréversibles.

QUAND LA SAPHENECTOMIE PEUT DEVENIR UN GESTE SIMPLE, SÛR, FAIBLEMENT AGREABLE...

E.VINCENTI, S.M.VOLPIN, U.BACCAGLINI, P.SORRENTINO, G.SPREAFICO
Istituto di Anestesiologia et Clinica Chirurgica I, Università di Padova, Italie

La saphenectomie est aujourd'hui un acte chirurgical se résolvant dans un milieu ambulatoire. Ce n'est pas seulement une question d'argent ou de reduction des listes d'attente, de personnel infirmier ou de rationalisation du travail. Mais, au contraire, il s'agit d'une nouvelle conception philosophique de l'assistance sanitaire: laisser au malade la possibilité de "se déplacer", de mener une vie active aussi sur la table operatoire où seulement la jambe à opérer reste immobile, parfaitement bloquée par une anesthésie sousarachnoidienne très particulière. Depuis le février 1987 jusqu'à l'octobre 1991, 323 patients, tous ambulatoires, âge moyen 42.6 ans (18-76), 78% f. et 22% h., ont été traités par une intervention chirurgicale personalisée (crossectomie, 34 cas; stripping long, 35; stripping court, 218; stripping de la petite saphène, 12; crossectomie + phlébectomie selon Müller, 24) juste après ponction sousarachnoidienne à L1-L2 ou L2-L3 et l'injection dans le décubitus homolateral de 0.5 ml de bupivacaine hyperbarique à l'1%. La mise en oeuvre de quelque précaution adaptée aux exigences de la saphenectomie (position, aiguille, modification de l'inclination de la table) a permis d'obtenir, après la première année, un taux de succès du 100% sans aucun desavantage intra et postopératoire, ainsi que la technique chirurgicale a assuré la réussite parfaite de l'intervention sans besoin, jamais, de retenir en hospital l'opéré. Des mots confidentiels, un milieu tranquille, la sympathie de l'équipe, font de la saphenectomie ambulatoire un geste presque agreable.

Phlébologie 92. Eds P. Raymond-Martimbeau, R. Prescott, M. Zummo.
John Libbey Eurotext, Paris © 1992, pp. 1024-1026

Twenty years of thread method of saphenectomy

B. Augusto Diaz, Karolina Diaz, Miguel Bermeo

Instituto de Angiología, cirugía vascular e impotencia sexual, Av. de la República 770 y Eloy Alfaro, Quito, Ecuador.

The thread method of saphenectomy is a non-traumatic and esthetic phleboextraction procedure that was invented by Dr. Jean Van der Strich and has been used in my country for more than 20 years with satisfactory results and associated to perforating veins sub-aponeurotic ligature and scaled varicotomies become a complete surgical treatment for essential varicose veins of the lowwer limbs.

Due to the disagreement among authors about the varicose veins classification and to get clearness to the clinical surgical treatment I will present to you three simple and practical classifications:

1. According the ethiology we divide: a) Those called essential or primary, which are more and most important. b) Post-thrombotic varicose veins. c) Varicose dilatations due to congenital anomalities or arterio-venous fistulae. d) Post-traumatic: brief and iatrogenic ones. (for b, c and d we know ethiological cause and we deduce logical treatment). For varices called essential the treatment would be performed according the venous wall dilatation degree and anatomo-topographic classification.

2. According anatomo-topographic location we have: a) of the axis insufficiency (internal and external saphenes) b) of anarchical location (depending on: perforant veins, communicating, sub-dermic and muscular veins. c) internal iliac dependant varicose veins, d) telangiestases varicose veins.

3. According venous dilatation degree they are divided in four groups: a) pre-varicose state with dilatation degree 1 and without damage of venous walls fibro-muscular elements, b) varicose state with dilatation degree 2 and little destruction of venous wall elements, c) Chronic venous insufficiency statement with dilatation degree 3 and 4 and great damage of the venous wall element and atrophy complications, and d) Telangiestasic venous dilatation. This third classification is conventional and subjective.

TREATMENT

We use for the varicose vein of the first group, without considering topographic location, clinical treatment elastic intermitent contention, phisiotherapy, acceptable life habits and weight within normal limits. Sometimes we use some phlebotonic drugs, specially derivated from extract of Castaño de Indias.

For the second group we use clinical treatment plus sclerosand treatment for anarchical location varicose veins.

For the third group we use surgery and for the fourth group we use esclerosant skirts and female hormones if they are required.

SURGICAL TECHNIQUE

After sistematical clinical evaluation and under loco-regional anesthesia by crural nerve blockage at the groin fold and infiltration of the internal saphene way we perform a little maleolar incision (internal), we look for the saphene vein and we bind four or five collateral veins.

Next, we introduce by the venous light an instrument called "stripper" which in almost 90% of the cases follows to the internal saphene light until its crook. We make a new incision parallel to the groin fold, we look for the saphenous crook and we perform a carefull ligature of collateral veins, then we make the saphenous crook ligature without leaving too long or too short necks. After we look for the stripper, which come to the superior top of the saphenous vein and we join its extreme with a thigh long piece of silk or nylon.

By distal saphenous extreme (maleolar) we straight the stripper leaving in its place the silk which later is joint to the crook's extreme of the saphenous vein, then we make an invagination of the vein and later it is carefully extracted until the ankle.. As you may see fleboextractor is only a simple metalic conductor.

Sometimes it could be necessary to return with the silk peforming a ligature at distal lower vein extreme and making the process of invagination and extraction indicated above. Sometimes it is necessary three or four very little supplementary incisions for anarchic and perforant varicose veins, which must be ligated.

We make an elastic compressive bandage or stocking and we leave the foot of the bed elevated. For external saphene we perform the same procedure taking care of its sub-fascial position and crook vein variations:

ADVANTAGES:

There are several advantages at the anesthesic, post-operatory, post-anestetic level as well as in surgical procedure.

This is an esthetic technique, performed by perfectly-hided incisions; but overall, the most important advantage is to be atraumatic, because vein extraction is performed by its endo vascular vein inside, in this way peri-venous integrity is guaranteed, and the canal left at this place, after vein extraction, usisng this method is reduced to the minimum, with blood loss and residual hematomas absence.

On the other hand, the traction over tissues is minimum and let us execute this intervention under local anesthesia.

CASUISTICS:

We have more than 12,000 cases operated in more than 20 years of work. Over 7,056 patients in which we perform 12,000 saphenectomies of which 10,512 are internal, 1,488 external saphene, mean 12.4% of the total of saphenectomies.

We have operated 342 patients with 4 operations each, 184 patients with 3 operations each, 3,551 patients with 2 operations each and 2,978 patients with just one operation each.

The maximum age was 96 years and the minimum 12, which give up an average of 48 years.

We have operated 3,846 male patients which mean 54.5% and 3,210 female patients, which mean 45.5%. My percentage is different over universal stadistics because this work has been performed over stadistics in Medical Centers as: Militar Hospital, Policlínico de la Policía Nacional, where patients are in its majority males. We have finished the surgical treatment with sclerosant skirts, in approximately 29% of operated patients. We use some substances as: Aetoxiesclerol, Maleato de Monoethanolamine, Yoduro de Sodio in diverse concentration as is required

We are suprised tolook that there are not to much complications; we have difficult cicatrization on 0.9%; skin necrosis on 0.3%, hematomas and equimosis in 2.8%, Venous residives in about 3%.

CONCLUSIONS:

This method seems to be very simple and satisfactory.

On mediat or immediate post-operatory phase we have not almost any residival veins which have appeared, discretely, in a long control period.

We obtain extraordinary esthetic results;

This is an atraumatic technique and well tolerated by patients.

By its mutiple advantages, local anesthesia do not permit us complications we could lament.

" LA CHIRURGIE DES VARICES SANS STRIPPING "

Dr.HORATIU ANGELESCU Bucarest Roumanie
Hôpital CFR Bucarest Roumanie.

Depuis plus de 28 ans (1962),nous applicons ce procédé original,fondé sur les données anato - miques fournies par:van LIMBORGH,DASELER,SHERMAN etc,. Nous commençons par un examen clinique effectué sur un malade en position debout,au cours du quel nous dessinons sur la peau l'emplacement des incisions.Nous ne recourons qu-exceptionellement aux examens paracliniques.

Notre technique trés minutieuse et peu traumatisante n'entraine pas de perte de sang.Elle est fondée sur des principes anatomo-physiologiques bien précis.Certes,le nombre des incisions est plus grand,mais elles disparaissent au fur et â mesure que le temps passe et le malade retire un bénéfice estetique.Le procédé peut etre appliquée aussi dans les syndromes dysembrioplastiques et les tromboses variqueuses !

La courte hospitalisation et la reduction du temps d' inaction rendet ce procédé très économique !!

L'absence de sclérotérapie complémentaire protège le malade de toute pigmentation cutanée et lui évite les quelques inconveniénts que peu engendrer,dans le domaine allergique ou anaphylactique,une scleroterapie.

L'opération peut être effectuée soit dans un hôpital soit dans un ambulatoire bien doté. (Tagesklinik .)

Phlébologie 92. Eds P. Raymond-Martimbeau, R. Prescott, M. Zummo.
John Libbey Eurotext, Paris © 1992, pp. 1028-1030

Crossectomie et stripping externe court selon Mayo sous anesthésie locale et ambulatoirement

Michel Gross

Avenue de la Gare, 10, 1003 Lausanne, Suisse.

In 1979 we started a new modality in phlebologic surgery,whose main aim was to prevent the so much feared scars, which in some cases caused a certain degree of invalidity and in some others they produced psychical disorders.
Trying to find a solution to this problem, we started with our team to carry out **"CROSECTOMY WITH ONE INCISION WITHOUT PHLEBOEXTRACTION"**.
Until 1985, we fulfilled only phleboextraction among those patients who had insufficient duct in all its extent, from its saphenous femoral joint to the internal malleolus.
Up to that date, out statistic data indicate: over 1260 patients surgically treated, only 25 were practised phleboextraction, representing 2% of the total number of operated on people.
We phlebologists, tireless fighters in bettering aesthetics, managed to avoid scars, so unpleasant for our patients,through microincision surgery, as well as discharges, wich similar to flare-ups appeared at different times after phleboextraction, beneath the incision at the level of the ankle.
Paraesthesias and anaesthesias so troublesome for certain operated on patients as consequence of traumatisms to the saphenous nerve or nervous fillets wich accompany the saphenous duct, have considerably decreased; then, if they exist during a crosectomy without phleboextraction and with microincision surgery, they would be the consequence of a technical mistake.
An important target pointed by ourselves was to keep the internal saphenous duct as an element for vascular replacement, demonstrating in several opportunities that after the surgical treatment, the remaining internal saphenous ducts work normally flowing into the profound venous system through Hunterians and Geniculars (This was shown through plebographic studies, fluxometric studies and ecco - doppler).

OPERATIVE TECHNIQUE

1.- We make a 2 to 4 cm. arciform incision over fold of the groin (Dr Odisios's technique). We try to reduce skin cutting Petrequin's fibres, following the subcutaneous vein, wich will lead to the internal saphena arch. We perform wide dissection of the femoral vein, from the crural arcade up till 1 cm. bellow the Allan Burns's ligament, wich is divided to avoid recidivation.

According to a statistical study by Dr. Odisio, there exists 34.3% of inflowing wich flow directly into the femoral vein.

2.- We proceed to the ligature of inflowing so as later we can bind up the internal saphena arch, dissecting its duct bellow the intersaphena, where we try to make the distal ligature.
Following, we start microsurgery of the varicose veins already marked; we do it wich scalpel Nr.11,performing 2 mm incisions, we make the venoextraction from distal to proximal avoiding phleboextraction.

COMMENTS

Until 1985 we had operated 1260 patients, out of wich only 25 were practised phleboextraction, in some cases bilateral, in some others unilateral, wich represented 2% of the operated patients in our casuistry, the rest were performed only internal saphena arch ligature and exeresis,through microsurgery of the superficial venous net. Out of the 1235 patients who presented partial insufficiency of the internal saphenous duct, 432 (35%) were practised resection of the insufficient sector, and the rest, 803 (65%) were not performed exeresis, the duct remaining "In -Situ".We had only to operate on again two patients because of insufficiency of the internal saphenous duct;both patients were pregnant after the surgical treatment.
The insufficiency of the above mentioned duct is done by reflux passed on through the hypogastric extrapelvics.
Until June 1990, 2165 patients were operated on, out of wich 1362 (62%) unilaterals, and 823 (38%) bilaterals.
Up till that date, 8 patients (7 female and 1 male) were operated on again for internal saphenous duct, from this group, two of them made their insufficiency through reflux passed on by the hypogastric extrapelvic inflowing, as consequence of gestation.A male and two female made it through reflux originated in the media Hunterian. Another one through insufficiency of the proximal perforans of the third upper part of the inner side of the leg, and two others through insufficiency of external saphena wich passed on reflux to the infrapatellar remaining internal saphenous duct.

CONCLUSION

With this technique, we achieved:

1.- To diminish varicose recidivation considerably.

2.- To keep to a great extent the internal saphenous duct partially, so important in view of possible arterial or venous by-pass.

3.- To reduce the possibilities of lymphatic and nervous injuries produced by the phleboextractor.

4.- To avoid antiaesthetic scars and infracicatricial shedding.

We have noticed that scars due to microincision disappear completely after a few months of the surgical treatment; only as a minimun, some pigmentation may remain; we have not seen keloid scars either.
With this technique we manage phlebopathy from the physiological point of view, without altering the fundamentals of every varices operation.

1.- To interrupt flux points.

2.- To resect the superficial varicose net.

STATISTIC DATA CORRESPONDING TO THE PERIOD MAY 1979-JUNE 1990

LIGATURE OF ARCH + F.E.	**=**	**25**	**(1.15%)**
LIGATURE OF ARCH + M.S.	**=**	**2140**	**(98.85%)**
TOTAL OF OPERATED ON PATIENS	**=**	**2165**	**(100.00%)**

BIBLIOGRAPHY

1.- ENRICE E., CALDEVILLA H,."FUNDAMENTOS Y MODIFICACIONES TECNICAS DE LA OPERACION DE COCKETT". Bol. y Trab. de la Soc. ARG. de Cirujanos, 35:7, 1974.

2.- GALOTTI, A."CIRUGIA CONSERVADORA DE LAS VENAS SAFENAS INTERNAS PARA SU EVENTUAL USO COMO PROTESIS".Rev. Arg. de Flebología.Vol. II, III, 1978.

3.- KAPLAN G, SCHAPIRA A,."SAFENECTOMIA CON UNA INCISION". Rev.Bras. de Ang. e Cir. Vas. Vol. 17,Nro.4 Dic. 1987.

4.- Odisio A,."VAR. DE LOS MIEMBROS INFERIORES".Akadia.1979.

Phlébologie 92. Eds P. Raymond-Martimbeau, R. Prescott, M. Zummo.
John Libbey Eurotext, Paris © 1992, pp. 1031-1032

Le clip saphène : résultats à moyen terme

J. Naouri, M. Schadeck, F.A. Allaert

École Européenne de Phlébologie, 6, rue Giordano Bruno, 75014 Paris, France.

La mise en place d'un clip sur un axe saphènien a d'abord pour but en évitant la section pariètale, de faciliter le phénomène de néo-vasculogénèse à partir des cellules endothéliales.
Après une étude exploratoire utilisant le doppler et l'échographie ou le dupplex scann parfaitement conduite, ce clip généralement doublé et disposé en quinconce est placé sur l'axe incontinent permettant ainsi de respecter les axes encore sains.
L'étude qui est ici proposée porte sur 65 patients revus à quatre ans regroupant 52 femmes pour 13 hommes, la moyenne d'âge étant de 41 ans avec des extrêmes de 14 et 68 ans.
Les principales indications se répartirent de a façon suivante :

- saphènes antèrieures isolées,
- grandes saphènes slérosrésistantes,
- récidives au scarpa post-stripping,
- grandes saphènes pendant la grossesse,
- divers .

Des reflux immédiats furent constatés chez 6 patients (26 %) dans le premier groupe, 4 patients (28,5 %) dans le second et 2 patients soit soit 25 %.
L'ensemble des reflux immédiats représente donc 12 patients soit 18,5 % .
Une seule néogénèse fut observée chez un patient préalablement déjà strippé.
Des reflux secondaires furent constatés dans 50 % des cas, lents, durables, non ou très peu significatifs.
La mise en place d'un clip n'apparaît donc pas d'une efficacité radicale et ne réalise donc qu'un barrage veineux incomplet. Celui-ci toutefois aisément compensé par une sclérose complémentaire généralement réalisée sous contrôle échographique.
Dans le cas de la récidive observée, les collatérales avaient en fait été sectionnées puis clipées.
D'autres paramètes comme l'âge ont été étudiés, montrant que les jeunes dont les saphènes ont encore des parois épaisses et musculeuses répondaient moins au traitement que es personnes plus âgées.

Globalement, les résultats à terme se révèlent donc excellents dans un confort indiscutable. Cet acte n'exclut pas bien sûr une surveillance régulière de la maladie variqueuse.

En conclusion, il apparaît que la mise en place d'un clip sur un axe saphènien incontinent ou ou branche récidivée, acte réalisé sous anesthésie locale, devait généralement être complété par une sclérothérapie secondaire, mais ne générait surtout aucune modification anatomique du système veineux traité .
Cet acte permet donc d'éviter la néo-vasculogénèse et devient particulièrement indiqué dans les maladies variqueuses à haut potentiel évolutif.

Phlébologie 92. Eds P. Raymond-Martimbeau, R. Prescott, M. Zummo.
John Libbey Eurotext, Paris © 1992, pp. 1033-1034

The clip saphène: Venous interruption on the saphenofemoral junction by clipping-in-continuity, a four-year follow-up

Lawrence L. Tretbar, M.D. FACS

Univ of MO Kansas City School of Medicine

This study evaluates the use of surgical hemostatic clips as a simple method of obliterating the saphenofemoral junction. Two objectives were identified: to determine whether the method would give a permanent obliteration of reflux at the junction; and whether this a traumatic approach might decrease the development of new veins at the site of surgery.

Methods and Material: 321 legs of 269 patients were studied over a four-year period. There were 247 women and 22 men in the group, whose ages ranged between 18 and 72 years.

Saphenofemoral incompetence was determined by Doppler examination in the standing position. Incompetence was defined as reflux lasting for one second or more using the augmentation technic.

To obliterate reflux standard titanium surgical hemostatic clips were placed over the saphenous junction and its tributaries. All operations were performed in the out-patient unit using local infiltration anesthesia without additional sedation. Operating time for the procedure was 30-45 minutes.

Truncal varicosities were treated either by injection sclerotherapy or by excision using a modified Muller technic.

Results: There were no major surgical complications, wound infections, DVT or scarring. A self-limiting, mild phlebitis developed in the long saphenous vein in 19 patients. However, the saphenous vein remains patent in all cases with no thrombosis even at the site of clipping.

One patient required re-exploration and clipping of a lateral tributary missed at the original operation.

The area has been free of reflux since that time.

All other junctions have been reflux-free. Because the vein is patent, blood refluxes slowly with augmentation down to the next perforating vein.

The most interesting finding is that in almost 2/3s of the cases of pregnancy-related saphenous incompetence, the vein becomes competent again after clipping. Apparently the vein shrinks enough that the valves are allowed to function again.

Phlébologie 92. Eds P. Raymond-Martimbeau, R. Prescott, M. Zummo.
John Libbey Eurotext, Paris © 1992, pp. 1035

Dispositif intraveineux d'obstruction ou de maintien

J.F. Van Cleef

45, rue de la Chaussée-d'Antin, 75009 Paris, France.

Les veines superficielles et profondes des membres inférieurs ont deux faces et deux bords.

Pour les veines superficielles l'axe préférentiel d'ap latissement de la lumière veineuse est parallèle à la surface de la peau. Les endoscopies veineuses dynamiques, réalisées avec JP. HUGENTOBLER, ont permis de vérifier que les bords libres valvulaires des bi-valves pariétales étaient bien parallèles à cet axe. Les commissures valvulaires sont sur les bords de la veine. Les incongruences pariéto- valvulaires sont les causes les plus fréquentes de reflux valvulaire. Dans la maladie valvulaire c'est la création d'un espace intercornéal ou commissural qui permet ce reflux.

Le dispositif intra veineux (DIV) proposé présente deux tiges parallèles, destinées à s'accrocher sur les bords de la veine, reliées par un écarteur, qui permet d'aplatir plus ou moins la lumière veineuse. Ce DIV est mis en place sous contrôle échographique en percutané. Sa pose peut être accompagnée d'injection de produits sclérosants.

Le DIV obstrue une veine ou diminue la surface de la section veineuse en l'aplatissant. Au niveau d'une bi-valve le DIV retend l'appareil et comble les deux espaces commissuraux sur les bords de la veine.

Il faudra plusieurs années pour connaitre le devenir de ce type de DIV.

Phlébologie 92. Eds P. Raymond-Martimbeau, R. Prescott, M. Zummo.
John Libbey Eurotext, Paris © 1992, pp. 1036-1038

Microphlebosuction : a new surgical technique

Miguel Eduardo Umansky, Saul Umansky, Ignacio Avila Bayon

Department of Phlebology, Clínicas Mepres. C/Rui Perez No.1.3P.Der. Avilés, 33400 Asturias, España.

SUMMARY.

Through this new technique which is carried out by combination of Phlebodestruction with the new Phlebocannulae, inspired on others which we published in 1969 and adapted to this operation, as well as the Aspirationby means of minimal puncturing, we achieved the Destruction and Extraction of lengths of veins, whether of the external or internal Saphenous Vein and/or collaterals under local anaesthetic, which allowed rapid walking after a brief period of observation, with virtually puntiform punctures. In this way significant cost savings are achieved by non-occupation of hospital beds, by reduced sick-leave as the patient is normally able to return to work within 24-48 hours of the operation.
From the Aesthetic point of view, it is superior to other surgical techniques, as no incisions are made and no scars are visible.
We therefore consider that this technique of Phlebodestruction and Extraction by Intraluminal and Extraluminal Aspiration, makes a contribution to the treatment of this venous pathology and whose consideration we recommend as it is in agreement with current trends towards reducing the agression towards tissue and it obtains excellent results from the Aesthetic and economic point of view.

INTRODUCTION.

In accordance with current evolution of medicine, seeking ever less damaging and aggresive techniques, and bearing in mind Aesthetic factors as part of a successful surgical procedure, we have developed a new technique of Phlebodestruction and Extraction of the vein by Aspiration by a novel Phlebocannulae based on the Phleboduretttes which we have designed and presented at various events since 1969. This can all be carried out under local anesthetic.
This technique, as well as cosmetic considerations, is also less expensive, as by avoiding hospitalisation; the costs of beds are saved and the patient may rapidly resume his employment, reducing sick leave.
It is evident that to carry out these and other advanced techniques which replace more primitives ones, a surgeon is required who is fully versed in Phlebological Techniques and their application in human beings and who respects the human body in the sense of "Curing without mutilating".

MATERIAL.

We have designed two models of Phlebocannulae:
1-Cannulae from 10 to 15 cms.in length with handle and a frontal bevelled cutting edge of 2-3 mm.diametre.
2-Cannulae from 10 to 15 cms. in length,also with handle but the point is blunt and side cutting through an orifice around whose distal edge of its periphery is a flap with a cutting edge.They are 2 or 3 mm.in diameter.
3-Conventional 1 atmosphere pressure equipment.

METHODS.

40 patients were selected,9 of whom had bilateral pathology,18 unilateral of internal or external Saphenae,6 for perforant insufficiency and 8 for simple asystematic collaterals.All of them were evaluated with a thorough clinical examination.functional tests and Fluxometric test using the Doppler effect.All of them were treated as out-patients under local anesthetic,Those exhibiting bilateral pathology were treated in two stages.
In Rectilinear Varices we shall use the Blunt Pointed Phlebocannulae with a side cutting orifice with a cutting flap in the distal part of this orifice.
In Cirsoid and/or Thrombosed varicoses we shall use the bevelled-edged Phlebocannulae.

OPERATING TECHNIQUES.

Presurgical preparation is carried out with the patient standing;the patient is operated on either prone or supine dending on the area to be treated.
The antisepsis of the zone,positioning of the sterile areas.The area is anesthetised with Mepivacaine Hidrochloride al 0.5%concentration or at 1%with Epinephrine in paralel to the vascular axis following its edges.The anaesthetic dose must not exceed 40 mls. at 1% or 80 mls. at 0.5%,with Epinephrine.In those cases where the internal or external Saphenous Vein had to be treated,a transcutaneous ligature in the distal area(towards the foot) is carried out with a triangular needle of 30 mms.and 3/8 of a circle,000 gut non reabsorbible, and from that an operation is undertaken to express or empty the vein towards the proximal area(Groin) positioning a second ligature in the area where the vein becomes insufficient;the most usual areas have been the 1/3 half of the thigh and the upper third of the calf.If the insuficiency is at the venous junction the technique and the ligature are direct following conventional practice.

Once the two ligatures has been effected,the Phlebocannula is introduced by transcutaneous intraluminal puncture,selecting the type of Canulae according to the type of vein to be treated.If it is linear, the Blunt-Pointed with the side hole cutting edge with a cutting flap is used,whereas if it is very sinuous,the frontal cutting edge type is used.
With the right hand movements are made to introduce and extract the Cannulae,which cuts with the edge,and aspirate,while the left hand accompanies these movements with a gentle pressure of the vein againts the cannullae so that the venous walls are allways in contact with the suction orifice and the cutting edge,thus avoiding the aspiration of blood.Each 10 or 15 cms.other puctures are peeformed,repeatingthe procedure as far as the ligatured areas.In the case of varices due to perforant insuficiency,double ligatures in the form of "X"are carried out,surrounding it,and then the varices produced by the ligatured perforants are destroyed and aspirated.Operation is concluded,withbandage Ligatures are removed on the 7th.day.Simple varices only Phlebosuction.

REFERENCES.

Altman Canestri.E.(1987).Tratamiento quirúrgico de las varices. Rev.Arg.de Flebología.V.I.

Altman Canestri.E.(1979).Cirugía Venosa Ambulatoria.Rev.Arg.de Flebología 2.172.

Hobbs.J.T.(1977).The tretment of Venous Disorders.Edit.MTP. Lancaster.England.

Pace F.(1991).Ligadura transcutánea ambulatoria de Varices Giganates.Revista Panamericana de Flebología.No2-36/40.

Simkin R.(1991).Varices,Ulceras y Angiodisplacias.Ed.López.Buenos Aires.

Sánchez C.(1988).Manual de Escleroterapia y Flebectomía Ambulatoria.Edit.Celsius.Buenos Aires.

Sánchez C.(1977).Uso de la Microcirugía en los tratamientos Flebológicos.Rev.Arg.De Flebología. 1.89.

Umansky S.(1969).Flebodisector cureta.Flebocuretage.Soc.Arg.de Cirujanos.30.9.

Van Cleef.J.F.(1988).La Phlebosuccion est elle possible?41.2. 287/295.

Phlébologie 92. Eds P. Raymond-Martimbeau, R. Prescott, M. Zummo.
John Libbey Eurotext, Paris © 1992, pp. 1039-1041

Réflexions sur les principes hémodynamiques sur lesquels se fonde la cure C.H.I.V.A.

M. Cappelli*, S. Ermini**, A. Turchi***, G. Bono*

** Studio flebologico, via Datini 46, Firenze, Italy. ** Studio flebologico, via Tizzano 18, Grassina, Firenze, Italy. *** 1° U.O. Chirurgia generale, Ospedale S.M. Annunziata, USL, 10/H Firenze, Italy.*

INTRODUCTION:

La cure C.H.I.V.A. du Docteur Claude Franceschi(1988) représente un nouveau type de traitement des varices. Le mot C.H.I.V.A. (Traitement Conservateur Hémodynamique de l'Insuffisance Veineuse en Ambulatoire) exprime la possibilité de corriger chirugicalement les altérations hémodynamiques présentes dans une maladie variqueuse tout en préservant au maximum le capital veineux superficiel. Tout cela est réalisable sous anesthésie légère, sans immobilisation, c'est la traduction du mot "ambulatoire".

Pourquoi conserver les varices ?.

L'avantage par rapport a un traitement démolitif est répresenté par la conservation du système saphenien (axes sapheniens et grosses collatérales) prédisposé au drainage de hautes quantités de sang étant en connexion avec les axes profonds par les perforantes qui permettent un rapide vidange du système.

D'autres arguments en faveur de la conservation des saphènes dérivent de l'étude écho-doppler des varices:

a) Ce qui souvent, par la simple inspection, est considéré comme une saphène variqueuse, n'est en fait q'une collatérale antérieure ou postérieure de cuisse dont le trajet est très proche de celui de la saphène. Celle-ci en fait se trouve en position profonde, dans un dédoublement du fascia superficiel et bien souvent, elle n'est pas atteinte elle-meme par la maladie variqueuse. Dans notre expérience, nous rencontrons ce cas de figure dans environs 40% des cas.

b) Par ailleurs, les saphènes de cuisse incontinentes sont souvent rectilignes et leur calibre dépasse rarement 10 mm, meme s'il y a de grosses varices plus bas au niveau de la jambe. Après une cure CHIVA, il y a toujours une réduction d'environ 50% après 6 mois à un an. Dans de telles conditions, ces saphènes ansi conservées peuvent etre utilisées pour les pontages artériels. A' signaler deux cas de patients dont les saphènes restaurées par CHIVA ont été utilisées pour un pontage.

PRINCIPES HÉMODYNAMIQUES

L'existence d'un reflux suppose l'existence d'un ou plusieurs points de réentrée du sang vers la profondeur au niveau des perforantes, ce que l'on nomme un SHUNT VEINO-VEINEUX ou circulation privée de Bassi (Bassi 1962 1985). Ce shunt veino-veineux caracteristique de la maladie variqueuse entraine une augmentation de pression à la marche et une réduction du drainage cutané.

L'interruption du shunt dans n'importe quel point de son cours comport une disparition du reflux. De cela l'affirmation qu'"**IL N'EXISTE PAS DE REFLUX S'IL N'Y A PAS LA POSSIBILITE' DE RÉENTRÉE".**

Tout cela est verificable avec des tests simples exécuté avec un doppler continu, Prenons le cas d'une incontinence saphénienne avec reflux de la cross et la présence de perforantes incontinentes en bas.

La normalisation ou l'amélioration pendant la marche des valeurs de pression mesuréé avec la phlébodinamométrie peut etre obtenue supprimant le long reflux (preuve de Trendelenburg) on interrompt de tel façon le premier shunt veino-veineux qui origine de la cross. A cet effet, il suffit de fermer la jonction saphéno-fémorale au-dessus des collatérales de façon à ce que ces dernierès continuent à drainer une colonne de pression en position orthostatique qui maintiendrait la distension des varices. Il faut y associer la fragmentation de cet colonne de pression au moyenne de ligatures qui doivent etre effectuées non au hasard mais sous les perforantes incontinentes, en les utilisant comme réentrées c'est-à dire comme de vrais points d'aspiration dans le système veineux profond.

Comment une perforante incontinente peut-elle trouver une fonction de réentrée du sang dans le système veineux profond ?

Il existe à cela des arguments anatomiques et fonctionnels:

- ARGUMENTS ANATOMIQUES:

Echographiquement, on peut parfaitement démontrer que beaucoup de perforantes sont fermées pendant la contraction musculaire (Shafer 1975), laminées par les structures fasciales et musculaires et donc, qu'elles ne refluent pas pendant la phase systolique, et par contre qu'elles continuent à exercer leur fonction d'aspiration dans la phase de diastole musculaire (Cappelli 1991).

- ARGUMENTS FONCTIONNELS:

La preuve de Perthes et les études de Bjordal(1981) démontrent comme l'apport de sang qui vient aspiré pendant la diastole est nettement supérieur à celle refluent au débout de la phase systolique. C'en est une démonstration le fait que les varices essentielles se vident avec la marche une fois supprimé le reflux long. En effet, pour la loi de conservation de l'energie, quand augmente la vitesse du sang dans un vaisseau la pression latéral se réduit en expliquant de cette façon comment le débit dans une perforante meme incontinente peut etre orienté vers les axes profonds déjà dans la phase terminale de la systole, moment dans le quel le sang acquit l'energie cinetique maximum.Tels éventes peuvent etre confirmés soit avec le duplex-scanner, mais beacoup mieux avec la doppler couleur. La lois de Pascal qui pourrait expliquer un reflux systolique important dans une perforante incontinente est employé seulement dans le cas d'un quadre obstruitif ou restrictif des axes profonds en aval de l'embouchement de la perforant. En tout cas l'apport refluent ou débout de la phase systolique, meme s'il n'est pas rilevant, peut donner origine à un autre shunt avec la réentrée en bas. La ligature du tronc sous la perforante incontinente,interrompant la circulation privée, originante de celle-ci, limite son reflux. La déconnection des collatérales variqueuses et la ligature en-dessous des perforantes incontinentes créent également une diminution de la compliance du système veineux et une augmentation parallèle de la résistivité du réseau superficielle qui autolimite le reflux et privilègie une fois de plus la fonction d'aspiration vers le système veineux profond.

La démonstration de tout cela est constituée du fait que les segments variqueux des malades opérés selon une strategie Hémodynamique se vident complètement quand le malade commence un soulèvement sur la pointes des piedes.

Donc résumons:

1) **LA DECONNECTION DES SHUNTS VEINO-VEINEUX**

2) **LA FRAGMENTATION DE LA COLONNE DE PRESSION IDROSTATIQUE RESPECTANT LES PERFORANTES ET EXALTANT COMME CELA LA LEUR PHYSIOLOGIQUE FONCTION DE RÉENTRÉE COSTITUENT LES DEUX PRINCIPES HEMODYNAMIQUES FONDAMENTAUX DE LA CURE CHIVA.**

Une approche hémodynamique de la maladie variqueuse nécessite une étude précise anatomique et fonctionelle des varices qui ne peut se faire que grace à l'instrumentation écho-doppler. De cet étude est née une classification des shunts veino-veineux selon Franceschi(1988), modifiée récement par la Docteur Marc Bailly. L'évaluation hémodynamique pré-opératoire par examen clinique et écho-doppler du patient doit repérer les perforantes qui seront "terminalisées", c'est à dire utilisées comme réentrées. En effet, c'est à une point essentiel, toutes les perforantes n'ont pas un débit suffisant pour drainer le sang vers le résau profond. Il exist donc des tests de compression mise au point pour évaluer la fonction hémodynamique des perforantes. A la suite de cet étude écho-doppler,un marquage sur la peau du patient est effectué, guidant ainsi les points d'intervention pour le chirugien. Après l'intervention beacoup de varices auront disparu et les varices restantes se videront à la marche pour disparaitre définitivement dans l'espace de quelques mois. Nos controles sont effectués à 3 mois et 6 mois et annuellement. On peut prévoir de temps à autre la nécessité de revenir sur des points oubliés lors de la première cartographie. C'est le cas en particulier, pour les grosses varices ou' il est préférable d'oeuvrer degré par degré. Le malade doit donc etre prévenu de la nécessité d'intervenir souvent en plusieurs fois sous anesthésie locale.

La CHIVA est une méthode qui fait appel à une interprétation logique de données hémodynamiques recqueillies par explorations fonctionnelles et le bon sens doit toujours prévaloir dans son application.

BIBLIOGRAPHIE

1. **BASSI G.: Le varici degli arti inferiori Minerva Medica Torino 1962.**
2. **Bassi G.: Compendio di Terapia Flebologica Minerva Medica Torino 1985**
3. **Bjordal R. I.: Circulation patterns in incompetent perforaiting veins of the calf in venous dysfunction. da: PERFORAITING VEINS di MAY R. e coll. pag 71 - 88 Urban e Schwarzenberg. Munchen Wien Baltimore. 1981**
4. **Bjordal R. I.: The clinical implication and therapeutical consequences of the observed hemodynamic patterns. da : PERFORAITING VEINS di MAY R. e coll. pag 89 - 93 Urban e Schwarzenberg. Munchen Wien Baltimore. 1981**
5. **CAPPELLI M. TURCHI A. ERMINI S.: Considerazioni sul ruolo fisiopatologico delle perforanti nella varicosi essenziale quale presupposto alla concezione terapeutica dell'intervento CHIVA. Ospedali d'Italia Chirurgia volume XLIV NOV-DIC 1991 n° 6 pag 425-438**
6. **Franceschi C.: Theorie et pratique de la cure C.H.I.V.A. Editions de l'Armançon 1988.**

Phlébologie 92. Eds P. Raymond-Martimbeau, R. Prescott, M. Zummo.
John Libbey Eurotext, Paris © 1992, pp. 1042-1044

Bases théoriques et stratégiques de la cure CHIVA (cure conservatrice et hémodynamique de l'insuffisance veineuse en ambulatoire)

Claude Franceschi

CEEM, 12, avenue de Wagram, 75008 Paris, France.

A/FONDEMENTS THEORIQUES DE LA CURE CHIVA

La théorie comme la pratique de la cure CHIVA (Conservatrice et Hémodynamique de l'Insuffisance Veineuse en Ambulatoire) telle que nous la proposons,(4) reposent les cinq arguments suivants.

1-LA PRESSION HYDROSTATIQUE.)

En orthostatisme immobile, l'atteinte pariétale primitive ou secondaire, aboutit par l'hypotonie qui en résulte,à la séquestration avec stase de volumes sanguins importants ,chute du débit de drainage dans les voies profondes,malgré une pression physiologique dans cette posture(3,5).

Cette pression (90 mmHg à la cheville) en position debout immobile, égale chez le sujet normal et le sujet pathologique,est pour l'essentiel constituée par la pression hydrostatique (hauteur du poids de la colonne d'eau entre le coeur et la cheville). L'autre composante revient à la pression résiduelle (pression artérielle réduite de la chute de pression par perte de charge dans la micro-circulation).

Si le sujet pathologique vient à être allongé, la dilatation et la stase se réduisent considérablement, par le simple fait que la pression hydrostatique a été notablement réduite.Ce fait souligne le caractère déterminant de la pression hydrostatique pour que se manifestent les anomalies pariéto-valvulaires, au point que l'on ne peut plus parler de varices lorsque le sujet est couché, mais seulement lorsqu'il est debout.

Si l'on fractionne la colonne de pression hydrostatique par un garrot veineux posé sur la partie proximale de la veine variqueuse pendant que le sujet est couché, la veine se regonfle nettement moins vite dès que le sujet est remis en position debout que s'il ne portait ce garrot (épreuve de TRENDELENBOURG)

Ces constations impliquent simplement que la veine variqueuse

2-POMPE VALVUO-MUSCULAIRE ET SHUNTS VEINO-VEINEUX.

Chez le sujet normal, la reprise de la marche après une période d'orthostatisme immobile prolongée et souvent mal tolérée corrige rapidement l'excès de stase , par la mise en marche des pompes valvulo-musculaires éfficaces qui augmentent le débit de drainage et réduit la pression superficielle.L'effet de ces pompes augmente le gradient de pression motrice entre les secteurs superficiel et profond. Il en va tout autrement chez le sujet variqueux .Lors de

elle fonctionne correctement par elle-même, ne peut plus assurer un drainage unidirectionnel, superficiel vers le profond en raison de l'incontinence valvulaire,qui permet la création d'un véritable volume mort circulant en circuit fermé (shunts veino-veineux ou circulation privée de BASSI)(1).Si l'on pose un garrot sur la partie proximale de la varice , et que le sujet reprend la marche, on voit la varice réduire de calibre et la pression baisser (épreuve de Perthes), car ce garrot, fractionne certes la colonne de pression hydrostatique, mais déconnecte les shunts veino-veineux qui s'opposaient aux effets bénéfiques de la pompe valvulo-musculaire(3,5).
Ces constations montrent que la pompe valvulo-musculaire permet de réduire le calibre et la pression des varices, pour peu que soient interrompus les shunts veino-veineux.

3-GRADIENTS DE PRESSION STATIQUE ET DE PRESSION MOTRICE.

Ainsi,le fractionnement de la colonne de pression hydrostatique et l'interruption des shunts veino-veineux aboutissent à une réduction de la pression physiologique et à l'unidirectionnalité des flux de drainage en orthostatisme immobile et à la marche.Mais à cela, s'ajoute un autre phénomène. En effet, bien qu'unidirectionnels(sans reflux profond-superficiel), ces flux de drainage sont rétrogrades (de haut en bas, contrairement au drainage physiologique de bas en haut). Cette particularité est avantageuse pour l'efficacité du drainage (débit élevé et pression basse),car ici la gravité joue un rôle favorisant , contrairement à ce qui se passe chez le sujet normal.Les gradients de pression hydrostatique et de pression motrice sont de même sens alors qu'ils s'opposent chez le sujet sain.

4-INTERACTION PARIETO-VALVULAIRE ET HEMODYNAMIQUE.

Quelque soit la cause première,anomalie pariéto-valvulaire primaire,destruction valvulaire après thrombose,agression mécanique (orthostatisme immobile prolongé,port de charges lourdes) , hypotonie pariéto-valvulaire transitoire (imprégnation hormonale), pression résiduelle excessive (shunt artério-veineux permanent ou transitoire), la maladie aura tendance à se développer en raison de la compromission d'un drainage correct en débit et en pression.Les altérations hémodynamiques et pariéto-valvulaires rétro-agissent défavorablement l'une sur l'autre en un véritable cercle vicieux. La correction hémodynamique par la réduction de la pression hydrostatique à des valeurs infra-physiologiques et la déconnexion des shunts veineux, doit aboutir à rompre, voire inverser ce cercle vicieux. Ainsi, la maladie variqueuse ne s'exprime plus si les conditions hémodynamiques sont favorablement modifiées.

5-CONSERVATION OU DESTRUCTION DES VEINES SUPERFICIELLES

La destruction ou l' oblitération d'une veine superficielle, compromet le drainage des territoires qui en dépendent.La pression résiduelle s'élève en amont, ouvrant des shunts artério-veineux, qui élèvent à leur tour cette pression résiduelle.Cet effet sera d'autant plus important que les voies collatérales suppléantes seront pauvres, compromettant la trophicité tissulaire, dilatant excessivement des petites veines collatérales qui deviendront incontinentes par décoaptation valvulaire , créant les conditions d'évolutivité variqueuse. C'est pourquoi , la préservation des voies de drainage, même préalablement variqueuses, mais hémodynamiquement corrigées, devrait sinon diminuer le risque spontané d'évolutivité variqueuse,tout au moins ne pas créer les conditions d'évolutivité liées à leur destruction.Cette destruction intéresse souvent les voies lymphatiques adjacentes

,dont les effets sur l'économie circulatoires peuvent être préjudiciables.De plus,cette destruction entraîne une réduction du capital d'autogreffes lorsqu'elle concerne les troncs principaux de la saphène interne notamment.

B/LA STRATEGIE DE LA CURE CHIVA.

Nous avons vu que la seule atteinte pariéto-valvulaire ne suffit pas à déterminer la maladie variqueuse. Il en constitue une condition nécessaire mais non suffisante. Il faut de plus, pour que la maladie s'exprime que soit remplie une autre condition nécessaire bien que non suffisante, un désordre hémodynamique. Corriger l'une ou l'autre de ces conditions aboutit à la non expression de la maladie. Si l'on ne peut pas corriger la première par régénération du tonus pariétal (indirectement amélioré par la contention) et du jeu valvulaire,il est possible aujourd'hui de corriger la deuxième,à savoir le désordre hémodynamique .Ainsi,la stratégie de la cure CHIVA consiste à appliquer à chaque cas particulier les principes hémodynamiques de fractionnement de la colonne de pression,de déconnexion des shunts veineux et de conservation des voies de drainage.

1/LE FRACTIONNEMENT DE LA COLONNE DE PRESSION

Les axes incontinents seront interrompus au moins au tiers supérieur de cuisse et au tiers supérieur de jambe, en des sites qui ne compromettent pas le drainage , c'est-à-dire

-au-dessous d'une collatérale drainante,

-au-dessous d'une perforante refluante ou non, pour peu que cette dernière se jette dans un jeu valvulo-musculaire profond aspirant et efficace ou bien

-au raz de l'abouchement d'une crosse incontinente.

2/LA DECONNEXION DES SHUNTS VEINO-VEINEUX(FIG.4)

La déconnexion des shunts veino-veineux profond-superficiels, consiste à ouvrir la boucle profond-superficiel-profond en interrompant les axes superficiels incontinents

-immédiatement au-dessous des perforantes incontinentes et qui reçoivent des branches descendantes

-au niveau des perforantes incontinentes qui ne reçoivent pas de branche descendantes ,

-au niveau des crosses incontinentes .

3/LA CONSERVATION DES VOIES DE DRAINAGE

La conservation des voies de drainage doit assurer la perméabilité de veines à débit suffisant et à basse pression.
A cette fin, elles doivent se jeter dans une pompe valvulo-musculaire la plus efficace possible , par des perforantes valvulées ou non mais de calibre suffisant.

BIBLIOGRAPHIE

1 BASSI G Traitement de l'insuffisance des veines perforantes. Phlébologie,1965; 18:194

2 BJORDAL I The role of perforating vessels in varicose desease in Superficial and deep venous desease of the lower limb. M. TESI, J.A DORMANDY, 1 vol., Turin, Panminerva Medica, 1984, p. 91-97.

3 BJORDAL I "Pressure and flow measurements in venous insufficiency of the legs"; In controversies in the management venous desorders . Butterworths, 1989.

4 FRANCESCHI C. Théorie et pratique de la cure conservatrice et hémodynamique de l'insuffisance veineuse en ambulatoire. 1 Vol., Armançon Ed., 1988. 21390 PRECY-SOUS-THIL

5 NICOLAIDES A.N., ZOKOWSKI A.J. The value of dynamic venous measurements. World J. Surg.,1986; 54: 919-924.

Phlébologie 92. Eds P. Raymond-Martimbeau, R. Prescott, M. Zummo.
John Libbey Eurotext, Paris © 1992, pp. 1045-1047

Traitement des ulcères veineux par la technique CHIVA : résultats préliminaires

A. Bahnini, C. Franceschi, X. Mouren, E. Kieffer

Dr. Bahnini Service de Chirurgie Vasculaire, Groupe Hospitalier Pitié-Salpêtrière, 83, Boulevard de l'hôpital, 75013 Paris, France.

Les ulcères veineux résistants au traitement médical habituel constituent un des problèmes les plus difficiles à résoudre en pratique phlébologique. Ils concernent le plus souvent des patients âgés pour lesquels il s'agit d'une véritable infirmité.

La Cure Conservatrice Hémodynamique de l'Insuffisance Veineuse en Ambulatoire (CHIVA) consiste après réalisation d'une cartographie hémodynamique de la circulation veineuse des membres inférieurs à interrompre sélectivement le réseau veineux superficiel à des endroits pré-déterminés afin de drainer les segments intermédiaires dans des segments veineux continents et de soulager ainsi l'hyperpression veineuse distale des membres inférieurs. Il nous a semblé que le meilleur moyen de juger de l'efficacité de la cure CHIVA était de l'appliquer à des patients ayant des ulcères veineux chroniques résistants au traitement médical, la cicatrisation de l'ulcère servant de critère d'efficacité de la méthode.

Matériel et méthodes

De mars 1989 à avril 1991, 18 malades (12 hommes, 6 femmes), (âge moyen 61,8 ans) ont été opérés sous anesthésie locale pour des ulcères veineux chroniques concernant 21 membres inférieurs par la technique CHIVA. Tous les malades avaient une dermo-épidermite scléreuse et un oedème des membres atteints, 2 avaient également un eczéma variqueux, et 4 une infection locale sévère. Tous avaient des ulcères évoluant depuis plus de 3 mois sans tendance à la cicatrisation malgré un traitement médical bien conduit associant désinfection locale, soins locaux et contention élastique. 12 malades avaient des ulcères évoluant depuis plus d'un an et 5 malades avaient des ulcères évoluant depuis plus de 10 ans (extrêmes : 5 mois - 43 ans). Deux patients avaient déjà eu dans leurs antécédents une chirurgie veineuse d'exérèse (stripping) pour ulcère.

La taille des ulcères allait de 2 cm2 à 20 cm2 et 3 malades avaient une lésion artérielle associée (occlusion fémoro-poplitée traitée par pontage fémoro-poplité chez un patient, sténose du carrefour aortique avec oblitération iliaque gauche et sténose iliaque droite chez un patient et une occlusion fémorale superficielle chez un patient).

Tous les malades ont eu un bilan écho-doppler complet avec doppler pulsé du système veineux en position debout, couché et après activation de la pompe musculaire. Tous les malades ont eu également une exploration du système veineux iliaque et cave inférieur.

Tous les malades avaient une insuffisance veineuse superficielle. Chez 11 d'entre eux, il y avait également une insuffisance veineuse profonde (thrombose veineuse profonde, incontinence veineuse profonde ou association des deux).

L'intervention a consisté en une cure CHIVA sous anesthésie locale associée à une diaz-analgésie légère. Le traitement a consisté en la section-ligature des troncs veineux superficiels aux endroits précis repérés par l'écho doppler. En cas d'hypodermite sévère, et de nécessité d'abord dans la zone d'hypodermite, il a d'abord été procédé à une chirurgie haute permettant d'améliorer l'état trophique de la partie basse de la jambe. Secondairement, à un mois ou deux d'intervalle, était réalisé le complément chirurgical à la partie basse de la jambe dans une zone cutanée qui s'était assouplie grâce au traitement antérieur.

Résultats

Sur les 21 membres opérés, 4 ont eu deux interventions successives. La cicatrisation a été obtenue en 1 mois ou moins pour 12 membres (57 %) et en moins de 3 mois pour 6 membres (28,5 %). 3 ulcères (14,5 %) n'étaient pas complètement guéris respectivement à 4, 6 et 9 mois malgré une amélioration locale notable.

Le suivi moyen a été de 9,3 mois (3-20 mois). Aucun des 18 ulcères cicatrisés n'a récidivé pendant cette période. Tous les malades ont vu une régression très nette des troubles trophiques cutanés avec un assouplissement de la peau, et une disparition ou une amélioration importante de l'oedème. Les 3 ulcères qui n'ont pas cicatrisés à 4, 6 et 9 mois siégeaient tous les 3 sur des membres atteints d'insuffisance veineuse profonde sévère.

En conclusion, la cure CHIVA semble très efficace dans l'obtention d'une cicatrisation rapide des ulcères veineux des membres inférieurs. Cette cicatrisation est obtenue au prix d'une agression chirurgicale mineure, l'intervention se déroulant en ambulatoire sous anesthésie locale. Cette technique peut donc s'appliquer très facilement aux personnes âgées et fragiles. L'existence d'un ulcère veineux des membres inférieurs d'évolution chronique, résistant au traitement médical bien conduit, impose à notre sens une étude hémodynamique complète par écho-doppler pulsé et la réalisation si elle est techniquement possible d'une cure CHIVA.

REFERENCE

FRANCESCHI C. - Théorie et pratique de la Cure Conservatrice et Hémodynamique de l'Insuffisance Veineuse en Ambulatoire. Précy-sous-Thyl. Editions de l'Armançon 1988.

Phlébologie 92. Eds P. Raymond-Martimbeau, R. Prescott, M. Zummo.
John Libbey Eurotext, Paris © 1992, pp. 1048-1050

Contrôles de la cure CHIVA à 1 an à propos de 1047 cas

Dr. Patrier, Dr. d'Argentre, Dr. Artru, Dr. Dumas, Dr. Fima, Dr. Grandjean, Dr. Joly, Dr. Pinto

Clinique Sainte-Croix, 28, chemin de la Solitude, 72016 Le Mans Cedex. Clinique de Pontlieue, 13, place Adrien-Tironneau, 72019 Le Mans Cedex. Centre d'Angéiologie, 1, rue Girard, 72000 Le Mans, France.

L'étude a porté sur 1047 membres, entre 1989 et 1991. Il s'agit soit d'une première intervention soit de récidive post-stripping.
Tous ont été opérés selon les principes décrit par Claude Franceschi, par cure CHIVA, sous anesthésie locale, en ambulatoire par une équipe homogène de 5 angéiologues et 3 chirurgiens vasculaires, dans une unité de lieu et de temps. L'équipe ayant effectué à ce jour plus de 5000 interventions CHIVA.

LES RESULTATS

1) Patients :

- 82 % de femmes, 18 % d'hommes.
- âgés de : 0 %<20 ans, 4 % entre 20-30ans, 21 % de 30 à 40 ans, 23 % de 40 à 50 ans, 26 % de 50 à 60 ans, 21 % de 60 à 70 ans, 3 % de 70 à 80 ans, et 0,2 % de plus de 80 ans.
- 1ère intervention 92 %
- Récidive post-stripping 8 %

2) Les territoires atteints :

SI 79 % ; SE 5 % ; SA 3 % ; SI + SE 4 % ; SI + SA 6 % ; autres 3 %.

3) La stratégie et chirurgie :

- CHIVA type 1 99,5 % - type 2 0,5 %
- Shunt type 1 92 % - type 1 + 2 8 %
- Geste sur crosse SI = 92 % ligature ; 8 % ligature résection.
- Geste sur Tronc SI = crural seul 2 % ; crural et jambier 0,4 % ; jambier seul 36 %.
- Geste sur Tronc SE 4 %;
- Geste sur branche = crurale seule 5 % ; crurale et jambière 38 % ; jambière seule 48 %.; aucune 8 %.
- Phlébectomie = aucune 78 % des cas ; limitée 11,5 % ; étendue 9,5 %.

4) Traitement associé :

- Rien 27 %
- HBPM seule 21 %
- AINS seul 41 %
- HBPM - AINS 9,5 %

5) Complications :

- Hématome 3% ; infections 0,5 % ; désunion 0,3 % ; paresthésies SI - SE 0,6 %

6) Contrôle à J5 - J10 :

- CHIVA fonctionnel 83,5 % ; Non fonctionnel 16,5 %
- T.V.P. # 0,001 % (1 cas)
- T.V.S. aucune 75 % ; limitée cul de sac 13 % ; étendues et segmentaires 12 %.

7) Contrôle à J90 :

7.1 : CHIVA fonctionnel 98 % Non fonctionnel 2 %

7.2 : Gestes complémentaires :

. Sclérose 19 %

. Ligature sur tronc SI 0,3 % ; ligature sur branche 9 % ; phlébectomies 1 %.

7.3 : Sur les signes cliniques (1= Aggravation, 2 = Sans changement, 3 = Amélioration légère, 4 = Amélioration franche, 5 = Satisfaction complète).

Moyenne des avis du patient, du chirurgien vasculaire et de l'angéiologue.

	Esthétique	Télangiectasies	Douleur	Oedème
1	2	24,7	0,4	2,8
2	3,5	62,3	2	3,8
3	15	10	6	9,7
4	60,9	2,75	36	29,7
5	18,3	0	55,4	53,8

	Eczéma	Hypodermite	Ulcère
1	3,6	2,9	10,5
2	3,6	2,9	10,5
3	20	35,2	0
4	16,3	52,9	10,5
5	56,3	5,8	68,4

8) Contrôle à J365 :

8.1 : CHIVA fonctionnel 98,6 % Non fonctionnel 1,4 %

8.2 : Gestes complémentaires :

. Ligature sur tronc 2 %

. Ligature sur branches 3,2 %

. Phlébectomie 1 %

. Sclérothérapie 8,5 %

	Esthétique	Télangiectasies	Douleur	Oedème
1	0,5	8,4	0,46	0,3
2	2,2	71,5	1,3	1
3	14,9	10,53	3,6	1,3
4	57,5	7,3	21,8	23,1
5	24,7	2,1	72,5	74,1

	Eczéma	Hypodermite	Ulcère
1	0	0	8,3
2	2,7	0	0
3	10,8	16,6	0
4	13,5	62,5	16,6
5	72,9	20,8	75

COMMENTAIRE

Les résultats d'ensemble ont modifié nos habitudes.
Actuellement après plus de 5000 CHIVA faites.

- Notre équipe réalise actuellement plus de 90 % de cure CHIVA contre moins de 10 % pour les autres techniques (stripping ou autres).
- Les problèmes de T.V.S. semblent résolus par une indication plus large des anticoagulants HBPM à dose préventive, une reprise très rapide de la marche, l'expérience de l'équipe médicale et paramédicale (% TVS $<$ 1 - 2 %).
- Le problème esthétique :

- Nous faisons plus fréquemment phlébectomie sur
- segment se drainant mal.
- Shunt 1 + 2 plus fréquent.
- Ligature des perforantes refluentes isolées.

CONCLUSION

Tous les problèmes ne sont évidemment pas résolus mais le plus grand mérite de la cure CHIVA proposée par Claude Franceschi, est de nous avoir fait réfléchir sur notre pratique phlébologique, et de nous avoir conduit à former des équipes médico-chirurgicales complémentaires, parlant de même langage ; afin de proposer d'un commun accord la meilleure stratégie thérapeutique possible pour chaque patient en fonction de la clinique et du bilan écho-doppler ; et non plus sur des shémas pré-établis.

CHIVA - La technique chirurgicale - Notre expérience après quatre années

M. Blandamura, P. Santoro

Fondazione Internazionale Di Angiologia, Roma

Les auteurs décrivent la technique chirurgicale de ligature de la crosse et des ramifications périphériques. Ils analysent les avantages et les désavantages de l'emploi des matériels divers pour interrompre la crosse saphène interne (clips, fil réabsorbible et non, clips avec possibilité de ligature). On reporte les cas de réouverture de la crosse, en analysant les causes relatives et en référant sur les modifications techniques adoptées pour surmonter le problème. Nous reportons notre propre expérience pour optimiser les résultats esthétiques, en plus de ceux fonctionnels (pas d'usage de catgut au niveau de la jambe, microincisions, emploi de sparadrap pour fermer les incisions).

Conservative hemodynamic surgery of varices

Dr. Lucio Consiglio, Giorgi Giorgio (Cortona), Farina M. Angelo (Caserta)

The authors, after having discussed the physiopathological bases and their relative corrections to achieve recovery from the varicose disease of the lower limbs, illustrate the equipment which is necessary in order to perform a correct "CHIVA" technique (chirurgie hemodynamique insuffisance veineuse ambulatoire). The video shows the performance of two CHIVA cartographies in two patients, one of whom will later be operated. The operation, carried out under local anesthesia, mainly consists of a double closing of the saphenofemoral cross and the following section binding of the varicose branches immediately below the incontinent perforating veins. The immediate effectiveness of the operation is then shown.

Phlébologie 92. Eds P. Raymond-Martimbeau, R. Prescott, M. Zummo.
John Libbey Eurotext, Paris © 1992, pp. 1052-1054

Valvuloplastie-Chiva-saphènectomie

Vincenzo D'Agata, Dario Danieli, Leonarda Perrone, Nizar Sacran, Francesco Dall'Antonia

Dipartimento di Chirurgia Generale 1, Ospedale Civile di Vincenza, Italia.

The development of multiple applied techniques in the treatment of varicose veins in the legs has taken place, due to a growth in the knowledge of phisiopathology and the application of the eco-Doppler investigation procedure; however traditional surgery still maintains an important role.

Recently various authors have discussed an alternative to the surgical removal of the long saphenous vein. Multiple surgical techniques have been developed, over the last few years, to be carried out when there is a long femorosaphenic reflux caused by the dilation of the long saphenous vein at the cross, and due to the uinefficiency of the valves.

Kisner,May,Taheri,Ferris, et al have proposed various techniques for direct repair of the venous valve and autotransplant of valvular venous segments in the subinguinal region. Other authors are now proposing the use of prosthetic materials, Wnich are applied externally and wound round the saphenic cross at the ostial valve in order yto stop it leaking.

The treatment of this pathology is carried out in our surgical department. Without having to admit the patient, with a superficial local anaesthetic.

The technique consists of isolating the saphenous and collateral veins at the cross,cutting the pudendal or the circumflex iliac vein about 5 cm. from the cross and opening it wide, and winding it round the saphenous vein like a bandage where the dilation has taken place and the valves are not working.

The size of the saphenous vein is reduced by stitching the collateral vein with P.T.F.E. to the saphenous vein. This establishs contact and so stops the leaking in the tract which has been narrowed in the saphena.

The end result is a bandage of about one centimetre which wraps the saphena at the cross in the femoral vein. In the tract of the saphena where internally, according to edwards Anatomical Studies in 1937

-1940 and Cotton in 1961 on 200 patients with essential varices,98% present valvular plant.
In fact,at this point, during the operation when a patient is asked to cough or push, as if moving his bowels, it can be clearly seen that the saphena doesn't dilate as it did before the technique had been carried out.
In post operative check ups the plebectasie from the long saphena are Eco-Doppler shows the dissappearence of the long femorosaphenic reflux. In our case histories there was no record of complications either during or in the immediate post-operative period.
The valvuloplasty which is not in opposition to Saphenectomie or Chiva but an alternative way of recupating the saphena, in all those cases where the disease of the vein is not diffused but is limited to a restricted area; Valvuloplasty together with the phelbectomy and the tie-ing of any eventual perforated veins or collateral dilated veins, is carried out.
Observation is still taking place at the moment we can however refer to the experience at a distance of three years, with regard to two hundred patients.
The later clinical check ups will tell us how much the external valvular plasty sapheno-femoral has been able to bring closer together the plaps of the valves and modify the pressure inside the vein and so has been able yto block the natural deterioration of the vein walls in the varicous vein syndrome.

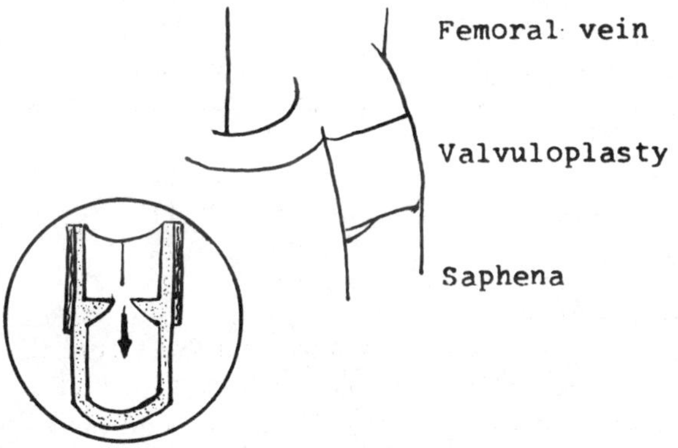

REFERENCES

Belcaro,G.,e coll.,(1989):Plication of the sapheno-femoral junction. An alternative to ligation. Phlebologie 89 - A.Davy,Stemmer R.,Eds. 1989 John Libbey Eurotex Ltd 990-991

Camilli,S.,e coll.,(1988): La venoplastica esterna nella terapia del l'insufficienza venosa profonda primitiva. Atti XXVI° Congr.L.S.C., Milano - Monduzzi ed. Bologna, Cardiovasc.Surg. II°:IX°, 833

Corcos,L.,e coll.,(1990): Chirurgia conservativa e ricostruttiva. IX Riunioni Fiorentine di Aggiornamento in Angiologia, Firenze. Abstracts S.I.F.L. Cortona 1990

Eriksson,I.,(1990): Reconstructive surgery for dup vein valve incompetence in the lowerlimb, Eur.J.Vasc.Surg., 4, 211, 1990

Franceschi,C.,(1988): Theorie et pratique de la cure conservatrice et l'insuffisance veineuse en ambulatoire. Ed.de l'Armacon 21390 Precy-sous-Thil

Kistner,R.L.,(1975):Surgical repair of the incompetent femoral vein valve.,Arch.Surg. 110, 1336,

May, R.,(1978):La chirurgia delle vene degli arti inferiori e del bacino. Ed.Piccin, Padova

Nicolades,A., e coll.,(1990): Progressi nella diagnostica venosa non invasiva. Stampa Medica, 490/97 45-51

Taheri,S.A.,Lazar,L.,Elias,S.,(1982): Status of vein valve transplantation after 12 mouths. Arch.Surg. 117,1313

Zamboni,P.,e coll.,(1989):Valvuloplastica venosa nell'insufficienza ostiale della vena safena magna.Tecnica originale.Atti delle Giornate Flebologiche Algheresi.

Chiva - résultats au cours de quatre années sur 1415 interventions

S. Mandolesi, M. Marchetti

Fondazione Internazionale Di Angiologia Roma

L'expérience italienne commence à partir de 1987 et pendant ces années elle a enregistré une augmentation exponentielle due à la diffusion que la Société italienne Opérateurs CHIVA (SIOC), née en 1989, a donné à cette méthodique au cours des trois dernières années. On présente les résultats cliniques et émodynamiques sur 1415 interventions que notre groupe a suivi pendant ces années. Tous les patients ont été opérés en anesthésie locale et en régime ambulatoire; par la suite, on a pratiqué une thérapie avec de l'héparine calcique. Les patients ont été contrôlés de la façon suivante dans la période postopératoire: après 10 jours - après 3 mois - après 1 an et par la suite tous les ans. Pour 85% les résultats cliniques ont été bons, tandis que pour 14.5% ils se sont avérés inchangés et pour 0,5% pires. On analyse en détail, au point de vue clinique et émodynamique, les complications, les récidives et les insuccès.

Phlébologie 92. Eds P. Raymond-Martimbeau, R. Prescott, M. Zummo.
John Libbey Eurotext, Paris © 1992, pp. 1056-1061

CHIVA : analyse critique

Claude Garde

93, avenue du Bac, 94210 La Varenne Saint-Hilaire, France.

La Méthode CHIVA pas plus que les autres méthodes ne vous permettra d'atteindre le nirvana dans le traitement des varices. Aucune d'ailleurs ne le permet , une complémentarité est obligatoire pour obtenir une certaine sénérité...intellectuelle et une réponse aux demandes de nos patients.

La méthode CHIVA, imaginée par le Docteur FRANCESCHI pour répondre aux critères modernes de tous traitements répond-t-elle aux questions suivantes:

- Prévient-elle de la récidive variqueuse?
- Donne-t-elle un résultat esthétiquement satisfaisant et répondant aux demandes des patients?
- Est-elle sans risque et sans complication?
- Est-elle légère à mettre en place?

METHODE CLASSIQUE (Schéma N° 1)

Le but des méthodes classiques est simple : Il consiste à empêcher le gradient de pression profondeur/surface et haut/bas de refluer dans le réseau superficiel par des perforantes devenues incompétentes, la plus haute située étant la crosse saphène interne pour le territoire interne, la crosse saphène externe pour le territoire externe, et, à stopper la dilatation des veines superficielles par le gradient haut/ bas en les supprimant. on empêche alors le système profond de se déverser dans le réseau superficiel. L'évacuation sus-aponévrotique se fait par les perforantes compétentes et le gradient <u>instantané</u> lié au travail musculaire qui, aspire le sang dans les voies profondes. Devant le même cas pathologique, la méthode CHIVA procède d'un raisonnement opposé .

(Shéma N°2)

Le but n'est pas de supprimer les réflux et les veines incompétentes, mais de les "vidanger" dans le système veineux profond. Pour ce faire (schéma 2) la saphène interne incompétente est ligaturée à plusieurs niveaux :

- d'abord au niveau de la crosse, en laissant quelques veines afférentes qui assureront une circulation sanguine, puis sous chaque perforante. Ainsi le flux du sang superficiel sera aspiré par le gradient de pression induit par la pompe musculaire.

- Les branches de la saphène sont elles aussi déconnectées afin de stopper les shunt veino-veineux et de réinjecter le sang dans les voies profondes.

<u>Ainsi</u> les branches, la saphène, et, donc tout le réseau superficiel, vont se vidanger en profondeur. Les veines, sans tension pariétale, vont retrouver un calibre normal et "disparaitre" en quelques mois.

<u>ANALYSE CRITIQUE</u> :

Toute mécanique dite "dynamique" a besoin de mouvement. Pendant l'activité musculaire normale (marche, course ect..) les troncs profonds vidangent les troncs superficiels. Si l'on pratique une phlébographie dynamique en injectant un produit de contraste de même viscosité que le sang dans une veine superficielle, on peut apprécier cette aspiration par les troncs profonds .

(Shéma N°3) (Schéma 4)

Mais que se passe-t-il en station debout immobile?

Pendant le repos musculaire et sans activité les valvules perdent partiellement leur compétence et le flux sanguin va progressivement stagner dans les pieds aussi bien au niveau superficiel que profond.

Il y a aussi une augmentation de pression et de la stase même chez les sujets normaux en position debout. Cette pression chute immédiatement après quelques pas chez les sujets sains.

Chez un sujet ayant subi une CHIVA , le système veineux superficiel va surcharger d'autant la pression sur les troncs profonds. Il y a alors majoration de la stase veineuse profonde. Ceci explique pourquoi la CHIVA n'est pas appropriée aux personnes travaillant debout immobile ou piétinant mais aussi pourquoi les signes fonctionnels (lourdeurs,douleurs,ect...) persistent dans ce cas après traitement par CHIVA.

Une autre limite à apporter à la CHIVA est la difficulté qu'il y a à associer une autre technique et particulièrement la sclérothérapie.

(Schéma N°5)

Quand le patient vient d'être opéré, le réseau superficiel est incompétent. Dans ce cas le flux sanguin se dirige normalement vers la profondeur. Mais il faut se souvenir que le premier but de la CHIVA est de faire chuter la tension pariétale, afin que le vaisseau, progressivement, retrouve une part de sa compétence.

Sur le plan hémodynamique, cette compétence constitue un frein circulatoire et va induire un bas débit avec parfois un arrêt circulatoire sans stase.

Ceci ne semble pas un problème, mais si pour une raison esthétique ou fonctionnelle on doit associer une autre thérapeutique et particulièrement la sclérothérapie, il y a un risque dans ce cas d'engendrer une thrombose de la CHIVA. Le résultat de la sclérothérapie sera par ailleurs imprévisible, le liquide sclérosant pouvant stagner ou fuser dans les branches non prévues.

(Schéma N°6)

Il faut se souvenir enfin que le réseau veineux n'est pas un système terminal, mais au contraire un véritable réseau en mailles de filet.
(Schéma N°7)

Ainsi le système veineux profond est connecté à la fois avec les saphènes, mais aussi,avec les branches et les branches de branche. Cela n'est pas d'emblée une contre-indication à la cure CHIVA qui permet un écoulement du flux comme sur les marches d'un escalier vers les troncs profonds,mais il faut tempérer cette méthode par deux ecueils:
(Schéma N°8)

- 1) La néogénèse autour des ligatures et des ligature-sections qui organise autour d'un processus cicatriciel classique, un nouveau reflux.
- 2) Mais aussi il faut se souvenir que les méthodes non invasives,clefs de voûte de la CHIVA, ne permettent pas de découvrir toutes les "mailles" du réseau, surtout si elles sont inférieures à 2mms.

Une autre contre-indication à la CHIVA apparait donc ainsi: les patients présentant un potentiel évolutif marqué ou un réseau complexe risqueront une récidive rapide avec possible réapparition de reflux longs.

INDICATIONS LOGIQUES DE LA CHIVA.

La CHIVA est une méthode logique. Bien indiquée, bien investiguée, bien appliquée elle doit, dans un certain nombre de cas donner des résultats supérieurs aux autres méthodes.

- Les sujets pratiquant une activité sportive,notamment,des sports d'endurance, plus généralement les sujets actifs et jeunes. Pour eux, la pompe musculaire permet de faire fonctionner le mécanisme.
- On peut aussi la proposer aux patients présentant une varicose peu évoluée et dont la cartographie variqueuse reste simple, surtout s'ils n'ont pas une potentialité évolutive marquée.
- Par contre: cette méthode donnera des résultats plus discutables chez les sujets travaillant debout,piétinant,sédentaires,à fortiori âgés.

- Elle sera une raison à éviter chez les sujets présentant une varicose complexe et évoluée, une récidive surtout si elle est post-chirurgicale.

- Elle sera contre-indiquée en cas d'insuffisance veineuse profonde et bien sur en présence d'un syndrome post phlébitique.

- Il conviendra en outre de prévenir le patient qu'elle n'entraine pas systématiquement la disparition de la varicose et par conséquent elle sera à éviter si le primum movens est complètement esthétique.

<u>CONCLUSION</u>: La CHIVA répond-t-elle aux critères de toutes thérapeutiques modernes?

Prévient-elle la récidive? C'eût été le cas si elle prenait en compte les fondements même de la maladie. Elle prétent soigner l'insuffisance veineuse alors qu'elle ne traite en fait , comme les autres d'ailleurs, que la maladie variqueuse. Elle ne prévient pas la récidive comme l'atteste le recul que l'on a actuellement sur la méthode.

<u>EST-ELLE ESTHETIQUE?</u> Oui, si l'on considère la taille et le nombre des incisions pratiqués. Non, si l'on souhaite une disparition quasi complète des varices.

<u>EST-ELLE AMBULATOIRE?</u> Oui, car tous les gestes sont pratiqués sous anesthésie locale.

<u>EST-ELLE NON DANGEUREUSE ET DENUEE DE COMPLICATIONS?</u> Oui, si l'on considère que le séul risque est la transformation du CHIVA en CIVA ou l'association ligature/thrombose et à terme ligature/sclérose.

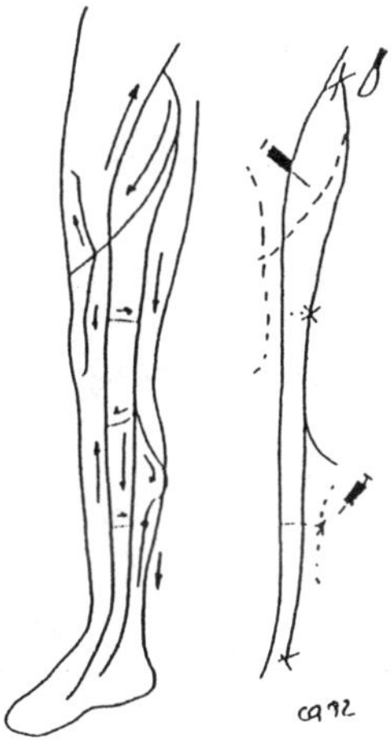

(Sçhéma N° 1)

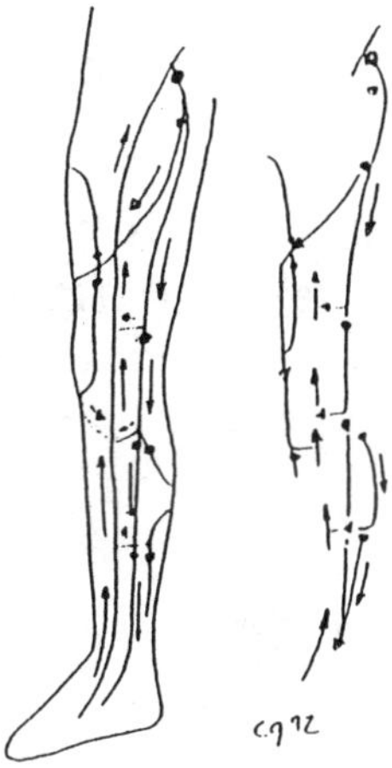

(Shéma N°2)

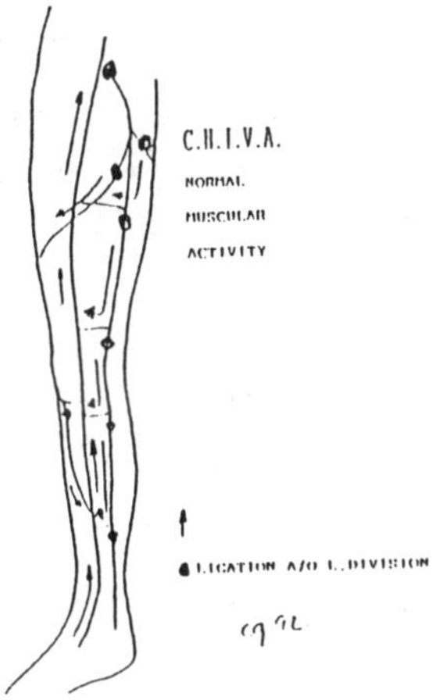

(Shéma N°3)

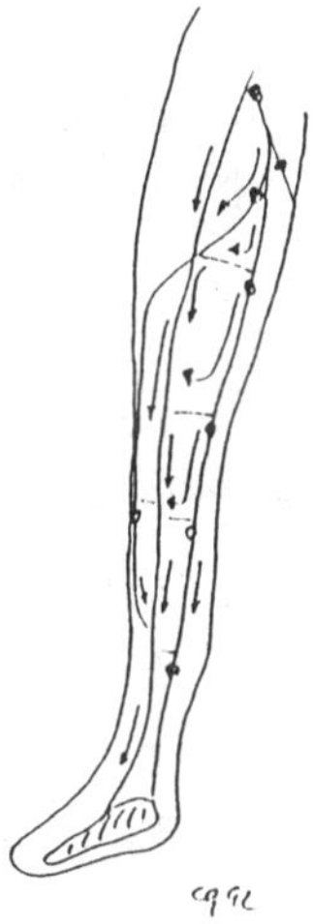

(Schéma 4)

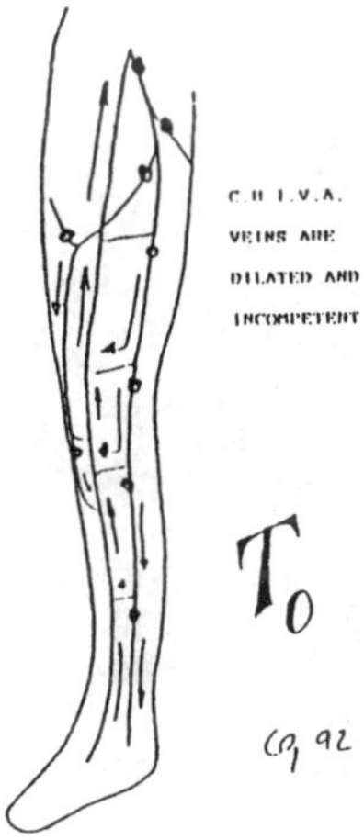

(Schéma N°5)

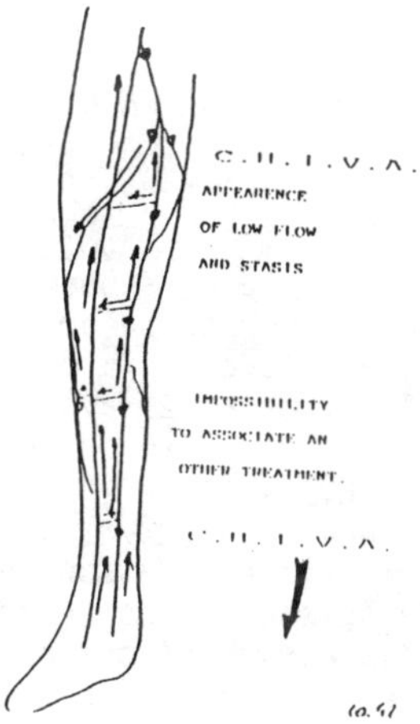

(Schéma N°6)

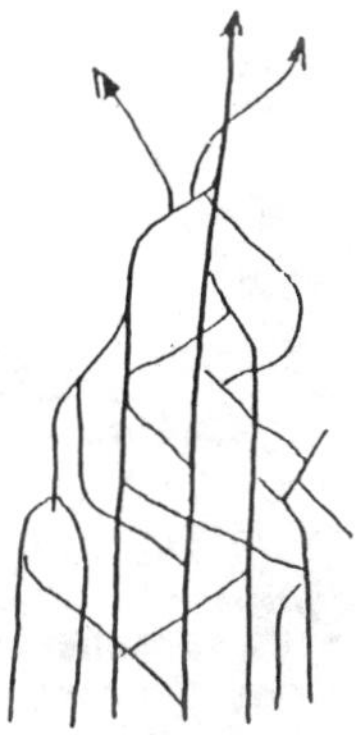

(Schéma N°7)

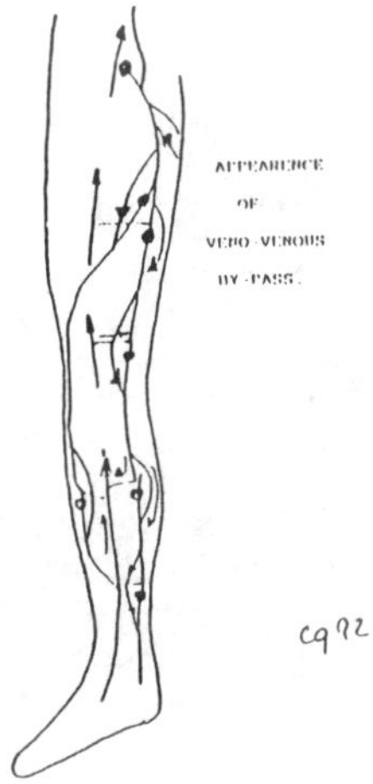

(Schéma N°8)

Phlébologie 92. Eds P. Raymond-Martimbeau, R. Prescott, M. Zummo.
John Libbey Eurotext, Paris © 1992, pp. 1062

Crossectomie et stripping externe court selon Mayo sous anesthésie locale et ambulatoirement

Michel Gross

Avenue de la Gare, 10, 1003 Lausanne, Suisse

Historique

Au 7ème siècle après Jésus-Christ, Paul d'Egine pratique l'excision, entre deux ligatures, de la saphène interne, et cela au tiers moyen de la cuisse, soit au-dessous de la 2ème perforante de Dodd.
En 1896, Moore de Melbourne pratique la crossectomie qu'il réalise ambulatoirement.
En 1906, Mayo de Rochester USA élimine la saphène interne par stripping externe.
En 1907, Babcock invente le stripping interne.
En 1950, Ryckaert de Bruxelles pratique ambulatoirement la crossectomie et le stripping externe.

Technique

Après avoir marqué avec précision le trajet de la veine saphène interne, nous anesthésions son parcours, et particulièrement la région où se situe la crosse.
Par une incision paralabiale et verticale, nous abordons la crosse de la saphène interne que nous lions, à ras de la veine fémorale, après avoir lié et sectionné toutes les collatérales. Le stripper de Mayo modifié, présentant un rebord tranchant, nous permet ensuite de stripper la saphène interne jusqu'en-dessous du genou et de la sectionner sans ouvrir la peau. Nous ressortons ensuite le stripper avec le segment crural de la saphène interne sur laquelle sont branchés les fragments des collatérales et des perforantes de suisse. Après fermeture de la plaie sus-inguino-crurale, nous pratiquons une compression et demandons au patient de marcher vigoureusement et immédiatement après l'intervention.
Les détails de la technique sont illustrés par la vidéo-cassette projetée lors du Congrès.

Conclusion

Le stripping externe de la saphène interne sous anesthésie locale et ambulatoirement écarte au maximum les inconvénients et dangers inhérents à une intervention analogue effectuée sous anesthésie générale entraînant un alitement.

Par cette technique, nous ménageons le nerf saphène interne qui est très vulnérable dans son trajet jambier, nous favorisons la marche immédiate, ce qui constitue la meilleure prophylaxie anti-thrombo-embolique, et, nous éliminons les risques de récidives puisque toutes les tuniques de la veine ont été enlevées par le stripper externe.

Stripping court - Préambule à la phlébectomie de Muller

Dr. Pierre-Marie Noël de la Pâquerie

Les améliorations de l'anesthésie locale ainsi que celles apportées par les techniques chirurgicales, aidées par la recherche écho-doppler des reflux veineux superficiels, ont permis le développement du traitement des varices totalement en ambulatoire et sans hospitalisation.

Actuellement, la majeure partie des patients peuvent traiter leurs varices sans recourir à l'hospitalisation et sans aucun risque pour leur santé.

Grâce au Docteur VAN DER STRICH et au Docteur MULLER, le traitement ambulatoire des varices était déjà partiellement codifié.

Notre expérience dans plus de 1000 cas nous permet, hors hospitalisation, de combiner le stripping court en préambule aux phlébectomies de Müller, complétées de scléroses ou plutôt de microscléroses. Dans la mesure où il existe au doppler une nette incontinence ostiale de crosse de grande saphène, on peut recourir au stripping et ce, strictement sous anesthésie locale grâce à l'application de blocs réfrigérants complétée de Xylocaine sous cutanée.

Dans le mesure où toutes les conditions de sécurité sont requises, le patient, dans une ambiance dédramatisée, peut alors voir traiter son incontinence ostiale avec sa portion saphène de cuisse. La pose de blocs réfrigérants assure une cryo-anesthésie qui rend l'injection de Xylocaine sous cutanée indolore.

Un contact permanent de confiance entre le phlébo-chirurgie et le patient permet un stripping court classique.

Les incisions ont été préalablement déterminées à l'écho-doppler, ce qui permet des cicatrices minimes d'autant que ces dernières sont assurées par des sujets intra-dermiques.

Médicalement et socialement, le traitement ambulatoire des varices présente ces avantages:

* de concilier un geste radical avec la dédramatisation et l'esthétisme de l'intervention;
* le patient conserve ses activités;
* nous n'avons pas noté de complications majeures, donc aucun risque pour le patient;
* le résultat esthétique et cosmétique est très intéressant;
* absence des répercutions financières non négligeable

Phlébologie 92. Eds P. Raymond-Martimbeau, R. Prescott, M. Zummo.
John Libbey Eurotext, Paris © 1992, pp. 1064-1066

Ambulatory stripping

Jean Van der Stricht

Faculté de Médecine, Université de Bruxelles, Hopital Molière, Longchamp, Belgique.

By saphenectomy I mean the pulling out either of the whole Long Saphenous Vein from the groin to below the internal malleolus or of the Short Saphenous Vein from the popliteal junction to the external malleolus.

I perform this operation in accordance with a well runned technique I have already described in 1962. It is mainly based on two features:
- 1° local anaesthesia exclusively.
- 2° removal of the vein by invagination.

I recall schematically (fig.1-2) the technique, already detailed in my previous publications (4) or taken up by other authrors (1-2-3).

By the invagination technique, tne turned inside out vein slides into its perivascular sheath. So, the removal of the venous trunk cannot drag down any nerve or other close tissues, as it may occur by the classical internal (BABCOCK) or external stripping (MAYO). Local anaesthesia avoids any vital risk. Moreover both invagination and local anaesthesia avoid morbidity such as haemorrhage and hematomas. Consequently, if a saphenous vein has to be removed ambulatorily I believe preference should be given to this atraumatic technique of stripping.

The question is whather saphenous vein must be stripped ambulatorily. It is to say, releasing from hospital and return home in the first hours following the operation.

A proper full saphenectomy is more than a suprafacial phlebectomy. The sapheno-femoral junction and especially the sapheno-popliteal junction are subfacial and close to arteries, nerves, lymphatics. It is not a "minor " surgery

So the strict rules of surgery must be respected. Therefore it must be performed in hospital and benefit from the substructures and equipment of an operating room.

That seems unquestionable but what about releasing the patient just after his operation ?

What are the advantages of releasing him without hospitalization a day or two ?

Obviously it reduces the patient's expenses. It avoids psychological trouble of an instable or aged patient. Finally it reduces the congestion of hospitals and the expenses of the Social Security.

What are the disadvantages ? In my opinion home coming urges patient to underestimate the seriousness of his treatment and not to take the postoperative orders into account.

The outcome of any surgical procedure depends on the quality of postoperative care. In the present case, special care has to be taken seeing Saphenectomy is a procedure performed on the lower limb where high venous pressure has to be avoided at any time to prevent oedema.

Complications of a well performed stripping are rare. Small bleeding or pain may occur in the first hours. They are not serious in hospital where the appropriate measures are taken automatically.

The same minor complications at home create patient's and his relatives ' anxiety. Soon the small complications trigger off an escalation of iatrogenic pathology that finally will cost the patient and the Society much more than the few expenses of two days hospitalization.

Unquestionably, the pitfalls of ambulatory surgery can be reduced by a sound organisation of homecare. But it also has its price and despite everything a small pourcentage of failures is always unavoidable.

A method may be applauded because it ensures 95% of success. It can also be criticized and rejected for the 5% failures, whereas even I% failure in the treatment of a disease as mild as the varicose one is too much !

It is why I never practise real ambulatory surgery and prefer, after stripping, to allow the patient to get up for a short period of active walking the very day of the operation but in hospital itself.

So, in my opinion ambulatory saphenectomy is quite feasible technically nevertheless it is not really useful for the patient.

References .

1/ BERGAN J.J. and YAO J. Venous disorders
Ed. Saunders I99I Pages 212 - 213

2/ PATEL J. et LEGER L. Nouveau traité de Technique Chirurgicale
Ed. Masson I970 Pages 540 - 542

3/ PERRIN M. Insuffisance Veineuse chronique des membres inférieurs
Ed. Mc. Graw-Hill Paris I990 Page 47

4/ van der STRICHT J. Saphenectomie par invagination sur fil
Presse Médicale Paris I963/2I Pages I08I - I082

Stripping by invagination technique.

(J. van der Stricht)

Fig. 1

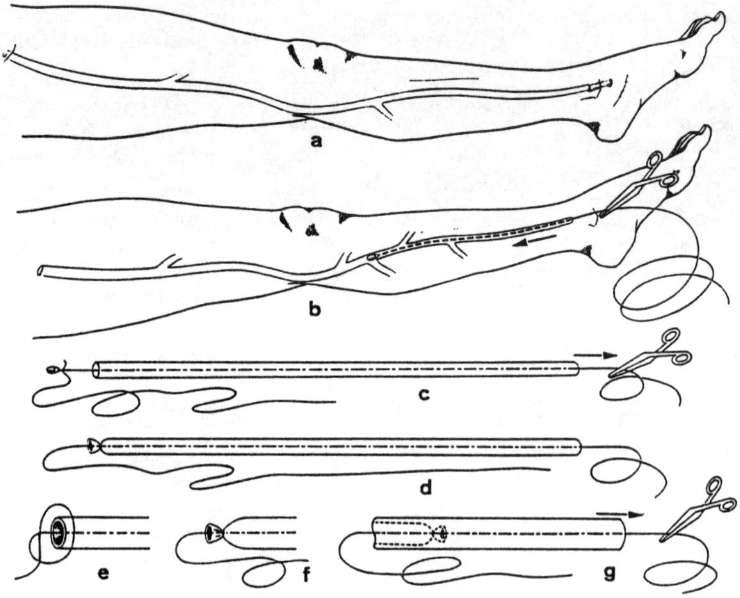

– *Stripping par invagination selon* Van der Stricht.

Fig. 2

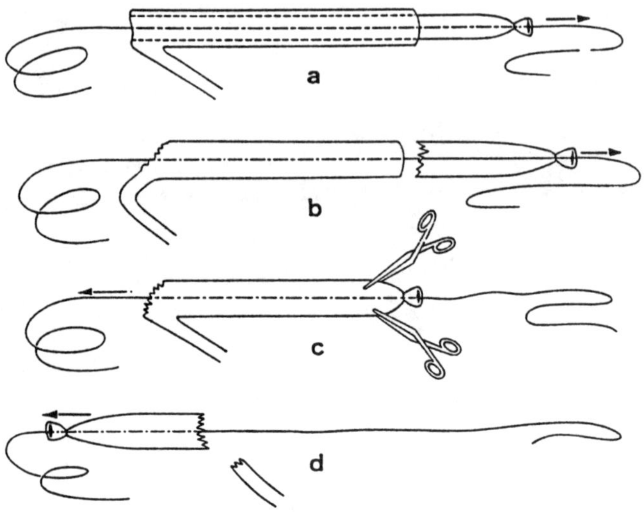

– *Reprise en sens inverse en cas de rupture de la veine.*

An other intraluminal stripping technique

Docteur Paul Albert Ouvry

Clinique Saint-Pierre, 76200 Dieppe, France

When in a young adult progressive dilatation of the long saphenous vein and its branches is caused primarily by an incompetent sapheno femoral junction, a flush ligation and a short stripping are first indicated.

The intraluminal invagination technique described for stripping by Keller before 1910 and by Van der Stricht in 1962 has been modified by the author. In his modification a gauze strip, 5 to 10 cm in width, is inserted with the invagination so that the risk of breaking and tearing the vein is decreased. The author describes directing the stripper in the long saphenous vein from groin to the upper leg. This stripper is then attached to a gauze strip with fishline. A 10-cm wide strip is used for large saphenous veins and a 5-cm strip for moderate saphenous veins. As the vein is stripped, the gauze strip remains in the venous pathway until the very end of the operation. In this way, it aids in hemostasis, decreasing hematoma formation. Residual varicose veins untreated by stripping technique are then treated by sclerotherapy beginning 3 weeks after the operation. 100 cases of invagination technique are reported.

Phlébologie 92. Eds P. Raymond-Martimbeau, R. Prescott, M. Zummo.
John Libbey Eurotext, Paris © 1992, pp. 1068

D'autres armes thérapeutiques dans le traitement chirurgical de la maladie variqueuse essentielle. Le stripping par invagination sur fil

Gérard Lange

Tours, France.

Le film qui est présenté décrit sur un mode parfois humoristique une technique datant d'une vingtaine d'années environ, reprise et modernisée par de nombreux angéiologues français, depuis quelques années.

On y insiste de manière didactique sur la préparation et la réalisation technique de l'intervention, dont le but essentiel est de réaliser un traitement purement ambulatoire de certaines phases de la maladie variqueuse essentielle.

L'anesthésie est strictement locale, et la technique peut être réalisée dans un cabinet d'angéiologie équipé de manière sommaire mais efficace sur le plan chirurgical et de la réanimation.

Il s'agit d'une intervention qu'on peut qualifier de micro-chirurgie (puisqu'elle nécessite parfois l'utilisation de lunettes grossissantes pour les veines de très petit calibre) et qui permet une déambulation immédiate et une reprise de travail soit dans la journée soit le lendemain de l'intervention.

La mise en évidence des résultats immédiats et à moyen terme, donne une idée vraisemblable de cette technique.

Phlébologie 92. Eds P. Raymond-Martimbeau, R. Prescott, M. Zummo.
John Libbey Eurotext, Paris © 1992, pp. 1069-1071

Proximal long saphenous vein stripping as office procedure

Stefano Ricci, Mihael Georgiev

Corso Trieste 123, 00198 Rome, Italy.

High ligation, division and stripping of the thigh portion of the long saphenous vein (LSV) ("short stripping") as described by Crossetti (2) is a part of the radical office-based varicose vein surgery previously described (6). The decision to strip the LSV is essentialy clinical: a Doppler-incompetent but not dilated LSV is not necessarily removed (7). As a rule we perform the LSV stripping as a last operation: all other varicose veins are removed first by the Müller's technique ("office phlebectomy") (5,6).

Marking

The LSV is identified in the standing position by careful palpation and percussion (Doppler assisted if needed) and its course marked on the skin with 7% $KMnO_4$. This is done prior to the removal of any varicose vein. A separate (transverse) sign is placed over the most dilated, superficial and best palpable sites; these are often the points of confluence of perforators and large collaterals, where - if needed - the LSV is more easily retrieved by a separate incision.

Anesthesia

A total of 80-100 ml of mepivacaine 0.4% with epinephrine 1:500 000 in saline are employed for local infiltration anesthesia: 20 ml for the groin infiltration and the rest along the LSV. While this amount and type of anesthesia is sufficient in most cases, some patients may experience discomfort or pain during the LSV dissection or because of the traction of a large perforating or collateral vein; in such case additional anesthetic may be injected under the guide of the tip of the stripper. In some cases, i.e. very anxious or oversensitive patients, we found it helpful to add a self-administered inhalation sedation-analgesia with nitrous oxyde/ oxygen, as widely used in dental practice (3).

High Ligation And Division Of The LSV ("Crossectomy")

The patient is operated in a supine Trendelenburg position, with the knee bent and the limb externaly rotated for optimal groin and medial thigh exposure.

A 3-cm incision at the groin crease (previously marked) is sufficient in most cases and heals fast with best cosmetic results. With the edges of the incision retracted by an assistant, the fatty and fibrous layers of the subcutaneous tissues are divided and retracted until the LSV is seen; the latter is then pulled up with a forceps to allow a Mayo's dissecting scissors to be passed under the vein, which is thus elevated and then divided between two haemostatic forceps. The proximal segment of the LSV is pulled up, all collaterals joining it ligated and divided until the exposure of the sapheno-femoral junction. The proximal stump is then doubly ligated: a 3-0 catgut ligature is placed as close to the femoral vein as possible and a second transfixion ligature with 3-0 catgut is placed just distal to the first one; the residual free stump is cut off.

LSV Stripping

The distal segment of the LSV is dissected downwards from the surrounding subcutaneous fat as much as possible. The constant postero-medial thigh vein is usualy exposed, ligated and divided. The LSV is then passed through the ring of the Mayo's external phlebo-extractor (4). While the LSV is kept under traction, the ring stripper is pushed downwards along the LSV, dissecting the latter from the surrounding tissues. A large collateral or the Dodd's perforator usually stop the progression of the stripper, which is then changed with the Corcos' external phlebo-extractor (1) (the tip of this instrument is not a ring but a cylinder with a cutting edge). This stripper usually cuts off the collateral and perforating veins and permits to dissect the LSV down to the point it has been ligated and divided during the previous operation; the LSV is then pulled out from the groin incision. If not previously divided, the LSV is simply cut at the knee level with the edge of the stripper or with a hypodermic needle, thus avoiding an incision. In about one half of the cases the groin incision is the only one needed; when the LSV ruptures or is cut at a higher level by the stripper, it must be retrieved from a small separate incision which heals without suture.

Immediately after the extraction of the LSV a firm gauze cylinder is repeatedly rolled from the knee up along the LSV mark in order to express any blood clots through the groin incision, and an adhesive bandage is applied on the thigh. Only then is the groin incision closed with a single intradermal absorbable suture with 3-0 catgut. Firm gauze or cotton pads are applied for selective compression over the groin an over the course of the LSV and then a firm adhesive bandage is applied. on the entire limb. Once bandaged thi limb, the patient resumes gradually the upright position and after ½ to 1 hour of walking exercise is allowed to leave the office.

This bandage is kept in place for one week, at the end of which the patient is seen again and the bandage removed. If there is no edema, induration, haematoma or tenderness along the course of the LSV, all that is needed is few weeks of 15-18-mm graduated elastic stocking. In the presence of the abovementioned lesions, 30-40-mm stocking (Sigvaris 504) or adhesive (or non-adhesive) compressive bandage is applied and worn until the latter subside.

Discussion And Conclusions

The above described LSV stripping is part of the radical office-based varicose vein surgery performed in our office (6). When more operations are needed on the same limb, these are performed at separate sessions 2-7 days apart. We found it advantageous to first remove all varicose veins with the Müller's technique and perform the LSV stripping - when needed - as a last stage. This major procedure (LSV stripping) is thus performed on a less tense patient (past experience), on a limb without varicose veins (no haemorrhage) and with the LSV itself reduced in volume because isolated and compressed by the bandage of the previous operation.

The local infiltration anesthesia (with or without inhalation sedation-analgesia) permits immediate deambulation thus making it possible to perform LSV stripping as a truly office procedure. Epinephrine infiltration, Trendelenburg position, emotional stress, previous removal of the varicose veins and immediate bandaging all make this operation nearlya"bloodless" procedure.

Complications are both infrequent and mild and in our long experience occur at a rather constant rate. During 1990 141 LSV stripping operations were performed in patients who previously had one or more Müller's operations. There were three cases of groin haematoma (2.1%), one of wound infection (0.7%), one of lymphocele at knee level (0.7%) and one of persisting foot edema of lymphatic type (0.7%)(6).

References

1. Corcos L. (1989) Structure and use of the external phlebo-extractor. Phlebology, 4:275.
2. Crossetti JP and Müller R. (1972) Traitement radical ambulatoire des varices. Proceedings of the 8th International and 19th Brazilian Congress of Angiology. p.439.
3. Langa WB. (1976) Relative analgesia in dental practice: inhalation analgesia and sedation with nitrous oxide. Philadelphia: WB Saunders.
4. Mayo CH. (1906) Treatment of varicose veins. Surg Gynecol Obstet, 2:385.
5. Müller R. (1966) Traitement des varices par la phlébectomie ambulatoire. Phlébologie, 19:277.
6. Ricci S and Georgiev M. (1992) Office Varicose Vein Surgery Under Local Anestesia. J Dermatol Surg Oncol 18:55.
7. Trendelenburg F. (1890) Uber die Unterbindung der Vena saphena magna bei Unterschenkelvarizen. Beiträge zur Klinische Chirurgie, 7:199.

Varizenchirugie - A simple method for the presentation of the Crosse

D. Dagmar Berg

To avoid with a maximum of security a "Rezidiv" in "Varizenchirugie" it is necessary to tie up all the sidebranches directly on the Crosse and to remove the "V.saphena" as near as possible to the entrance into the "V.femoralis".

For this reason, after opening the groin, we start slinging the "V.saphena" with three treads. The further preparation of the sidebranches exist each time one thread is placed underneath one sidebranch and the sidebranch is alloyed simultaneously with a separate thread.

With this technique it is extremely important to look for the "V.epigastrica superior" at the mouth of the "V.saphena magna" into the "V.femoralis", to tie it up and to carry on underneath this veine with the guided thread. Afterwards the Crosse can be alloyed directly at the mouth. For security the second thread is layed on top of the first knot. Hereafter by a separate cut either in the area of the knuckle or underneath the knee-joint one looks for the "V.saphena magna" and one pushes the "Nabastoff-probe" up to the groin.

The third thread now serves as a support and one can open the "V.saphena magna", the probe is going to come out and is fixed with the third thread.

The probe still lying down, afterwards with the help of very small cuts of a size of a millimeter it is looked after "Perforansvenen" which can be drawn out without ligature.

The suture of the skin has to be closed; the packing by lifting up the leg is followed and in the end the "V.saphena magna" Will be drawn out in completely.

With this very careful treatment it is possible to avoid bloodloosing and the time of the operation will be minimised. In the meantime 15,000 operations of this kind have been prooved very successful.

Phlébologie 92. Eds P. Raymond-Martimbeau, R. Prescott, M. Zummo.
John Libbey Eurotext, Paris © 1992, pp. 1073-1075

Stripping court de la grande saphène au moyen de la seule incision inguinale

P. Sorrentino, G. Spreafico*, C. Castoro, P. Borelli, F. Schwan, E. Vincenti, U. Baccaglini

*Clinica Chirurgica I, University de Padova, Italy. * Presidio Ospedaliero Dolo, Venezia, Italy.*

Selon le concept de base qui caracterise la phlebologie moderne, la cause des varices essentielles des membres inferieurs reside dans un reflux ostial (1). En outre, dans 30% des cas, le reflux n'interesse pas la saphene dans sa totalite mais au niveau de la jambe les branches collaterales, anterieure et/ou posterieure, seulement sont impliquees (3). Cette donnee est confirmee par l'etude pre-operatoire effectuee avec doppler: 41,7% des patients presentaient la saphene de jambe indemne avec varices a charge de la veine de Leonardo et/ou de la collaterale anterieure. C'est sur ce fondement que se base le choix de regler la longueur du stripping sur le niveau du reflux constate a l'examen Doppler (5).
La preservation de la saphene de jambe reduit, en effet, la possibilite de lesions du nerf saphenien (1) et permet de conserver une veine qui pourra etre utilisee dans le futur pour la reconstruction arterielle permettant ainsi d'atteindre la radicalite therapeutique avec un acte chirurgique minime.

MATERIEL ET METHODE

De Janvier a Juillet 1991, 87 patients ont passe un stripping court de la veine grande saphene a-travers l'utilisation de stripper externe de Mayo que nous avons modifie et incision inguinale unique. Il s'agissait de 71 femmes (82%) et 16 hommes ages de 45 ans en moyenne (de 18 a 71 ans).
Tous les patients, avant l'operation, ont ete examines avec doppler CW et plethysmographie a lumiere reflex.
Le Doppler mettait en evidence une incontinence de la crosse saphenofemorale avec reflux tout au long du cours de la veine grande saphene dans 58 cas (67%) alors que dans les 29 cas restants (33%) la veine grande saphene de jambe etait continente et le reflux interessait une ou chaque collaterale de jambe.
Nous avons effectue:
- une sclerotherapie pre-operatoire des varices de jambe, a-travers technique a partir du bas selon Sigg, dans 22 cas (25,3%);
- une sclerotherapie post-operatoire des varices residuelles de jambe dans 46 cas (52,8%);
- aucune therapie sclerosante dans les 19 cas restants.

Pour tous les cas une anesthesie subaracnoide superselective a ete utilisee.
La crossectomie a ete effectuee a-travers une petite incision inguinale.
La technique du stripping que nous adoptons remonte a celle esoveineuse proposee par Mayo en 1906 (5) qui n'eut pas beaucoup de succes et qui fut abandonnee tres vite. La cause de cet insucces est due au fait qu'elle fut consideree par la plupart particulierement brutale et sanglante. Cela etait du certainement au type d'instrument utilise en tant que stripper.
Pour cette raison nous avons tout d'abord modifie le stripper de Mayo: la modification consiste dans la mise en axe (90 degres par rapport a la tige de support au lieu des 60 degres du stripper de Mayo) de la bague que nous avons rendue cylindrique avec extremite distale legerement arrondie.
L'instrument, ainsi modifie, permet de reduire les espaces morts dans la progression de l'instrument, grace egalement aux divers calibres que nous avons predisposes pour l'adapter au mieux au calibre de la veine. La modification successive consiste dans la creation d'un mecanisme qui permet de sectionner la veine a son extremite distale avec un simple mouvement de rotation de la poignee sans necessite d'effectuer une contre-incision.
La section et le stripping de la veine sont precedes par l'introduction dans le lumen veineux d'un stripper interne rigide qui est retire de quelques centimetres seulement au moment de la coupe: il represente une garantie contre la rupture accidentelle de la veine dans un point non desire. Dans le cas d'operation d' un patient non traite preventivement avec sclerotherapie, la sonde crio peut etre utilisee pour congeler la veine sous le genou avant la section afin de reduire ainsi le saignement durant l'operation.
A la fin de l'operation, la jambe est bandee avec des bandes adhesives a allongement court. Le pansement est ote apres 7 jours lorsque les points de suture cutanes sont enleves.

RESULTATS

Tous les patients qui ont subi une operation sont restes a l'hopital en moyenne 4 heures et, en aucun cas, l'hospitalisation a ete necessaire. Les complications ont ete minimes. Le risque de varicophlebite des branches residuelles de jambe, qui peut se developper dans les patients soumis a stripping selectif de la grande saphene non sclerosee en precedence (3% de l'ensemble de nos cas), n'est pas present dans la totalite des patients soumis a sclerose pre-operatoire a partir du bas.
Nous n'avons eu aucun cas de suppuration de la blessure inguinale alors que dans 2 cas (2,2%) il y a eu une lyponecrose du tissu souscutane a attribuer, vraisemblablement a une utilisation excessive de l'electrobistouri dans l'hemostase des vaisseaux sous-cutanes. Dans 2 cas nous avons remarque un hematome de cuisse qui a ete gueri avec therapie conservative. Nous n'avons remarque aucun hematome de jambe. Dans ce groupe de patients nous avons eu 2 (2,2%) parestesies residuelles de jambe dues a lesion du nerf saphenien; sur la base de l'ensemble de nos cas, parmi tous les patients soumis a stripping court les parestesies sont restees dans le 0,88% des cas malgre que la section de la veine ait eu lieu toujours au troisieme superieur de jambe; ceci est du au fait que probablement il y a des variantes anatomiques du cours du nerf qui le font passer en connexion avec la grande saphene meme au niveau du genou.

Une pigmentation de la peau au-dessus de la varice a ete notee sur 6 des patients (27,2%) traites avec sclerotherapie pre-operatoire. Des telangiectasies residuelles se sont developpees sur 4 patients (4,6%) au long du cours de la veine strippee. Ceci est du probablement au microtraumatisme effectue par le cylindre du stripper externe sur le tissu sous-cutane.

DISCUSSION

Sur la base des resultats preliminaires de notre experience, le stripping selectif de la veine grande saphene avec la technique de Mayo modifiee est une operation fiable avec complications negligeables.

Grace a l'enveinage de la veine par incision inguinale seulement, l'operation est particulierement esthetique et par consequent plus appreciee par le patient.

Vu le follow up tres court (max. 18 mois - min. 12 mois) il n'est pas possible d'exprimer une opinion sur le pourcentage de recidive variqueuse dans ce groupe selectionne de patients.

BIBLIOGRAPHIE

COX S.J. ET AL. (1974): Saphenous nerve injury caused by stripping of the long saphenous vein. Br Med J., 1-415.

DE GROOT W.P. (1989): Treatment of varicose veins: modern concept and methods. J. Dermatol Surg. Oncol., 15-191.

KENICHI KOYANO ET AL. (1988): Selective stripping operation based on Doppler ultrasonic findings for primary varicose veins of the lower extremities. Surgery, 103-615.

MAYO C.H. (1906): Treatment of varicose veins. Surg. Gynecol. Obstet., 2 : 385-387.

RIVLIN S. (1975): The surgical cure of primary varicose veins. Br J Surg, 62-913.

Phlébologie 92. Eds P. Raymond-Martimbeau, R. Prescott, M. Zummo.
John Libbey Eurotext, Paris © 1992, pp. 1076-1078

Outpatient surgery of the great saphenous vein : about 311 cases

P. Sorrentino, G. Spreafico, P. Borelli, P. Pavei, , F. Schwan, A. Stellio, U. Baccaglini

Clinica Chirurgica I, University of Padova, Italy, Presidio Ospedaliero Dolo, Venezia, Italy.

Primary varicose veins of the inferior limbs are a frequent pathology. The alternative possibility of an ambulatory treatment is getting more and more interesting if we consider the lack of beds in the big hospitals and the increasing sanitary expenditure.
As regards the surgery of varicose veins of the inferior limbs, the Royal College of Surgeons of England (2) confirmed in 1985 that all the operations for varicose veins can be ambulatory performed for the patients in good general health.
Our experience in the outpatient surgery of the great saphenous vein is hereinafter described.

PATIENTS AND METHODS

Between February 1987 and October 1991, 311 patients underwent ambulatory surgery of safenectomy.
68 men and 243 women between 18 and 76 of age (42 on average) were studied. All patients have been examined with Doppler and pletismography study before surgery.
We made crossectomy with short stripping of the saphenous vein in 218 cases; one groin cut only, using modified Mayo's stripper, in 87 cases; crossectomy with long stripping in 35 cases; crossectomy with Muller's phlebectomy in 24 cases.
Three anaesthesia types have been used:
- in 166 cases we used superselective subaracnoidale anaesthesia by injection of 0,5 ml of hyperbaric bupivacain 1% at level L1-L2 or L2-L3 with a 25G spinal needle.
- in 65 cases we used local anaesthesia.
- in 45 cases we used Propofol in addition to local infiltration.
- in 35 cases we used Winnie's technique with a "3 in 1" block of the femoral, the otturatoric and the lateral cutaneous nerve by infiltration of 30 ml of Carbocain 1,5% at the groing (4).

The first step of surgery consists in crossectomy. When the crossectomy is completed, the stripping is obtained by the invagination stripping by thread described by Van der Stricht (3) or with external stripper of Mayo modified by us.

The stripping level is based on the length of reflux, evaluated through Doppler study.
At the end of surgery, an elastic compression with adhesive bendages is applied and they are removed, together with the points of cutaneous suture, after 7 days.

RESULTS

On average, the patients stay in hospital 4 hours and only 4 patients couldn't be discharged from Hospital within 12 hours.
We observed minimum of complications. In 9 cases (3%) there was an event of varicophlebitis due to the residual varicose veins of the lower leg which was managed within few days only by elastocompression. No case of wound infection.
The main cause of postoperative complications was the spinal anaesthesia; we observed, in 21 cases (13%) amongst 166 patients with subaracnoidal anaesthesia, an important cefalea which has been spontaneously resolved after 3-4 days. This complication was observed in the first year only and was due to the first needle type that we used.
One month after surgery, 219 patients (70,5%) asked for sclerotherapy of the remaining varicose veins of the lower limb.

DISCUSSION

The varicose veins of the lower limbs demonstrate a highly frequent pathology. Our experience, according to similar one in bibliography (1) demonstrates the possibility of ambulatory surgery of this pathology in day-hospital without hospitalization with the relevant advantages both for the patient and for the hospital structure.
The pre-operative study must be complete as well as accurate and surgery must be performed in a scrupulous way in order to reduce complications.
The different techniques of anaesthesia allow an immediate postoperative deambulation so reducing the risk of hematoms or faerful deep venous thromboses.
As per our experience, ambulatory surgery results completely reliable with an incidence of negligible minor complications.
According to the literature, the result of outpatient surgery is the same of traditional hospital one.
Patients well accept ambulatory surgery because the contact with the hospital structure is less traumatic and the immediate return to his normal life is possible.
The economic advantages of outpatient surgery are obviously evident with respect to the hospitalization.
The ambulatory surgery can be only performed with a qualified organization. Surgery is only a component of this service.
All diagnostic and therapeutic assistance must be assured to the patients from the ambulatory structure. Surgery must be performed with maximum accuracy and adequate post-operative assistance. At home the patient can contact in any moment, through a direct telephone number, the medical staff.
Ambulatory surgery is not a minor surgery but it means aboveall a total improvement of assistance.

REFERENCES

BISHOP C.R. ET AL. (1986): Outpatients varicose veins surgery under local anaesthesia. Br J Surg, 73-821.

ROYAL COLLEGE OF SURGEONS OF ENGLAND (July, 1985): Commission of the prevision of surgical services-guidelines for day case surgery.

VAN DER STRICHT H.R. (1963): Safenectomie par invagination sur fil La Presse Medicale, 71-1081.

WINNIE A.P. ET AL. (1973): The inguinal paravascular technique of lumbar plexus anaesthesia: the "3 in 1" block. Aneasth. Analg. 6-989.

Phlébologie 92. Eds P. Raymond-Martimbeau, R. Prescott, M. Zummo.
John Libbey Eurotext, Paris © 1992, pp. 1079-1080

Le maintien du flux de la saphène interne avec l'abolition de l'incontinence ostiale par crossectomie

G. Cantelli*, A. Vannuzzi**, A. Pieri**

** Istituto Nazionale Riposo e Cura per Anziani, I.N.R.C.A., Centro di chirurgia, Ospedale Poggiosecco, via Incontri 30, 50139 Firenze, Italy. ** Centro traumatologico ortopedico, C.T.O., Servizio di Diagnostica angiologica, Largo Pelagi 1, Firenze, Italy.*

Chez des patients présentant une incontinence de l'ostio-saphène-fémorale, des perforantes de cuisse et avec tronc saphénien très altéré, l'intervention d'élection est le stripping . Mais lorsqu'on se trouve face à une incontinence isolée de l'ostio-saphène-fémorale avec début de varices de jambe, ce type d'opération chirurgicale est , à notre avis,excessif.

Notre intention est de corriger le reflux ostial de façon définitive par une crossectomie tout en maintenant accessible la veine saphène interne de façon à garder disponible un réseau de compensation valable en cas d'une éventuelle thrombose veineuse profonde à charge de la veine poplitée et/ou de la veine fémorale superficielle limitativement au tiers inférieur de la cuisse. Ce genre de pathologie se rencontre fréquemment suite à des fractures de la jambe et à des interventions orthopédiques. Travaillant dans un service de diagnostic angiologique d'un hôpital de traumatologie orthopédique, il nous a été donné constamment de relever , à l'examen doppler pratiqué sur des patients affectés de thrombose poplitée ou à charge de la fémorale superficielle, une activation marquée de la saphène interne qui présentait un flux spontané très rapide et non modulé par les actes respiratoires. Une telle situation peut être reproduite chez des individus bien portants en exécutant une compression manuelle sur le réseau profond jusqu'au tiers moyen de la cuisse.

20 patients (18 femmes et 2 hommes), âgés de 20 à 72 ans, ont été soumis, en cabinet de consultation, à une légature de la saphène interne au ras de la fémorale avec sectionnement des collatérales de la crosse en anesthésie locale. Tous présentaient une insuffisance de l'ostio-saphène-fémorale, démontrée par examen clinique et instrumental, avec tronc saphénien en bonnes conditions mais avec varices à charge des collatérales de jambe.
Comme prophylaxie d'éventuelles thrombo-phlébites, nous avons administré aux patients une dose journalière de 200 mgr d'eparansolfate pendant les dix jours qui ont précédé et suivi l'intervention au terme de laquelle nous avons invité les patients à marcher après avoir enfiler un bas mono-collant de 2ème classe de contention . Dans aucun des cas nous n'avons relevé de complications post-opératoires, ni précoces,ni tardives . Après quarante jours, 16 patients ont

été soumis à une thérapie sclérosante des varices de jambe restantes par doses légères de trombovar ou de atossisclerol ; chez les 4 autres patients, aucune thérapie sclérosante complémentaire n'a été nécessaire.

Cette méthode a donné de bons résultats tant du point de vue fonctionnel qu'esthétique. En effet, tous les patients ont obtenu un net bienfait grâce à l'intervention et à la thérapie sclérosante complémentaire avec disparition des troubles qu'ils accusaient auparavant tels que sensation de lourdeur et douleur; en outre, toutes les varices de jambe qui représentaient un préjudice esthétique, surtout pour les plus jeunes femmes, ont disparu .
Au bout d'un, puis de trois mois (après l'intervention) nous avons soumis tous les patients à un contrôle doppler et nous avons vérifié l'accès du tronc de la saphène interne en dépit de la suppression du reflux ostial par crossectomie.

Par conséquent, nous pouvons affirmer qu'avec cette méthode, la saphène interne reste disponible pour remplir la fonction de réseau de compensation en cas de thrombose profonde de la jambe et du tiers inférieur de la cuisse.
En effet, chez un patient en position penchée, si l'on pose la sonde doppler sur la saphène interne au niveau du condyle médiant du fémur et si l'on exécute une compression digitale de la veine poplitée de façon à lui provoquer une sténose, nous relevons, chez les patients soumis à une crossectomie, une activation de la saphène interne analogue à celle qui se vérifie chez les patients non opérés.

Dans cette optique donc, il nous semble intéressant qu'une simple intervention comme la crossectomie , certes qui n'est pas nouvelle comme technique et qui est sans prétention hémodynamique, mais qui peut être pratiquée en cabinet de consultation sous anesthésie locale , puisse résoudre, du point de vue esthétique et fonctionnel, des situations qui ne sont pas particulièrement avancées tout en garantissant la disponibilité d'une veine très utile en cas d'oblitération du réseau profond.

Références

Benhamou,A.C.(1990): La chirurgie de la saphène interne . In " La maladie variqueuse ". pp 91-94

Dauzat,M.(1988): Ultrasonografia vascolare, ed. Piccin, pp 359-369

Davy, A .: Examen clinique d'un malade atteint de varices. In "La maladie variqueuse"." Benhamou A.C. pp 25-28

Ouvry,P.A.: Les strippings par invagination sur mèches calibrées. Extrait de phlébologie n° 4/1989 pp. 599-604

Ouvry, P.A. Davy, A.: De la vanité des incisions multiples dans la chirurgie des varices. Communication à la Soc. française de Phlébologie,1982;35 (4)pp.851

Perrin,M.: L'insuffisance veineuse chronique des membres inférieurs.pp.41-46(1990)

Pieri, A.,Benelli L. ,Vannuzzi A.,de Saint Pierre G. : Test indiretto di pervietà della vena femorale superficiale. In communicazione della riunione della sezione tosco-umbra della Società italiana di patologia vascolare.Dic. 1991 p. 103

Pieri A. , Benelli L., Vannuzzi A., Duranti : La sindrome delle"varici senza varici" in idem p. 111

Tournay et coll. (1976) : La sclérose des varices. Expansion scientifique française

Vaughan Ruckley, C. : Surgical management of venous desease. Test Atlante (1988) p.21 pp. 38-47

Phlébologie 92. Eds P. Raymond-Martimbeau, R. Prescott, M. Zummo.
John Libbey Eurotext, Paris © 1992, pp. 1081-1082

Should we strip the long saphenous vein ? A randomized controlled trial

S. Sarin, J.H. Scurr, P.D. Coleridge Smith

Department of Surgery, University College and Middlesex School of Medicine, The Middlesex Hospital, London, W1N 8AA, UK.

Saphenofemoral junction (SFJ) ligation alone combined with multiple avulsions in the treatment of primary long saphenous vein (LSV) varicosities will not result in adequate treatment of contributory mid-thigh perforating veins which may explain the high incidence of recurrance following this procedure. The aim of this study was to investigate whether the addition of above knee LSV stripping to the procedure would reduce the incidence of reflux in residual veins.

105 limbs of 69 informed and consenting patients (Median age 50 years (IQR 41-62), M:F=19:50) with primary SFJ reflux and LSV varicosities were randomized at operation to either SFJ ligation and above knee LSV stripping or to SFJ ligation alone combined, in all limbs, with multiple avulsions. Pre operative assessment by Duplex Scanning and photoplethysmography was compared to post operative assessment (undertaken 3 months after surgery).

RESULTS	**Pre-operative**		**Post-operative**		
	SFJ&LSV Reflux	**Thigh Perforators**	**SFJ Reflux**	**LSV Reflux**	**Residual Thigh Preforators**
AK Stripping(n=49)	49	9	0	9	2
No Stripping(n=56)	56	8	1*	25+1*	6

Following treatment, more LSVs demonstrated reflux in the group that had been randomized to SFJ ligation alone ($\chi^2=7.5$, $p<0.01$). 95% refilling times were improved in both groups following treatment (Wilcoxons Rank Sum Test, SFJ ligation+AK stripping $p<0.001$ and SFJ ligation alone $p<0.001$), though were significantly higher in those limbs without residual reflux (Mann Whitney U Test $p<0.05$).

We have shown that in a large proportion of cases sapheno-femoral junction ligation combined with multiple avulsion of varicosities fails prevent venous reflux and fails to normalize venous function. In contrast, ligation of the sapheno-femoral junction and multiple avulsion of varicosities combined with stripping of the long saphenous vein to the upper calf results in fewer veins with residual reflux and a better functional outcome. We suggest that, in limbs shown to have primary SFJ reflux, SFJ ligation combined with above knee stripping of the LSV is preferable to SFJ ligation alone because of a lower incidence of reflux in the residual segments of the LSV which may lead to recurrance of varicosities.

Phlébologie 92. Eds P. Raymond-Martimbeau, R. Prescott, M. Zummo.
John Libbey Eurotext, Paris © 1992, pp. 1083-1085

Surgical treatment for varicose veins of the legs using intraoperative angioscopy

Shunichi Hoshino, Hirono Satokawa, Takashi Ono, Tsuguo Igari

Department of Cardiovascular Surgery, Fukushima Medical College, 1 Hikarigaoka, Fukushima, 960-12, Japan.

Introduction

The conventional treatments of the primary varicose veins with vein valve reflux in the legs are high ligation with or without stripping procedure or sclerotherapy. In those treatments, there is the disadvantage that the long saphenous vein is not available for coronary bypass, peripheral vascular bypass or other surgery. To preserve the long saphenous vein and to prevent the vein valve reflux effectively, we applied the angioscopy to evaluate the morphology of the incompetent vein valve and try to repair vein valve reflux under direct observation during surgery.

Materials and Methods

A total of 65 limbs, 41 cases of the primary varicose veins were operated upon using angioscopy in the Department of Cardiovascular Surgery in Fukushima Medical College from 1989 to 1992. Ten cases were male and 31 cases female. Ages ranged from 37 to 71, averaging 51 ± 10 years old. An angioscope (Olympus, PF type 28) was used and the angioscopic pictures were recorded with a VTR seytem. The long saphenous vein was exposed at the saphenofemoral junction and the angioscope was inserted into vein from its branch. Heparin added saline solution was flushed by hand from the flush lumen of the angioscope to observe the vein valves clearly.

Type	Angioscopic findings	
Type I	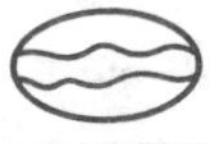	wide separation between the cusps atrophy of the cusps
Type II	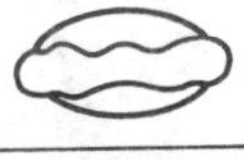	dilatation, depression of the commissure wide separation between the cusps
Type III	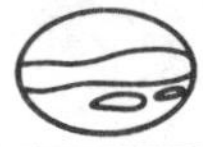	perforation of the cusp monocusp

Fig. 1. Classification of the incompetent venous valve

Results

1. Angioscopic findings of the incomeptent vein valves.

Intraoperative angioscopic observation of the incompetent vein valves was performed for vein valves of the primary varicose vein in the lower extremities. Incompetent valve were classified into three types as illustrated in Fig 1. Separations and atrophy of the cups were observed in type I (45%),

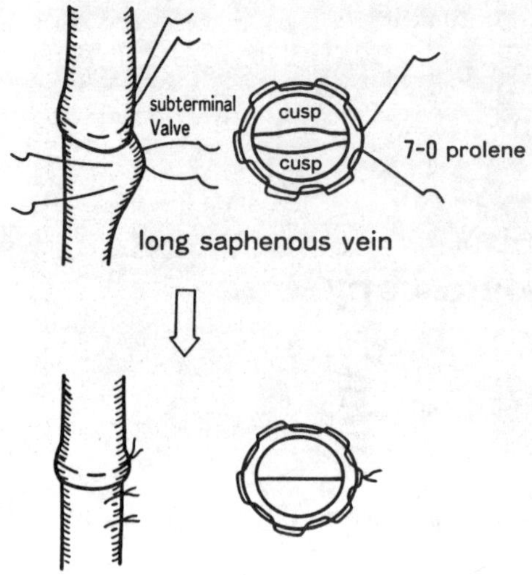

Fig. 2..Annuloplasty for vein valve

dilatation and depression were mainly in type Ⅱ(46%) and perforations, destructions and monocusps were classified as type Ⅲ(9%).

2. Annuloplasty for the vein valve reflux.

According to the angioscopic findings of the incompetent vein valve, several operative procedures were performed on 29 limbs in 24 cases. Among these cases, annuloplasty was performed in 27 limbs, valvuloplasty and vein segment transposition were performed on one limb each.

The annuloplasty as illustrated in Fig 2 was performed in the subterminal valves of the long saphenous vein. In type I, the annuloplasty was successful in all cases. However, in Type Ⅱ and Ⅲ, there were some technical difficulties in diminising the reflux in some cases which were ultimately performed with the conventional stripping procedure. Angioscopy was effective to determine the degree and tightness of the annuloplasty during surgery.

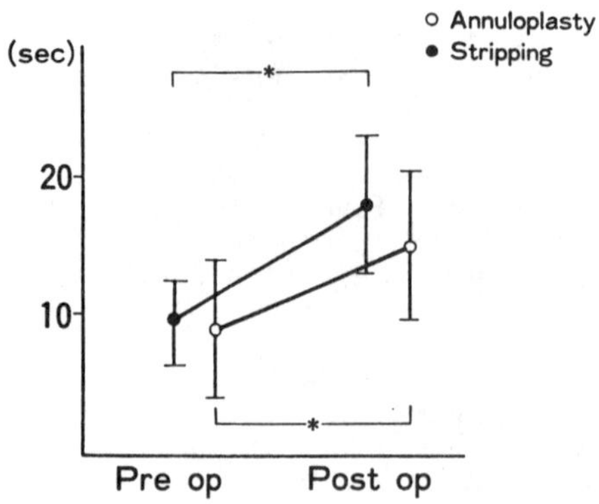

Fig. 3. Refilling time

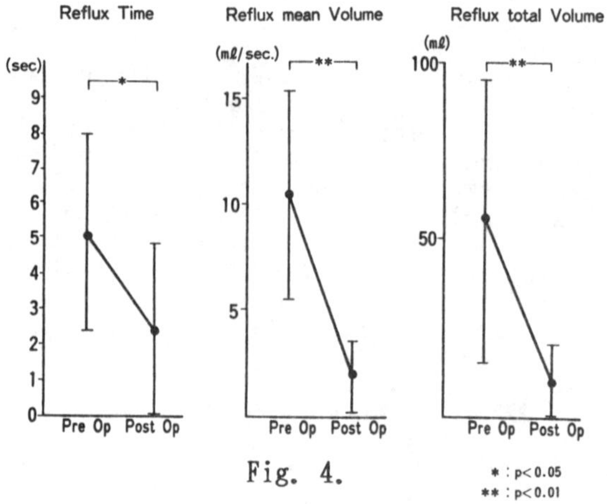

Fig. 4.

Refilling time after annuloplasty was measured by means of photoplethysmography. Refilling time was elongated from 9.3 ± 4.2 sec to 14.9 ± 4.3 sec ($p<0.01$) after the annuloplasty. These results were very similar to the results obtained with the stripping procedure as shown in Fig. 3.

Venous reflux of the subterminal valve was examined by duplex scanning after the annuloplasty. Reflux time decreased from 5.1 ± 2.8 sec to 2.4 ± 2.6 sec postoperatively ($p<0.05$). Reflux mean volume (mean reflux velocity × venous area) decreased from 10.7 ± 5.1 ml/sec to 2.1 ± 2.2 ml/sec ($p<0.01$) and reflux total volume (reflux mean volume × reflux time) decreased from 55.7 ± 40.3 ml to 10.0 ± 12.1 ml ($p<0.01$) postoperatively as shown in Fig 4.

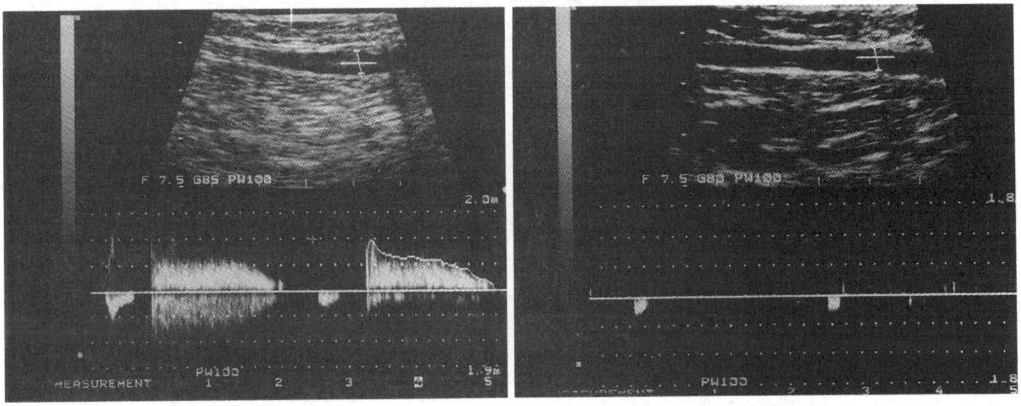

before annuloplasty after annuloplasty

Fig. 5.

In the 2~28 months (mean 11 months) postoperative follow up period, repaired valve function was observed by duplex scanning (Fig.5). Recurrence of slight vein valve reflux and dilatation of the vein were observed in 7 out of 27 limbs (29 %). However, in other 22 limbs (71 %) of the annuloplasty, there were no vein valve reflux, or redo cases.

Summary

Many surgical techniques have been tried to prevent vein valve reflux, including vein segment transposition, vein valve transplantation and valve direct plastic surgery. However, it is difficult to evaluate the efficacy of complete prevention of vein valve reflux during surgery, therefore, we applied angioscopy to observe directly the adaptation of the vein cusp and could decide on the most appropriate degree and tightness of the annuloplasty.

References

Banjo, A.O. (1987) : Comparative study of the distribution of venous valves in the lower extremities of black africans and caucasians : Pathogenetic correlates of prevalence of primary varicose veins in the two races. Anat. Rec., , 217: 407-412.

Belcaro, G.V. (1989) : Plication of the sapheno-femoral junction : An alternatiove to ligation. Acta. Chir. Belg., 89 : 305-308.

Cotton, L.T. (1961) : Varicose veins : Gross anatomy and development. Br. J. Surg., , 48: 589 -598.

Gottlob, R. and May, R. (1984) : Venous valves - Morphlogy Function Radiology Surgery (3rd ed.). Wien, New York, , Springer-Verlag, p.25-33.

Kistner, R.L. (1975) : Surgical repair of the incompetent femoral vein valve. Arch. Surg., , 110: 1336-1342.

Queral, L.A., Whitehouse, W.M., et al. (1980) : Surgical correction of chronic deep venous insufficiency by valvular trasposition. Surgery, 87: 688-695.

Raju, S. (1985) : Valvuloplasty and valve transfer. Inter. Angio., , 4: 419-424.

Taheri, S.A., Lazar, L., et al. (1982) : Surgical treatment of postphlebitic syndrome with vein valve transplant. Am. J. Surg., 144: 221-224.

Takamoto, S., Houjyo, H., et al. (1988) : Duplex scanning studies of saphenous valvuloplasty combined with stripping for varicose vein. J.J. C.V.S., 17 : 499-501.

Phlébologie 92. Eds P. Raymond-Martimbeau, R. Prescott, M. Zummo.
John Libbey Eurotext, Paris © 1992, pp. 1086

Diagnosis and treatment of incompetent cockett perforator veins by endoscopy : present state

Reinhard H. Fischer

Schreinerstr. 7, CH-9000 St-Gallen, Switzerland.

This is a perivenous endoscopy of the Cockett veins performed in the cleft between the fascia cruris and the flexor muscles. The method has the advantage that diagnosis and treatment of incompetent perforators can be done at the same time. In addition large incisions in the distal skin which often presents with trophic changes can be avoided. However the bloodless limb technique is a prerequisite and therefore regional or general anesthesia is necessary. As any other endoscopy also endoscopy of the perforator veins on Lintons line has to be learned and performed very carefully. And as other endoscopies it has its complications.

This endoscopy can be done by three different techniques: First: The Cockett veins are inspected and treated simply through an endoscopy tube with direct vision like in sigmoidoscopy (Fischer, 1991). Second: In addition, an angulated optic system is used (Hauer, 1988). Third: In addition to the tube and the angulated optic system the surgeon makes use of a video system (Sattler 1991). In each of these techniques the endoscopy is done through a small incision on the inside of the proximal leg. All three techniques have their advantages and disadvantages. It depends on the education and the situation of the surgeon which of these techniques will be the most suitable for him.

The author has developped the first of the three techniques. It is at the same time the simplest one. Few instruments are necessary and the endoscopy can be done in a short time. During the period of time selected for this study we have operated upon 1280 legs. In 462 of them endoscopy was used. 354 of the 462 presented with one or several incompetent perforator veins on Lintons line. The total number of incompetent perforator veins diagnosed and dissected was 480 .

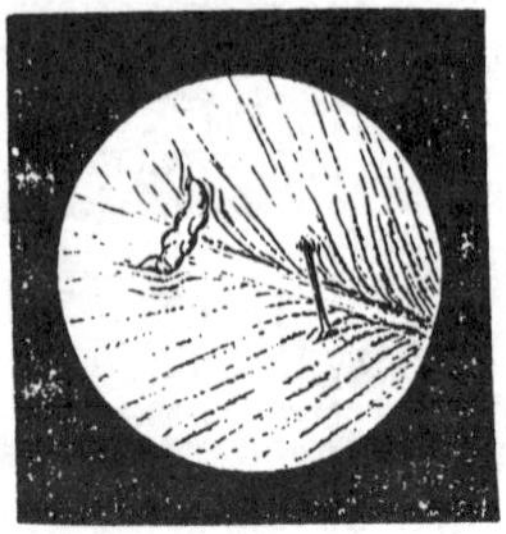

Fig. When performing the endoscopy the surgeon sees above the fascia cruris and below the flexor muscles. It is here, on Lintons line or better Lintons lane, that the perforators cross the cleft formed by the structures mentioned above. Usually it is easy to recognise whether the perforating vein is incompetent (left) or competent (right). Incompetent perforators then are dissected endoscopically.

References

Fischer R: Erfahrungen mit der endoskopischen Perforantensanierung (EPS) . Phlebologie 1992 (im Druck).Hauer G, Wisser I, Deiler S: Subfasziale endoskopische Diszision der Perforansvenen. In: Brunner U (Hrsg) Der Unterschenkel. Aktuelle Probleme in der Angiologie, Huber Bern Stuttgart Toronto 1988: 187-92.Sattler G, Bramann M, Hagedorn M: Weiterentwicklung der endoskopischen Perforansvenendiscision mit Hilfe einer Stablinsenoptik. 31. Kongress der Deutschen Gesellschaft für Phlebologie 1991 Frankfurt.

Phlébologie 92. Eds P. Raymond-Martimbeau, R. Prescott, M. Zummo.
John Libbey Eurotext, Paris © 1992, pp. 1087-1088

Endoscopic subfascial dissection of perforating veins (video film)

Michael Jugenheimer

Department of General and Abdominal Surgery, Marienhospital, Zeise 4, 5100 Aachen-Burtscheid, Germany.

Subfascial elimination of incompetent perforating veins is the most effective therapeutic principle in the treatment of trophic skin disorders associated with varicosis.We report in a video film about a new endoscopic technique, which allows subfascial coagulation and sectioning of all perforating veins with minor trauma and with direct view control.The requirements for a differentiated surgical therapy are knowledge of the anatomy and the underlying patho-physiological changes,which are demonstrated in the video film.
After a explanation of the importance of the perforating veins in the lower leg the video showes the necessary preoperatives diagnostic and their performances.
Indications for the method in the therapeutical concept in treatment of primary varicosis are incompetent perforating veins or the combination with a trunk varicosis.

The new method and the varices stripping are both demonstrated in all details.The advantages of the new method are discussed at the end from the video film.

Production: Fa.Richard Wolf GmbH,7134 Knittlingen,GERMANY

System : U-matic NTSC

Language : English

Run Time : 15 min

Phlébologie 92. Eds P. Raymond-Martimbeau, R. Prescott, M. Zummo.
John Libbey Eurotext, Paris © 1992, pp. 1089-1091

Endoscopic perforating vein dissection and paratibial fasciotomy for the treatment of the venous ulcer

Gerhard Sattler, Klio Mössler, Manfred Hagedorn

Department of Dermatology, Städtische Kliniken Darmstadt, Heidelberger Landstr. 379, 6100 Darmstadt 13, Germany.

The surgical treatment of chronic venous incompetence requires the removal of all insufficient sections of veins, and in particular the surgical therapy of incompetent perforating veins will be presented in this paper.

The importance of incompetent perforating veins of the lower leg for the development of lipodermatosclerosis and leg ulcers has been discussed for more than 30 years by specialists including Bassi (1981), Bernink (1981), Cockett ((1955), Dodd and Cockett (1976), Linton (1938) and May (1981). Since the rejection of Linton`s radical leg operation, nowadays incompetent perforating veins are treated either by a selective percutaneous method involving multiple skin incisions or by a non selective perforating vein dissection with or without an additional paratibial fasciotomy.

The selective perforating vein dissection requires an exact preoperative location of the incompetent perforating veins. The phlebography is the most important examination image producing method along with the clinical examination including palpation and Doppler ultrasound. Light reflection rheography, measurement of the veneous pressure during and after ankle leverage and Duplex ultrasound are further examination methods.

In spite of thorough preoperative examination often we could not identify our intraoperative prepared section of vessels as a perforating vein. Furthermore, during the postoperative check we found in a lot of cases a considerable amount of early recidivism, so called pseudorecidivism.

Since we have been using the endoscopic procedure we have found that incompetent perforating veins are best visualized intraoperatively. Only with the endoscopic technique is the high ligation of the perforating veins possible, i.e. the dissection of the perforators in the subfascial space.

Similar to described methods from Hauer (1987; 1988) and Fischer (1992) of endoscopic perforating vein dissection we use a 30 cm long 1 cm in diameter thick endoscope with a rod-lense optical system and a working channel for endoscopic forceps, scissors and hooks.

In order to accomplish a necessary bloodlessness a roll-compression sleeve described by Löfquist (1988) is rolled over the extremities. Then a 2 cm wide skin incision follows on the middle calf and then a 1 cm wide fascial incision. After a short and blunt dissection of the subfascial space, the endoscope is inserted and is pushed forward to the retromalleolar region. The operation is monitored by means of a video camera.

During the retraction of the endoscope, we see the appearance of perforating veins before they transverse the fascia (Fig. 1A). The dissection is carried out with electric forceps. Then it is possible to dissect the perforating vein with the endoscopic scissors (Fig. 1B). With this procedure it is possible to inspect thoroughly the subfascial space ot the medial calf especially in the region of the medial ridge of the tibia.

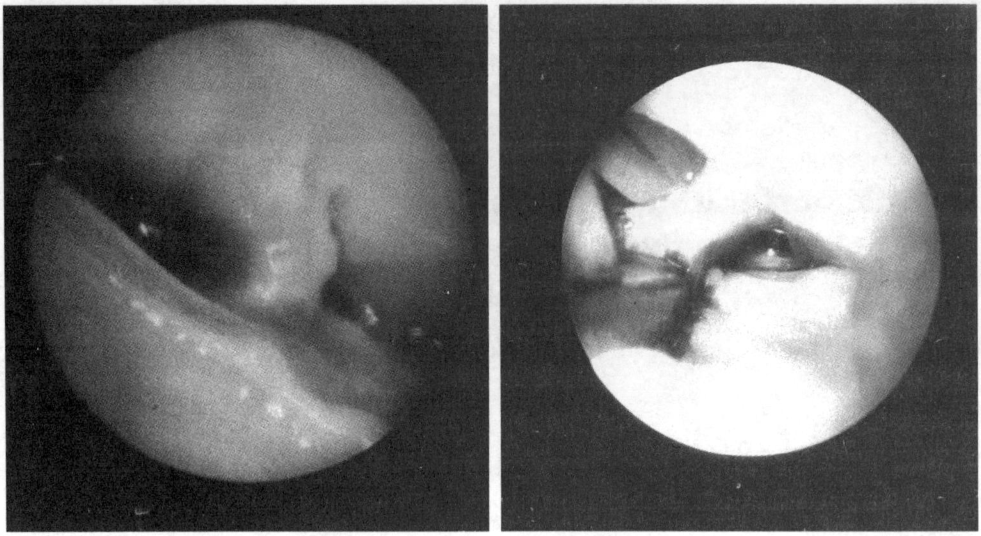

Fig. 1. Intraoperative view of incompetent perforating vein in the subfasical space (**A**). Dissection of incompetent perforating vein by means of the endoscopic scissors (**B**)

A concentration of perforating veins has been described by Staubesand, Schäfer and many others. Our intraoperative observation enforces these statements. Only few perforating veins cross the subfascial space horizontally in Linton`s line. Our observations show that many perforating veins originating medial from the ridge of the tibia run in a dome shaped course before they leave the fascia completely. In order not to miss those it is necessary to inspect carefully the medial edge of the tibia.

At the end of the operation we apply a compression bandage, and we remove the roll-compression sleeve.

Due to the anatomical description we were treating trunks of vessels including arteries and nerves next to the incompetent perforating vein. So we were aiming to prepare and separate the accompanying nerve before we coagulate and dissect the perforating vein. Since this modification we have hardly seen any cases of paraesthesia.

In summary 6 main points to note:

1. only one skin incision
2. none or hardly any hematoma
3. selective targeted dissection
4. dissection of the perforating vein before a possible branching
5. visually controlled procedure
6. protection of the accompanying arteries and nerves of the perforating veins

Until now we have performed more than 70 endoscopic procedures. Our experience shows that this method is extremely sparing and less traumatising for the patient and at the same time completely effective in the cure of incompetent perforating veins.

Further to this endoscopic procedure we have developed with the support of STORZ Company an endoscopic folding knife which enables visually controlled antegrade performance of a paratibial fasciotomy. The extent of the paratibial fasciotomy can be individually performed from distal to proximal and can be limited to the lipodermatosclerotic part of the fascia.

REFERENCES

Bassi, G. (1981): Klinische Bedeutung insuffizienter Venae perforantes. In Venae perforantes. Symposion der Österreichischen Gesellschaft für Angiologie, eds R. May, H. Partsch and J. Staubesand, pp. 110-113. München, Wien, Baltimore: Urban & Schwarzenberg.

Bernink, B.P: (1981): Die physiologische Venenklappe. Einige Konsequenzen für die Pathophysiologie der Venae perforantes. In Venae perforantes. Symposion der Österreichischen Gesellschaft für Angiologie, eds R. May, H. Partsch and J. Staubesand, pp. 138-143. München, Wien, Baltimore: Urban & Schwarzenberg.

Cockett, F.B. (1955): The pathology and treatment of venous ulcers of the leg. British J. Surgery. Vol. 43: 260.

Dodd, H., and Cockett, F.B. (1956): The pathology and surgery of the veins of the lower limb. Livingstone, Edinburgh, London. 1. Aufl. 1956. Churchill Livingstone, Edingburgh, London, New York. 2. Aufl. 1976.

Fischer, R. (1992): Erfahrungen mit der endoskopischen Perforantensanierung (EPS). Phlebol. (In press).

Hauer, G. (1987): Operationstechnik der endoskopischen subfascialen Discision der Perforansvenen. Chirurg 58: 172-175.

Hauer, G. & Gaitzsch, A. (1988): Endoskopische Perforansdissektion. Langenbecks Arch. Chir. Suppl. 2: 57-160.

Linton, R.R. (1938): The communicating veins of the lower leg and the operative technique for their ligation. Ann. Surg. 107: 582.

Löfqvist , J. (1988): Chirurgie in Blutleere mit Rollmanschetten. Chirurg 59: 853-854.

Sattler, G., Mössler, K., Hagedorn, M. (1992): Weiterentwicklung der endoskopischen Perforansvenendiszision mit Hilfe einer Stablinsenoptik. Hautarzt. (In press).

The posterior approach and the videoendoscopic treatment for subfascial ligation of incompetent perforating veins of the leg.

VIANI MP, PINTO A, MARUOTTI RA
Divisione di Chirurgia - Ospedale "C. Cantù"
Abbiategrasso - Milano- Italy

The role of incompetent perforating veins of the leg in chronic venous disease is well established.

When conservative therapy has failed, surgery is indicated. In uncomplicated cases, subfascial ligation through multiple small incisions is the procedure of choice. In case of severe dermatitis or ulcer the choice of surgical intervention is still debated. Subfascial dissection of perforating veins through a long medial incision (Linton operation) or posterior incision of the leg (Felder operation) have been described (1, 2). Recently endoscopic subfascial discission of perforating veins (ESDP) has been introduced by Hauer (3, 4).

CLINICAL DATA

From January 1989 to July 1992, out of 308 patients submitted to venous surgery, 20 patients (6.5 %) (7 males, 13 females) underwent subfascial ligation of incompetent perforating veins. All patients were affected by severe dermatitis of the lower limbs and incompetence of perforating veins of the leg, 6 patients by venous malleolar ulcer, 3 by post-phlebitic syndrome with perimalleolar ulceration. All patients were submitted to doppler sonography, 14 to strain-gauge plethysmography and 12 to ascending phlebography. Cultures were obtained from all ulcers before surgery. In 15 patients subfascial ligation of perforating veins was performed through a posterior midline incision (Felder intervention). From February 1992 we started our experience with endoscopic subfascial discission of perforating veins (ESDP) of the leg. During this period 5 patients were submitted to ESDP. Greater saphenous vein removal in 15 patients, lesser saphenous vein stripping in 2 and re-exploration of sapheno-femoral junction in 2 cases were associated.

RESULTS

We had no mortality, deep venous thrombosis, compartimental syndrome or sural lesion. The main complication was infection of the surgical incision (2 patients). In the last five patients submitted to ESDP no complications were registered. Medium follow-up was 20.9 months. In 2 out 3 patients affected by post-phlebitic malleolar ulcer and submitted to Felder intervention, ulceration doesn't heal after a 6 months follow-up In one case ulcer healed after three months. In all patients affected by venous ulcer ulceration healed in one-two months.

COMMENTS

The posterior approach for subfascial ligation of perforating veins of the leg is the best surgica' procedure in patients with severe dermatitis or venous ulcer. Compared to Linton intervention or multiple surgical incisions, Felder technique offers several advantages: operative exposure is superior because medial and lateral perforating veins are easily identified and severed, post-operative infection and recurrent ulceration are lower. Main contraindications to the Felder intervention are severe arterial insufficiency, cause the possibility of skin necrosis and absence of a patent deep venous system. In case of post-phlebitic syndrome the intervention seems to be uneffective.

Surgical technique. The incision is extended from the Achilles tendon to the medium third of the leg. If necessary, the lesser saphenous vein is ligated and stripped through a short incision in the popliteal space. The deep fascia is incised the whole lengh of the skin incision. Careful isolation and preservation of the sural nerve is mandatory. The dissection allows a superb exposure of the perforating veins emerging from the deep calf muscles. The incompetent perforating vein are easily interrupted with hemoclips and then divided.

The main complication of Felder intervention is represented by post-operative infection, ranging from 4 to 24% (5). Recurrence of ulcer ranges from 4 to 16.6% (5).

Felder intervention allows an excellent regression of chronic dermatitis and ulceration and offers good long term results. This technique transforms the subfascial ligation of perforating veins in a rapid and simple surgical exercise.

In the last years advances in endoscopic techniques have allowed the development of endoscopic surgical treatment for various affections. Endoscopic subfascial discission for the treatment of incompetent perforating veins of the legs (ESDP) was introduced by Hauer in 1985 (3, 4).

Surgical technique. Through a small medial cutaneous incision of the leg, a cold light operating tube is inserted

under the fascia allowing insertion of an operating telescope. A dissecting forceps, inserted through the instrument channel of the telescope, allows isolation and bipolar coagulation of the perforating veins. An endoscopic scissors allows the severing of the coagulated vein.
Compared to traditional surgery, the videoendoscopic discission of perforating veins of the leg (ESDP) offers several advantages (6). The risk of wound infection, skin necrosis, sural nerve lesions and compartimental syndrome are avoided. Moreover small incision allows cosmetic preservation, rapid disappearance of pain and reduction of the hospitalization time.
The tecnique has the same indications of traditional surgical treatment: 1) incompetent perforating veins with serious skin lesions 2) recurrent varicose ulcers after medical and elastocompressive therapy. Previous non-recanalized deep venous thrombosis and post-phlebitic syndrome are the main contraindications.

REFERENCES

1. Linton RR
The communicating veins of the lower leg and the operative technique for their ligation.
Ann Surg 1938; 107: 582-593

2. Felder DA, Murphy TO, Ring DM
A posterior subfascial approach to the communicating veins of the leg.
Surg Gyn Obst 1955; 100 : 730-734

3. Hauer G.
Die endoscopische subfaszialeDiszision der Perforans venen vorlaufig Mitteilung
VASA, 1985; 59 61

4. Hauer G. Barkun J. Wisser I, Diller S.
Endoscopic subfascial dissection of perforating veins.
Surgical Endoscopy 1988; 2: 5-12

5. Viani MP, Pinto A, Maruotti RA
La legatura sottofasciale delle vene perforanti della gamba per via posteriore
Chirurgia 1991; 3: 118-123

6 Maruotti RA, Viani MP, Pinto A
Legatura endoscopica delle vene perforanti della gamba per il trattamento delle ulcere e delle dermatiti da stasi venosa
Chirurgia 1992; 5: 180-184

Phlébologie 92. Eds P. Raymond-Martimbeau, R. Prescott, M. Zummo.
John Libbey Eurotext, Paris © 1992, pp. 1095-1097

Le « phlebo-kit » : vers un pansement logique, standardisé pour la chirurgie veineuse des membres inférieurs

P.L. Choukroun

141, avenue Émile Zola, 75015 Paris, France.

Le problème du pansement post-opératoire après chirurgie veineuse des membres inférieurs se pose dans la pratique de façon quotidienne et nous n'avons que rarement constaté un consensus sur ses modalités.

Ceci nous a amenés à nous poser la question suivante :

QUELLES QUALITES DOIT-ON EXIGER DU PANSEMENT POST-OPERATOIRE ?

1/- LA COMPRESSION : elle est nécessaire pour parfaire ou pérenniser l'hémostase après Eveinage Saphénien ou Phlébectomie.
Elle se doit donc d'être ELASTIQUE, bien sûr, mais à la fois sélective et quantifiable :

- Sélective : évitant la compression trop forte au niveau du creux poplité et de la région de l'anneau du 3ème adducteur,
  - plus forte au niveau de la jambe que de la cuisse,
  - couvrant enfin le triangle de Scarpa et la région trochantérienne, zone où souvent ont été pratiquées des phlébectomies des veines pelviennes, indépendantes des crosses saphéniennes.
- Quantifiable, par étalonnage des bandes.

2/- L'INNOCUITE : nous avons tous observé des phlyctènes, des ecchymoses dessinant le trajet des bandes, des sparadraps ou même des compresses lorsqu'est appliquée une élasto-compression inadéquate.

3/- L'ASEPTIE : ceci est évident puisque ce pansement est posé en milieu stérile quelque que soit le geste chirurgical.

4/- LE MINIMUM DE GENE ET D'ENTRAVE, à la toilette quotidienne, à la marche et à la reprise précoce des activités, à l'heure de la chirurgie ambulatoire.

5/- LA FACILITE DE POSE et aussi de "dépose" si nécessaire.

6/- LE COUT MODÉRÉ et si possible son remboursement partiel ou total par les organismes sociaux.

7/- LE CARACTERE STANDARD, facile à prescrire en fonction du sexe, de la taille ou de la configuration corporelle du patient.

8/- ENFIN L'ELEGANCE (pourquoi pas ?) dans le choix des couleurs et des matériaux.

Forts de notre expérience de chirurgie phlébologique et ayant eu à colliger les résultats de plus de 6800 cas de soins post-opératoires chez des patients opérés par une équipe homogène au sein de la Société Européenne de Phlébectomie (en fait 4 opérateurs principaux), nous avons été amenés à utiliser un pansement standardisé que nous proposons.

CE COFFRET, QUE NOUS AVONS NOMME "PHLEBO-KIT" COMPORTE TROIS ELEMENTS :

1/- UN HEMI-COLLANT DROIT OU GAUCHE DE CONTENTION FORCE II (46 à 100 CN/cm² ou 15 à 20 mmHg) :

- Cet élément doit couvrir la face antérieure de la cuisse et le trochanter assurant une compression sur le triangle de Scarpa, l'incision inguinale et les éventuelles micro-incisions de phlébectomies au niveau des veines pelviennes et obturatrices, responsables de varicose de jambe ou de cuisse.
- Il assure une compression progressive plus forte à la jambe qu'au niveau de la cuisse. Nous le préférons "pied fermé" pour deux raisons :
  - éviter la striction annulaire au niveau des orteils constatée souvent avec les collants "pied ouvert",
  - permettre la déambulation normale sans adjonction d'une chaussette ou d'un bas pendant les 5 à 7 premiers jours.

  Certes on pourrait reprocher à ceci une surveillance plus difficile de la coloration et de la chaleur des orteils, ce qui est vrai, mais en pratique peu gênant.
- Enfin, conçu selon les normes de fabrication, ce collant est moins compressif au creux poplité et à l'anneau du 3ème adducteur, protégeant la voie veineuse profonde.

2/- UNE BANDE ELASTO-COMPRESSIVE ETALONNEE DE FORCE II (46 à 100 CN/cm² ou 15 à 20 mmHg) :

- L'élasticité des bandes proposées dans le commerce peut être uni ou multi-sens. Nous préférons, comme bien des phlébologues, les bandes dont l'élasticité s'exerce uniquement dans le sens de la longueur car souvent les stries cutanées ecchymotiques sont dessinées sur les bords de la bande dont la striction est plus forte au milieu dans le cas de "multi-sens".
- L'étalonnage doit être facile à lire permettant de doser la compression et éventuellement de surdoser légèrement si, localement, un point est particulièrement hémorragique, quitte à la dérouler 2 à 3 heures plus tard pour la reposer avec une compression plus douce une fois l'hémostase contrôlée par épreuve de marche.

3/- UN COLLANT DE CONTENTION DE CLASSE I, 70 deniers (10 à 15 mmHg) pour les Phlébo-kits "femmes" ou des bas-jarrets pour les Phlébo-kits "hommes".

DEPUIS DEUX ANS, NOUS UTILISONS CE MATERIEL SELON LE PROTOCOLE SUIVANT :

- J O = Jour de l'intervention : toutes les incisions supérieures à 3 mm sont fermées, soit par fil monobrin 5/0, soit par fines agrafes métalliques. Aucun pansement collé ou non n'est appliqué.
  L'hémicollant stérile est posé directement sur la peau, le membre inférieur étant surélevé.
  Puis la bande élastique unisens est enroulée jusqu'à l'aine, modéré-

ment serrée et fixée par des sparadraps.
Si le patient sort le jour même, il est prévenu de la nécessité de surélever les membres inférieurs pendant la première nuit.
Une épreuve de marche est effectuée avant la sortie vérifiant l'absence de saignement notable à travers le pansement.

- J 1 = 24 à 36 heures plus tard : ablation de la bande.
  Le seul hémicollant est laissé en place pendant 5 jours, permettant marche, toilette et activité normale.

- J 5 = Ablation des fils ou agrafes.
  Le port, uniquement DIURNE, d'un collant de contention de force I, ou de bas-jarrets pour les hommes, est conseillé pour trois semaines.

Ce protocole constitue une simplification, une durée de compression suffisante, et donne pleine satisfaction chez tous nos opérés.

La fabrication de ce "Phlébo-kit" est en route. Des problèmes de standardisation, de choix des couleurs et de matériaux, ainsi que de stérilisation, trouveront leur solution très prochainement.
Cependant, toute méthode est perfectible ...
La parole est maintenant à ceux de nos lecteurs qui voudraient bien nous suivre dans cette voie et, bien sûr, à nos partenaires fabricants de matériel qui voudraient bien concourir à l'amélioration des pansements post-opératoires.

La place de la chirurgie itérative dans le traitement des varices

M. Perrin, J.M. Bayon, J.P. Gobin

9 Cour Général Giraud, France

Quelle attitude adopter devant un mauvais résultat après chirurgie des varices? Quels examens doit-on entreprendre? Quelle thérapeutique conseiller?

L'examen clinique reste fondamental. Il permet le plus souvent d'éliminer les causes non veineuses. L'étiologie veineuse affirmée, nous réalisons en complément un Duplex-Scanner et parfois une PPG.

a) Le bilan révèle des varices sans point de fuite important entre réseau veineux profond et superficiel. Traitement: Sclérothérapie, plus rarement phlébectomie.

b) Le bilan révèle la persistance d'un point de fuite important entre réseau veineux profond et superficiel. La réintervention pour supprimer ce point de fuite est la règle, complétée par sclérothérapie. Elle est précédée d'une phlébographie poplitée dynamique.

c) Une 3ième éventualité ne doit pas être oubliée. Le mauvais résultat après chirurgie des varices peut être lié au fait qu'on n'était pas en présence de varices primitives mais secondaires (maladie post-thrombotique, insuffisance valvulaire profonde primitive, etc...). Des traitements spécifiques peuvent alors être proposés.

Phlébologie 92. Eds P. Raymond-Martimbeau, R. Prescott, M. Zummo.
John Libbey Eurotext, Paris © 1992, pp. 1099-1101

Surgical management of varicose veins in the elderly with chronic arterial disease

Bruno Gossetti, Luigi Irace, Roberto Gattuso, Ombretta Martinelli, Fabrizio Benedetti-Valentini

2nd Chair of Vascular Surgery, (Head : Prof. F. Benedetti-Valentini), « La Sapienza » University of Rome, Italy.

SUMMARY

Primitive and/or secondary varicose veins and/or their complications in the elderly population are a particular problem since the surgical indications and techniques are not yet estabilished and since associated disease like coronary lesions, hypertension, diabetes, pulmonary obstructive disease, arterial disease etc make it difficult to choose the surgical approach.
In this study we have evaluated the indications and venous surgical procedures carried out in the last ten years in a group of 18 patients aged from 62 to 83 years in whom venous and arterial disease were coexisting. Those patients presented varices with oedema and eczema/dermatosis in one case, phlebitis of the long saphenous vein and its branches in two and ulcers of various sizes in the remaining 15, six of whom with postphlebitic syndrome. Arterial symptoms were claudication in three patients an rest pain in 15. In the three patients with claudication arterial repair was not advised because of their long walking distance and obstruction of the superficial femoral artery and good collateral supply. Of the 15 patients with rest pain 11 were unoperable and 4 had a failure of an arterial repair. Twelve patients were operated upon by stripping of the long saphenous vein and ligature of the incompetent perforating veins and six were submitted only to selective suprafascial ligature of perforators. Epidural anesthesia was used in the first group and local anesthesia in the second one. Limb conditions were assessed postoperatively by clinical means and non invasive tests. Walking distance remained unchanged in the three claudicants and surgical wounds healed promptly. Arterial disease did not seem to affect negatively the results of venous surgery. Venous surgery improved limb condition in 15 cases (83.4%) leaving the remaining three (16.6%) unchanged. Stripping of long saphenous vein and ligature of perforators is advisable in selected elderly patients with chronic arterial disease of the lower limbs.

The coexistence of a venous disease of the lower limbs, cararacterized by primary and/or secondary varicose veins and/or

their related complications and by postphlebitic syndrome, with chronic arterial disease represents a particular problem particularly in the elderly population since the surgical indications and techniques are not yet established. Moreover, it is not well known, untill now, how those disease can affect the evolution and the prognosis of each other and the outcome of the surgical procedures carried out either on the venous or on the arterial side.
In this study we have evaluated retrospectively the indications and the venous surgical procedures carried out in a group of 18 patients with a mean age of 72 ys, in whom venous and arterial disease were coexisting.

CASE MATERIAL

In the last ten years 18 patients who suffered for venous disorders and for a coexisting chronic arterial obstructive disease of the lower limbs were submitted to venous surgery. The patient's age ranged from 62 to 83 years with a mean of 72.
In all those patients the preoperative studies included ultrasound investigations (Doppler waveform analysis, segmental pressures measurement, Duplex scanning), plebography and arteriography either conventional or digital.
The venous pathology was characterized by varices with oedema and eczema/dermatosis in one case, phlebitis of the long saphenous vein and its branches in two and ulcer of various size in the remaining 15, six of whom suffered for a postphlebitic syndrome. The arterial symptoms were a reduction of the walking distance in three patients and rest pain in the remaining 15. No arterial surgical reconstruction was attempted in the three claudicants because of a wide walking distance and because the angiographic findings showed only an obstruction of the superficial femoral artery and a good collateral supply. In 11 cases there was no possibility of reconstructions and in the remaining 4 an unsuccessfull bypass had been previously attempted.
Twelve patients were operated upon by stripping of the long saphenous vein and ligature of the incompetent perforating veins and six were submitted only to selective suprafascial ligature of the perforators. We choosed to have an epidural anesthesia in all the patients of the first group and local anesthesia in the second one. This choice was justified by the high risk condition of the patients related to coronary and/or pulmonary obstrucive disease, hypertension and diabetes.
All the patients in the postoperative period and during the follow-up (mean time 3 years) were assessed by clinical means and ultrasound investigations.
There were no improvements in the arterial symptoms. In 15 cases (83%) a healing of the throphic lesions was observed and the conditions of the limb was positively improved. In three cases no beneficial effect was obtained (16.6).

DISCUSSION

This study performed in patients with coexisting arterial and venous disease of the lower limbs allow us the following considerations: 1) the presence of a chronic obstructive arterial disease does not seem to affect negatively the venous surgery since the surgical wounds healed promptly as did the throphic lesions; 2) it must be emphasized that the venous surgery did not cause any complication and allowed the healing of leg ulcers with significant improvement of the limb conditions either in patients just submitted to an unsuccessfull arterial reconstruction either in unoperable ones; 3) epidural or local anesthesia seems to be the right choice in those selected patients who must be submitted to venous surgery; 4) stripping of the long saphenous vein and suprafascial ligature of the perforators is advisable in selected elderly patients with chronic arterial disease of the lower limbs.

REFERENCES

Browse N.L. (1986): The etiology of venous ulceration. World J.Surg. ;10:938

Kluken N. (1986) : Problems in the differential diagnosis of lower leg ulcers by vascular disorders. In Negus D., Janet G. edt Phlebology '85. Londra Libbey J.Ldt ;554

Summer D.S. (1989): Haemodinamics and pathophisiology of venous disease. In Vascular Surgery, Rutherford R.B. edt. pgg:1483. W.B. Saunders company U.S.A.

Nicolaides A.N.(1989): Diagnostic evaluation of patients with chronic venous insufficiency. In Vascular Surgery, Rutherford R.B. edt. pgg:1583. W.B. Saunders company U.S.A.

Silver D., Cikrit D. (1989): Operative management of perforators vein incompetence. In Vascular Surgery, Rutherford R.B. edt. pgg: 1608. W.B. Saunders company U.S.A.

Sidney R.(1989): Surgical techniques in the treatment of varicose veins. In Vascular surgical tecniques: an atlas; Greenhalgh R.G. Edt. pagg: 374. W.B.Saunders company London.

Cockett F.B. (1989): Ligation of perforating veins. In Vascular surgical tecniques: an atlas; Greenhalgh R.G. Edt. pagg: 392. W.B.Saunders company London.

Phlébologie 92. Eds P. Raymond-Martimbeau, R. Prescott, M. Zummo.
John Libbey Eurotext, Paris © 1992, pp. 1102-1104

The management of injuries to major veins

Francesco Pollice*, J.B. Murphy

* *Department of Cardiovascular Surgery, University of Bari, Italy.*

A review was made of the hospital records of all patients with blunt extremity vascular injury admitted to department of Cardiovascular Surgery,University of Bari,Italy between 1 January 1972 and 31March 1991.Over this interval,62 patients presented with blunt vascular injuries to 63 extremities.Patients ranged from 11 to 74 years of age(mean age,31).The majority(87%)were men.Thirty-seven per cent of these patients sustained multisystem trauma;40% suffered extremity injury alone.Forty-seven per cent of the group were hemodynamically unstable on hospital admission.Forty-seven injuries(76%)resulted from motor vehicle accidents,including automobile,motorcycle and pedestrian accidents.Crushing forces were responsible for nine extremity injuries,falls for three injuries and explosions were responsible for two injuries.Twenty-two patients sustained blunt trauma to major extremity veins.All but one had damage to a major extremity artery.

RESULTS

Upper Extremity. Nine of 25 patients with upper-extremity vascular trauma sustained damage to major veins.Multisystem trauma was present in five of these nine patients.Seven venous disruptions resulted from motor vehicle accidents,one from a crush injury and one from a fall.All patients had concomitant arterial injury and venous damage was discovered during evaluation or treatment of the arterial trauma. Eight patients sustained injury to the brachial vein and one patient experienced distal axillary vein disruption.Massive soft-tissue trauma was seen in 67% of the extremities with venous injury,versus 25% of those with arterial injury alone.Fractures or dislocations were present in eight of the nine upper extremities with arteriovenous injury and in 12 of the 16 extremities with arterial injury alone.Seventy-five per cent of the extremities with arteriovenous damage had concomitant nerve injury,versus a 63% incidence in extremities with arterial trauma alone.Two patients had venous repair by lateral suture and two had saphenous vein interposition grafts.Five patients underwent venous ligation.All patients had appropriate arterial reconstruction.Fasciotomy was used in two of the four patients undergoing venous repair.Systemic anticoagulation was used in three of the four patients with venous reconstruction.Neither anticoagulation nor fasciotomy was used in patients with venous ligation.No amputation were required in the patients with vein injury.However,significant edema occurred in four of the extremities,including three in the venous repair group.The mode of therapy of the venous injury did not influence the rates of subsequent infection or persistent neurologic deficit.

Lower Extremity. Twelve of 38 patients with blunt lower extremity vascular trauma sustained wounds of major veins.Nine of the 12 patients experienced multisystem trauma.All but one patient with venous disruption sustained damage to a major artery.Six venous injuries were due to motor vehicle accidents,three to crush injuries,one to a fall,one to a blast injury and one was of unstated etiology.Major soft-tissue damage occurred in 67% of the patients with venous damage,compared with a 46% incidence in patients sustaining only arterial trauma.Fewer nerve injuries were seen in the patients with venous damage than in those without venous injury(17 vs.46%).Ninety-five per cent of the patients with venous trauma and 96% with only arterial injury,had associated fractures.Seven patients sustained injury to the common femoral vein.Six of these patients had associated femoral arterial damage.Five traumatized veins were ligated.All five patients developed massive edema of the extremity postoperatively.Two patients had persistent edema,two would have required amputation for ischemia had they not succumbed to other injuries and one patient ultimately was free of edema.Two damaged common femoral veins were repaired with autogenous vein interposition graft.One venous repair and the associated arterial repair were unsuccessful,leading to hip disarticulation owing to ischemia and sepsis 9 days postinjury.The popliteal vein was injured and successfully repaired in two patients.One patient,who required vein graft for repair,underwent amputation 3 days postoperatively owing to failure of the associated arterial reconstruction.One saphenous and one superficial femoral vein were repaired primarily without morbidity.Another patient with avulsion of the posterior tibial vein required amputation following venous ligation and repair of associated arterial injuries.Postoperative anticoagulation was used in two of the six patients with lower extremity venous repairs,neither of whom had significant postoperative edema.Two of the remaining four patients required amputation.Fasciotomy of the lower leg was performed in five of the six patients with venous repair.Overall,seven patients with major injuries to the venous system of the lower extremity had ligation or documented unsuccessful repair.Six of these seven patients had postoperative edema or vascular compromise.Among five patients with successful venous repair,none had significant edema.

DISCUSSION

The recognition and management of blunt extremity venous injury remain a challenge.Such patients frequently have sustained multisystem trauma,as was the case in 37% of the patients in our series.The need to treat life-threatening conditions can delay diagnosis of blunt extremity vascular damage.Even when attention is turned to the injured extremity,major venous injuries can easily be overlooked.The majority of our patients had venous disruption discovered at the time of operation for arterial injury. Rich proposed the use of Doppler studies in the recognition of penetrating venous injuries.However,this diagnostic modality would be difficult to apply in blunt trauma.The luxury of a defined area of trauma,which often occurs with stab or gunshot wounds,is usually absent in blunt extremity injury.Not infrequently,for example,the bluntly traumatized extremity is injured at multiple levels.In addition, the swelling associated with fractures or soft-tissue damage mimics the expanding hematoma which is a frequent clue to vascular trauma.Bleeding from open fractures may mask the steady flow of dark blood from a venous disruption,which may be the only clue to the presence of a major venous injury.Hence,there are many reasons that delayed recognition of major venous injuries of the extremity is common.Even after establishing the diagnosis of major extremity venous trauma,the management remains controversial.Although venous ligation may be required to control exsanguinating hemorrhage in the patient with other life-threatening injuries,there are significant sequelae following the interruption of major extremity veins.Data from the literature suggest that post-ligation complications are much more common with venous injury in the lower extremity that the upper extremity.[1]Ligation after penetrating injuries of veins in the lower limb has consistently resulted in a higher rate of edema than that following repair.[2]Despite the small sample size,our experience suggests that repair is preferable to ligation for blunt lower extremity venous damage.The rationale for venous repair is the prevention of venous insufficiency,a common late complication of venous trauma.In addition,the repair of a major extremity vein,when the associated artery is also injured,may be extremely important to the success of arterial repair.Hobson and coworkers[3]reported that femoral arterial blood flow in dogs is decreased significantly for 24 hours following ligation of the femoral vein.The arterial blood flow returned to control levels by 72 hours.Although the limb blood flow following femoral venous ligation was sufficient to maintain the patency of arterial anastomoses in dogs,Hobson and associates postulated that in the clinical situation the decreased arterial flow following venous interruption could contribute to extremity ischemia and decreased graft patency.Sullivan[4] attributed the failure of popliteal artery repair in several patients with penetrating injuries to ligation of the popliteal vein.Such a phenomenon would be even more likely in the face of the massive soft-tissue injury frequently seen in blunt trauma.Thus,these data lend further support to the concept of repair of lower extremity venous injuries whenever possible.The use of a distal arteriovenous fistula to increase flow into a venous graft and improve patency rates is controversial.[5] No arteriovenous fistulae were performed in our patients.As reported by Rich,recanalization of thrombosed vein grafts can occur.This phenomenon may obviate the need for distal arteriovenous fistulae in the face of venous repair. The incidence of edema following venous injury in the lower limb in our series is considerably higher than that previously reported after penetrating venous trauma.Fractures,massive soft-tissue injury and concomitant arterial injuries occur more frequently in blunt trauma. The accompanying destruction of lymphatic and collateral venous drainage increases the likelihood of postinjury edema and ischemia.When venous insufficiency develops following venous ligation or failed venous repair,delayed in situ venous reconstruction has been advised by Hobson and associates.If successful,this approach may avoid the complication of chronic venous stasis.Deep vein thrombophlebitis and pulmonary embolism,cited in many reports as a concern following either repair or ligation of venous injury,was not seen in our series.[4,5] Massive blunt trauma to the extremity commonly leads to the development of compartment syndromes.Fasciotomy should be strongly considered in any patients with blunt vascular trauma,particularly in the lower limb.The liberal use of fasciotomy in the present series probably prevented the development of compartment syndromes following vascular repair.The use of systemic anticoagulation in patients with blunt venous injury should be judicious.Often,these patients have closed head injuries or other organ damage and systemic heparinization might be ill advised.In our limited experience with anticoagulation in blunt extremity venous injury,we have used subcutaneous heparin and intravenous low molecular weight Dextran.Our results suggest that this treatment may be beneficial following venous injury in the lower,but not be upper extremity.

CONCLUSION

The vein of the upper extremity can be safely ligated without increasing morbidity.In the lower extremity,however,morbidity in the form of marked postoperative edema may be avoided by successful venous repair.The use of a saphenous vein interposition graft may be required.Venous ligation has had acceptable rates of limb salvage following penetrating injuries.The long-term morbidity associated with blunt extremity venous injury,however,demands a more aggressive approach to venous repair whenever possible.

REFERENCES

1. AGARWAL N.,SHAH P.M.,CLAUSS R.H. et al.:Experiences with 115 civilian venous injuries.J. Trauma. 22:827-832, 1982.
2. BLUMOFF R.L.,POWELL T.,JOHNSON G.:Femoral venous trauma in a university referral center.J. Trauma. 22: 703-705, 1982.
3. HOBSON R.W.,HOWARD E.W.,WRIGHT C.B. et al:Hemodynamics of canine femoral venous ligation:Significance in combined arterial and venous injuries. Surgery. 74: 824-829, 1973.
4. RICH N.M., SULLIVAN W.G.: Clinical recanalization of an autogenous vein graft in the popliteal vein. J. Trauma. 12: 919-920, 1972.
5. SCHRAMEK A., HASHMONAI M.,FARBSTEIN J. et al: Reconstructive surgery in major vein injuries in the extremities. J. Trauma. 15: 816-822, 1975.

The hidden problem: "Cinderella" SSV. Efficient diagnosis and surgical treatment of sapheno-popliteal insufficiency. Report on 100 operations.

H.-J. Schubert

Schlobklinik Abtsee, 8229 Laufen /Salzach, FRG

The problem: Often overlooked and functionally misunderstood (HODDS 1905, SCHUBERT 1991, et al.), the sort saphenous vein (SSV) with its tributaries is still the "cinderella" of leg varicosities. Even if routinely explored and treated, high rates of failures in diagnosis and surgical treatment are seen, mainly due to a false and multiple surgical strategy. Wide variation patterns of the sapheno-popliteal junction and multiple erratic communicating veins (e.g. GIACOMINI) to the long saphenous, superficial or deep femoral veins, gastroenemius veins and others contribute to disappointing results. **Methods:** From July 1987 to April 1992 in two institutions (Chirurgische Tagesklinik Traunreut, a freestanding polyvalent surgicenter and Schlobklinik Abtsee, 32-bed vein clinic) in all 665 radical varicose vein operations have been performed by one surgeon and his team. Out of these, 100 partial or total stripping procedures have been undertaken for sapheno-popliteal incompetencies (15%) due to the SSV or its tributaries. **The solution:** Besides clinical investigation, doppler, photoplethysmography, strain-gauge plethysmography diagnostic efforts had to be necessarily completed by lateral SSV-phlebography using VALSALVA-maneuver. Just recently we started CDFI. Only adequate demonstration of SP-junction and variable tributaries guaranteed successful and efficient surgery. No thrombosis or deep wound infection occurred. Recurrence and re-operation rate run up to no more than about 7%. Prolonged edema and repeated swelling of the lower leg within half a year postoperatively was noticed in about 13%, mainly after total SSV-strippings. The first analysis of pre-, intra- and postoperative documentation seems to confirm, that subtile preoperative assessment should include special x-ray scrutiny to improve therapeutical results in often overlooked SSV-varicosities. At present there is no furnished proof, that abandoning and replacing phlebography in favour of CDFI will be the right way to solve the often hidden problem of SSV and erratic veins. Especially in younger women painful lower leg syndrome can only be treated efficiently after exact phlebography, which is even mandatory prior to re-operations in recurrences.

Phlébologie 92. Eds P. Raymond-Martimbeau, R. Prescott, M. Zummo.
John Libbey Eurotext, Paris © 1992, pp. 1106-1107

Surgical treatment of gastrocnemial veins

Thiery Leon

Department of Phlebology, Institut Moderne, Koningin Fabiolalaan 57, 9000 Gent, Belgium.

Long ago we began to study the Gastrocnemial veins, becoming aware of their importance in venous pathology. In Milano, Italy, at the 5th Congress of the Union (1974) we explained our results of some 600 operations. Three years later, in Buenos Aïres, more up to date and detailed information was provided. Actually the number of operations exceeds by far 15000, and we are convinced of the impact of Gastrocnemial and Solear insufficiency on superficial venous pathology, and the need of surgical treatment.

The Triceps Surae is a triple muscle : 1 Solear and 2 Gastrocnemial.
The Triceps muscle is a blood sponge, where all venulae empty into intramuscular collectors. The reservoirs have a flimsy but elastic wall with many valves, (The valves close to the Peroneal or Posterior Tibial vein is of utmost importance) It stretches so easily, that the contents hardly has any effect on internal pressure. The revervoirs combine pooling and blood pressure regulation functions.

The Triceps contraction has also a pumping effect , shifting the contents of the reservoirs into the deep veins. Solear and Gastrocnemial veins, are connected with eachother , this coupling explains the surgical treatment and the good results.

A good pump requires perfect valves and strong muscles.
While walking , the venous sponge empties into the muscular reservoirs, who drain into the deep veins . The valves guide and regulate the venous flow avoiding any reflux.
Calf-pump function is perfect when muscles are strong , valves opening and closing

properly, veins and reservoirs large and without any internal or external obstruction or compression.
Weak muscles (flat feet - static insufficiency of the knee - ankylosis - arthosis) or avalvulation (as a result of thrombosis or external compression) reduce pump function. Post-Tibial and Peroneal veins are part of the calf pump, squeezed together and emptied against the Post-Tibial muscle by any contraction of the Triceps Surae.

Gastrocnemial veins are linked to the superficial veins of the calf and to the Popliteal vein . Their particular structure can explain most of the pathology.

Inside the muscle, these veins are shaped like 4 or 5 fingerlike reservoirs. Appearing at the muscle rim all 5 Gastrocnemial veins reunite to enter the Popliteal vein at the external and internal side. This is a short distance, hardly one or two cm.,but a difficult and unyielding passage since the branches of the Posterior Tibiae nerve tend to block the passage, squeezing the Gastrocnemial vein, and reducing considerably the outflow. Thence a residu distends the Gastrocnemial veins, destroys the valves, each muscle contraction pumping blood in the superficial network of the calf.

To Summarize : Varicose Gastrocnemial veins develop 1) everytime valve destruction allows reflux out of the Poplitial vein, or 2° when outflow in that vein is reduced by external compression. Overfilling or poor drainage produces always varicose veins of the calf , spreading upwards to the Saphenous vein.

The Solear reservoirs are bigger, than the Gastrocnemial.
Three small preforating veins connect them with the deep system and the superficial network of the internal ankle region.

When these preforating veins become incontinent, deep vein pressure is transmitted through the facia in the subcutateous tissu : oedema, dermatosclerosis, artrophie blanche, ulcera shall develop.

Solear and Gastrocnemial veins, when sufficient, have a completely different symptomatology. But Solear and Gastrocnemial veins have many communications and through these connections the bloodvolume can move from one into the other.
This explains that calf pump function is improving after resection of the Gastrocnemial verices, that resection of one of this varicose muscle-veins is not irrational and never disabling.

Phlébologie 92. Eds P. Raymond-Martimbeau, R. Prescott, M. Zummo.
John Libbey Eurotext, Paris © 1992, pp. 1108-1109

Surgical treatment of insufficient gastrocnemial and solear veins

Leon Thiery

Institut Moderne, Koningin Fabiolalaan 57, 9000 Gent, Belgium.

The construction, the proportions and size of the muscular veins in the calf suggest other functions than simple venous drainage.
They probably have, up to a certain degree, a pooling function.
The thin and elastic wall can distend easily and adapt to a varying volume.
Located in the core of the muscle they function as the chambers of the calf pump.
In our experience, gastrocnemial veins distend frequently, bringing about typical symptoms.
Gastrocnemial insufficiency is a common syndrome in modern society incomoding mainly young female who take the pil since several years.
It is often the beginning of a superficial varicosis.
The clinical diagnosis is easy, provided the doctor is aware of the probability of the syndrome and informed of its symptoms.
A conservative treatment can eventualy relieve the discomfort for a long period if the treatment is never stopped.
When improvement is poor or none, we ask for a selective phlebography to recheck and reaffirm the diagnosis. In our opinion the information of the phlebography is crucial in deciding an operation.
Duplex imaging, although non invasive and more functional can not reveal the exact number of gastrocnemial veins neither their exact localization or degree of enlargement in the calf, details that are essential for surgery.
Phlebography and duplex give different but complimentary information.
Promoting a surgical treatment for gastrocnemial insufficiency some 25 years ago, brought forth quite a lot of excitêmentand critic.
The argument always being that gastrocnemial veins, as a part of the calf pump, are so important you ought never touch them, let stay eliminate them.
Up to now we operated + 15.000 gastrocnemial veins, by far the highest recorded amount. Most of them were followed up every 2 or 3 year.
We never had any trouble disposing of medial or both gastrocnemial veins.
When a vein becomes very large and valveless we call it a varicose vein. As already said, gastrocnemial veins become very often insufficient for many reasons. Two important causes being avalvula-

tion and external nervous compression.
After many years of permanent distension deep inside the muscle, the hypertension spreads into the superficial network of the calf where varicose veins develop.
Varicose veins, whether superficial or deep must be eradicated.
With enlarged gastrocnemial veins, the calf pump is working poorly and breaking down more and more.
The abnormal high intramuscular tension,as a result of the distension of the deep veins,is also a serious nuisance since capillary and venular flow depend heavily on environamental tissue pressure.
Muscle atrophy and neuromyositis will develop gradualy.
Moreover, many connections exist between muscular veins of the triceps surae. The elimination of a defective and faulty section will improve, not worsen, the function of the leg pump.
Persistant pain, continuing degradation of the pump function or neuromyositis are the main reasons to decide a surgical treatment.
The operation must be performed in the popliteal space always, in the calf sometimes.
Surgery on deep veins, especialy in the knee, is dangerous and delicate and must be performed by trained vascular surgeons only.
The results are gratifying : debilitation, lassitude and pain disappear progressively in the first months.
Never we had any serious trouble (oedema - thrombosis - trofic changes or lasting pain).
Unsatisfactory results, mainly in the beginning period, were the result of a technical blunder.
Venous anatomy is very variable and inconstant especialy in the popliteal region, no wonder that one of the many gastrocnemial veins might be overlooked.
The cosmetic results are perfect when intradermal suture is used and mostly invisible as far as the quality of the skin permits.

Early operation of the primary varicosis of the long saphenous vein

Ludwig Metz, Joachim Neugeoauer

Clinic of Vascular Surgery

The severity of a primary varicosis of the long saphenous vein correlates often with the severity of an insufficiency of the deep veins in our clinical and angiographic diagnosis. Pro- and postoperative phlebodynamometry could verify this coexistence.

So the definition of primary varicosis loses its validity, according to which the deep vein show no changes. In our experience the insufficiency of the long saphenous vein might cause the development of an insufficiency of the deep vein.

Therefore we recommend the early operation of the insufficient long saphenous vein, in order to prevent the development of insufficiency of the deep veins.

Phlébologie 92. Eds P. Raymond-Martimbeau, R. Prescott, M. Zummo.
John Libbey Eurotext, Paris © 1992, pp. 1111-1113

Warren's shunt preventing oesophageal bleeding recurrences

Dino De Anna, Paolo Zamboni, Vincenzo Gasbarro, Carlo Feo, Vittorio Bresadola, Gian Carlo Pansini, Rossana Berta, Giuseppe Fiorentini, Alberto Liboni, Fabrizio Bresadola*

*Department of Surgery, the University of Ferrara, 44100 Ferrara, Italy. *Department of Surgery, the University of Udine, 35100 Udine, Italy.*

INTRODUCTION

The oesophageal varices haemorrhage represents the most severe cirrhosis complication. We have treated with a Warren' s spleenal-renal shunt the portal hypertension in patients who had acute episodes of bleeding varices just treated with endoscopic scleroterapy. We thought that this choice could give us the best long distance results for the alcoholic cirrhosis because of the frequent relapse in potus.

SURGICAL TECHNIQUE

The rationale of the selective Warren' s distal spleenal-renal shunt (D.S.R.S.) is to deconnect the right districict, mesenteric-portal with hepatopetal flow, from the left district, the splenic one, to decompress the venous oesophagus-gastric siphon maintaining an adequate perfusion of the liver.

In the film we present are illustrated the fundamental technical aspects for a good exit of the intervention. These aspects can be outlined as follows:

- median laparotomy;
- omental vessels venous pressure measurement;
- eventual intraoperative portography;
- inframesocolic approach;
- skeletonization of the left renal and spermatic veins and ligature of the inferior surrenalic vein;
- section of the splenic vein at its confluence with the inferior mesenteric vein, ligature of the spleenal-pancreatic vessels

- to performe the spleenal-renal T-L anastomosis at the surrenalic ostium and always below the origin of the spermatic veins anyway;
- ligature of the vessels of the gastro-colic legament;
- ligature of the right gastroepiploic vein;
- double interruption of the stomachic coronary;
- final mesurament of the pressure values;
- retroperitoneal parasuture drainage;

We generally evaluate the functionality of the anastomosis in the first days after the intervention by the means of ecotomography; before patient discharge and 60 days within the intervention by selective angiography of the celiac tripode .The medium and long term control investigations are the oesophagogastroscopy and renal/hepatic lab.ex..

DISCUSSION

The D.S.R.S. guarantees an efficient detension of the oesophago-gastro-splenic syphon, maintaining a good portal perfusion due to the mesenteric hypertension. Thus, besides a valid prevention of the varices bleeding, the D.S.R.S. assures an hepatic metabolic compensation status, lowering the risk of an hepatic encephalopathy.

We have treated with an elective surgical intervention oesophageal varices that had bleeded and had been already unsuccesfully treated with scleroterapy.

Our experience started two years ago and has not produced definitive data but the high live quality observed in the operated patients encourages this approach.

We would like to underline a few points that we consider fundamental for successfull operation.

First of all the ligature of the spleenal-pancreatic vessels up to the splenic ilum associated, according to some authors to the spleenal-colic deconnection in order to guarantee the complete divertion from the mesenteric-portal axis

The T-L spleenal-renal anastomosis has to be executed at the surrenalic ostium level and, in any case, below the origin of the spermatic vein to allow to the reflux renal flow in case of an anastomotic thrombosis.

The ligature and section of the gastro-colic ligament, the interruption of the right gastro-epiploic, piloric and stomachic coronary veins, eventually guided by an intraoperative portography, represent the final, but not less important, time of the intervention.

REFERENCES

CARNEIRO D' ALBUQUERQUE L.A., GAMA RODRIGUES J. OLIVEIRA ET AL. (1990):
A simplified technique for splenopancreatic disconnection with distal splenorenal shunt.
Surg.Gyn.Obstet., 4, 355.

WARREN W.D., ZEPPA R., FOMON J.J. (1967):
Selective transplenic decompression of esophageal varices by DSRS.
Ann. Surg., 166, 437.

RISALITI A., TERROSU G., CARCOFORO P., DE ANNA D., BRESADOLA F. ET.AL.:
Atti del congresso nazion ale dellla Società Italiana di Flebolinfologia Clinica e Sperimentale.
Nuzzaci G. editor. Firenze, 10-12 dicembre 1990.

Phlébologie 92. Eds P. Raymond-Martimbeau, R. Prescott, M. Zummo.
John Libbey Eurotext, Paris © 1992, pp. 1114-1116

Hepatic vein reconstruction in hepatectomy

Satoshi Nakamura, Shukichi Sakaguchi, Takachi Hachiya, Hiroyuki Konno, Kennichi Koyano, Shozo Baba

Second Department of Surgery, Hamamatsu University School of Medicine, 3600 Handa-cho, Hamamatsu 431-31, Japan.

When a tumor is adjacent to or invades the hepatic vein trunk, resection of the trunk is necessary. However, subsequent congestion of the remnant liver is often a problem. The liver function of patients in whom the hepatic vein was removed did not improve postoperatively and two of them had hepatic failure after surgery and one of the two patients died on 14th postoperative day. Therefore, in patients who require the function of all their remnant liver segments, the hepatic vein should be reconstructed. However, there were no reports on this procedure until our article in 1990 (1).

Patients and methods

Eight patients underwent hepatic vein reconstruction in hepatectomy. Four patients had hepatocellular carcinoma, three had hepatic metastases from colorectal carcinoma and one had cholangiocellular carcinoma. In 6 patients, the right, middle and left hepatic veins were reconstructed with autogenous saphenous vein, superficial femoral vein, or external iliac vein. Reconstruction was performed by patch angioplasty in one patient and by direct end-to-end anastomosis in one. Interrupted sutures using 6-0 monofilament nylon were done in anastomosis. The donor site of external iliac vein was reconstructed using a ringed expanded polytetrafluoloetylene graft. Postoperative heparin therapy was only used in the first two patients.

Results

All patients survived without any complications due to hepatic vein reconstruction. Postoperative liver function of the patients with hepatic vein reconstruction was significantly better than that of the patients in whom reconstruction was not done.

Hepatic venography was performed one month after surgery in all patients. The reconstructed right hepatic vein was patent in all 4 patients (Fig. 1, 2), but the saphenous vein graft to the middle hepatic vein and the external iliac vein graft to the left hepatic veinwere both occluded, possibly because of inappropriate graft selection. One of the two patients had a postoperative

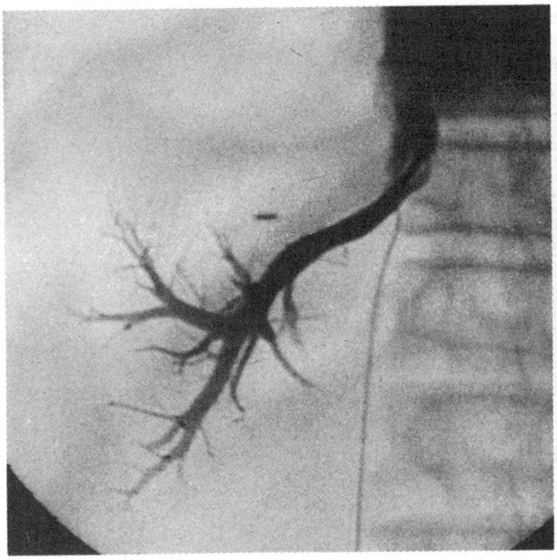

Fig. 1 Right hepatic vein was reconstructed. There was no stenosis.

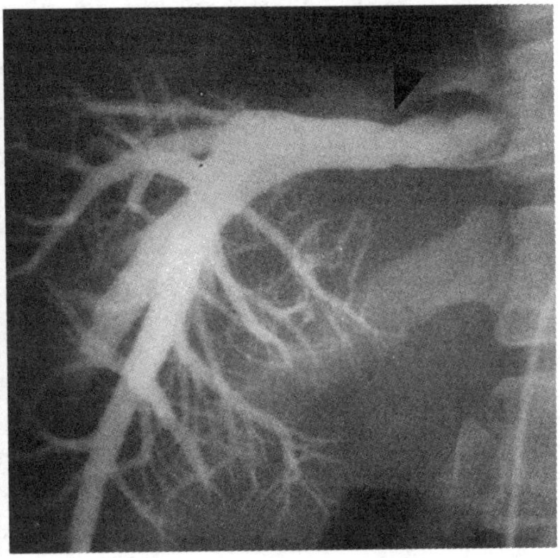

Fig. 2 Right hepatic vein was directly anastomosed in an end-to-end manner (arrow head).

complication of small biliary fistula. The patency rate was 6/8 (75%) (Table 1). The 7 patients are alive without recurrence of carcinoma after 8-42 months.

Discussion

There is some controversy on the indications for this procedure. Ou and Herman (2) stated in 1987 that hepatic vein ligation is a safe procedure which permits the preservation of the drained liver segments. However, this may only be true in patients with sufficient collateral flow via the inferior right hepatic veins. As confirmed by our animal experiments and clinical studies of postoperative liver functions (3), reconstruction of the right hepatic vein trunk is required in patients with small or poorly developed inferior right hepatic veins. A thick inferior right hepatic vein is present only in 20-24% of humans according to anatomic studies (4, 5).

The proper material for hepatic vein grafting should be chosen according to the diameter of the vessel to be reconstructed. A great saphenous vein was considered to be unsuitable as a graft for interposition of a hepatic vein. The external iliac vein may be used for a right hepatic vein graft. A superficial femoral vein has an appropriate size as a graft for the left or middle hepatic vein. Selection of an optimal sized graft is the most important point in hepatic vein reconstruction. Inflammation due to biliary fistula or retrograde infection along the drainage tube may cause stenosis or occlusion of a graft.

A direct end-to-end anastomosis of the right hepatic vein was possible by sufficient mobilizing the right lobe when resection of a 2-cm segment of this vein was performed. A patch graft was also useful in a case with short invasion to the hepatic vein. It is necessary to simplify the technique of hepatic vein reconstruction as possible.

Table 1. Details in hepatic vein reconstruction

Pts. No.	Primary liver disease	Liver tumor	Hepatic resection	Autograft	Patency
1.	B type LC	HCC	S VII+VIII	Rt. external iliac vein	P
2.	None	MLC	S IVs + right lobe	Rt. great saphenous vein	O
3.	B type LC	HCC	S VII+VIII	Patch graft of great saphenous vein	P
4.	CAH	MLC	S II	Rt. external iliac vein	O
5.	None	MLC	S VII+VIII	Direct anastomosis	P
6.	B type LC	HCC	S VII+VIII	superficial femoral vein	P
7.	CAH	HCC	Partial resection of S V,VI,VII,VIII	superficial femoral vein	P
8.	CAH	CCC	S VII+VIII + IVs	superficial femoral vein	P

Abbreviations: HCC: hepatocellular carcinoma, CCC: cholangiocellular carcinoma, MLC: metastatic liver carcinoma, LC: liver cirrhosis, CAH: chronic active hepatitis, S: segment, IVs: superior part of the fourth segment.

In conclusion, one-month patency rate of the reconstructed hepatic veins was 75%. A vein graft is necessary in most of patients who have hepatic vein reconstruction. Selection of an optimal graft is very important in order to get a good long-term patency rate after this procedure. Hepatic vein reconstruction for patients with cancer at the confluence of the hepatic vein and inferior vena cava is a new addition to routine hepatectomy which helps to both preserve remnant liver function.

Reference

1. Nakamura S, Sakaguchi S, Kitazawa T, Suzuki S, Koyano K, Muro H. Hepatic vein reconstruction for preserving remnant liver function. Arch Surg, 1990; 125:1455-9.
2. Ou QJ, Herman RE. Hepatic vein ligation and preservation of liver segments in major resections. Arch Surg, 1987; 122: 1198-200.
3. Kitazawa T, Nakamura S, Muro H. Clinical and experimental studies on ligation of the draining vein in the remnant liver during hepatectomy. J Jpn Surg Soc 1988; 89:863-70.
4. Nakamura S, Tsuzuki T. Surgical anatomy of the hepatic veins and the inferior vena cava. Surg Gynecol Obstet, 1981; 152: 43-50.
5. Couinaud C. Le foie. Etudes anatomicales et chirurgicales. Paris: Masson & Cie, 1957.

Phlébologie 92. Eds P. Raymond-Martimbeau, R. Prescott, M. Zummo.
John Libbey Eurotext, Paris © 1992, pp. 1117-1119

Diseases of superior vena cava. Surgical approach

A. Sortini, V. Gasbarro, D. De Anna , S. Occhionorelli, G. Fiorentini, M. Santini, I. Donini

Institute of Clinical Surgery, University of Ferrara, Italy. Corso Giovecca 203, 44100 Ferrara, Italy.

SUMMARY

The Authors report on their experience of surgical diseases of superior vena cava consisting in 12 cases. They discuss about the diagnostic value of T.C., venography end particularly mediastinoscopy. The last one is able to define histological features of the neoplastic lesions conducing to a superior vena cava syndrome.At the end, after a discussion on surgical approach in treatment of cases observed, the AA. underline the considerable value of the pathology considered even if a rare one.

Key words: mediastinum, superior vena cava, mediastinoscopy.

INTRODUCTION

Mediastinal physiopathology is based on the alterations of one or more mediastinic functions and has as its main cause a compressive mechanic factor. The dislocation of the various organs of the mediastinum induces a series of symptoms which costitute the mediastinal syndrome. This presents different aspects according to which organ is initially affected by the pathologic process and in relation to the degree and the nature of the secondary alterations of the nearly organs. As is known, the veins are easily compressible in such a measure as to obstruct and sometimes to interrupt the blood flow towards the heart (1). The superior vena cava syndrome (S.V.C.) constitutes one of the most characteristic aspects of the mediastinal pathology its surgical interest however, is as today somewhat limited becouse of its pathological rarity, for the frequent difficulty of of a correct diagnostic (2) and therapeutic approach, and for the presence of many centers, which being specialized in this type of pathology, resolve the almost totality of the cases.

PHYSIOPATHOGENISIS AND PHISIOPATHOLOGY

The accepted causes of the S.V.C. syndrome are (3):
A) Thrombosis of intraluminal or parietal cause.
It is noted today that the principal cause of vena cava thrombosis is iatrogenic, that is due to the intravenous introduction of foreing bodies such as infusion catheters, Swan-Ganz probes, cardiac pace-maker catheters, peritoneal jugular shunts. Frequent also is thrombosis of the axillosubclavian venous axis extended sometimes to the S.V.C.. We must also cite Bechet's disease characterized by a primitive fibrosis of the tunica intima, essential or secondary, which leads to S.V.C. thrombosis (4,5,6,7).
B) Primitive lesions of the vasal wall.

These are either rare tumors often asyptomatic, which rise from the vena cava wall (hemangiosarcoma and leiomyosarcoma) or aneurysms of a dysmorphic nature.
C) Benign external compressions.
Refering to all of those benign neoformations of mediastinal origin, that is, thymomas, dysembryomas and thymic cysts, endothoracic thyroid goiters. To mention also, compressions of the vena cava determined by mediastinal lymphodenomegalys (ex. Tubercolosis and Sarcoidosis) of aneurysmal pathology of the large vessels and of rarae post-traumatic mediastinal hematomas.
D) Direct traumas of the S.V.C.
In this group we include lesions caused by cutting arms or firing weapons and iatrogenic lesions represented by cavo-atrial disinserrtion during sternotomy.
E) Malign mediastinal-pulmonary neoformations.
This is without doubt the most serious and frequent cause of S.V.C. pathologys and is represented by all primitive mediastinal tumors recognized with increasing frequency as being neoformations of pulmonary origin and of all lymphoadenopaties both primitive and secondary. The clinical origin, usually stealthy, is characterized by the appearance after a certain period, of pathognomonic symptoms caused by a progressive obstacle of the venous drainage from the body's upper parts with the beginning of a collateral circulation which bypassed the venous obstruction.
The compression of the S.V.C. may occur above the outlet of the Azygos vein, and in this case the neck, face and upper limb veins have a characteristic turgor,with the typical "mantle" edema: the collateral circlein this case is costituted by the intercostal and vertebral veins. If, instead, the caval compression is under the outlet of the Azygos vein, the circulation inverts in this, and the blood is thus inverted to the inferior vena cava through the lumbar veins. If then the obstruction is situated at the same level of the Azygos vein's outlet, the principal collateral circulation is blocked easily, cAusing a decompensation of the mediastinal syndrome: in this case however, the superficial communication between S.V.C. and I.V.C. is secured through the epigastric and mammary veins and the lateral thoracic and abdominal vains.

MATERIALS AND METHODS

We have observed 12 cases of S.V.C. pathology so divided:
-5 cases due to compression and/or infiltration of broncopulmonary neoplasms.
-2 cases due to compressions from metastatic mediastinal lymphonodes which derive from bronchial cancer.
-2 cases due to venous compression from primitive mediastinal neoformations (a cyst and a thymoma).
-2 cases of venous thrombosis from phlebitis caused by catheterization
-1 case of thrombosis caused by a parietal trauma from a firearm.
In all of the cases the diagnostic course included a phlebography, in 8 cases a mediastinoscopy was performed which permitted us, in 6 cases, to identify the histological type of the primitive and secondary neoplasms.
In 7 patients we performed a mediastinal C.T..

DISCUSSION

Our survey, although limited, agrees with the data reported in literature and permits us to make some general considerations:
- The extreme rarity of the pathology in question seems confirmed, being equal in our experience to 1% of all surgical pathology of the thorax.
The diagnosis of the S.V.C. syndrome is directed towards the identification of the primitive morbid condition. Towards this purpose our diagnostic approach always includes a venous angiography which shows the site of the venous obstruction and the filling up of the numerous collateral veins.
Often a C.T. is executed. Due to the fact that more than 3/4 of these patients have malignant tumors, histological diagnosis is often usefull: in this case a mediastinoscope is necessary to clarify the histological type in the pathological

prcess. It is also true that in case of stenosis of S.V.C. obstruction, an important venous stasis may exist in which a sanguinary diagnostic method such as a mediastinoscope is contraindicated.
Nontheless, we are covinced of the usefulness of this type of investigation even at deprice of notable anxiety during the operation.
- A surgical treatment is rarely indicated in this group of patient as the lesions are usually inoperable (8). In our survey 8 patients equal to 66% of the total group have been operated: in 2 cases the primitive mediastinal mass has been removed; in 3 cases a pulmonary exeresis with mediastinal lymphadenectomy has been performed; 3 explorative thoracotomies have been performed.
- We registered a mitigation of caval compressions symptoms in only 5 cases (41.6%) even though our results remined after a certain time in only 3 patients (a case of a tumor of bronchial origin and two mediastinal masses).
- The 5 cases operated without a symptomatological remission died a short time after the operation; the 4 cases which were not operated instead, had the following conclusions: a patient with a grave inoperable bronchial tumor died after only three months, while two cases of iatrogenic caval thrombosis from catheters and one case of caval thrombosis caused by a firearm are alive and are in seemingly good health although the signs of insufficient venous drainage to the upper districts of the body are still present in various degrees.
- Up untill now we have done no surgical intervention of the superior vena cava.
Concluding, we can affirm that the S.V.C. pathology, although rare, presents notable diagnostic and therapeutic possibilities which require a close collaboration between the surgeon, the thoracic endoscopist and the radiologist (9,10,11).

REFERENCES

1) CERRINA J., GRATEAU G., PIETTE J.C., GODEAU P., MERLIER M.(1986): "Mediastinite fibrose dite idiopatique". Chirurgie, 112, 367.
2) CARLENS E.(1959): "Mediastinoscopy". Dis. Chest., 36:343.
3) EFFLER D.B., GROVES L.K.(1962): "Superior vena cava obstruction". J. Thorac. Cardiovasc. Surg., 43, 574.
4) DARTEVELLE P., LEVASSEUR P., ROJAS-MIRANDA A., LE BRIGAND H., MERLIER M.(1982): "Aspects chirurgicaux actuelles des syndromes caves superieurs". Rev. Practicien., 32, 409.
5) DUNDAR S., YAZICI H.(1982): "Superior vena cava syndrome in Bechèt's syndrome". Vasc. Surg., 18, 28.
6) GAILLARD J., PRADIES F., MOREAU J.C.(1979): "Pathologie non tumorale et non ganglionaire du mediastin". Encycl. Med. Chir.(Paris-France) Poumon, 1979, 6047-B-50, 4-6p.
7) MONTGOMERY J.H., D'SOUZA V.J., DYER R.B., FORMANEK A.G., PRABHU S.H.(1985): "Non surgical treatment of the superior vena cava syndrome". Am. J. Cardiol., 56, 829.
8) SANTIAGO S.M., WILLIAMS A.J.(1986): "Acute superior vena cava syndrome after Swan-Ganz catheterization". Chest., 89, 319.
9) SCHERK J.P., KERSTEIN M.B., STANSEL H.C.(1974): " The current status of vena cava replacement". Surgery, 76, 209.
10) STANFORD W., DOTTY D.B.(1986): "The role of venography and surgery in the management of patients with superior vena cava obstruction". Ann. Thorac. Surg., 41, 158.
11) STANFORD W., JOLLES H., ELL S., CHIU L.C.(1987): "Superior vena cava obstruction: a venographic classification". Am. J. Roentgenol., 148, 259.

Phlébologie 92. Eds P. Raymond-Martimbeau, R. Prescott, M. Zummo.
John Libbey Eurotext, Paris © 1992, pp. 1120-1121

Global surgical treatment in phlebopathic-obese woman

G. Amisano, P. Milone, M. Bormioli, P. Celoria, F. Morino

Istituto di Clinica Chirurgica Generale e Terapia Chirurgica, Torino Casa di Cura Privata Eporediese S.p.A., Via Castiglia, 27, Ivrea, Italy.

The indications to surgical treatment by vertical gastroplasty according to Mason for morbid obesity are represented by a body weight greater than 80% of the ideal body weight calculated according to Lorenz, resistence to all types of medical and dietary therapies, exogenous obesity, paying further attention to the psychological stability and general conditions of the patient. Alcoholism, drug dependence, psychosis, peptic ulcers and other eventual concomitant pathologies are absolute controindications. The surgical intervention consists in creating a small gastric pouch realized with a double line of suture between the anterior and posterior gastric walls for a lenght of about 9cm, parallel to the small curvature. The passage between the two cavities so obtained is calibrated with a ribbon of Dacron: the resulting pouch has a capacity inferior to 50cc.

The early sensation of satiety is the fundamental basis of the reduction of the quantity of food entake, thus leading to a weight loss not correlated to malabsorption.

The case examined concerns a 31 years old white female affected by varices of lower limbs, weighting 120 Kg at a height of 166cm.

The first part of the surgical treatment consisted in Mason's gastroplasty; after three years the patient obtained a steady weight loss of about 30 Kg; she then underwent abdominal lipectomy in order to correct residual cutaneus ptosis.

Eight months later we intervent in a combined way with lipoaspiratio according to Illoux (to define those areas in which the adipose panniculum was still represented in an excessive manner)and bilateral saphenectomy according to Hardiller-Amisano, after Doppler cw evolution.

The goal of the surgical treatment of varices is to obtain a good functional result, avoiding complications and recurrences without forgetting the esthetic component.

The incision for the crossectomy is made at 1cm above inguinal line: the scar will be then covered by pubic hair.

The G. Saphena is prepared according to the digitoclasic technique of Hardiller-Amisano thus saving the limphatics; the vein is then freed from perivenous structures and then sectioned after legature.

The cross is then finished with the search a section of the collaterals and the

accessory saphena. The G. Saphena is then finally tied-up at its origin which is correspondant to the white-line. We proced with the preparation of the G. Saphena at the malleolare site. The insufficient collaterals are then interrupted.
The stripping is perfectioned applying to the head of the stripper a pad wetted with a coagulating solution that will be removed after we wrapped the leg.
The coutaneus sutures are then carried out by intradermic technique.
Few months later the patient underwent lipectomy of the thighs in order to eliminated excessive volume.
The long term control has been satisfactory from the clinical and estethical point of view, all of this comforts and stimulates the patient in mantaining the results so achieved.

Treatment of postphlebitic syndrome with valves transplantation

Mackiewicz Zygmunt, Molski Stanislaw, Jundzill Wieslaw

Department of General and Vascular Surgery,
Medical Academy of Bydgoszcz

The aim of the study was the estimation of transplantation of brachial vein with two sufficient valves to popliteal vein in patient with grade II of postphlebitic syndrome.

The basic method of objective results was photo-plethysmography venous refilling time. The strain gauge plethysmography Digitmatic 2000 was used.

The operation was performed in ten patients.

In eight the improvement was observed. The elongation of plethysmography refilling time was noted in all patients but in two patients was shorter then ten seconds. The follow-up study was from one to twenty two months.

B.
TECHNIQUE ASSOCIÉES
COMBINED TECHNIQUES

LONG TERM FOLLOW-UP TREATMENT FOR VARICOSE VEINS

JA Dormandy, A Loh, J Evans, H Hutflesz, RS Taylor

Vascular Unit, St. George's Hospital, London

363 legs were treated in one clinic for varicose veins either by surgery or by compression sclerotherapy and were followed up for a minimum of 5 years (mean 9 years and 2 months). The patients were treated by injection sclerotherapy if there was no evidence of long or short saphenous reflux and the varicosities were confined to below the knee. All patients were seen at yearly intervals and success of treatment determined by a standardized questionnaire and examination by a doctor.

Patients treated by disconnection of the sapheno-femoral junction and stripping with or without local ties had the highest proportion of success (91%) at end of follow-up, although 28% of these patients required further procedures during the follow-up period. Similar patients whose long saphenous vein was not stripped had an 84% final success rate but 43% had required further treatment during follow-up.

28% of patients were judged suitable for sclerotherapy alone at presentation but only 55% of these were deemed to be successful at follow-up in the absence of subsequent treatment. A further 27% had a satisfactory result after a later surgical procedure.

Several conclusions can be drawn from a detailed analysis of this long term follow-up but perhaps the most important is that the selection of patients for sclerotherapy alone has to be even stricter than in this series.

Phlébologie 92. Eds P. Raymond-Martimbeau, R. Prescott, M. Zummo.
John Libbey Eurotext, Paris © 1992, pp. 1126-1128

Cross-sectomy, elastocompression and sclerotherapy in out-patient treatment of varicous veins of the lower limbs

Luis Burgoa, Loredana Burgoa

Private Practice Ponte S. Pietro (B.G.), Italy.

Summary

We think it's possible to have good phisiophatological and aesthetic results by treating patients with varicous veins of the lower limbs without admission to Hospital.
Accurate dissection of the sapheno femoral venous junction, ligature of all collaterals of the great saphenous vein and ligature and section of the former vein at the triangle of scarpa, immediatelly followed by elastocompression with elastic stockings and subsequently (after 6/8 weeks) sclerotherapy.
All these procedures with some skill and experience risolvs brightly these problems in out patients.
Since November 90 to October 91, from a numerous group of examined patients, we chose 45 in whom these procedure was applid.

From November 1990 to October 1991 45 patients who bearers of essential varices of the lower limbs were examined. They received outpatient treatment in the form of cross-sectomy, elasto compression and at a later point sclerotherapy. 10% of the patients were male, the age average of forty years, some patients (20%) had already undergone sclerotherapy but only on small veins and telangiectasis. Besides the typical symptomatology for varices (oedematous limbs, a feeling of heaviness and heat in the legs, especially after a period of time in orthostatism and prevalently in summer and so on) all patients had swollen varices, some more so than others, with dilation of the saphena and the collaterals concerned.
In all patients the Doppler Fluximetry was used to study the deep veins that should be pervious; and the continence or not of the saphenous-femoral valve.
The suggestion to tie the great saphena and the collaterals at the Scarpas triangulous springs from the incontinence of the above mentioned valve.
Therapy.- Besides the standard measures of hygiene and prophylaxis (keeping legs in a raised position, avoiding the heat and sedentary activities so that the muscular pump for the legs could be kept active) the carefully screened patients

underwent outpatient treatment. This involves local anaesthetic, approximately 10 cc. of carbocaina 1%, applied to the groin near the saphenous femoral inlet, followed by an incision of 3-4 cm., then a complete dissection of the cross and the tyng of all collaterals with rapidly reabsorbable thread.
The saphena is then tied both in the proximal direction at the precise point of the femoral attachment and distally with non-reabsorbable thread and then cut between the two ligatures.
Immediately afterwards elasto compression is applied to the upper thigh by means of an elastic stocking with 30-40 mm. Hg of compression at the ankle which decreases in the cranial direction. In these cases the stocking was compound of Polyamid 70%; Elastan 30% (Medi) and was worn for approximately 2-3 months.
After about 6-8 weeks, a period during wich the calibre of the varicose veins diminishes so that they become flabby and consequently less visible, the sclerotherapy session begin-the number of these session, the quantity injected, the concentration of the liquid and other less important variants will differ-followed by adhesive elasto compression, directed at times with sponges, especially on the most swollen veins.
12 ÷ 13 weeks after cross-sectomy, but always based on the calibre, number and extent of the varicose veins, they completely disappeared. The results are excellent both from a physiopathological stand point (there's no longer a reflux from the femoral vein to the saphenous vein) and from an aesthetic one since the limb bears no sign of scars. Moreover, the fact that the patient is never disabled and can lead a normal life whether in the family, at work, socially, except for the first hours immediately after cross-sectomy.
Only rarely, and then only when there is a marked dilation of the veins, does any residual thrombus form, and in this case it can be easily sucked out by means of a needle and syringe.
In cases where big insufficient perforant leg veins are present, it has been possible to sclerose the perforant itself, but this requires paying particular attention to the directed compression. Thus the fibrosis of the perforant, insufficient vein is obtained.
The only precaution needed to avoid possible damage to deep circulation (deep vein thrombosis) is to make the patient walk at length immediately after sclerotherapy.
In one case we had to resort to a surgical ligature of the perforant vein which had not been closed by sclerotherapy.
In conclusion we think that this is an excellent technique that avoids hospitalization, operating theatre stress and the relative morbility which are a consequence of different kinds of surgical treatment.

References

Apicella F. Lombardi A. (1990): Crossectomy and sclerotherapy for treatment of varices of lower limbs out patient surgery. Abstracts V.European American Simposium on venous diseases. 4,B3.

Holme, J.B. ' et al ' (1989): The anatomic relationship between the long saphenous vein and the saphenous nerve. Phlebology digest. 3, 16-17.

Jospeh G.Sladen. (1983): Compression sclerotherapy: preparation, technique, complications, and results. Am.J Surg. 146, 228-230.

Kerner, J. ' et al ' (1989): Functional effects of different steps in the course of sclerotherapy. Phebology digest. 2, 28-29.
Korstanje, M.J. Neumann, H.A.M. (1991): Compression therapy with elastic stocking. Phlebology digest. 2, 21-22.
Patel, J. Leger L. (1973): Nouveau traitè de technique chirurgicale.5,513-516.

Phlébologie 92. Eds P. Raymond-Martimbeau, R. Prescott, M. Zummo.
John Libbey Eurotext, Paris © 1992, pp. 1129-1131

Comparison of truncal varicosity ablation after saphenofemoral interruption: excision vs sclerotherapy

Lawrence L. Tretbar, M.D. FACS

Univ of MO Kansas City School of Medicine

This study compares two methods of treating varicose veins which originate from an incompetent long saphenous. Each treatment method is combined with surgical interruption of the saphenofemoral junction.

Methods and Materials: During the past four years a consecutive group of patients with varicose veins were studied. All had truncal varicosities caused by incompetence of the long saphenous vein at the saphenofemoral junction. None were associated with DVT.

There were 269 patients with 320 legs treated. Of this group there were 247 women and 22 men. Their ages ranged between 18 and 72 years.

Saphenous incompetence was determined by Doppler examination with the patient in the standing position. Incompetence was defined as reflux lasting for a second or longer as determined by augmentation.

All patients were treated with venous interruption of the saphenofemoral junction by clipping-in-continuity. Standard surgical titanium hemostatic clips were used to obliterate the saphenofemoral junction and its tributaries without transecting or removing the veins.

For the first two years of the study the truncal varices were treated with injection sclerotherapy alone. This encompassed 154 legs of 127 patients.

During the last 2 years all major varices have been excises by a micro-avulsion technic with sclerotherapy reserved for small residual veins. There were 166 legs of 142 patients in this group.

Surgery was performed in the out-patient unit under local infiltration anesthesia without additional sedation. Operating time for the saphenofemoral clipping was 30-45 minutes. A modified Muller technic was used for the excisions and required an additional 69-90 minutes of operating time.

Sodium tetradecyl sulfate was utilized for the sclerotherapy in all cases. In most instances 2-4 mls of a .75-1% solution were used during 2-3 injection sessions. The legs were wrapped during the day for a week following each injection visit.

Results: There were no major complications, DVTs, infections, skin sloughs, prolonged pigmentation or scarring, from surgical clipping and excisions nor from sclerotherapy.

Sclerotherapy Group: All sclerotherapy patients have been followed from 2-4 years. In about half, 72 legs, the truncal varices were 1.5 cm or smaller in diameter. All of these varices treated with injection/compression sclerotherapy have remained closed.

In the remaining 82 legs, where the varices were more than 1.5 cm in diameter, all treated veins remained closed for at least 1 year. However, 22 legs have shown opening of sclerotherapy treated veins after 1 year.

In 8 of these 22 legs the recurrences were associated with the appearance of nearby incompetent perforating veins, usually in the low thigh. All recurrences were successfully retreated either by reinjections or with surgical excision.

Excisional Group: These 142 patients have been followed from 1-2 years. The results of treatment have remained excellent. Treatment results are the same regardless of the size of the varices.

Regardless of treatment method, 8% of the legs have developed new small distal varices. It is suggested that these veins may have already been damaged by the venous hypertension of the saphenous vein but had not yet dilated at the time of treatment. They were all successfully treated with injections.

Conclusions: Both methods of treating varicose veins have been successful after interruption of the saphenofemoral junction. However, the injection technic used may not be adequate for some varices larger that 1.5 cm. Unfortunately it was not possible to determine which of the larger varices would and which would not respond, Therefore surgical excision appears to give a more permanent treatment in all cases.

No new veins have been found to grow around the operative site.

These data show that clipping-in-continuity of the saphenofemoral junction is a safe, effective and permanent method of interrupting venous reflux. In fact it allows many incompetent veins to establishment prograde flow and normalize function.

Phlébologie 92. Eds P. Raymond-Martimbeau, R. Prescott, M. Zummo.
John Libbey Eurotext, Paris © 1992, pp. 1132-1134

Valeur de l'association chirurgie itérative-sclérothérapie post-opératoire après échec du traitement chirurgical dans les varices des membres inférieurs

Michel Perrin, Jean-Pierre Gobin*, Catherine Grossetete*, Franck Henri**, Madeleine Lepretre*

*Chirurgie Vasculaire et * Phlébologie, Lyon, France. ** Laboratoire Beaufour, Paris, France.*

Entre Janvier 1985 et Décembre 1986, 105 malades (145 membres inférieurs) avaient bénéficié d'une chirurgie itérative suivie de sclérothérapie.
Le but de cette étude rétrospective est l'analyse des résultats fournis par cette association thérapeutique entre la 5ème et la 6ème année, l'enquête ayant été réalisée entre Janvier et Juin 1992.
La décision thérapeutique avait été prise d'un commun accord entre chirurgien et phlébologues au vu du mauvais résultat fourni par l'intervention initiale suivie ou non d'une sclérothérapie.
Il s'agit donc d'un groupe sélectionné pour lequel le critère de décision était essentiellement représenté par la persistance d'un point de fuite pathologique majeur entre réseau veineux profond et réseau veineux superficiel.
L'examen clinique avait été complété par un examen Doppler directionnel et dans 80 % des cas par une phlébographie poplitée dynamique.
La chirurgie itérative a été réalisée par un seul chirurgien (MP) alors que la sclérothérapie a été effectuée par 19 phlébologues.
Dans un premier temps, les malades ont été divisés en deux groupes :
Le premier rassemble les malades pour lesquels le diagnostic de varices essentielles a été retenu (85 %), le second groupe les patients chez lesquels une lésion du réseau veineux profond a été identifiée avant la réintervention (15 %) : Syndrome post-thrombotique ou Insuffisance Valvulaire Profonde Primitive.
Les patients ont ensuite été répartis en trois groupes :
. Le premier rassemble les malades chez lesquels l'intervention initiale comportait une erreur chirurgicale technique (crossectomie SI ou SE incomplète dans la majorité des cas).
. Le second réunit les malades chez lesquels l'intervention première comportait une erreur tactique (réseau saphénien pathologique non traité).
. Le troisième rassemble les patients dont la maladie variqueuse avait évolué dans un territoire non pathologique lors de l'intervention initiale.
Nous sommes bien conscients que la distinction entre second et troisième groupe n'est pas toujours facile à déterminer et comporte obligatoirement un certain nombre d'erreurs.
Le pourcentage des groupes se répartit ainsi : (Groupe 1 : 73 %, Groupe 2 : 28 %, Groupe 3 : 12 %) en sachant qu'un malade peut appartenir à plusieurs groupes.

L'âge moyen lors de l'intervention première était de 39 ans (Extrêmes 34-80) avec un sex ratio de trois femmes pour un homme.
Au plan anatomique, 97 % des interventions premières avaient été réalisées sur la Veine Saphène Interne (VSI), 9 % sur la Veine Saphène Externe (VSE).
Après cette intervention première, 51 % des malades avaient eu une sclérothérapie complémentaire.
La symptomatologie qui a conduit les patients à se faire réopérer se répartit ainsi :

. 80 % présentaient des signes fonctionnels : Douleurs ou lourdeurs de jambe.
. 52 % avaient une motivation esthétique.
. 52 % présentaient un oedème.
. 10 % avaient un ulcère de jambe.

Environ la moitié des malades avaient un mauvais résultat des deux côtés. Lorsque celui-ci était unilatéral, il prédominait à gauche.
Les résultats fournis par l'intervention première avaient été considérés comme mauvais d'emblée dans 36 % des cas, progressivement dégradés dans 64 % des cas.
Le délai qui s'est écoulé entre l'intervention première et la réintervention a été en moyenne de 12 ans (Extrêmes 6 mois-22 ans). L'âge moyen au moment de la chirurgie itérative était de 51 ans.
Au plan technique, la réintervention a été entreprise :

. Dans 59 % des cas sur la VSI.
. Dans 24 % " " sur la VSE.
. Dans 17 % " " sur la VSI et la VSE.

Donc dans 41 % des cas, la chirurgie itérative a porté sur la VSE. Dans la grande majorité des cas, cette chirurgie de la VSE était liée à une erreur tactique (insuffisance SE non traitée) ou à une évolutivité de la maladie variqueuse.
83 % des patients ont bénéficié d'une sclérothérapie complémentaire après leur réintervention qui se répartit ainsi dans le temps :
60 % ont été sclérosés lors de l'année qui a suivi la réintervention. Cette sclérothérapie a été poursuivie pendant 3 ans dans 50 % des cas et dans 35 % des cas jusqu'à la 5ème année.
67 % des malades ont bénéficié d'un traitement phlébotonique per os après leur réintervention.
L'appréciation des résultats après chirurgie itérative suivie de sclérothérapie a été réalisée de la façon suivante :
- Un questionnaire détaillé a été adressé aux malades. Sur les 105 questionnaires envoyés (105 malades - 145 membres), nous avons eu une réponse dans 71 % des cas (74 malades sur 105 et 105 membres sur 145).
- Un examen clinique a été réalisé par un phlébologue n'ayant jamais traité le malade. 50 malades (66 membres) ont répondu au questionnaire et ont été réexaminés soit 45,5 % du collectif initial.
Les résultats fournis par cette enquête ont été jugés par les patients de la façon suivante :

. 67 % se déclarent améliorés.
. 18 % " " moyennement améliorés.
. 13 % " " inchangés.
. 2 % " " aggravés.

A la question posée : "Vous feriez-vous réopérer ?", 82 % ont répondu OUI.

Si on analyse les résultats en tenant compte de la symptomatologie, on relève que :

. 65 % des malades se déclarent améliorés au plan fonctionnel.
. 60 % " " " " " au plan de l'oedème.
. 68 % " " " " " au plan esthétique.

Aucun des malades présentant un ulcère n'a récidivé. Un seul patient qui n'avait pas d'ulcère avant l'intervention en a présenté un. Il s'agissait d'un syndrome post-thrombotique.
Quand les patients ont bénéficié d'un traitement phlébotonique complémentaire, celui-ci a été jugé efficace dans 67 % des cas.
Lorsque les résultats sont jugés par le phlébologue qui a revu le malade entre la 5ème et la 6ème année, ils se répartissent ainsi :
Au plan fonctionnel, 78 % de bon résultats, 12 % de résultats moyens, 10 % de mauvais résultats.
Au plan esthétique, 30,5 % de bons résultats, 52,2 % de résultats moyens, 17,3 % de mauvais résultats.

En conclusion, il apparait que le bénéfice de l'attitude thérapeutique que nous avons adoptée est globalement positif puisque 82 % des malades se déclarent satisfaits.
L'amélioration est nettement moins importante au plan esthétique lorsqu'elle est jugée par le phlébologue alors que pour le patient les résultats sont équivalents au plan esthétique et fonctionnel.
Une analyse statistique plus détaillée a fait l'objet d'une étude qui sera publiée ultérieurement.

Crossectomie-sclérothèrapie per-operatoire: évaluation morpho-fonctionnelle à distance.

O. Maleti; M. Collura; M. Lugli; M.P. Zauli-Sajani; A. Cavezzi; V. Carigi.

INSTITUT DE PATHOLOGIE CHIRURGICALE

UNIVERSITE' DES ETUDES DE MODENE

Dans la période Janvier 1986 et Janvier 1992, 572 petients d'age compris entre 18 et 78 ans ont été operés de crossectomie élargie, dont 438 femmes et 134 hommes. Le 65,73% de ces patients ont été soumis à sclérothérapie per-operatoire. La sclérothérapie a été effectuée en introduisant un cathéter à travers une contreincision à pointe et possé à l'interne de la jointure du genou, de sorte d'obtenir une distribution homogene du produit sur une veine vide à temp chirurgical terminé et membre bandé.
Le produit utilisé a été tetradecilsulfate de sodium à 1% dans une première série et solution iodée à 4% dans l'autre, en quantité de 3ml pour la première et 2ml pour la seconde.
L'injection a été faite en position de léger Trendelenburg, suivi aussitot par la deambulation du patient.
Une compression appropriée était préventivement appliquée sur le cours de la saphène.
L'application du Duplex Scanner au follow-up de ces patiens a permis une meilleure évaluation des résultats, en intégrant les données cliniques obtenus dans une première série. Le follow-up de 203 patients a permi de partager les patients memes en 4 sous-groupes:
-sclérose saphéienne persistente
-recanalisation saphénienne
- refflux en saphène de calibre reduit
-pérméabilité de la saphène sans reflux
concernant trois groupes cliniques divisée selon l'absence des symptomes subjectifs (35%), amélioration des symptomes sbjectifs (49%) et persistance des symptomes subjectifs (16%).

Intraoperative sclerotherapy by catheter - 32 months later

Johannes Kunze, Hermann Rudolphi, Sonja Robdeutscher-Borowka

The intraoperative sclerotherapy by catheter was done after crossectomy instead of stripping the main trunk of the long saphenous vein (LSV).

This treatment has been realized to 61 patients. The results and complications of this therapy have been documented during the operation as well as 1 week, 1 month and 12 months later. 52 patients could be investigated after 32 months.

The documentation contents facts of phlebitis, hyperpigmentations, pain, venous induration, disorder of sensitivity as well as examinations with the continuous-wave Doppler Ultrasound (cw DUS) and light reflexion rheography (LRR). Serious complications following the treatment have not been observed. The therapeutic effect was very good even if in 19% of the 52 patients there was a partial or complete reflux demonstrated with the cw DUS ad least after 32 months. But only 6 patients were not satisfied with the treatment because of recurrence (3) or rise (3) of new varicose veins. Overall the intraoperative sclerotherapy seems to be a good method to treat the varicose LSV without the serous complications, which could occur by stripping.

The operation can be performed under local anaesthesia, the patient can be mobilized immediately after surgery. There is very little trauma and no danger of sensory.

Phlébologie 92. Eds P. Raymond-Martimbeau, R. Prescott, M. Zummo.
John Libbey Eurotext, Paris © 1992, pp. 1136-1138

Intraoperative segmental sclerosation of varicose systems in the outpatients' sector by the air bloc catheter technique instead of stripping. A report on 7000 interventions

Herbert Ermisch

Phlebological Outpatients, Dr Ermisch, Franz-Liszt-Str. 5, 0-8020 Dresden, Germany.

The epifascial venous insufficiency of the lower limbs is characterized by pathological venous flow parameters within valve-insufficient trunk and lateral branch veins and by increased pressure transmissions into the postcapillary interstice. The time factor of these manifestations is determining for the severity of interstitial tissue changes occuring in the distal limb sections.

On the basis of purposeful interventions, phlebosurgery is in a position to remove this venous flow pathology and so change the degree of severity into the tolerable I or O stages. This should be done very early and before first decompensation symptoms arise.

As prevalency and incidence of this disease, however, overtax clinical and economic capacities, a solution is provided by shifting the operative therapy into the outpatients sector. --This was the reason why we investigated from 1960 to 1964 into operative techniques practicable on an outpatients basis and involving more benefits than disadvantages for the patient.

Crossectomy stripping methods (BABCOCK 1910), as predominantly applied in hospitals, are well known, but they require a regional or general anaesthesia. The varicose main streams are torn off the largely ramified lateral branch systems, intact vein segments are removed in an uncontrolled manner, haemorrhages and haematomae occur, and nerves are injured. Pre- and post-operative expenditures are high, and it takes several hours to reach postoperative walking ability.

This relatively rough method is less suitable for the outpatients sector.

In 1911-1929, UNGER repeatedly reported on an intraoperative sclerotherapy involving the use of ureteric catheters for varicectomy. We have revised, modernized, technically improved and updated this method and have operated on more than 7,000 limbs in outpatients practice.

After crossectomy of the vv. saphena magna or/and parva, the insufficient trunk and lateral branches are not extracted, but sclerosed by means of a catheter which has been inserted in these systems. This procedure can take place under local anaesthesia, it is less strenuous for the patient, it is gentle, harmless and involves lower technical and personnel expenditures. --Crossectomy of the v. saphena magna requires 30 millilitres of 0.5-per-cent lidocaine in inguinal infiltration, the v. saphena parva needs about 15 millilitres for eliminating pains. Similar to a venae sectio, the varicose venous trunks are laid bare somewhat above the affluents with the catheter then being introduced into the varix systems. An air-bloc injection initiates a desired thrombotic process eventually blocking these epifascial varicosities. This segmental sclerosation is free from pain, and there are only 0.2 to 0.5 millilitres of a 3-per-cent obliteration agent (aethoxysclerol) in the form of foam required. The maximum obliteration agent quantity consumed during an operative procedure thus is 2 to 2.5 millilitres. It is of course necessary to expose and ligate penetrating veins prior to sclerosation.

After the wound has been closed and an appropriate bandage applied, the patient gets up from the operating table, gets dressed and has himself taken home by car. The patient is also given written instructions on his or her postoperative behavior, and arrangements are made with the family physician about the care during the next few days.

The long-term results of this phlebosurgery refer to the criterion of effectiveness, and a comparison can be drawn between 1,290 limbs after stripping and a group of 2,700 limbs after crossectomy with sclerosation. --The total number comprises 1,930 stripping cases and more than 7,000 sclerosing interventions.--

Relapses are unavoidable and shall not be hidden:

--- The overall recidivity frequency is 5.3 per cent for the stripping group and 6.6 per cent for the sclerosation group.

--- The evaluation of the sclerosation group shows the following results:

2.8 per cent	Relapses of v. saphena magna or parva = incomplete crossectomies
2.4 per cent	Relapses by penetrating veins = cannot be influenced
5.3 per cent	Relapses from lateral branch systems = insufficient after-care
0.4 per cent	Ulcus cruris relapses due to the haemodynamic pathology

Further recidivity analyses confirmed that a variety of new secondary symptoms can arise from incomplete elimination of the flow pathology. In this regard, it is necessary to emphasize the importance of a postoperative treatment lasting several months to allow operative insufficiencies to be recognized and eliminated as early as possible.

An economic consideration to conclude:
Under the assumption of a 7 days' stay in hospital and an even very low daily rate of 200 deutschmarks (= 138 Canadian dollars), 7,000 phlebosurgical interventions in the outpatients sector would make up for 49,000 bed days at an expense of altogether 9.8 millions of deutschmarks (= 6.76 millions of Canadian dollars).

REFERENCES

Babcock, W.R. (1907): Extraction for the removal of varicose veins. *J.amer.med.Assoc. 1907*
Bericht Chirurg 1910, 1339
New York med. J. 1907 86, 253

Dodd, H., and Cockett, F.B. (1956): The Pathology and Surgery of the veins of the lower limb. *E. + S. Livingston Lfd. Edinburgh + London*

Ermisch, H. (1984): Intraoperative Sklerotherapie statt Stripping, Bericht über 2 700 Eingriffe. *Z. ärztl. Fortbild.* 78, 327-328

Keller, W.L. (1924): Combined exstirpation and obliteration in the treatment of varicose veins. *Ann. Surg. No. 6* 79, 907-912

Unger, F. (1911): Einiges über Krampfadern. *Bln. klin. Wschr.*

Unger, F. (1927): Zur Technik der Varizenbehandlung. *Bln. Ges. Chir.*
(1927): *Ref. Zbl. Chir. Nr. 51,* 3273, 3287
(1929): *Bln. Ges. Chir.*
(1930): *Zbl. Chir.* 3, 159

C.
RÉSULTATS
RESULTS

Phlébologie 92. Eds P. Raymond-Martimbeau, R. Prescott, M. Zummo.
John Libbey Eurotext, Paris © 1992, pp. 1141-1143

The results of « limited stripping » of long saphenous vein connected with the local varicotomy and perforators ligation : comparison with group after Babcock procedure

Jacek Gawrychowski[1], Ryszard Zbroński[2]

[1] Department and Clinic of Thoracic Surgery of Silesian Medical Academy (Head : Prof. dr. Med. Kazimierz Czyżewski), 41-800 Zabrze ul. 3-go Maja 13/15, Poland. [2] II Department and Clinic of the General Surgery and Vessels of Silesian Medical Academy (Head : Prof. dr. med. Marian Pardela), « Medservice »-private ambulatory (Krystyna Twardowska-Saucha), Poland.

Surgery is advisable when there is proximal incompetence of either the long or short saphenous vein (4,6,8). None of the treatment of methods is ideal,but in the case of varicose veins related to long saphenous incompetence flush ligation and stripping is commonly recomended (8). There are controversies on what kind of stripping is a better procedure either the long one from ankle to groin or the short one - from the upper third of the calf to groin (6,8).We have tried to answer for this question.

MATERIAL AND METHODS

We compared two groups of patients treated because of varicosity as well as functional trouble before and after surgical cure.
The first group (n=38, in 41 legs) following sapheno - femoral flush ligation with division and ligation of groin tributaries we underwent "*limited stripping*" (*Negus* procedure (8)), while second one (n=20) was operated by the *Babcock* technique.
After stripping in both groups we performed subfascial perforating vein ligation and local varicosity.For the estimation of the results we were consulting reasons as follows: functional troubles (pain,heaviness),neurological complications (*saphenous* or *suralis nn.*trauma), and aesthetic.Areas of sensory impairment were detected by simple neurological tests in all patients.Moreover we were measuring the speed of conductivity in *n. suralis*.

RESULTS

There were no significant differences between the age and sex rations of the patients in both groups.In the *table* 1 we present kinds of troubles before and after operation procedure in these groups.We must underline that nearly 90% of patients came to us with the pain in their legs.Moreover, before operation 29,3% of patients suffered from oedema,27,6% from heaviness and 22% have had trombophlebitis.The results were considered "*excellent*" when the limb was wholly free from symptoms,without any signs of residual superficial varices or of persisting perforator insufficiency. It was classed as "*good*" in wholly asymptomatic patients

Kinds of operation		Kinds of troubles				
		pain	heaviness	oedema	trombophlebitis	neurological troubles
Babcock procedure n=20 legs	before	19	6	3	6	3
	after	2	2	0	0	11
"limited stripping" n=41 legs	before	36	10	14	7	3
	after	3	2	1	0	5

tabl.1 *Comparison of kinds of troubles before and after varicose surgery by Babcock and "limited stripping" procedures.*

showing no sings of perforator insufficiency,but who sufferd from a residual varix or varices either left at the operation or formed later.The results were noted as "*fair*" in patients whose condition improved, but who still had symptoms consisting of persistent oedema,pain,or feeling of heaviness in the leg or large superficial veins.The results were termed as "*poor*" when the patient did not feel any improvement when large varices persisted or when pronounced symptoms were present (3).According to this classification we present results of the operation procedure in both groups in *table* 2.After stripping no nerve tissue was seen attached to any of the stripped long saphenous veins.

Kinds of operation	Results of surgical procedure			
	excellent	good	fair	poor
m.Babcock n = 20 legs (1987-1990)	9	9	2	0
"limited stripping n=41 legs (1991)	27	11	3	0

tabl.2 *Results of surgical procedure after Babcock and "limited stripping" operation.*

We may say,difference of results in "*excellent*" groups (45% vs 66%) depends on the uneven time between the operation and the examination.On average 2,6 years after *Babcock* procedure,follow--up of 11 legs out of 20 (55%) showed areas of sensory impairment.The various areas of sensory loss extended from the regions of medial malleolus upwards on to the medial aspect of the legs.Mean areas of sensory loss were 33,3cm^2(range 5 to 120 cm^2).After limited stripping we have observed sensory loss in five (12,2%) patients,mean 31 cm^2 (range 5 to 80 cm^2).Moreover in 50% of patients after Babcock procedure and in 17% after "*limited stripping*" following subfascial ligation of perforating veins or stripping we noted slightly lower speed of conductivity (range 0,3 till 4,3m)s).Five cases in the both groups were noted as "*fair*" results. None of them were recorded when superficial insufficiency was present alone.All were coupled with moderate or severe insufficiency of perforating veins.

DISCUSSION

In the early period surgery gives range 60 up till more than 90% satisfactory results (3,5,9),in our material as well.The long saphenous vein is usually only dilated and incompetent to the upper third of the calf, at which point it is joined by the major calf tributaries (8).The perforating veins in the lower part of the leg do not join directly with the long saphenous vein,but via the loops of the posterior arch vein.The saphenous nerv lies deep to the long saphenous vein at knee level and is separated from it by subcutaneous fat (1,8).Below the knee it becomes progresively closer to the vein.Loesions of nerve branches by the stripper head is therefore difficult to avoid. Incidence of pain,paresthesia or sensory loss caused by saphenous nerve damaged after *Babcock* procedure is reported ranging 23-58% (1,8),but after "*limited stripping* 4,2%. Sensory impairment, transient or permanent, depends on trauma saphenous or suralis nerves caused by the passage of the stripper or by the dissection of the saphenous vein at the ankle (1,7). For majority of patients stripping of the lower saphenous vein is unnecessary as the future source of veins to harvest for coronary vessel replacement if needed (2).

The present investigation has shown:

1-radical operation by the *short stripping* up to 1/3 upper calf gives,similar good results of the cure,as the *Babcock* procedure

2-all worse results were connected with moderate or severe perforating veins insufficiency,

3-the limited stripping operation effectively removes proximal long saphenous veins and avoids neurological complication of stripping to the ankle

REFERENCE

Cox S.J.,Wellwood J.M.et al.,(1974):Saphenous nerve injury caused by stripping of the long saphenous vein.*Br.Med.Journal* 1,415-417

McFarlane R.,Godwin R.J. et al.(1985): A varicose vein and coronary artery bypass surgery compatible? *Lancet*, 19,859

Hager K.(1966):Five year results of radical surgery for superficial varices with or without coexistent perforator insufficiency, *Acta Chir.Scand.*131,38-49.

Hobbs J.T.(1974):Surgery and sclerotherapy in the treatment of variecose veins.*Arch.Surg.*109,793-796.

Hobbs J.T.1977:A random trial of the treatment of varicose veins by surgery and sclerotherapy.In:*The treatment of venous disorders* ed. J.T.Hobbs pp.195-207.Lancaster:M.T.P.Press Ltd.

Large J.1990:The treatment of varicose veins:a personal review. *Phlebology* 5,141-146.

Miliken J.C.,Dinn E.,et al.(1986):A simple Doppler technique for the rapid diagnosis of significant saphenofemoral reflux. *Phlebology* 1,125-128.

Negus D.(1986):Should the incompetent saphenous vein be stripped to the ankle? *Phlebology* 1,33-36.

Trempe J.(1991):Long-term results of sclerotherapy and surgical treatment of the varicose short saphenous vein.*J.Dermatol. Surg.Oncol.* 17,597-600.

Phlébologie 92. Eds P. Raymond-Martimbeau, R. Prescott, M. Zummo.
John Libbey Eurotext, Paris © 1992, pp. 1144-1147

Résultats bénéfiques de l'élastocompression sur la cicatrisation dans la chirurgie des varices. À propos de 1 000 cas

William Taieb

9, rue de Turin, 75008 Paris, France.

L'un des buts de la chirurgie des varices est d'assurer un résultat esthétique.Le temps des incisions "balafres" est révolu.

Nos patients sont maintenant,capables d'assumer leur maladie variqueuse,leurs suites opèratoires,mais sont trés exigeants sur la qualité esthétique de leur résultat post-opèratoire.

Le but de ce travail est mettre en évidence le role de la contention post -opèratoire,afin d'en déterminer ses limites.

PROTOCOLE OPERATOIRE :

L'élasto-compression comprend 2 phases:

-La mise en place de bandes Elastiques,stériles,à la fin de l'intervention,portées pendant 3 à 4jours,

-puis relayées par un collant,ou des bas à varice,pendant un mois.

Les incisions des Scarpa sont refermées par surjet intradermique de Monofil,et les incisions de phlébectomie sont recouvertes de pansement,y compris les incisions des chevilles,en cas d'éveinage.

RESULTATS

AUCUNE CICATRICE CHELOIDE N'A ETE RETROUVEE.

1/ <u>Incidence sur le délai de cicatrisation:</u>

-Temps moyen à la jambe,à la cheville,au pied : 5 jours,

quel que soit l'état cutané antérieur.(Eczéma).
-Disparition des cicatrices au 1r mois postopèratoire.

<u>2/Incidence de la longueur de la cicatrice :</u>

La compression favorise le rapprochement des berges,qui ont été parfois agrandies ,de dedans en dehors,pour extraire de grosses varices.

<u>3/ Incidence des zones d'intervention :</u>

Meilleurs résultats à la cheville et au genou:
Effet " massage" bénéfique de l'élastocompression sur les zones mobiles.

<u>4/ Incidence sur les cicatrices inflammatoires:</u>
Elles ne sont pas sensibles à l'élasto-compression.
L'adjonction de corticoides locaux,ou de gels anti-inflammatoires est obligatoire,pour éviter l'apparition secondaire de cicatrices hyperpigmentées.

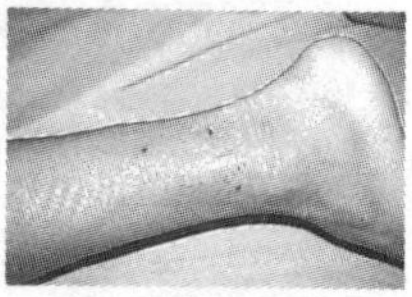

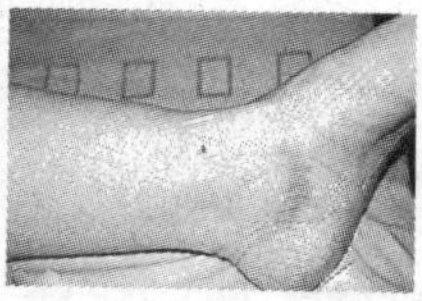

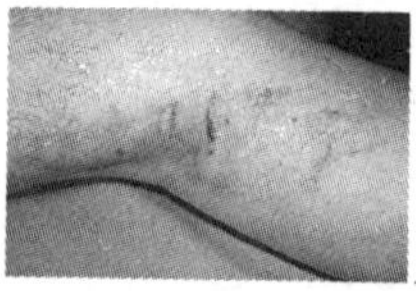

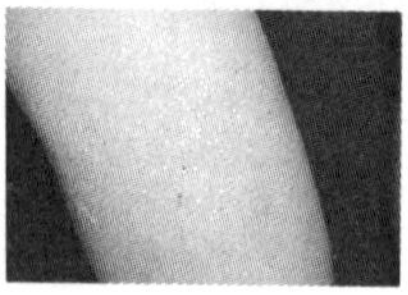

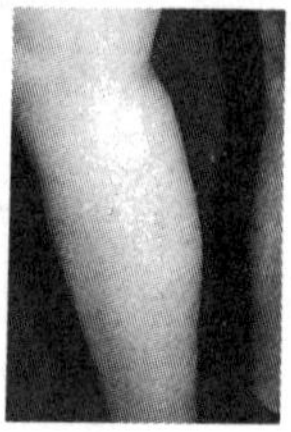

DISCUSSION :

Certes,les incisions sont minimes.

L'absence de compression ne jouerait peut-être pas sur la qualité du résultat esthétique. Le fait d'extraire les varices de dedans en dehors,doit favoriser une cicatrisation plus rapide.

Une étude en double aveugle serait justifiée.

Un étalonnage précis permettra de moduler tel ou tel aspect de cette thérapeutique adjuvante,qu'est l'élasto-compression.

Conclusion :

L'association Mini-incisions Elastocompression post-opèratoire permet actuellement de garantir un résultat esthétique tout à fait satisfaisant,à savoir:

-Absence de chéloides,

-Invisibilité des cicatrices,au premier mois post-opèratoire,

-Mais elle ne garantit pas contre l'hyperpigmentation,ni contre l'inflammation.

CHIRURGIE DE L`INSUFFISANCE DE SAPHÈNES ET DE PERFORANTES

J. Mazuch, Ľ. Machan, J. Pelč, K. Géč

Service de chirurgie, Hôpital régional, Lučenec
Chef Doc. MUDr. J. Mazuch, DrSc., Tchécoslovaquie

Le but de la chirurgie est de supprimer radicalment les troubles hémodynamiques et l`insuffisance veineuse chronique. Il faut donc de supprimer tous les points de reflux au niveau des crosses saphènes internes au scarpa, des crosses saphènes externes dans le creux poplitée, soit au niveau des perforantes incontinentes. Notre statistique porte sur 1455 interventions chirurgicales pour les varices des membres inferieurs avec l`insuffisance veineuse chronique au niveau des saphènes et des perforantes. Nos résultats élognés après intervention chirurgicale sont satisfaisants. Nous avons réussi les bons résultats dans 93,5 % des cas avec le recul moyen de 8,7 ans. Les récidives nous avons constaté dans 6,2 % des cas.

Functional and aesthetic valuation after surgical treatment of varicose veins of lower limbs

Prof. F.Sciannameo,dr. D. Alberti,dr. P. Ronca

Università degli studi di Perugia
Istituto di Patologia chirurgica (R) sede in Terni

For an objective valuation of the results after surgical treatment of varicose veins of lower limbs,a simple method is proposed.
For each patient,a final score is obtained by the overall valuation of functional and aesthetic parameters,summarized in a table easy to fill in.
The subjects analized to obtain this score are:improvement of subjective symptoms,clinical and instrumental results and personal degree of satisfaction expressed by the patient.
It is so possible to deduce objective and compareble results of the surgical treatment and better analize its efficacy.
An experience of 850 patients,affected by varicose veins of lower limbs and undergone surgical treatment in our Institut from january 1988 to december 1991 is reported.
In all these patients we performed a detailed valuation of preoperatory and postoperatory functional and aesthetic parameters and expressed a final score.

SAPHÉNECTOMIE EN AMBULATOIRE, RÉSULTATS

CHRISTIAN CHOUINARD, MD, FRCP(S),
CENTRE HOSPITALIER GOUIN-ROSEMONT,
MONTREAL, CANADA.

Je présente les résultats de 500 strippings consécutifs où j'ai employé en majeure partie le stripping invaginant avec phlébectomies associées. Les résultats sont colligés à partir de réponses des malades à un questionnaire auquel ils ont été soumis.

Sont donc présentés des données anthropométriques, raisons de consultation, types de chirurgie, types d'anesthésie, séjour hospitalier, convalescence, survenue de complications et infections et évaluation globale du patient.

Le faible taux de complications et le peu d'effets indésirables sur la vie sociale nous encourage à continuer ce type de chirurgie.

Phlébologie 92. Eds P. Raymond-Martimbeau, R. Prescott, M. Zummo.
John Libbey Eurotext, Paris © 1992, pp. 1150-1152

Étude sur 1500 strippings saphène interne longs sous anesthésie locale ambulatoire

Denis Creton

Espace Chirurgicale Ambroise Paré, 54100 Nancy

Le choix, dans le traitement des varices, d'une exérèse chirurgicale des sources de reflux, des différentes voies de transmission du reflux, ainsi que l'exérèse des varices, nous a conduit à associer, depuis 1987, au sein d'une même intervention , la crossectomie, le stripping saphène interne long et l'ensemble des phlébectomies ambulatoires.
Après 5 années d'expérience et la réalisation de 2000 strippings saphène interne longs et phlébectomies ambulatoires complètes , nous avons pu ,sans réduire la qualité de l'exérèse, atteindre un minimum d'agressions chirurgicales par l'anesthésie locale et, la chirurgie ambulatoire.

I Matériel d'étude

. Ces 4 années d'expérience ont été divisées en 5 périodes successives comportant un même nombre d'interventions (670 en moyenne) et, parmi celles-ci, ont été étudiées les interventions ayant comporté un stripping saphène interne long en plus des phlébectomies ambulatoires complètes. Les patients étaient porteurs de varices essentielles , ils ont tous été revus au moins 21 jours après l'intervention.

II La technique utilisée a été identique.

. L'anesthésie locale réalisée par :

- un bloc crural avec repérage du nerf crural et de ses branches par électrostimulation et ,
- injection d'anesthésique local sous cutanée dans les zones cutanées dépassant la surface d'anesthésie du bloc crural
- l'anesthésique utilisé a été, tout d'abord , la MEPIVACAINE 1% ou 0,5 % , puis la LIDOCAINE non adrénalinée à 1%.

. L'intervention associe :

- crossectomie par une incision haute et interne dans le triangle pubien
- stripping saphène interne long par invagination
- phlébectomies ambulatoires de Muller réalisées complétement.
- crossectomie et stripping saphène externe invaginant , si nécessaire;

. Double contention,

- pansement chirurgical stérile, fixe élastique pour 5 jours,
- bande élastique amovible pour l'orthostatisme et la marche.

III Evolution des indications.

L'analyse de ces 5 périodes traduit une évolution des indications et des techniques opératoires, en effet :

. Sur le même nombre d'interventions, le pourcentage de strippings saphène interne longs diminue régulièrement au profit d'interventions atypiques plus adaptées aux troubles hémodynamiques mieux explorés actuellement (stripping partiel haut ou bas , hémicrossectomie, phébectomies ambulatoires simples, pathologie saphène externe isolée).
Il y a 5 ans, le stripping saphène interne long était pratiqué dans 96 % des interventions, actuellement il fait partie de l'intervention dans seulement 66 % des cas. Cette évolution traduit une meilleure connaissance de l'hémodynamique veineuse superficielle.
. La proportion de strippings saphène interne longs fait sous anesthésie locale est passée en 4 ans de 43 % à 89 % .
- L'obésité et l'importance des varices ne sont pas des contre indications anatomiques à l'anesthésie locale. En effet, nos indications extrêmes concernant le poids atteignent 160 kg et 130 incisions pour l'importance des varices.
- Les contre-indications psychologiques sont aussi largement réduites grace à l'usage plus large de médications adjuvantes.
MIDAZOLAN (1 à 2 mg d'HYPNOVEL) ALFENTANYL (1/2 à 1 mg de RAPIFFEN) ou ATROPINE 1 mg, qui sont des produits à durée d'action très courte qui ne compromettent pas la chirurgie ambulatoire;
Durant les premières périodes du libre choix du mode d'anesthésie par la patients , l'usage de ces drogues représentait 5 %, actuellement l'extension très large et dirigiste de l'anesthésie locale nous fait utiliser ces drogues dans presque 30 % des cas. Cela représente le pourcentage de patients qui n'aurait pas choisi spontanément l'anesthésie locale.
Malgré l'extension des indications le nombre de patients satisfaits du confort de l'anesthésie locale reste identique (95 %).

. La proportion d'ambulatoire parmi les strippings saphène interne longs sous anesthésie locale est régulièrement croissante, paraissant atteindre un maximum de 90 % . Cette limite est due à plusieurs facteurs que l'on retrouvent dans la même proportion sur les deux dernières périodes.

1° L'anesthésie locale n'est pas prévue pour être faite en ambulatoire ,il s'agit de
- Problèmes médicaux annexes : diabète, anticoagulation, bilan d'autres affections, troubles de la crase sanguine, affections intercurrentes , thrombose saphène.
- Problèmes extra médicaux. Troubles psychiques, déficit socio familial, transports, intempéries, confort personnel, éloignement du domicile .

2° l'anesthésie locale prévue pour être ambulatoire doit être annulée. Une fois la mauvaise hémostase de l'artère honteuse externe nous a conduits à réintervenir une heure après l'intervention. Une fois un bloc crural d'une durée de 9 heures a interdit le départ du centre. Parmi ces patients hospitalisés en post opératoire, on trouve souvent des patients de plus de 60 ans, présentant d'importantes varices (plus de 40 incisions) , présentant des troubles trophiques cutanés ou opérés tard dans la journée.
Le volume maximum d'anesthésique local injecté est certainement responsable, par la vasoplégie, des malaises ou fatigue post opératoires qui interdisent le retour à domicile.
Cette limite , 5 % des patients, peut être considérée comme un échec de ce type d'intervention prévue en ambulatoire.

IV Analyse des paramètres de l'intervention

. Le volume moyen d'anesthésique utilisé par intervention est de 42 ml pour la MEPIVACAINE, de 44 ml pour la LIDOCAINE avec des extrêmes allant de 20 à 60 pour la MEPIVACAINE et, de 20 à 80 pour la XILOCAINE. 10 ml suffisent pour obtenir un bloc crural complet.
La MEPIVACAINE a le double avantage d'être plus puissante donc d'induire une analgésie plus profonde et plus confortable pour le patient , mais aussi de pouvoir être utilisée avec la même efficacité que la LIDOCAINE à une concentration deux fois moindre, ce qui permet d'augmenter la surface cutanée de l'anesthésie sans augmenter le volume d'injection.
La MEPIVACAINE a été utilisée pour 772 interventions et la LIDOCAINE pour 990 interventions.

. Le type de stripping a toujours été, de principe, un stripping par invagination de haut en bas.

- Dans 70 % des cas, le stripping invaginant a été complet soit de haut en bas, soit de bas en haut, soit en deux parties de haut en bas et de bas en haut avec rupture sous le genou.

- Dans 28 % des cas, le stripping invaginant a été considéré comme incomplet, présentant à la partie moyenne du membre une partie de la veine saphène interne télescopée sur le strippeur entre les deux parties , haute et basse, invaginées.

- Dans 2% des cas, le stripping invaginant trop insuffisant a dû être complété par un stripping complémentaire de type BABCOCK.

Une incision intermédiaire ne dépassant pas 6 mm a été nécessaire dans 14 % des cas.

Nous avons associé dans le même temps opératoire une crossectomie saphène ou/et un stripping saphène externe par invagination long ou court dans environ 6 % des cas.

V Analyse du risque embolique

. On attribue le peu de risque thrombo embolique de l'anesthésie locale à l'absence de vasoplégie et à une accélération concomitante de la circulation profonde.

Le peu de risques thrombo emboliques est conforté par la prescription systématique d'héparine de bas poids moléculaire, moyennant quoi nous n'avons eu aucun accident thrombo embolique sur les 1500 interventions réalisées en ambulatoire.

Le seul accident thrombo embolique concernait une patiente , jeune (25 ans) sans aucune anomalie de l'hémostase, présentant de très importantes varices (70 incisions), intervention longue (1 H 45), patiente hospitalisée et alitée pratiquement 48 heures durant son intervention sous anesthésie locale ; la projection embolique vérifiée 8 jours après , traitée et surveillée n'a laissé aucune séquelle . 2,5 pour mille parmi les hospitalisés.

VI Conclusion

L'étude de cette série permet de montrer que la chirurgie d'exérèse des varices évolue et que le stripping n'est plus le pivot central de l'intervention.

La chirurgie d'exérèse variqueuse, grâce au stripping par invagination, avec bloc crural et la technique de Muller, atteint un niveau minimum d'agression, puisqu'aujourd'hui l'anesthésie locale est réalisable dans tous les cas sans exeption et l'intervention dans 90 % des cas en ambulatoire.

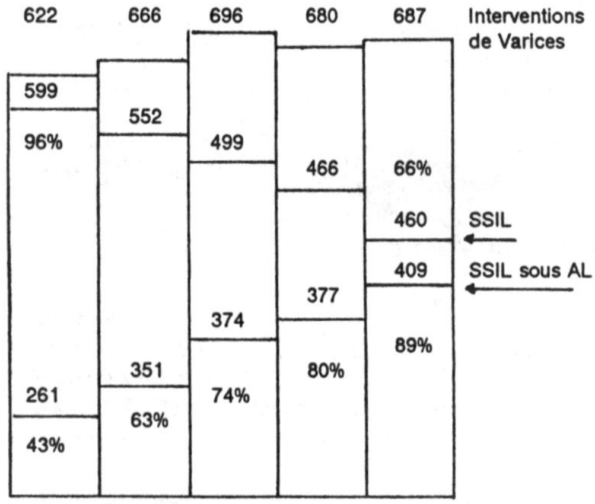

Pourcentage de stripping saphène interne long sous AL

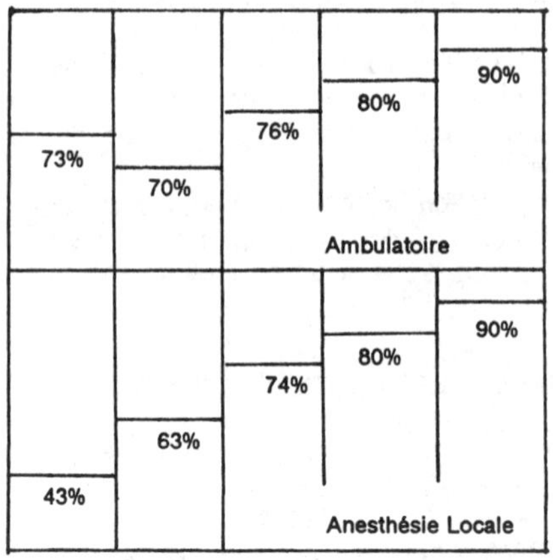

Pourcentage de stripping ambulatoire

Phlébologie 92. Eds P. Raymond-Martimbeau, R. Prescott, M. Zummo.
John Libbey Eurotext, Paris © 1992, pp. 1153-1155

Effects of surgery and compression bandaging on transcutaneous oxygen in limbs with venous hypertension

James P. Travers, Katherine L. Dalziel*, Geoffrey S. Makin**

*Department of Human Morphology, * Department of Dermatology and ** Department of Surgery, University Hospital, Queen's Medical Centre, Nottingham, NG7 2UH, UK.*

SUMMARY

Longstanding venous hypertension is associated with lipodermatosclerosis (LDS) which in turn leads to decreased oxygen transport to the overlying skin and venous ulceration. We measure transcutaneous oxygen content (TcPO2) of skin above the medial malleolus in patients with unilateral varicose veins with and without LDS. Pre-operative measurements showed a significant decrease in TcPO2 in limbs affected by LDS ($p < 0.01$) compared to control limbs. Surgical removal of varicose veins in 9 patients with LDS significantly increased TcPO2 in affected legs ($p < 0.02$) 12 months after operation.

Treatment of venous ulceration in 27 patients with compression bandaging significantly increased TcPO2 levels ($p < 0.01$) at the ulcer edge with ulcer healing.

Correction of venous hypertension by surgery or compression bandaging is associated with improved skin oxygenation in patients with LDS and ulceration.

INTRODUCTION

The mechanism of venous ulceration is not established. Recent theories suggest an oxygen diffusion block to skin by fibrin cuff deposition (Burnand et al., 1976) or white cell trapping (Coleridge-Smith et al., 1988). Transcutaneous oxygen levels are decreased at the ulcer edges suggesting a pathological barrier (Mani et al., 1989).

We investigate the effect of surgery and compression of varicose veins on skin TcPO2 above the ankle.

METHOD

Patients with unilateral long saphenous varicosis were placed into two groups, those with (n = 9, mean age 57 ± 3 years) and without LDS (n = 12, mean age 47 ± 4 years) with the contralateral limb used as control. Those with ankle systolic indices less than 0.9 (Doppler studies) were excluded. TcPO2 measurements using the TCM2 apparatus,

Fig.1.

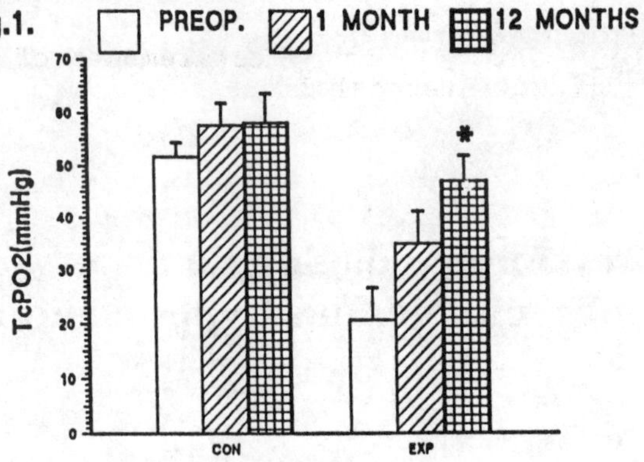

* = *Significant to Exp.preop at p<0.02*

TcPO2 control/exptl.limbs at 0,1,12 months postoperatively

Fig.2.

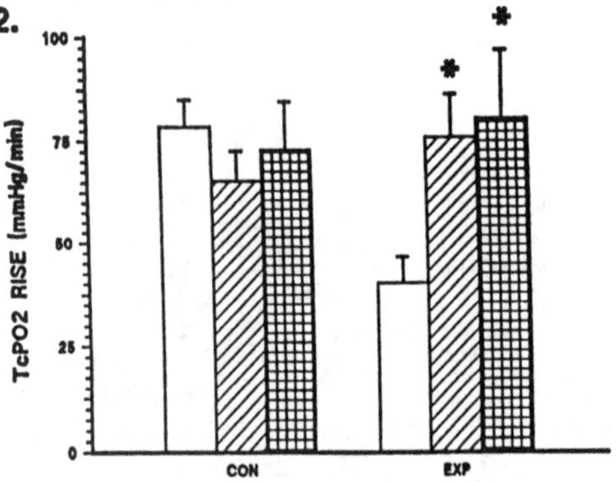

* = *Significant to Exp.Preop. at p<0.02*

TcPO2 rate of rise in control/exptl limbs at 0,1,12 months postop.

Fig.3.

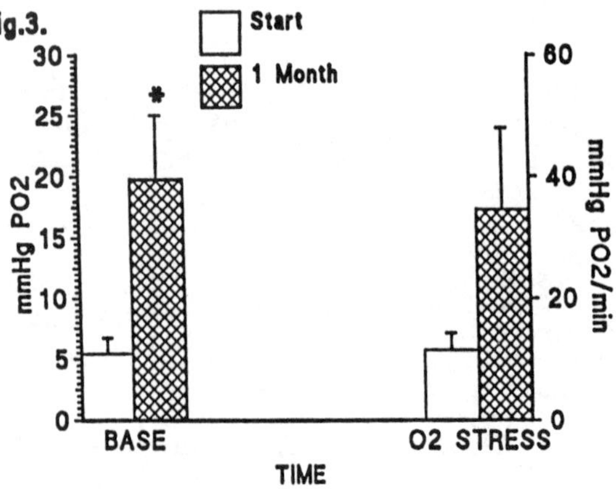

**=Significant to start at p<0.01%*

TcPO2+rate of rise(O2 stress) following compression bandaging

(Radiometer, Copenhagen) with electrode temperatures at 44°C, were taken with the patient semi-recumbent at 20°C at 5 cm above the medial malleolus on both control and experimental limbs. Measurements of chest TcPO2 were taken at the left third intercostal space.

TcPO2 readings following stress testing were also assessed using 100% oxygen inhalation, (15 l/minute) for 5 minutes and rate of rise estimated. Readings were performed pre-operatively, 1 month and 12 months post-operatively. Twenty seven patients with venous ulcers (mean age 58 ± 5 years) had TcPO2 readings taken as above, before compression bandaging using either Tensopress (Smith and Nephew) or Panelast Acryl (Lohmann) and after 1 month of treatment.

RESULTS

TcPO2 was significantly lower pre-operatively in limbs with LDS as compared to controls ($p < 0.01$). Surgery significantly improved TcPO2 levels in limbs affected by LDS after 12 months (Fig. 1, $p < 0.02$) and after oxygen stress testing (Fig. 2, $p < 0.02$). Compression bandaging improved TcPO2 in limbs affected by ulceration at rest (Fig. 3, $p < 0.01$) after 1 month's treatment.

DISCUSSION

This study shows that TcPO2 is decreased in limbs affected by LDS but improved following surgical correction of venous hypertension. External compression improves skin oxygenation adjacent to ulcers. We postulate that reversal of venous hypertension by surgery or compression, whether by aiding recovery of capillary function (Curri et al., 1989) and accelerating fibrin cuff resorption, leads to better skin oxygenation and prevention of venous ulceration.

REFERENCES

Burnand, K.G., Clemenson, G., Whimpster, I. & Browse, N.L. (1976): Extravascular fibrin deposition in response to venous hypertension: the cause of venous ulcers. Br. J. Surg. 63, 660-661.

Coleridge-Smith, P.D., Thomas, P., Scurr, J.H. & Dormandy, J.A. (1988): Causes of venous ulceration: a new hypothesis. Brit. Med. J. 296, 1726-1727.

Curri, S.B., Annoni, F., Pabisch, S., De Stefano, A., & Montorsi, W. (1989): Changes of cutaneous microcirculation from elasto-compression in chronic venous insufficiency. In Phlebologie '89, ed. A. Davy & R. Stemmer, pp. 852-854. London: John Libbey & Co Ltd.

Mani, R., White, J.E., Barrett, D.F. & Weaver, P.W. (1989): Tissue oxygenation, venous ulcers and fibrin cuffs. J. Roy. Soc. Med. 82, 345-346.

Phlébologie 92. Eds P. Raymond-Martimbeau, R. Prescott, M. Zummo.
John Libbey Eurotext, Paris © 1992, pp. 1156-1158

Long-term results of the selective varicose vein surgery

Svatopluk Kaspar, Voboril Zbynek

Department of Surgery, Faculty of Medecine, Charles University, Hradec Králové, Czechoslovakia.

INTRODUCTION

Surgical removal of varicose veins remains the treatment of choice in the carefully selected patients. Radical surgery often includes total ankle-to-groin stripping of the long saphenous vein /LSV/.Since the veins of the lower extremity were discovered as being the ideal arterial reconstructive substitute, surgeons called up to treat truncal varicose veins are facing an intellectual conflict, stirred up by the antagonism between removal of incompetent venous channels in order to ensure maximal long-term results on one hand, and the quest for maximal preservation of these most valuable spare parts on the other. Contrary to a frequent opinion, long saphenous veins of some varicose patients are suitable for arterial bypass. Further more, limited stripping of the LSV may reduce risk of damage to the saphenous nerve.
The aim of our study was to assess the possibilities and results of preservation of the normal long saphenous veins and to determine the risk of nervous lesions after varicose veins operations.

MATERIAL AND METHODS

Our stúdy comprised 159 limbs operated on consecutively from November 1986 through April 1988 in our department. There were 40 men and 65 women, totally 105 patients with primary varicose veins.
According to the clinical preoperative investigation, varicosities were classified into seven types. In type 1 reverse flow goes down from the groin through the saphenous trunk until it reaches the proximal part of the lower leg. Anterior and posterior branches of the lower leg are affected too. Type 2 involves incompetence of the saphenofemoral junction and varicosities of the tributaries of the groin. There is no reverse flow in the long saphenous trunk. In type 3 reverse flow goes down until it encounters the thigh. Type 4 involves the abnormalities of the short saphenous vein, the long saphenous trunk in not touched. In type 5 the entire long saphenous trunk is afflicted from the groin to the ankle. Type 6 shows reflux over the saphenofemoral junction but there are no excessive varicose changes of the saphenous trunk. The LSV acts only as a conduit for the reflux into the distal varicosities. In type 7 varicose veins receive reflux from incompetent perforators. The main trunk is not involved.
The selective operation was performed in most cases. Only type 5 required removal of the entire long saphenous vein.

RESULTS

In about one third of the entire group /51 limbs/ the long saphenous vein was completely removed, but in the remainder, the outstanding effect of this procedure was found /34 to 100 percent of the vein preservation/. Totally, with this concept, 46 per cent of the quality venous material were spared.
The results of the treatment were assessed in the period ranging from 3,5 to 5 years. Total of 149 limbs /these are 94 per cent from the whole series /in 100 patients were examined. There were 38 men and 62 women. It means that our group consisted in quite important part from the male population. Complications, current complaints and residual varicosities were recorded and graded according to current classification /Hamilton Jakobsen, 1979/.
In the group of patients, treated selectively, 100 limbs were examined. Results reported by patients were satisfactory in 97 per cent, unsatisfactory in 3 per cent. The observer, closely following his guide lines, found 88 per cent of results beeing satisfactory and 12 per cent unsatisfactory.
In the group of patients treated by the total stripping of the LSV /49 limbs examined/, 90 per cent of patients found the final results satisfactory and 10 per cent unsatisfactory ones. Observer assessment was satisfactory in only 71 per cent and unsatisfactory in 29 per cent.
The limbs were assessed for presence or absence of valve incompetence by testing with 8 MHz directional Doppler ultrasonic instrument. In the standart stripping operation group /49 limbs/ the reflux from the area of high saphenal ligation was observed once, from the incompetent thigh perforator four times, from the leg perforator four times and in the area of the short saphenous vein four times. Only two limbs /that are 4 per cent/ required further surgical treatment.
In the selectively operated on patients /100 limbs/ a certain degree of reverse flow was detected in substantial part of the group /39 limbs/. But no relationship was observed between the degree of reflux and the results of patient and observer assessment because only 8 limbs required additional surgical correction /8 per cent/. Five of them were classified as type 6 with the femoral part of the LSV left in place. So we think now that this part of the vein should be removed in majority of cases. Severe, long-lasting neurological complications assessed by the patient /paresthesiae, pain etc./ were noted. The standart operations with total long saphenal stripping were followed by these complication in more than 8 per cent, selective treatment in only 2 per cent.

DISCUSSION

A logic policy in the treatment of the varicose veins is to remove only the diseased portions of the veins and to preserve as much healthy material as possible /Melliere et al., 1991/. In recent years, the concept of complete stripping of the LSV has been questioned. According to Goren and Yellin /1990/, the classical high saphenous ligation was needed in only 64 per cent of 230 varicose limbs. To avoid nerve injury, Rivlin /1975/ has recommended that the LSV should be stripped from 4 cm below the tibial tubercle to the groin. Stripping from this level, at which the saphenous nerve is not in intimate relationship with the vein, may achieve the benefits of stripping with a lower incidence of distressing side effects. But Almgren /1990/ showed that this partial stripping of the LSV cannot be recommended as standart routine procedure without close investigation of the vein. It resulted from our previous study /Kašpar and Suchý, 1991/ that with our concept 46 per cent of the venous material were spared.
The results of the long-term follow-up study showed satisfactory results in 88 per cent of limbs /observer assessment/ and 97 per cent of limbs /patient assessment/. The results were even better than in the group of patients treated by the standart stripping operation /71 and 90 per cent, respectively/.

CONCLUSION

It is unwise to treat patients with varicose veins without thinking about the possibility of atherosclerotic disease occuring later on. It is apparent, that it is possible to treat varices effectively and, at the same time, preserve undamaged major veins. A precise preoperative diagnosis is necessary in every case in order to individually tailor the therapeutic needs of each patient. The frequently and still practiced indiscriminate and blind ankle-to-groin stripping in cases of primary truncal varicose veins, should be avoided by all means. Selective varicose vein surgery has two main advantages: firstly, it preserves sufficient presumably normal vein; and, secondly, there is a significant reduction in the incidence of saphenous nerve damage. Thus, destructing treatments of saphenous veins should be only proposed to patients whose veins are obviously unsuitable for arterial bypass.

REFERENCES

Almgren, B. and Eriksson, I. (1990): Valvular incompetence in superficial, deep and perforator veins of limbs with varicose veins. Acta Chir. Scand.156, 69-74

Goren, G. and Yellin, A. E. (1990): Primary varicose veins: topographic and hemodynamic correlations. J. Cardiovasc. Surg. 31, 672-677

Hamilton Jakobsen, B. (1979): The value of different forms of treatment for varicose veins. Brit. J. Surg. 66, 182-184

Kašpar, S. and Suchý, T. (1991): Die Planung vor Varizenoperationen unter dem Gesichtspunkt einer möglichen späteren Gefässrekonstruktion. Vasomed Aktuell 11, 18-22

Melliere, D., Cales, B., Martin-Jonathan, C. and Schadeck, M. (1991): Nécéssité de concilier les objectifs du traitement des varices et de la chirurgie artérielle. Conséquences pratiques. J. Mal. Vasc. 16, 171-178

Rivlin, S. (1975): The surgical cure of primary varicose veins. Br. J. Surg. 62, 913-917

Lower limb thermometry after stripping

Molokia F., Naga R.

Fac. of Med. Alexandria Univ.

Thirty patients with uncomplicated primary varicose veins of the lower limbs, and the same number of age matched normal persons as controls, formed the material of the study. YST tele-thermometer have been used to measure skin temperature in all limbs before and after stripping. A spacial pattern of cutaneous hyper-thermia in primary varicose veins was found depending on the anatomical distribution and communications of the varices. A significant return to normal pattern of skin temperature in the diseased group was found after stripping. This simple, sheep and non-in vasive method can show the distribution of clinically occult varices especially in obese legs which then can be attached during surgery so to avoid recurrence of varices.

Phlébologie 92. Eds P. Raymond-Martimbeau, R. Prescott, M. Zummo.
John Libbey Eurotext, Paris © 1992, pp. 1160-1162

Assessment of the efficacy of surgery of internal saphenous with computer support

J. Talbot

Clinique médicale de Repentigny, 520, rue Notre-Dame, Repentigny, Québec, J6A 2T8, Canada.

The efficacy of surgery appears to be a parameter difficult to assess in previous studies (Perrin, 1990, Covo, 1991). We conducted a prospective study to validate a quantitative method for evaluating the efficacy of surgery in superficial venous disease.

PATIENTS AND METHODS

In order to test the usefulness of the method, we survey the following population:
- 102 legs, 84 patients,70 women, 14 men: mean age: 42 years
- primary internal saphenous insufficiency, with sapheno-femoral incompetence confirmed by 8 MHz pocket doppler
- 54 long strippings and afterward 48 short strippings were undergone. They were examined by the same observer pre-operatively and an average of 3.2 months post-operatively
- no evidence of associated deep venous disease assessed by clinical means and by duplex scan in severe cases
- no associated therapy

The proposed method is a computerized application of the concepts developped by Cornu-Thenar et al (1986): clinical quantification of varicose veins. Each lower limb is divided in seven sections: the thigh and the leg into 3 sections each, and the foot forming the seven section. The maximum diameter of the visible and palpable varices is measured with a rule in the internal saphenous territory. The length of the diseased veins is evaluated by the number of affected sections in the main stem and in the collaterals: that method is less fastidious then measuring the exact total length. The maximum diameter multiply by length gives a score which roughly estimate the surface, and has a high correlation coefficient (0.92) (Cornu-Thenar, 1991)

That procedure permit to quantify the <u>extent of the disease</u>. We have notice that:
- a score under 50 correspond to a light affliction usually localized to the leg

- a score from 50 to 100 correspond to a more extensive affliction localized to all the lower leg
- a score over 100 correspond to a widespread affliction with numerous collaterals or very large diameter vessels.

The severity of the disease comply with the standards of venous insufficiency suggested by an european-american comity (Porter et al. 1988) except for oedema, which is uneasy to computerized. The software used was a semi-relationnal database on Macintosh environnement: Filemaker Pro.

RESULTS

If we plot the extent and the severity of the disease on a table, we obtain the following datas:

Table 1: Extent of disease and severity of chronic venous insufficiency

	Venous insufficiency			
Extent	**stade 0**	**stade I**	**stade II**	**stade III**
light	8	48	2	0
moderate	5	27	3	1
severe	0	6	1	1

We compute the average score, before and after surgery: the difference calculated can be regarded as highly statistically significant.

Table 2: Validity of the method
(Paired Student's t test)

Type of surgery	n	mean score ±s.d.		p value
		before	after	
short strippings	48	46±26	12±14	< 0.0001
long strippings	54	58±36	10±13	< 0.0001
all strippings	102	52±32	11±14	< 0.0001

We defined conservatively as therapeutic success the disappearance of 2/3 of the previously observed varices, along the internal saphenous territory.
If we substract post-operative from pre-operative score, we obtain the following datas for all the strippings, for the long strippings and the short strippings.

Table 3: All strippings

Extent	Score	Success	
		n/tot	%
light	0-49	43/58	74
moderate	50-100	31/36	86
severe	>100	7/ 8	87
total		81/102	79

Table 4: Long strippings

Extent	Score	Success	
		n/tot	%
light	0-49	19/25	76
moderate	50-100	19/22	86
severe	>100	7/ 7	100
total		45/54	83

Table 5: Short strippings

Extent	Score	Success	
		n/tot	%
light	0-49	24/33	73
moderate	50-100	12/14	86
severe	>100	0/ 1	0
total		36/48	75

CONCLUSIONS

This quantitative method reflect, with statistical significance, the efficacy of surgery of superficial veins.
It appears that 3/4 of the observed legs presents lightly or moderately extensive disease, with minimal chronic venous insufficiency. Overall, the success rate, 3 months post-operatively, is increased, if the surgery is more extensive. However, if we exclude the severe cases, the success rate is identical for the long strippings and the short strippings. Finally, the results are better, if the disease is more extensive.

REFERENCES

1. Cornu-Thénar, A., De Vincenzi, I.& Maraval, M.(1991): Evaluation of different systems for clinical quantification of varicose veins. *J. Dermatolo. Surg. Oncol.* 17, 345-348.
2. Cornu-Thénard, A., Boivin, P., Parpex, P., Moulin, J.P., Schadeck M.& Valty J.(1986): Essai d'une quantification clinique des varices pour l'épidémiologie, la thérapeutique et l'informatique. *Phlébologie*, 39, 661-676.
3. Covo L.(1991): Sclérothérapie et maladie variqueuse: à quel stade?. *Phlébologie*, 44, 221-225.
4. Perrin M.(1990): *L'insuffisance veineuse chronique des membres inférieurs.* Medsi McGraw-Hill pp.87
5. Porter, J,W., Rutherford, R.B., Clagett, G.P.,Raju, S. & Zierler, R.E. (1988): Reporting standards in venous disease. *Journal of vascular surgery*, 8,172-181.

Phlébologie 92. Eds P. Raymond-Martimbeau, R. Prescott, M. Zummo.
John Libbey Eurotext, Paris © 1992, pp. 1163-1165

A new approach to minimize the pain after hemorrhoidectomy

Filippo La Torre, Attilio Nicastro, Stella Luigi Persico, Paolo Pontone

III Department of Surgery, University « La Sapienza », Rome, Italy.

INTRODUCTION

Hemorroidectomy has always been considered particularly painful immediately after surgery and this obviously leads many patiens to refuse it. Scientific research was therefore carried out to conceive, experiment and implement new techniques to help minimize the trauma and the surgical work on the anal region, which is rightfully considered the main cause of post-operative pain.The techniques in question are: 1) Rubber band ligations 2) Sclero therapy 3) Cryotherapy 4) Infrared photocoagulation. Anyway, a correct treatment of hemorroids is always based on the following parameters: - cost effectiveness (in relations to the length of the hospitalization); - radicalness of the treatment itself; - absence of post-operative symptomatic consequences; - absence of complications; - vaste scale feasibility.
Given these assumptions, the new methods of hemorroid treatment have several criticizable aspects as they can only be carried out on a limited number of selected cases, they are not radical and usually have complications.
For these reasons many surgeons still prefer the traditional techniques for the treatment of hemmorroids. In practice, however, it is observed that, whatever the treatment chosen, the post-operative period always entails important painful consequences for all patients. The aim of our study is that of facing and possibly eliminating the post-operative pain caused by radical hemorroidectomy, according to the general principles regulating the correct approach and treatment of hemorroids.

PATIENTS AND METHOD

Our study is based on 150 consecutive, active patients affected with II (32), III (77) and IV (41) hemorroids degree, who have been treated according to our protocol Careful evaluation and selection of patients represent the first step of our approach; the patients should be strongly motivated to undergo surgery and they receive full information about all the different aspect of the procedure. Thorough clinical assessment and instrumental investigation are required, including total colonscopy and anoscopy, this last examination being useful to rule out a chronic non-specific proctitis, which requires medical management before the operation. Our operative technique consists of open he,orrhoidectomy with high ligation of the vascular pedicle and careful preservation of at least 3 bridges of intact skin and mucosa. The procedure is completed by a left lateral internal sphincterotomy, accurate hemostasis, anesthetic infiltration (10-20 ml of 2% Carbocaina); only a small gauze (4X4 cm) is left in the anal canal. In the evening the patient is given only a mild sedative to guarantee adequate overnight rest. On the first post-operative day the patient is started on bland laxatives, anti-inflammatory and anti-edemigen drugs, sitz baths and capillary protectives, this therapy to be continued for at least 10 days. Following discharge on the second post-op day, the patient is seen again on day X, XX and XXX. Annual controls are then established. All the patients have been operated by the same surgeon (FLT) and in interviewed in the follow-up examinations by the same physician (AN).

R E S U L T S

In the immediate post-operative period 73.6% of patiens experienced a bothersome perineal sensation, 24% real discomfort, while only 2.4% complained of severe pain. Overall, 9 patients could not get adequate rest on the first night following the operation. Complete healing could be observed in 88.6% of cases on day XX and in all on day XXX. 65.4% of patients could attend regular working activity on day III; all patients could be back to work within day X, the delay being caused by a persistent perineal discomfort. While recurrent hemorrhoids were never observed, anal stenosis developed in 4 patients (2.6%), who had been operated upon because of recurrent IV degree hemorrhoids with mucosal prolapse (1pts) and IV degree hemorrhoids with mucosal prolapse (3pts); therefore, stenosis has been related to the surgical reduction of the prolapse; in both cases it has been successfully treated by utilizing anal dilatators.

D I S C U S S I O N

The eradication of post-operative pain was the main objective of our therapeutical protocol. It is clear that the psycholical attitude of the patients towards the operation plays a major role in inducing post-operative pain, rather than the surgical trauma itself: in our experience, only 4 out of 150 (2.6%) patients complained of severe pain. We would therefore affirm that it was particularly useful to inform all our patients about the different aspects of the surgical procedure. We also think it is very important to rule out chronic non-specific proctitis because, when associated with hemorroids, it can cause annoying post-operative troubles, such as tenesmus, itching, mucorrhea and rectal bleeding. Medical treatment is therefore necessary before the operation. In our therapeutical approach some important surgical aspects have also been taken into account, such as: reduced manipulation ot the anal canal with no forceful stretch, manteinance of mucocutaneous bridges, the lateral internal sphincterotomy. To reduce post operative pain and hence to accelerate the wound healing process, anestetic infiltration and avoidance of gross rectal essing are equally important. We do believe, however, that an accurate physical and psychological preparation of the patient to surgery is essential in order to obtain good results. As compared with alternative outpatient procedures which are normally used to treat Grade I and II hemorroids and whose radicality is somewhat questionable, or methods grants better results because it is cost effective, radical on the short and long term and it allowes a shorter hospitalization and as well as a prompt return to a regular working activity.

C O N C L U S I O N

The high incidence of hemorroids among the active young and adult population progre

ssively brought about the diffusion of outpatient methods of treatment.
As compared with traditional surgical operation, such newer techniques are undoubtedly cost effective and better accepted by the patient but they can only be used in selected cases and long term results are not always satisfactory.
Traditional methods have been therefore modified to obtain better results in the short term and a high degree of radicality and safety in the long term.

REFERENCES

1) F. La Torre et al.: Pain after Haemmorrhoidectomy Colo-Proctology, XIV(2): 107-109; 1992

2) G. Accarpio et al.: Outpatient Treatment of Haemorrhoids with a Combined Technique. Results and Complications in 2850 Cases. Colo-Proctology, XIV(2):110-111; 1992

3) Yadav S. et al.: Evaluation of proctoform as a post-operative analgesic in pattients undergoing haemorrhoidectomy. Br J Clin Pract 1984;38:414-5

4) Milligan ETC, Morgan CN, Jones LE.: Surgical anatomy of the anal canal and the operative treatment of haemorrhoids. Dis Colon Rectum 1985;28:620-8

5) Alexander RM.: A technique for avoiding mucosal stenosis and secondary hemorrhage after hemorrhoidectomy. Dis Colon Rectum 28:271-3; 1985

6) Traynor DJ. Carter AE. Cryotherapy for advance haemorrhoids: a prospective evaluation with 2- year follow-up. Br J Surg 1984; 71:287-9

7) Shemeish EI. Severe complication of rubber band ligation of internal hemorrhoids. Dis Colon Rectum 1987; 30:199-200.

EVALUATION DE LA THÉRAPEUTIQUE CHIRURGICALE À L'AIDE DE L'INFORMATIQUE

Jacques Talbot

Clinique médicale de Repentigny, 520, rue Notre-Dame, Repentigny, Québec, Canada J6A 2T8

Les difficultés d'évaluer la thérapeutique anti-variqueuse, en raison de séries difficilement comparables, seront évoquées. Une méthodologie faisant appel à l'informatique, permet de quantifier la surface atteinte et de proposer une méthode plus objective d'appréciation de l'étendue de la maladie. La sévérité de la pathologie sera appréciée selon la classification d'un comité américano-européen. Cette méthodologie sera expérimentée sur un modèle facilement accessible: les insuffisances de la saphène interne opérées de novo par stripping court ou long et revues en deçà d'un an, sans atteinte clinique du système profond. Les réussites, soit une diminution des 2/3 de la surface visible et palpable, se chiffrent à 76% pour les strippings courts, 84% pour les strippings longs et 80% dans l'ensemble. Ces résultats pour une chirurgie limitée, se situent en deça du taux de 95% évoqué dans la littérature, pour une chirurgie radicale. Cette méthodologie constitue une approche nouvelle et d'usage aisé d'évaluation de la thérapeutique chirurgicale.

D.
COMPLICATIONS
COMPLICATIONS

Phlébologie 92. Eds P. Raymond-Martimbeau, R. Prescott, M. Zummo.
John Libbey Eurotext, Paris © 1992, pp. 1169-1172

Venous thrombosis in association with deep and superficial venous surgery

John J. Bergan, M.D., F.A.C.S., Hon., F.R.C.S. (Eng.)

Venous thrombosis in association with direct venous surgery is uncommon. Similarly, it is rare in association with indirect treatment of chronic venous insufficiency by perforator disconnection as occurs in the treatment of postphlebitic syndrome. Patients undergoing venous surgery have the highest risk for deep venous thrombosis and pulmonary embolization. This is especially true if a previous episode of thromboembolic disease has been documented. Other elements such as age, obesity, presence or absence of diabetes and/or smoking play much less important roles. It is those patients with a history of previous thromboembolic disease who come to direct venous reconstruction or indirect venous disconnection. The apparent lack of danger of venous thrombosis in this population is unexplained.

Studies of outpatients with phlebographically proven acute deep venous thrombosis should give information on the relative frequency of coagulopathy in a non-hospitalized population. This has been done and documentation of the overall prevalence of deficiencies of antithrombin III, protein C, protein S, and plasminogen have been found in 8.3% (23 of 277 patients). When compared with age-matched and sex-matched controls without deep venous thrombosis, the results are striking. The latter group of individuals exhibited only 2.2% of isolated autogenous anticoagulant deficiencies (3 of 138 subjects). Thus it is clear that over 90% of patients with acute venous thrombosis occurring on an outpatient status will not exhibit a diagnosable coagulopathy (1).

Studies of the effects of operative stress on the coagulation profile are similarly nonrevealing. Such studies show that a number of coagulation parameters change as a result of surgical stress and that patients undergoing peripheral vascular surgery respond in a manner similar to those that do not. The trend towards increased coagulopathy occurs with an increased platelet count, increased factor VIII, increase in fibrinogen and thrombin generation index, as well as decrease in antithrombin III. Prothrombin activity does not change nor does the activated partial thromboplastin time (2). Thus, it is clear that just under 10% of patients studied on a non-hospitalized basis exhibit coagulation abnormalities and that normal patients undergoing surgical stress give evidence of coagulation changes towards coagulopathy.

Studies of patients with venous disease and venous ulceration have shown that abnormalities are present in these patients with regard to systemic fibrinolysis. Patients with venous disease have a prolonged euglobulin lysis time and elevated plasma fibrinogen levels. These patients have markedly elevated levels of total fibrin-related antigen and D-dimer which is the terminal degradation product of cross-linked fibrin. In contrast, the levels of D-monomer, the breakdown product of fibrinogen and non-cross-linked fibrin monomer are normal in venous disease patients. As might be expected, those patients with the most severe forms of chronic venous insufficiency and ulceration show the highest levels of D-dimer (3). Thus it is clearly shown that patients with venous disease have uniform evidence for enhanced fibrin formation. This is evidenced by the elevated levels of total fibrin-related antigen and D-dimer. Therefore, there is every reason to suspect that patients undergoing surgery for chronic venous insufficiency would be at high risk for new episodes of venous thromboembolic disease.

Physical changes occur in vein walls during general anesthesia and surgery. Using high-resolution ultrasound imaging of gastrocnemius and posterior tibial veins, the Middlesex Hospital (London) vascular group has shown 22 to 28% increase in venous distention by the end of operative procedures (4). Such distention is most prominent in the gastrocnemius veins but lesser distention was observed in posterior tibial veins. Infusion of as much as one liter of saline in addition to basal requirements exacerbated the distention to as much as 57% compared to 22% in the control group.

Thus, it is seen that intraoperative venous distention as documented, in association with other factors which lead to deep venous thrombosis should markedly elevate the risk for such phenomenon in patients with venous disease undergoing surgery. The unexplained fact remains. Patients with venous insufficiency sufficient to require superficial or deep surgery are not patients who exhibit deep venous thrombosis or thromboembolic complications. The reason for this fact is as yet unexplained.

REFERENCES

1. Heijboer H, Brandjes DPK, Buller HR, et al. Deficiencies of coagulation-inhibiting and fibrinolytic proteins in outpatients with deep vein thrombosis. N Eng J Med 1990; 323: 1511-16.
2. Collins GJ Jr, Barber JA, Zajtchuk R, et al. The effects of operative stress on the coagulation profile. Am J Surg 1977; 133:611-16.
3. Falanga V, Kruskal J, Franks JJ. Fibrin- and fibrinogen-related antigens in patients with venous disease and venous ulceration. Arch Dermatol 1991; 127:75-78.
4. Coleridge-Smith PD, Hasty JH, Scurr JH. Venous stasis and vein lumen changes during surgery. Br J Surg 1990; 77:1055-59.

ACCIDENTS ET COMPLICATIONS DANS LA CHIRURGIE DES VARICES DES MEMBRES INFERIEURES.

Dr.Aurel Mironiuc, Prof.Dr.Aurel Andercou, Dr.Sanda Radulescu

CLINICA CHIRURGIE NR.II, UNIVERSITATEA DE MEDICINA CLUJ, ROMANIA.

En étudiant 1000 patients opérés pour des varices des membres inférieures,nous avons constaté les accidents suivants:

2 cas (0,2%) avec lésion de veine fémorale, ce qui a nécessité d'être rémédié par reconstruction veineuse, 1 cas (0,1%) avec lésion d'artère réparée par des techniques d'hémostase et suture artérielle.

130 patients (13%) ont eu des complications post-opératoires de gravité différente: 3,5% oedèmes malléolaires, 3% hématomes de divers degrés 2,5% suppurations sous-cutanées, la nécrose des plaies gambières post-opératoires 0,8% cas, des plaies atones post-opératoires 0,6%, accumulation lymphatiques 0,1%, trombophlébites en 4% cas, embolies pulmonaires en 0,2% cas.

Les accidents et les complications locales prolongent le temps d'hospitalisation et retardent la reprise de l'activité. Les complications générales comprommettent le résultat post-opératoire et peuvent mettre en danger la vie du malade.

Phlébologie 92. Eds P. Raymond-Martimbeau, R. Prescott, M. Zummo.
John Libbey Eurotext, Paris © 1992, pp. 1174-1176

Saphenic neuropathy as consequence stripping of great saphenous vein

O.F. Cormaci, C. Germiglio, A. Grasso, C. Costanzo, S. Romeo

Cattedra e Scuola di Specializzazione in Chirurgia Vascolare (Direttore Prof. S. Romeo), Universita degli Studi di Catania, Italy.

INTRODUCTION

Saphenic neuropathy is a syndrome caused by a saphenous nerve's damage of various intensity it is often a consequence of surgical manipulations along nerve territory.

This sensorial nerve may be damaged hardly and definitely or only temporary.

So we distinguish: 1) neuropathies for irritation
2) neuropathies showing a deficit.

The former are due to a trauma along nerve passing, without anatomical irreversible damage but with cellular irritation (perinervous infiammation or infection light crashing by surgical instruments, formation of haematomas near nerve passing).

This brings to continous, abnormal fiber's stimulation and shows different symptomatology: from a simple tingling sensation to an "electric shock". The latter is a serious hyperestesy produced with a simple soft brushing with innervated cutaneous areas, so that also the contact with clothes is umbereable.

A greater damage con produce spontaneos pain of variable intensity.

The second neuropathies show themselves only after a damage totally or partially compromising sensorial conduction nerve function. They bring to a loss or reduction of sensitivity of interested cutaneos area.

Among other surgical manipulations, stripping of great saphenous vein is one of the most important causes of saphenous neuropathy.

In this research we noticed onset, type, seriousness, and course of internal saphenous neuropathy in patients surgically treated with great saphenous vein stripping. The complessive follow up is one year but for subjects submitted to surgical treatment in the last year, the follow up is relatively shortey but already sufficent to evaluate new surgical procedures in a more favorable developping of neurological complicances.

MATERIALS AND METHODS

From january 1989 to july 1991 we took into consideration in our operatory casistic, 263 patients who underwent surgical intervention of stripping of great saphenous vein with varicectomy according to Muller's tecnique. Since 63 patients were operated on both sides, the total number of operations was 326 and all stripping were done from distal to central side.

We did not consider all cases of stripping of little saphenous vein, of perforant ligature, in medial side of leg, of stripping of great saphenous vein in legs with serious lipodermatosclerosis or large phlebostatic ulcer.

In 1965 Garnjobst already observed saphenic neuropathies could arise after surgical manipulations on the medial face of the leg without saphenous stripping.

Each patient underwent a neurological consultation to establish subjective simptomatology so that we were able to distinguish between irritative in neuropathies (tingling, burning, hiperestesy like "electric shock" pain, frank pain), and deficitary neuropathies (light or severe hypoestesia, total anestesy) The basal control was detected after a week; the follow up was structured with 3 check up after one month, three months and one year.

In hypoanestesies we detected and measured the cutaneous areas near perimalleolar or anterotibial region their temporal evolution during the follow up as detected with a great care.

RESULTS

Irritative neuropathies were tingling in 156 cases (48%), burning in 117 (36%), hiperestesia in 19 (6%) light pain in 6 (1,8%) and frank pain in 6 (1,8%). During the follow up this complication reduced its incidence as shown in table I; after three months, these tedious sensations greatly improved or totally disappeared. In fact after at one year only tingling in 8 legs (3,3%) and hiperestesia in 2 legs (0,8%) remained.

After three months 221 patients only went under our check-up (totally 271 legs). After one year only 199 patients (totally 239). So we lost 64 subjects. Of course in most cases there was the association of these different particular neurological simptomatologies: often tingling and burning were both present; all cases of hyperestesies were associated with tingling.

Deficitary neuropathies

Follow up;	1 week	1 month	3 months	1 year
tingling	156(48%)	76(24%)	39(14%)	8(3,3%)
burning	117(36%)	43(13,8%)	21(7,8%)	3(1,2%)
hyperestesy	19(6%)	10(3,2%)	4(1,5%)	2(0,8%)
light pain	6(1,8%)	1(0,3%)	/	/
frank pain	6(1,8%)	2(0,6%)	/	/
Tot.legs (100%)	326	310	271	239

table I

Deficitary neuropathies were distributed in such a way: in basal control light hypoestesia was detected in 101 legs (31%), severe hypoestesia in 21 (6,5%), anestesy in 16 (4,9%). Unlike irritative neuropathies, the most severe deficitary alterations incidence remained unchanged after one year. In fact light hypoestesia was detected after one year in 19 legs only (7,9%) while severe hypoestesia and anestesia was still present in high percentage: 3,3% (for 8 legs) and 4,6% (for 11 legs) respectively (table II).

Irritative neuropathies

Follow up;	1 week	1 month	3 months	1 year
light hypoestesy	101(31%)	72(23%)	41(15%)	19(7,9%)
severe hypoestesy	21(6,5%)	17(5,4%)	19(7%)	8(3,3%)
anestesy	16(4,9%)	16(5,1%)	15(5,5%)	11(4,6%)
Tot.legs (100%)	326	310	271	239

table II

We also distinguished four classes of cutaneous extension of sensitivity loss as showed in table III (the first enclose those inferior of 10 cm2 and the fourth those superior to 120 cm2)

We noticed a meaningful tendency to reduction of the most limited neurologic damages while the most extensive remained unchanged about incidence. So cutaneous areas smaller than 10 cm2, affected by light hypoestesies decreased from 37 to 0. Those interesting cutaneous areas between 10 and 50 cm2 decreased from 52 to 14. On the other hand anestesy did not improve over one year even if its basal incidence was low.

Cutaneous area evolution about incidence of deficitary neuropathies

Extension	1 week	1 month	3 months	1 year
< 10 cm2	37	29	19	/
10-50 cm2	52	37	23	14
50-120 cm2	58	33	27	23
> 120 cm2	1	1	1	1

table III

DISCUSSION

In our casistic, irritative neuropathy was the most recurrent consequence of saphenous nerve damage. This is also the most easily improvable type of neurological complicance. On the contrary, deficitary neuropathies, more taedious for patients, are initially less recurrent but remained unchanged in further check-ups.

S.J.Cox in 1974 showed that saphenous neuropathy remained unalterated after 3 months both in absolute number or in their cutaneous extension, in legs exposed to a centripetal stripping. Each patient was himself control because only bilateral stripping were detected (one leg centripetal and the other centrifugal)

Cox asserted that stripper head gets entangled in inversed V of the last troncular bifurcation of saphenous nerve just near lateral face of grat saphenous vein causing its laceration.

On the contrary when stripper head runs in a centrifugal way, it will get over this obstacle producing a light and not ireversible damage.

Recently we have tried a surgical update technique by carrying out a stripper of great saphenous vein in a centrifugal way, down to subgenicular region only in order to avoid the passage of the stripper head in the lower part of the leg because the last part of great saphenous vein is invaginated on itself.

It is early to make a comparison between the two surgical methods about the incidence and the development of neurological complications, but first data are in accordance with Cox's hypotesis.

Absolute number of neurological damage is inferior. Among this irritative neuropathies, the type with the highest percentage of spontaneous improvement, are the most recurrent.

REFERENCES

1) COX J., WELLWOOD J.M., MARTIN A.: Saphenous nerve injury caused by stripping of long saphenous vein. Brit. Med. J. 1, 415, 1974.

2) ADAR R., MEYER E., ZWEIG A.: Saphenous neuralgia. A complication of Vascualr Reconstructions below the inguinal ligament. Ann. Surg. 190, 609,1979.

3) ENRIQUEZ A.A., BOYERO M.R., FERNANDEZ L.S.: Sindromes neuropaticos tras la cirurgia de varices en los miembros inferiores. Angiologia, 33, 79, 1981.

4) G.MARIANI, E.PATUZZO, R.MONACO, C.BAKARA, R.BOGGIANI, M.ANDREOLI, I.GIACOMINI.:Neuropatia safenica nelle flebopatie. Monduzzi Ed. IV Congresso Italiano della Societa' di Flebologia Clinica e Sperimentale. Napoli 30 Nov-3 Dic 1987.

5) COSTANZO C., CORMACI O.F., GRASSO A., ROMEO S.: In tema di chirurgia delle varici: una variante di tecnica allo stripping. In corso di stampa.

Phlébologie 92. Eds P. Raymond-Martimbeau, R. Prescott, M. Zummo.
John Libbey Eurotext, Paris © 1992, pp. 1177-1179

Venous complications in the treatment of chronic and acute pancreatitis

M. Ruzicka, P. Dite, H. Simonova, L. Veverkova

1st Surgical Clinic, Masaryk University, Brno. 3rd Medicine Clinic, Masaryk University, Brno, Czechoslovakia.

SUMMARY:

We report our experience with 28 patients operated on for diagnosis of chronic pancreatitis and 41 patients which underwent surgical therapy for acute necrotizing pancreatitis in the years 1985 - 1991. Of the 28 patients with chronic pancreatitis 4 had had haemorhage from injured venous wall during surgical procedure. The venous wall was sutured in 3 patients. In one case the replacing with 2 cm long graft from long saphenous vein was necessary.

Acute pancreatitis is dangerous for large necrosis of the peripancreatic tissue. One of the most dangerous complications is bleeding from necrotic vein, usually vein in the mesocolon or splenic vein. We have had 3 patients with these complications, two of them were succesfully operated on and bleeding was controled. But one patient died earlier than succesful surgical treatment could have been done.

Chronic pancreatic is defined by the presence of chronic inflammatory lesions characterized by the destruction of exocrine parenchyma and fibrosis.

In keeping with the Marseille - Rome meeting classification (1988) four main forms of chronic pancreatitis are distinguished:

1. Chronic obstructive pancreatitis

2. Chronic calcifying pancreatitis

3. Other poorly defined forms of chronic pancreatitis

4. Asymptomatic perilobular fibrosis

Standard pre-operative investigations are often not satisfactory in the definition of different forms of disease. To distinguish one form from another is often possible only on the basis of pathological dates. The diagnosis of different forms of chronic pancreatitis may be achieved by sonography, computerized tomopraphy and retrograde pancreatography. These are followed by investigation of exocrine and endocrine pancreatic function.

More surgical procedures are recommended for the treatment of chronic pancreatitis. Current surgical trends have veered away from distal pancreatectomies to proximal pancreatic resection because the main inflammatory mass is usualy in the head of the gland. Intractable, incapacitating pain arises especialy from:

- Duodenel stenosis

- Biliary obstruction

- Portal vein stenosis

- Perineural inflammation and proliferative neuropathy of splanchnic nerves

With resection of the head of the pancreas we solve also the source of patients compliants. Most patients were treated by Whippler's hemipancreatoduodenectomy. But we prefer now duodenum preserving pancreas head resection and pancreatogastroanastomosis.

28 operations were done with following procedures:-

Pancreatojejunoanostomosis Partington-Rochelle	: 07
Hemipancreatoduodenectomy Whipple	: 10
Duodenum preserving pancreas head resection	: 08
Distal pancreatic resection	: 02
Choledocho - duodenoanastomosis	: 01

It was stated that serious complications were in procedures with pancreas head resection. Superior mesenteric vein or portal vein was injured 4 times.

Large retropancreatic fibrosis was the reason of the injury. Operation technique is exceedingly difficult because of dense inflammatory adhesions around the pancreas. We noted 3 injuries of the venous wall 1/2 - 3 cm long and suture of the wall was necessary to control the bleeding. In 1 case 2 cm of the portal vein was replaced with the graft from long sophenous vein.

Acute pancreatitis is defind as a group of lesions generally considered to be reversible. Generally accepted is Ulm classification with 4 forms:

1. Interstitial edema

2. Pancreatic necrosis

3. Pancreatic or Peripancreatic abscess

4. Pancreatic pseudocyst

Acute pancreatitis is a disease with very fast progress and the investigations helping to confirm the form of acute pancreatitis is necessary to be without delay. Sonography and computerized tomography are often useful. Surgical procedure is mandatory in patients with pancreatic abscess in the acute phase of the disease, patients with persistent pseudocyst are indicated to drainage procedure electively. In the stage of abscess only debridement and drainage is usually performed. Repeated surgical procedures are often necessary to remove all necrotic tissue.

11 Patients with infected acute pancreatic abscess caused by acute pancreatitis were operated on in the years 1985 - 1991., most of them necessitated from 2 to 5 operations. Intraabdominal hemorrhage as a complication of acute pancreatitis occured in 3 patients. It is usually result of peripancreatic necrosis and abscess and in our patients recurred 2 - 3 days after previous debridement. It was every time serious bleeding, twice from the veins of the mesocolon and once from splenic vein. In two patients the bleeding was surgically controlled, one patient died.

Surgery of the pancreas is one of the most difficult parts of the abdominal surgery. Inflammation diseases of the pancreas can have different forms. These disease itself and surgical procedures on the pancreas can leed to life threatening massive venous bleeding and is necessary try to avoid these complications.

Phlébologie 92. Eds P. Raymond-Martimbeau, R. Prescott, M. Zummo.
John Libbey Eurotext, Paris © 1992, pp. 1180-1181

La thrombose veineuse profonde post-opératoire tardive

Raymond Benoit

Angiologue FMH, chemin Beau-Soleil 12, 1206 Genève, Suisse

La plupart des auteurs admettent que la majorité des thromboses veineuses profondes (TVP) post-opératoires se développent dans les 10 jours qui suivent l'intervention. Chacun sait également que le risque thrombo-embolique persiste bien au-delà de ces 10 jours, mais il existe peu d'études sur ce sujet.
Scurr et al. (1988) ont étudié l'incidence des TVP après la sortie de l'hôpital. Sur 57 patients de plus de 40 ans subissant une intervention chirurgicale abdominale majeure, 6 ont fait une TVP à l'hôpital. Les 51 patients restants ont été suivis jusqu'à 6 semaines après leur sortie, et la TVP (recherchée par le test au fibrinogène radio-marqué) a été retrouvée chez 13 d'entre eux, ainsi dans ce collectif les TVP post-opératoires furent deux fois plus fréquentes à domicile qu'en milieu hospitalier. Dans un étude récemment publiée, Huber et al. (1992) ont repris 28953 dossiers de la clinique de chirurgie digestive. Parmi ces malades, 90 (0.31 %) ont présenté une embolie pulmonaire (EP) durant le séjour hospitalier, dont 80 (0.42 %) pour les malades opérés et 10 (0.10 %) pour les autres. Dans les 30 jours suivant leur sortie de l'hôpital, 29 patients ont été réadmis pour EP, dont deux sont décédés. Le risque d'EP augmente ainsi de 30 % (0.54 % au total).

Actuellement, pour des raisons économiques surtout, les séjours hospitaliers tendent à devenir de plus en plus courts, et la chirurgie ambulatoire se développe beaucoup. Par conséquent, il est fort probable que les complications thrombo-emboliques se produiront plus fréquemment à domicile, entraînant un difficulté supplémentaire au diagnostic, d'autant plus que l'on est loin de la date de l'opération. Souvent frappé par les délais prolongés entre l'acte chirurgical et le moment du diagnostic de TVP, nous avons décidé d'entreprendre une étude permettant de préciser ce délai, ainsi que le moment de l'apparition des symptômes.

Patients et méthode

L'étude porte sur 31 patients consécutifs vus **ambulatoirement** en consultation d'angiologie pour une TVP et chez qui la récente intervention chirurgicale a été considérée comme étant la cause de la TVP. Il s'agit donc d'une sélection de patients par rapport au total des TVP vues durant cette période (79) pour 287 malades référés pou suspicion de TVP. Lorsque les renseignements n'étaient pas fournis par un médecin, les malades ont été interrogés sur le type de chirurgie, le genre et la durée de la prophylaxie, la longueur du séjour, la date de l'apparition des symptômes de TVP ou d'EP et leur évolution, et finalement le temps écoulé entre l'opération et le moment du diagnostic de TVP a été calculé.

Résultats

Le collectif est formé de 17 hommes et 14 femmes. L'âge moyen est 53.5 ans, dont 4 seulement ont moins de 40 ans. La durée du séjour est extrêmement variable, allant jusqu'à 3 mois, alors que 3 personnes ont été opérées ambulatoirement. le type de chirurgie est intéressant: l'orthopédie vient largement en tête avec 13 cas, puis l'urologie (4), les varices (3), l'abdominale (3), la liposuccion (3), et avec 1 TVP chacune la chirurgie cardiaque, vasculaire, thoracique, dermatologique, neurologique. La prophylaxie anti-thromboembolique est également trés variée, la préférence semble tout de même aller à l'héparine pour toute la durée du séjour. Six n'ont reçu aucune prophylaxie. Pour les facteurs de risque, relevons 4 cancers, 1 hémopathie, 4 femmes sous contraception orale, 4 antécédents de TVP, 1 phlébite superficielle, 1 polytraumatisé. Sur 31 TVP, 2 seulement étaient localisées aux veines jambières, toutes les autres touchaient au moins la veine poplitée, 4 atteignaient la veine iliaque, et 3 ont entraîné une EP certaine. Le membre inférieur droit était touché 13 fois, le gauche 18 (les TVP bilatérales n'ont pas été recherchées systématiquement). Le délai moyen entre l'opération et le début des symptômes est de 7.8 jours, entre l'opération et le moment où la TVP est diagnostiquée 46 jours (Fig.1).

Figure 1: Délai entre l'apparition des symptômes et le diagnostic de TVP

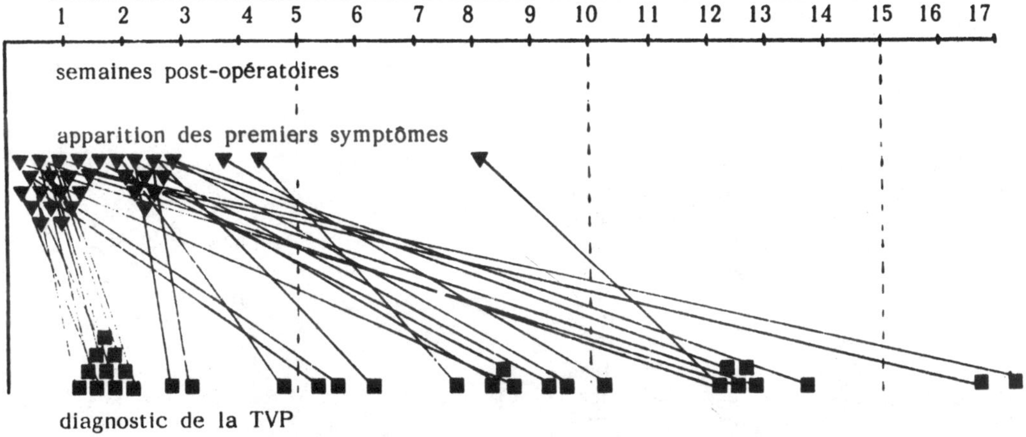

Discussion

Le fait le plus marquant est la disparité nette entre le début de l'apparition des symptômes de TVP (oedème ou douleur) et le moment où le diagnostic est enfin posé. Schématiquement, on peut dire que les symptômes surviennent en majorité dans les 10 jours post-opératoires, souvent déjà en clinique, alors que le diagnostic de TVP n'est formellement éclairci qu'après plus de 6 semaines. Ainsi, il semble que la TVP se forme généralement tôt, mais elle peut rester latente, ne s'exprimant clairement que plus tard, au moment de la mobilisation complète du malade. Pour éviter cet écueil, il faut proposer à nos malades une prophylaxie individualisée en fonction du risque opératoire, ainsi qu'une prolongation de la prophylaxie si le séjour hospitalier est court, ou si la mobilisation est imparfaite, ou encore dans les états hypercoagulables. Enfin, chose connue mais qui mérite d'être rappelée, la chirurgie orthopédique provoque davantage de complications thrombo-emboliques, et il est essentiel de poursuivre l'effort de formation des chirurgiens pour qu'ils sachent reconnaître et rechercher précocément la TVP et l'EP.

IATROGENIC INJURIES TO FEMORAL BLOOD VESSELS DURING VARICOSE VEINS SURGERY - CAUSES AND PREVENTION.

Georges JANTET
The Ealing Hospital, London, England

It is reported that 3-4% of all groin operations for varicose veins are associated with an injury to the femoral vein.
The Medical Defence Societies (of Great Britain) report 1-2 major blood vessel injury per year during varicose vein surgery.
One Defence Society says that 27% of all the complaints they receive following varicose vein surgery relate to damage to the femoral blood vessels which is the commonest single cause of reported complaint.
Most of these, often tragic, accidents are avoidable and indefensible, resulting in heavy claims for damages.
The types and causes of major vessel injuries are discussed and rules presented to avoid these accidents.

E.
RÉADIVES
RECURRENCE

Phlébologie 92. Eds P. Raymond-Martimbeau, R. Prescott, M. Zummo.
John Libbey Eurotext, Paris © 1992, pp. 1185

Video - varicographie as a useful help to avoid recidival problems in venous surgery

Andrew J. Megyeri M.D.

Vascular Surgical Ward, The Institute of the Hungarian State Railway, 1528 Szanatorium str. No. 2/A. Budapest, Hungary

The recurrent problems have a great importance in the field of the venous surgery, however most of the causes can be antedated to the time of the first operation. The main advantage of Video - varicographie that with its help you have the opportunity to avoid possibility of recidiva by understanding the problems of the venous system, one can find the low and high insuffitiency points of the Long Saphenous Vein. The correct solution during the operational procedures primary to ligate the ineffetive perforating veins. To find the perforating points the Video - varicographie gives you a great help. In some cases without its help you are not able to make the diagnoses. For instance : finding the Hach perforating vein. / Perf. vein of V.fem. prof./
During the evaluation you can use the advantages of the moving pictures, so the functional disturbances can be easily studied. In our practice the Video - varicographie is an indispensible help at most of the cases.

Phlébologie 92. Eds P. Raymond-Martimbeau, R. Prescott, M. Zummo.
John Libbey Eurotext, Paris © 1992, pp. 1186

Does long saphenous vein stripping prevent recurrence from perforating veins?

Lawrence L. Tretbar, M.D. FACS

Univ of MO Kansas City School of Medicine

144 legs of 86 patients were examined with Doppler ultrasound 2-41 years after stripping of the Long Saphenous Vein. The anatomic distribution of new varicose veins and recurring varicosities was noted.

The most significant finding was the development of new varicose veins from perforators along the stripping path in 88/144 legs. The origin of the varices were divided between thigh and upper calf perforators.

Major varices developed from previously operated saphenofemoral junctions in 28 legs. In a majority of these operations the groin incision was 2-3 cm below the crease.

Varicosities recurring at ligation sites were seen in 96 legs.

These findings challenge the traditional concept that stripping the LSV prevents the development of varicosities from perforators along the path of stripping. It also reiterates the necessity of a properly placed groin incision.

Phlébologie 92. Eds P. Raymond-Martimbeau, R. Prescott, M. Zummo.
John Libbey Eurotext, Paris © 1992, pp. 1187-1189

Recurrent varicose veins : an anatomical analysis

C.V. Ruckley, I. Beggs

Vascular Surgery Unit and Department of Radiology, Royal Infirmary, Edinburgh, Scotland.

The 1990 Lothian Surgical Audit (all general surgical units in one Health Board : population 750,000) documented 1014 varicose vein operations of which approximately 20% were for recurrent veins.

This is a preliminary report of an ongoing prospective study of a consecutive series of patients with recurrent varicose veins under the care of one surgeon (CVR). The overall aims of the study are:
(i) to analyse causes of recurrence in terms of anatomical findings.
(ii) to compare and correlate alternative methods of investigation and
(iii) to assess abnormalities of the deep venous system in this population.

This paper is confined to an analysis of the anatomical findings to date.

PATIENTS AND METHODS

The protocol of investigation comprises clinical assessment, Doppler examination, varicography, Duplex of the deep veins and anatomical assessment at the time of operation. The series currently numbers 117 patients, 146 legs with recurrent varices. Records were found to be incomplete in 5 and 50 legs have not yet undergone operation. This preliminary analysis is therefore based on 112 patients, 141 legs and 91 operations, the data being derived from the pre-operative Doppler examination and operative findings.

Of the 116 legs where there had been one or more previous operations in the groin 81(70%) still had detectable reflux at the sapheno-femoral junction on Doppler. Of the 70 legs having re-exploration at the groin 50 (71%) still had a patent sapheno-femoral junction. In all cases the patent sapheno-femoral junction connected through scar tissue to varying numbers of tributaries and in some also to residual long saphenous vein. Where the sapheno-femoral had been effectively obliterated the cause of recurrence was almost invariably a residual saphenous vein fed by one or more major thigh deep perforating veins. An intact saphenous vein in the thigh was found in 53 (74%) of 72 legs explored and of these 43 (81%) were also found to have one or more large thigh perforators.

Of the 12 legs where there had been previous short saphenous surgery 5(42%) were found on exploration to have an intact sapheno popliteal junction.

CONCLUSIONS

1. Recurrence of varicose veins remains a major surgical problem.
2. Patterns of recurrence well recognised by previous authors (Lofgren & Lofgren 1971; Shepherd 1978; Munn etal 1981) persist.
3. Recurrent varicose veins are associated predominantly with incompetence of the long saphenous system.
4. Two broad categories stand out:
(a) persisting patency at the sapheno-femoral junction.
(b) persisting reflux down the long saphenous vein stemming from incompetent thigh perforator(s).
5. These two causes of recurrence can be avoided by appropriate surgical technique at the primary operation ie. proper dissection at the sapheno-femoral junction and removal of the thigh segment

of the long saphenous vein.

REFERENCES

Lofgren E P, Lofgren K A. Recurrence of varicose veins after the stripping operation. Arch Surg 1971; 102: 111.

Sheppard M. A procedure for the prevention of recurrent saphenofemoral incompetence. Aust NZ J Surg 1978; 48: 322.

Munn S R, Morton J B, Macbeth W A G, McLeish A R. To strip or not to strip the long saphenous vein? A varicose veins trial. Br J Surg 1981; 68: 426.

RECURRENT VARICOSE VEINS: AN ANATOMO-CLINICAL REPORT

G.Scipioni - G.Perilli - A.Scipioni

Servizio di Flebologia Chirurgica Ospedale S.Eugenio Roma, Italia

We report 75 cases of recurrent varicose veins, who were divided into three groups:

1- in 24 patients, phlebography showed permanent or dynamic compression on popliteal vein, with perforating veins incompetence in the leg; no recurrent patology was found two years after popliteal vein blunt dissection and perforating vessels ligation.

2- 50% of recurrency was demostrated, after a two years follow up, in 14 patients with deep venous insufficiency, who underwent sclerotherapy, multiple phlebectomies and permanent elastic compression.

3- in 37 patients, with previous uncomplete surgery, submitted to radical surgery of saphenic crosse and phlebectomies, 27 (73%), were free from recurrencies after two years.

Therefore, an accurate preoperatory screening, allowes to prewiew any insufficient result.

LES RECIDIVES VARIEQUEUSE. Causes et localisation les plus frequentes, d'après notre experience

E. CERAUDO, M. R. DEL GOBBO*

I Service de Chirurgie.* Ambulatoire de Phlèbologie
Jesi - ITALIE

Pendant 8 ans nous avons soigné 47 patients atteints de rechutes variqueuses, dont seulement 9 avaient ètè operés précédemment chez nous. Les états variqueux intéressaient la veine de Leonardo, la veine anterieure de la jambe, la saphene accessoire de la cuisse, la veine de Giacomini, le veines périnealés et ils étaient causés par la manque de déconnexion des veines ostiales dans des patients opérés dans d'autres hopitaux, par le manque d'identification et traitement des perforantes du compartiment tibial antérieur. L'étude pré operatoire a été effectué par l'examen clinique, la vélocimétrie doppler, limitant la phlébografie à 7 cas seulement.
L'attitude thérapeutique a été conditionnée par le lieu des varices, par l'importance du reflux, par des états variqueux et par le désir manifeste de quelques patients d'avoir un traitement conservatoire. 22 patients aux varices dues à de modestes reflux ont été traités par sclérothérapie, parmi ces patients 4, dans des temps variables ont été soumis à une intervention ambulatoire de ligature. 9 patients ont voulu être traités par la contention elastique. 20 patients dont 4 avaient la sclérothérapie ont été soumis à une intervention ambulatoire de varicectomie avec mini incisions.

Varicose vein surgery recurrences and experiences in reoperations

S. Fontanyi, S. Berczvai, L. Helembai

Department of Surgery "A", Péterfy S. Hospital, Budapest, Hungary

The tactics and technique in varicose vein surgery may be perfected by analysis of recurrences and experiences in reoperations.

Material: 1043 extremities of 832 patients of whom 255 underwent reoperation. The steps of analysis:

I - Previous operation's assessment diagnostically by:

1. Vein percussion test: cross ligation, remnant segments
2. Fegan test: perforating vein localization
3. TPM / Toe-Plethysmometry: non-invasive venous pressure measurement to estimate deep venous system
4. Blood oxymetry: av microshunts demonstration
5. Phlebography: in dubious deep vein patency

II - Prereoperative findings documentation on fotos / percussion lines, scars, perforating veins / and summarizing tables

III - Previous operation's assessment during reoperation regarding:

1. Cross ligation quality
2. Remnant truncs and segments
3. Short saphenous vein
4. Perforating veins location

IV - Reoperation's findings illustration on sketches, tables

V - Obtaining experiences by comparison pre- and post-reoperative documentations, helping for perfection in diagnostics, operative and reoperative tactics and technique.

Phlébologie 92. Eds P. Raymond-Martimbeau, R. Prescott, M. Zummo.
John Libbey Eurotext, Paris © 1992, pp. 1192-1194

Nouvelle incidence anatomique dans les récidives de crossectomies saphènes internes : à propos de 300 cas

William Taieb

9, rue de Turin, 75008 Paris, France.

Bien que la crossectomie saphène interne soit un geste de base de la chirurgie des varices, une étude rétrospective des Rédux de Varices,nous a permis de mettre en évidence un nouvel élément où une faute technique initiale pourrait être plus souvent en cause,en grande partie grace à l'échographie.

PROTOCOLE OPERATOIRE :

La "Crossectomie de base",consiste en une section au ras de la veine fémorale de l'ostium de la saphène interne,en laissant un moignon si possible inexistant,avec ligatures de toutes les collatérales visibles,s'abouchant dans celle-ci.
Pour nous,ce geste est insuffisant,car toute la veine fémorale doit être explorée,sur toutes ses faces.

RESULTATS :

Les 300 interventions pour récidive se répartissent ainsi:
-Interventions bilatérales : 98 cas,donc196 interventions,
-Interventions unilatérales : 104 interventions.

La reprise consiste en une dissection étendue du carrefour fémoral artériel et veineux.
Une fois repèré le moignon de la néocrosse saphène ,une nouvelle crossectomie est effectuée.
La veine fémorale est disséquée sur 2 à 3 centimètres,au dessus et en dessous de la néo crosse,non seulement sa face antérieure,ses faces latérales ,mais aussi sa face postérieure.

Les résultats tardifs feront l'objet d'une publication ultérieure.

N.B

Ce qui est vrai pour la saphène interne l'est encore plus pour **la saphène externe**,où les variations anatomiques de la terminaison de la crosse ,dépistées par échographie,sont trés fréquentes,et expliquent le grand nombre de récidives ,à ce niveau.

Elles feront l'objet d'une communication ultérieure;

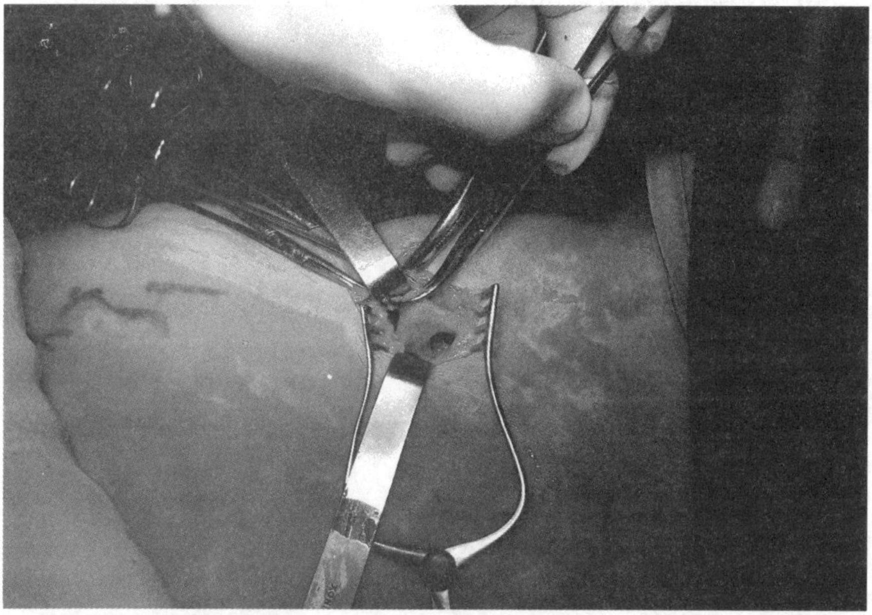

DISCUSSION :

Pourquoi une telle dissection,aussi étendue?

1/Si l'on admet la théorie de COGET et MERLEN sur les récidives post-opèratoires,fondées sur des raisons mécaniques,liées à la faiblesse de la paroi veineuse,
2/ la saphène interne est l'une des rares veines de la face antérieure de la veine fémorale,

on peut tenter une hypothèse etiologique:
Les veines ,en général les circonflexes,s'abouchant à plein canal,à la face postérieure de la veine fémorale,créent un hyperdébit en regard du moignon fragile de la crossectomie (photos).
L'échographie pré-opèratoire permet de retrouver ces collatérales,dans la plupart des cas.

CONCLUSION :

Une des hypothèses étiologiques sur l'apparition d'une néo crosse saphène interne pourrait être, dans 70 % des cas, l'existence de veines postérieures de la veine fémorale(le plus souvent les circonflexes) créant un hyper débit localisé qui accentue la fragilité d'une zone de moignon de crossectomie.

References :

Bassi G.,(1967), in "les Varices des membres inférieurs" Ed.DOIN.

Phlébologie 92. Eds P. Raymond-Martimbeau, R. Prescott, M. Zummo.
John Libbey Eurotext, Paris © 1992, pp. 1195-1197

Re-exploration of the sapheno-femoral junction in recurrent varicose veins : properties of Li's technique

Pietro Belardi, Germano Lucertini

Cattedra di Chirurgia Vascolare, Università degli Studi di Genova, Viale Benedetto XV, 10 16132 Genova, Italy.

The excellent management of varicose veins requires correct diagnosis and accurate treatment . Lack of the former and/or the latter carry out relentlessly unsatisfactory results. This consideration is related particularly to valvular incompetence of the sapheno-femoral junction. Such finding is the more often observed change in varicose veins.
Recurrent varicose veins are often caused by incorrect treatment of the sapheno-femoral junction (1 2), although the importance of the adequate great saphenous vein treatment has been widely stressed.
Recurrence dependent from the sapheno-femoral junction valvular incompetence requires surgical treatment at that site.
Re-exploration of the sapheno-femoral junction is not easy problem. It must ensure removal of venous reflux among scar tissue. Thereafter it exposes to risk of blood vessels and lymphatic lesions.
Aim of the present study is evaluation of a surgical technique, described by Li (3), for re-exploration of the sapheno-femoral junction.

Material and methods

Since January 1978 to December 1990 96 lower limbs with recurrent varicose veins for incorrect treatment of the sapheno-femoral junction were operated upon. The patients studied were 87, 24 males and 63 females, age ranging from 32 to 74 years (mean 48). Valvular incompetence of communicating veins (at the thigh and/ or the calf) and/or of lesser saphenous vein was associated with the one of the sapheno-femoral junction in some legs. The cases were evaluated by careful clinical evaluation, quite always by Doppler C.W. too and sometimes by ascending phlebography. Only the cases with recurrence of primary varicose veins entered this series; the ones of postthrombotic syndrome or primary deep venous insufficiency were excluded.
Surgical treatment was constituted by re-exploration of the sapheno-femoral junction (in 18 patients bilaterally at the same time) and other surgical procedures according to pathophysiological conditions of each case.
The surgical technique performed for re-exploration of the sapheno-femoral junction was described by Li (3). This procedure requires incision in the groin crease as for projection of femoral vessels and therefore laterally extended as to ligation of the saphenofemoral junction (Fig. 1A). Approach to the stump of the great saphenous vein is led by dissection

of subcutaneous tissue, opening of fascia and exposition of common femoral artery, easily identifiable (Fig. 1B). Dissection is carried on from this vessel medially to join common femoral vein above and below the saphenofemoral junction (Fig. 1C). Finally, the stump of the great saphenous vein is reached superficially. As rule, ligation of the stump is performed close to the common femoral vein. Ligation and division of all tributaries also must be executed (Fig. 1D).

Patients can be operated upon under general, spinal or local anaesthesia.

Early mobilisation (during the same day or the one after surgery) and physiotherapy are utilised as measures for prophylaxis of deep venous thrombosis.

Results were assessed according to correction of venous reflux at the inguinal level, further recurrence of varicose veins in the upper thigh, postoperative complications and cosmetic outcome.

Follow-up ranges from 1 to 12 years.

Results

Operative mortality was 0%.

Results were functionally positive in 93/96 (97%) cases. Recurrence of the sapheno-femoral reflux was never observed. In 3/96 (3%) legs recurrence of varicose veins in the upper thigh occurs some years after surgery. It was due to the incompetence of communicating vein in the upper or middle thigh, as showed by varicography.

Surgical operation was complicated only in 6/96 (6%) cases. In all cases postoperative complication was lymphorrhoea, always recovered. Lesions of femoral vessels, hematoma, infection and deep venous thrombosis were never observed.

Cosmetic results were satisfactory. The incision resulted masked in the inguinal crease.

Discussion

Re-exploration of the sapheno-femoral junction for recurrent varicose veins pursues definitive correction of the sapheno-femoral junction reflux as fundamental aim. This goal can be difficult to be reached in scar tissue. Moreover high risk of lesion of femoral vessels, lymphatic trunks, lymph nodes and minor vessels is present.

Common characteristic of all techniques for approach to the sapheno-femoral junction is dissection through uninjured area to avoid scar. Beyond this property, the technique described by Li shows other very important characters. Among these, skin incision in the groin crease and common femoral artery as easily available mark are to be considered. The former allows to mask well surgical wound. The latter makes sure and easy the approach to the sapheno-femoral junction. Common femoral artery is available mark because pulsating vessel.

Our experience with the described technique yielded very satisfactory results. It confirms the known properties of this surgical procedure. According to our experience, we can stress easy approach to the sapheno-femoral junction, lesser surgical injury and excellent functional results. These characters allow correction of the sapheno-femoral reflux and avoid important complications. With regard to these, it must emphasise that complications were less than 6% in our own experience and were constituted always by lymphatic problems. Everywhere these can occur after all techniques for re-exploration of the sapheno-femoral junction.

Difficulty or impossibility of ligation and division of all great saphenous vein tributaries has not to be missed. This is due to strong scar tissue encasing veins. Thereafter persistent reflux in untreated tributaries (particularly superficial epigastric and iliac circumflex veins)

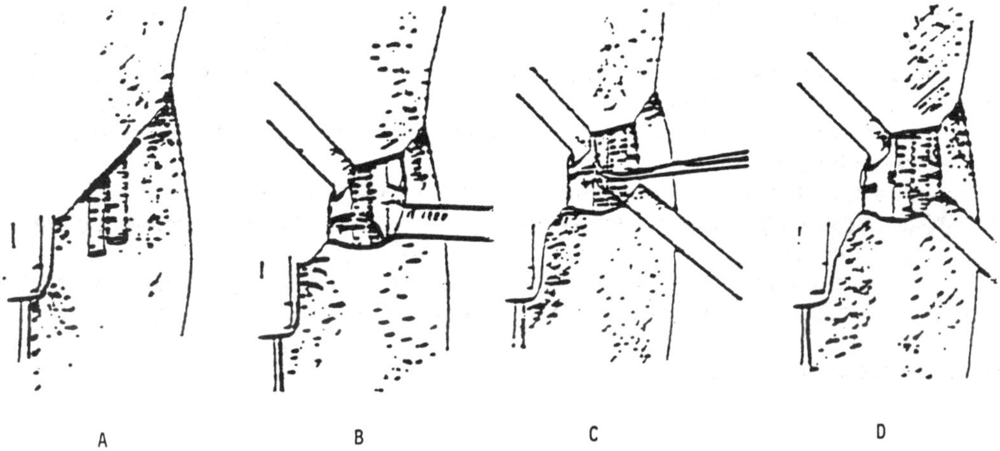

Fig. 1. The technique described by Li for re-exploration of the sapheno-femoral junction. A: Skin incision in the groin crease. B: Exposition of the common femoral artery. C: Exposition of the common femoral vein and ligation of the sapheno-femoral junction. D: Ligation of all great saphenous vein tributaries.

produces further recurrence of varicose veins in the upper thigh (4). Other cause of further recurrent varicose veins is constituted by progression of the venous disease. An example of this occurrence is the incompetence of a communicating vein in the upper thigh, as well as demonstrated by varicography (5). This event is rare indeed. It was observed only in 3% of our series.

In conclusion, we consider the lateral approach described by Li the optional procedure for the troublesome problem of the sapheno-femoral junction re-exploration.

References

1. Juhan C, Haupert S, Miltgen G, Barthelemy P, Eklof B. recurrent varicose veins. Phlebology 1990; 5: 201-211.

2. Lofgren EP, Lofgren KA. Recurrence of varicose veins after the stripping operation. Arch Surg 1971; 102: 111-114.

3. Li AKC. A technique for re-exploration of the sapheno-femoral junction for recurrent varicose veins. Br J Surg 1975; 62: 745-746.

4. Hobbs JT. Can we prevent recurrence of varicose veins? In: Greenhalgh RM, Jamieson CW, Nicolaides AN, eds. Vascular Surgery. Issues in current practice. London: Grune and Stratton, 1986: 355-373.

5. Starnes HF, Vallance R, Hamilton DNH. Recurrent varicose veins: a radiological approach to investigation. Clin Radiol 1984; 35: 95-99.

Phlébologie 92. Eds P. Raymond-Martimbeau, R. Prescott, M. Zummo.
John Libbey Eurotext, Paris © 1992, pp. 1198-1200

Les récidives variqueuses de l'aine

Claude Elbaz

70, rue Michel-Ange, 75016 Paris, France.

INTRODUCTION :

Les récidives post-chirurgicales des varices trouvent essentiellement leur origine dans la région de l'aine, plus rarement au niveau de la fosse poplitée et des perforantes cruro-jambières : dans une étude portant sur 436 récidives opérées entre 1964 et 1986 (4), nous avions comptabilisé 263 malades présentant un redux dont l'origine se situait au niveau de l'aine. Pour l'essentiel, il était imputable à une crosse restante de la saphène interne, autrement dit à une malfaçon opératoire qui laissait en place les conditions idéales d'une récidive.
Le développement des investigations invasives (phlébographie et varicographie) et surtout non invasives (échographie et doppler couleur) ont permis de mieux connaitre l'histoire naturelle de ces récidives.

MATERIEL ET METHODES :

L'étude de nos dossiers portant sur les trois dernières années (1989 à 1991) nous a permis d'affiner nos connaissances sur l'étiologie des redux de l'aine. Pendant cette période, nous avons opéré 1 533 malades parmi lesquels 240 présentaient une récidive post-chirurgicale, soit 16% du total des varices opérées. Ce pourcentage se retrouve dans les statistiques de HOBBS (7), 10% à 6 ans, ROYLE (12), 18% à 5 ans, et LOFGREN (9), 15% à 10 ans. Sur 240 récidives, 162 se situent au niveau de l'aine, associées ou non à d'autres localisations. Sur 162 malades, nous retrouvons 44 hommes et 118 femmes. L'âge moyen est de 49,2; avec des extrêmes de 24 à 70 ans.

ANALYSE DES RECIDIVES :

L'analyse des récidives s'établit comme suit :

1° Crosses restantes de saphène ou néo-crosse.................... 147
2° Varices périnéales.. 15 dont 7 isolées
3° Collatérales de la saphène.................................... 12 dont 5 isolées.

1° Récidives par crosse restante ou par néo-crosse.

Elles représentent l'essentiel des causes de récidives de l'aine. Jusqu'à ces dernières années, une confusion nosologique existait entre ces deux termes qui désignent deux notions entièrement distinctes.

a) La crosse restante est la conséquence d'une malfaçon opératoire qui a laissé en place une crosse de 2 à 3 cm avec ses collatérales à partir desquelles s'est développée rapidement une néo-saphène interne ou un réseau réalimentant une saphène non strippée. Cliniquement, le diagnostic est évident devant une cicatrice trop basse et la perception d'une crosse tendue. Il est confirmé par l'échographie/doppler. Plus rarement, il peut s'agir d'une deuxième crosse ou d'une saphène accessoire négligée.
b) La récidive par néovascularisation s'effectue à partir d'un thrombus au niveau duquel s'organise une vasculo-génèse donnant naissance à un réseau de néo-vaisseaux fragiles, tortueux, s'anastomosant, d'une part à la veine fémorale, d'autre part au réseau veineux superficiel et constituant une néo-saphène dont les méandres apparaissent sur le trajet de la saphène précedemment

strippée. Cette cause de récidive évoquée par TRENDELENBURG a été récemment réhabilitée par GLASS (6). Mais OLIVIER (10) la décrivait parfaitement dès 1965 grâce à des observations documentées par la phlébographie et l'histologie. Cette néo-vascularisation se développe dans un tissu scléro-cicatriciel dense qui capitonne la lame cellulo-lymphatique sur la fémorale et rend la dissection difficile et parfois dangereuse. Elle peut prendre l'aspect d'un cavernome : 31 cas dont 16 hommes et 15 femmes. Ces cavernomes sont l'expression d'une potentialité évolutive particulièrement vive faisant qualifier les varicoses de "malignes".

Au total, cette classification nosologique est parfois difficile à établir à l'examen de certains dossiers et il arrive que l'on hésite à cataloguer une crosse restante ou une néo-crosse en dépit des explorations et de l'examen histologique.

2° Récidives par les collatérales de la saphène.

La sous-cutanée abdominale ou la veine circonflexe peuvent réalimenter une volumineuse "écharpe" antérieure de cuisse. L'éventualité est relativement rare quand elle est seule en cause et elle est bien matérialisée par une varicographie. Encore faut-il s'assurer d'une absence de perforante de cuisse.

3° Récidives par les veines périnéo-vulvaires.

Sur des varices vues en première main, elles existent une fois sur dix et ne doivent pas être méconnues car elles constituent une voie de dérivation autonome ne passant pas par le carrefour saphéno-fémoral. Nous avons relevé 15 cas de récidives imputables à des varices périnéales remontant à travers le plancher pelvien jusqu'aux veines pelviennes et spécialement les veines hypogastriques, les veines ovariennes et le pédicule lombo-ovarien. Cliniquement, ces varices peuvent entrainer des troubles gynécologiques (dyspareunies, douleurs post-coïtales, syndrome congestif pelvien) bien individualisés par certains auteurs (7). La varicographie et surtout la phlébographie sélective de la veine lombo-ovarienne gauche mettent en évidence des ectasies importantes des veines ovariennes et un reflux vers les veines périnéo-vulvaires. La suppression par phlébectomies ou sclérose peut suffire. Mais, l'existence d'une symptomatologie gynécologique associée justifie la résection du pédicule lombo-ovarien que nous avons pratiqué cinq fois avec succès par voie sous-péritonéale.

PREVENTION DES RECIDIVES.

De nombreuses récidives seraient évitées si la chirurgie de la saphène était correctement exécutée. Elle implique la résection de la crosse au ras de la veine fémorale associée à la ligature de toutes ses collatérales sans oublier une crosse surnuméraire ou une collatérale s'abouchant séparément dans la veine fémorale. Le stripping de la saphène interne est la règle ainsi que le stripping d'une saphène accessoire ou d'une saphène antérieure de cuisse.

Le risque de récidive par néovascularisation est grandement évité en interposant une ou des barrières entre la veine fémorale et les veines superficielles : la fermeture soigneuse du foramen ovale est faite systématiquement depuis plus de 25 ans. Son utilité vient d'être rappelée par GLASS (6). Lorsque la fermeture de cette fenêtre aponévrotique n'est pas satisfaisante, on peut y adjoindre la mobilisation de l'aponévrose du pectiné proposé par SHEPPARD (13). Nous utilisons depuis plus de 10 ans un tulle de Mersylène auquel nous préférons un treillis résorbable de Polyglactine (Vicryl).

TRAITEMENT DES RECIDIVES.

La voie d'abord se fait, soit par une incision verticale externe (1), soit en prolongeant en dehors l'incision primitive (8) : dans les deux cas, on aborde d'abord l'artère fémorale puis la veine fémorale et la jonction saphéno-fémorale . Nous préférons utiliser une incision qui reprend la cicatrice primitive et qui est prolongée en dedans en crosse de hockey, ce qui nous permet d'aborder directement la veine fémorale. Dans toutes les techniques, on doit éviter de passer dans le bloc scléro-cicatriciel et passer en dessous de la lame cellulo-lymphatique en restant au contact du fascia superficialis. La crosse restante ou la néo-crosse est isolée et sectionnée au ras de la veine fémorale. Le foramen ovale est soigneusement fermé au fil non résorbable. On termine par une révision complète du triangle de SCARPA en poussant la dissection jusqu'à l'arcade crurale de façon à supprimer des petites crosses accessoires. On finit par la mise en place d'un treillis de Vicryl.

CONCLUSIONS.

1° La maladie variqueuse est une maladie évolutive qui doit inciter à la prudence et à l'humilité.
2° Les récidives de l'aine sont dues essentiellement à une crosse restante imputable à une malfaçon opératoire ou à une néo-crosse consécutive à une néovascularisation.
3° Les varices périnéales constituent une voie de récidive non négligeable et pouvant provenir d'un reflux des varices pelviennes.
4° La phlébographie et surtout l'écho/doppler couleur sont des investigations indispensables.
5° L'intervention requiert une grande expérience chirurgicale et ne doit pas être confiée à un débutant. (COCKETT).

REFERENCES.

1° DARKES S. (1991) : Recurrent varicose veins in BERGAN JJ, YAO JST eds , venous disorders - 250-257.
2° DOOD H. , COCKETT B. (1976) : The patology and surgery of the veins of the lower limb - Churchill Livingston eds - 144-154.
3° ELBAZ Cl. (1975) : Chirurgie itérative dans les récidives après opération pour varices essentielles . Journal de Chirurgie. 565-575.
4° ELBAZ Cl. (1989) : Recurrence of varicose veins following surgery. Vascular Surgery 23. 90-94.
5° FRILEUX C., WALIGORA J. (1967) : La chirurgie itérative dans les varices essentielles des membres inférieurs. Analyse de 230 observations de récidives post-opératoires. Mem. Ac. Chir. 93. 270.
6° GLASS GM. (1989) : Prevention of recurrent sapheno femoral incompetence after surgery for varicose veins. Br. J. Surg. 76. 1210.
7° HOBBS J. (1991) : The treatment of vulvual and pelvic varices in BERGAN JJ, YAO JST eds, venous disorders. 250-257.
8° LI AKC (1975) : A technique for a reexploration of the sapheno-femoral junction for recurrent varicose veins. Br. J. Surg. 62. 745-746.
9° LOFGREN EP. (1985) : Treatment of the long saphenous varicosities and their recurrence. A long term follow up in BERGAN JJ, YAO JST eds, Surgery of the veins. GRUNE and STRATTON. 285-299.
10° OLIVIER Cl. et all (1966) : Les réinterventions pour varices essentielles des membres inférieurs. Presse Médicale 74. 1355-1360.
11° OLIVIER Cl. (1975) : Le traitement chirurgical des récidives après opération pour varices essentielles. Journ. Chir. 109. 565-575.
12° ROYLE JP. (1986) : Recurrent varicose veins. World Surg. 10. 944-958.
13° SHEPPARD M. (1975) : The incidence, diagnosis and management of sapheno femoral junction for recurrent varicose veins. Br. J. Surg. 62. 745-746.

Les veines jumelles internes et le traitement des varices du creux poplite

Ph. Blanchemaison, Ph. Gorny

Centre de Phlébologie Ambulatoire (CPA) - Paris, France

Les causes anatomiques de récidives du creux poplité sont connues: persistance d'un site de reflux associée à la saphène externe, malfaçon chirurgicale, ligature trop à distance de la veine profonde.

Deux mécanismes hémodynamiques de récidive post-chirurgicale des varices du creux poplité peuvent être imputées à une pathologie des veines jumelles internes:

1. Les perforantes de la face interne du mollet, centrées sur les veines jumelles sont siège d'un reflux lors de la contraction musculaire, avec phénomène de blow-out visible en endoscopie.

2. D'autre part, les récidives post-crossectomies saphènes externes peuvent être liées à une ectasie des veines jumelles, venant mettre en surcharge, lors d'efforts musculaires, les perforantes du creux poplité.

XV.
TRAITEMENT CHIRURGICALE RECONSTRUCTIF
RECONSTRUCTIVE SURGICAL TREATMENT

A. Veines profondes / *Deep veins*

Phlébologie 92. Eds P. Raymond-Martimbeau, R. Prescott, M. Zummo.
John Libbey Eurotext, Paris © 1992, pp. 1207-1208

Microsurgical correction of portal hypertension

V. Krylov, M. Fachratov, K. Abalmasov, J. Abramov, S. Norkusiev

Moscow, Russia.

The distal spleno-renal porto caval anastomoses cause a large operative trauma to the patient, are technically difficult, have post operative complications and a high mortality rate. These were among the reasons to find another way of helping the patients.

Between 1989-1991 we investigated 67 patients aged between 15-69 years of age (44 men and 23 women) with endoscopy, ultrasound examination, radionuclear and angiography investigations. 47 of these patients were operated on. According to the level of the blockage they were divided into categories; 37 intrahepatic, 7 extrahepatic portal hypertension, 3 mixed form. The indications for microsurgical porto-caval anastomosis were:

- The risico of the bleeding from the varicosed oesophageal veins.
- Transitory or stable ascites and the repeated bleeding after previously performed operations.

The variant of the porto-caval operation with microsurgery depends on the characteristic of the portal blockage, the amount of portal hepatic blood flow, also on the surgical possibilities to make the bypass. Out of the 37 operations in the intrahepatic form of the portal hypertension. In 16 patients we made the microsurgical omphalo-saphenous shunt, in 21 patients omento-epigastric and omento-saphenous bypasses. In cases of the recanalised umbilical vein we performed extraperitoneal porto-caval omphalo-saphenous bypass.

Clinical investigation together with haemodynamic testing showed that the omphalo-saphenous bypass in severe patients is a less traumatic operation. They effectively control the portal hypertension. The microsurgical omento-epigastric bypass is indicated also in intrahepatic blockage with the lower amount of the portal hepatic blood flow when it is necessary to eliminate the danger of the bleeding from the varicosed oesophageal veins with preservation of the portal hepatic perfusion. In such cases we also performed the omento-saphenous shunts with the transposition of the vein mobilising the greater omentum, if the porto hepatic blood flow remained within 700-900ml/minute. If it was not possible to rotate a part of the greater omentum we made a new modification of the microsurgical omento-saphenous reversed bypass which was carried out in seven patients with very good haemodynamic effect. We considered this method specially indicated in extra hepatic form of the portal hypertension. In 7 patients with imminent oesophageal bleeding and in the presence of the transitory or stable ascites we performed microsurgical omento-systemic bypass together with the creation of the lympho-nodulo-venous anastomosis with the lower epigastric veins. That was the bypass between the lower epigastric vein and the vein of the greater omentum.

The study of the remote results of the microsurgical correction in portal hypertension showed usefulness of these new methods in surgical correction of the portal hypertension.

Rational Approach to Venous Reconstructive Surgery

Seshadri Raju, M.D.

University of Mississippi Medical Center

Chronic venous insufficiency may be due to obstruction, reflux or a combination. Measurement of arm/foot venous pressure differential and foot venous pressure elevation with reactive hyperemia can diagnose and grade obstruction. Venous bypass is not indicated even when a venographic obstruction is identified when the resting pressure gradient is normal (Grades I and II obstructions). Bypasses performed for Grades III and IV obstructions should be adequate in size for the anatomic location. In general, the saphenous vein is inadequate in the Palma position and a larger prosthetic bypass is preferred. Femoral venous obstructions are generally well compensated from a large profunda popliteal connection. Crural obstructions are occasionally quite hemodynamically severe and may benefit from a perforator bypass. Bypasses performed in the postphlebitic extremity are not durable.

Cryptogenic valve reflux can be corrected by the valvuloplasty procedure which is more durable than either the axillary vein transfer or Kistner segment transfer techniques. External valvuloplasty techniques include the imbrication method and the application of a Dacron or PTFE sleeve in situ. Utilizing a combination of the above techniques, multiple valve reconstructions as a one-stage procedure can be carried out repairing the superficial femoral, profunda, posterior tibial and the peroneal valves. The surgical approach to combined obstruction and reflux remains undetermined. Preliminary experience indicates that the success rate with an anti-reflux valve reconstruction procedure in this setting is less than that seen in cryptogenic reflux. A modified Linton procedure has approximately a 50% success rate in the presence of combined venous pathology.

Phlébologie 92. Eds P. Raymond-Martimbeau, R. Prescott, M. Zummo.
John Libbey Eurotext, Paris © 1992, pp. 1210-1211

Hemodynamic and anatomic follow-up of deep venous valvular reconstruction by valvuloplasty and axillary vein to popliteal vein valve transplant

Thomas F. O'Donnell, Jr., M.D.

New England Medical Center

To treat patients surgically with stage III and advanced stage II chronic venous insufficiency, the deep venous system must be reconstructed. Valvular incompetence is the cause of deep venous insufficiency in excess of 90% of patients. In patients with primary valvular incompetence (30-60% of patients with deep venous valvular malfunction) the valve itself may be repaired either by a direct open technique or, more recently, by angioscopic methods. The remainder of patients with post-thrombotic damage of the valves, however, require transplantation of a functioning valve as there is no remaining valve structures to repair. The purpose of this presentation will be to review our experience with the pre- and post-operative evaluation of these two procedures.

Indications: We restrict deep venous valvular reconstructive procedures to patients with stage III CVI and rarely for advances stage II disease.

Preoperative Evaluation: Patients undergo hemodynamic assessment by air plethysmography (APG) with measurements of venous filling index and ejection fraction as well as determination of valve closure time by duplex scanning after the method of von Bemmelen. Ascending and descending phlebography is then performed.

Procedure: The patient's pathology can generally be determined by preoperative studies, but if there is any question, intraoperative angioscopy allows the differentiation of post-thrombotic from primary valvular incompetence. For primary valvular incompetence, valve repair is performed under a closed angioscopic guidance technique. For post thrombotic valvular damage, the axillary vein, containing at least one functioning valve is transplanted to the above knee popliteal vein.

Postoperative care: Patients are placed in intermittent pneumatic compression devices to increase venous flow across the reconstruction, and are anticoagulated with heparin which is converted to coumadin.

Postoperative Findings: Nine limbs underwent vein valvuloplasty and 15 limbs axillary vein valve transplant. There was one recurrence of ulcer in the transplant group, but there was no recurrence in the vein valve transplant group.

Postoperative hemodynamic studies revealed a reduction in venous filling index in both the transplant and valvuloplasty group, but ejection fraction was unchanged from pre-op. All segments were patent by ascending phlebography and duplex scan in the follow-up.

Venous reconstructive surgery is an effective method for managing Stage III disease.

Phlébologie 92. Eds P. Raymond-Martimbeau, R. Prescott, M. Zummo.
John Libbey Eurotext, Paris © 1992, pp. 1212-1216

Résultats de la chirurgie restauratrice dans les reflux veineux profonds

Michel Perrin, Jean-Marc Bayon, Pédro Castells-Ferrer, Bernard Hiltbrand

Unité de Pathologie Vasculaire Jean Kunlin, Clinique du Grand Large, 69154 Decines-Charpieu Cedex, France.

Entre 1984 et 1991, nous avons réalisé quatre vingt treize interventions pour reflux de la voie veineuse profonde à l'étage sous-inguinal.
Au plan étiologique, on relève cinquante (54 %) syndromes post-thrombotiques (SPT), trente sept (40 %) insuffisances valvulaires profondes primitives (IVPP), trois syndromes de KLIPPEL-TRENAUNAY. Dans trois cas, le doute persistait entre SPT et IVPP.
Au plan clinique, on notait 53 ulcères récidivants (57 %), 79 hypodermites sévères (84 %) et 14 oedèmes isolés.
Au plan hémodynamique, le bilan pré-opératoire comportait en règle : Un examen Doppler directionnel ou un écho-Doppler, une photoplethysmographie (PPG), une mesure dynamique des pressions (MDPV), une phlébographie ascendante et une phlébographie fémorale.
Les résultats s'établissaient ainsi : Le temps de retour veineux (PPG - MDPV) était inférieur à 12" avec garrot. La baisse de la pression veineuse après manoeuvre dynamique avec garrot était inférieure à 30 % du chiffre initial. L'index de reflux poplité (Duplex-Scanner) était supérieur à 0,50 (moyenne 1,2). Le reflux dans la voie veineuse profonde était du grade 4 défini par KISTNER (Phlébographie fémorale).
Au plan technique, il a été réalisé : 46 Valvuloplasties, 26 Transplantations, 12 Transpositions, 9 Interventions de PSATHAKIS.
Préalablement à la chirurgie anti-reflux de la voie veineuse profonde, les malades avaient été traités de façon conservatrice (contention) et pour un certain nombre d'entr'eux une chirurgie de l'insuffisance veineuse superficielle (46 fois) ou des perforantes (5 fois) avait été réalisée. Ces thérapeutiques s'étaient traduites par un échec au plan clinique.
Il importe également de noter que lorsque le bilan pré-opératoire a révélé une insuffisance veineuse superficielle et (ou) un reflux par les perforantes, ces troubles physiopathologiques ont été corrigés chirurgicalement quelques jours avant le geste de chirurgie restauratrice de la voie profonde (33 strippings, 41 ligatures des perforantes).
Il apparait cependant qu'au plan hémodynamique l'insuffisance veineuse superficielle jouait un rôle modeste puisque le temps de retour veineux n'était amélioré en moyenne que de 2 secondes par la mise en place d'un garrot. 62 malades bénéficient d'un recul de 2 ans à 7 ans (moyenne 44 mois).

Les résultats fournis par les valvuloplasties réalisées essentiellement dans les IVPP (79 % des cas) peuvent être considérés comme excellents dans 80 % des cas au plan clinique et hémodynamique.
Ces résultats sont conformes à ceux publiés par les autres équipes (1, 2, 3, 4).
A l'inverse, Transplantations, Transpositions et interventions de PSATHAKIS ont été entreprises dans presque tous les cas pour des SPT (91 % des cas). Nous avons eu un nombre important de thromboses post-opératoires (38 %). Les résultats satisfaisants au plan clinique sont décevants au plan hémodynamique.
Ces résultats sont nettement moins favorables que ceux publiés par certaines équipes nord-américaines (1, 5, 6) mais correspondent à ceux rapportés par d'autres auteurs (2, 4).
Il nous apparait licite de conclure au vu de cette étude rétrospective que:
- Dans les IVPP, la Valvuloplastie représente une intervention efficace qui doit être proposée dans les IVPP non contrôlées par la contention.
- Dans les SPT, la chirurgie du reflux veineux profond doit être réservée aux cas particulièrement sévères.

REFERENCES

1 KISTNER R.L. and FERRIS E.B.
Femoral vein reconstruction in the management of chronic venous insufficiency.
Arch. Surg., 1982 ; 117 : 1571-79.

2 RAJU S. and FREDERICKS R.
Valve reconstruction procedures for non obstructive venous insufficiency. Rationale techniques and results in 107 procedures with 2 to 8 years follow-up.
J. Vasc. Surg., 1988 ; 7 : 301-310.

3 SOTTIURAI V.S.
Technique in direct venous valvuloplasty.
J. Vasc. Surg. 1988 ; 8 : 646-48.

4 ERIKSSON I.
Vein valve surgery for deep valvular incompetence. In : Controversies in the management of venous disorders.
B. EKLOF, J.E. GJORES, O. THULESIUS, D. BERGQVIST.
Butterworths. 1989 ; 267-79.

5 TAHERI S.A., HEFFNER R., MEENAGHAN M.D. and al.
Technique and results of venous valve transplantation. In : Surgery of the Veins.
J.J. BERGAN and J.S.T. YAO. ORLANDO.
GRUNE and STRATTON. 1985 ; 219-31.

6 O'DONNEL T.F., MACKEY M.C., SHEPAR A.D.
Clinical, hemodynamic and anatomic follow-up of direct venous reconstruction.
Arch. Surg., 1987 ; 122 : 474-82.

Intraoperative evaluative method of deep venous valvuloplasty for primary valvular incompetence
-reference to supravalvular hydrostatic pressure method-

Naoki Konagai, Y. Obitsu, H. Fukushima, S. Ishimaru, K. Furukawa

The 2nd Department of Surgery, Tokyo Medical College, 6-7-1 Nishishinjuku, Shinjuku, Tokyo 160, Japan

INTRODUCTION

We have performed saphenous vein stripping and perforating vein ligation to varicose veins, but have experienced several cases of recurrent varicose veins and venous ulcers at long-term postoperative days. So we conducted retrograde phlebography (RPG) before operation, valvuloplasty was done to the case with significant deep venous valve reflux. And the observation of the valve cusp by fiberoptic angioscopy and the measuring of supravalvular hydrostatic pressure (SVH pressure) were performed for intraoperative evaluation. Herein we report our study results.

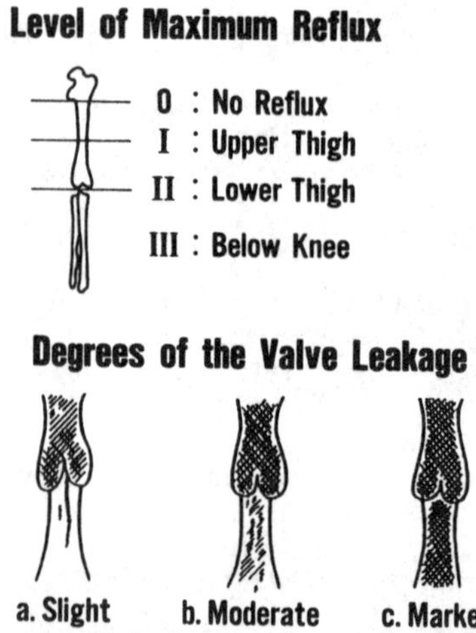

Fig.1 : Functional integrity of the venous valve was classified according to the level of maximum reflux and the degree of valve leakage.

MATERIALS AND METHODS

From August 1990 to the present, we conducted RPG on 110 cases who were admitted to our hospital for surgical treatment of varicose veins. The common femoral vein was punctured with 21G-elastic needle. Contrast medium was injected into the vein at 60° semi-upright position with the Valsalva maneuver. Functional integrity of the valve was graded based on the level of maximum reflux (0, I, II, III) and the contrast degree of valve reflux (a, b, c).(Fig. 1) The indications for plasty were limited to IIIb reflux with skin changes or IIIc reflux, and in result, we performed valvuloplasty on 25 cases (25 legs).

The present study was done on 25 subjects, 15 males and 10 females, average age was 57 years old. Prior to surgery, 10 of these subjects were grade IIIb and 15 were IIIc.

Surgery was done under systemic heparinization, and a fiberoptic angioscopy was inserted via the saphenous vein influx to observe the valve while it was being flushed with saline solution. Saline solution leaking toward the peripheral region was drained through an incision made in the peripheral vessel. In 14 of the cases we recently treated, we inserted an elastic tube in the upper part of the valve via the saphenous vein influx, and filled the vein and tube with saline solution, and measured the following parameters (SVH method):

1) height to which saline solution in a tube set upright finally fell to,
2) time required for the saline solution to reach its final height,
3) falling velocity.

Measurement were made in accordance with SVH method (Fig. 2) before and after valvuloplasty. For valvuloplasty, a longitudinal venotomy was made on the central side of the valve, and the redundant valve cusps were plicated to each commissures using 7-0 monofilament sutures. Stripping and ligation were then performed, but heparin was not generally neutralized.

RESULTS

(1) Fiberoptic angioscopy

In the venous valve where reflux occurred, two redundant valve cusps were observed undulating from the force of saline solution flushing. After valvuloplasty, valve cusps were re-strained.

(2) SVH method

Final height (SVH pressure) was significantly elevated ($p<0.001$), going from 8.9 ± 7.8cmH$_2$O before plasty to 18.3 ± 7.0cmH$_2$O after; this indicated that the valve had incurred higher pressure. Falling time increased significantly ($p<0.01$) from 13.7 ± 5.2sec to 18.3 ± 7.0sec. Falling velocity also significantly dropped ($p<0.01$) from 3.9 ± 2.8cm/sec to 2.1 ± 1.5cm/sec.

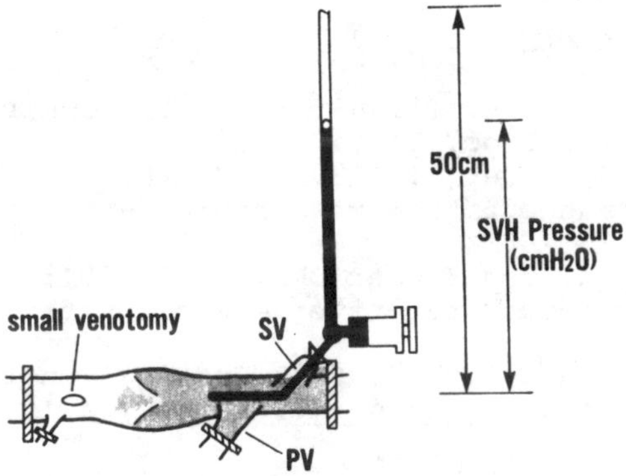

Fig.2 : SVH pressure is expressed in centimeters of water.
SV : Saphenous vein. PV : Profunda vein.

(3) Postoperative RPG

In 2 cases RPG findings did not change, but in all other cases RPG findings improved after valvuloplasty (Fig. 3).

DISCUSSION

Valvuloplasty is surgical procedure for primary valvular incompetence. There are several approaches to venotomy, including vertical incision via the commissure (Kistner, 1968), transversal incision on the central side of the valve (Raju, 1988), and a combination of the two (Koyano, 1990). We attempted vertical incision not via the commissure but on the central side of the valves, obtaining a satisfactory field of vision.

Intraoperative evaluation can include blood pressure measurements in the dorsal vein of foot (Sottiurai, 1991), strip tests, and others. We studied venous blood pressure directly applied to the valve. SVH pressure (final height) reflected the highest pressure (threshold) in the upper part of the valve, which prevented reflux. SVH pressure significantly elevated by valvuloplasty, and it indicate quantitative improvement in valve function.

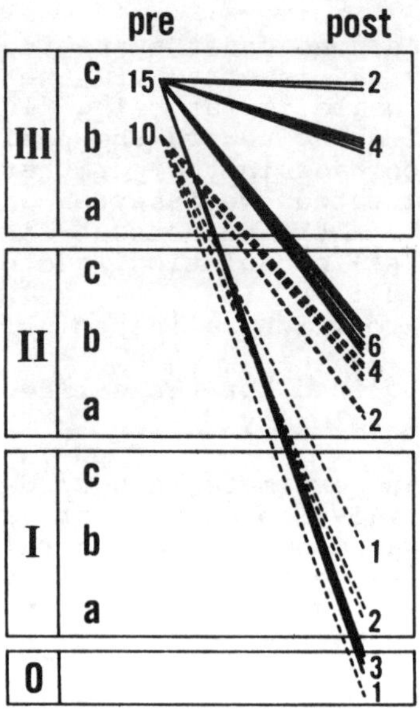

Fig.3 :
Results of retrograde phrebography.
(Pre and Post valvuloplasty)

As valvuloplasty carries the risk of postoperative thrombo-obstruction, there are not reports like ours on valvuloplasty done to prevent the recurrence of varicose veins. Although we only conducted perioperative systemic heparinization and did not perform postoperative anticoagulation therapy, we encountered no postoperative thrombo-obstruction. We have not obtained the long-term postoperative results, but the results from this study suggest that conducting valvuloplasty in addition to the conventional stripping or ligation is significant for preventing the recurrence of varicosis or ulcers.

REFERENCES

Kistner, R.L. (1988): Surgical repair of a venous valve. Straub Clin. Proc. 34: 41-43.

Koyano, K. et al.(1990): Valvuloplasty and vein segment transportation in chronic venous insufficiency. Jpn. J. Phlebol. 1: 33-40.

Raju, S. and Fredericks, R. (1988): Valve reconstruction procedure for nonobstructive venous insufficiency. J. Vasc. Surg. 7: 301-309.

Sottiurai, V.S. (1991): Surgical correction of recurrent venous ulcer. J. Card. Surg. 32: 104-109.

Phlébologie 92. Eds P. Raymond-Martimbeau, R. Prescott, M. Zummo.
John Libbey Eurotext, Paris © 1992, pp. 1217

Incorporation pattern of alloplastic protheses

G. Dasbach, K.M. Müller

Institut für Pathologie, BG-Krankenanstalten « Bergmannsheil », Universitätsklinik, 4630 Bochum 1, Germany.

Within histological, immunohistochemical, immunofluorescence and electronmicroscopical methods we analyzed the incorporation pattern of 50 prostheses, made of Teflon and Dacron.
The duration of the implantation periods ranged from 30 minutes up to 10 years. The findings show a different transprosthetic organization and degradation of the material by cells and components of the extracellular matrix. The results of the investigation could demonstrate reasons for different complications after vascular reconstruction.

VENOUS RECONSTRUCTION IN THE TREATMENT OF POST-PHLEBITIC ULCER.

FUAD AL ASSAL; A.C.S. GOMES; RICARDO AL ASSAL.

PUC UNIVERSITY MEDICAL SCHOOL . CAMPINAS - BRAZIL.

PATIENT: - 60 years old, had hip replacement and acute deep venous thrombosis 10 years ago. Right leg ulcer since 9 years. Conservative therapy and saphenectomy without sucess. After phlebography and venous pressure study, Venous Reconstruction with contralateral saphena was done. Video shows aspects of leg ulcer and phlebography with recanalized limb veins.

SURGERY: - Incision on left groin for discovery of saphena. Retrograde injection of saline for competency test of saphena. Saphena dissection and excision from groin to upper third of leg. Careful preparation of saphena. Incision at right groin Dissection of femoral artery and vein (common and deep). Incision at distal third of thigh. Discovery of popliteal artery and vein. Oblique section of popliteal vein. Anastomosis of its distal stumps with saphena graft, using interrupted sutures with prolene 5.0 or 6.0. Graft is passed under Sartorius to groin. Oblique section of graft and end to side anastomosis with common femoral vein, with similar technique.

Our experience in P.T. venous surgery

O. Dall'Aglio, M. Zurita, M. Julis

Universidad Nacional De La Plata

From 1970 to the actuality, we totalized 136 surgeries. The total was divided according to the pathology in Avalvulation and Persitent occlusion of the deep venous system (P.O.D.V.S.)

In Avalvulation, until 1981, we made 18 indirect surgeries. From 1981 in advance, we made four kind of direct surgeries:

- Venous valve transplantation 39
- Venous transposition 12
- Venous valvuloplasty 05
- Combinated procedures 01
- Miscellaneous: Other procedures 04 ... totalizing 61

In P.O.D.V.S.: we divided our experience in four groups:

- Group I:29
- Group II:15
- Group III:10
- Group IV:03 ... totalizing 57

We'll show our experience at more than 10 years.

Phlébologie 92. Eds P. Raymond-Martimbeau, R. Prescott, M. Zummo.
John Libbey Eurotext, Paris © 1992, pp. 1219-1221

Post-thrombotic syndrome venous valve transplantation : surgical procedures

Osvaldo Dall' Aglio, *et al.*

Department of Vascular Surgery, Universidad Nacional de la Plata, Clínica Avenida, calle 11 n° 1018, La Plata, Provincia de Buenos Aires, CP 1900, Argentina.

It is a known fact that,in a venous thrombosis,if a timely **treat** -ment - has no been undertaken,lives a post thrombotic syndrome due-to: Persistent occlution of the deep venous sistem,...or

Avalvulation,becouse of valv digestion during the process of clot reabsortion

...,both producing distal venous hipertention

Avalvulation can be total or partial (proximal or distal)

In the surgical evolution of P.T.S.treatment,we consider two ages

-From 1970 to 1981,we made indirect surgical procedures(Psathakis)

-From 1981 in advance,we are making five different direct surgical procedures:Venous Transplant

Venous Transposition

Venous Valvuloplasty

Combinated procedures

Other procedures

in this paper,we are going to talk only about Venous transplantation

The first who made a venous valv transplant was Fuadd Al Assad , from Brasil in 1976;posteriorly it was well diffused by S.Tahery,from Buffalo U.S.in 1981,in the International Vascular Symposium of London We were listening and from that,we consider that the venous valv - transplant age was began.

So,in 1981 Tahery spoke about two-centimeter brachial vein transplant in femoral position and,in end to end venous anastomosis.In the same year,we propouse:five-to-eight-centimeter superficial vein (saphenous,cephalic or basilic) transplanted at both femoral and popliteal level,tricompartimented the system in order to be congruent - with the phisiopathology.In our first successful surgery,we made - double transplant at both,femoral and popliteal level(four by pass) becouse of the hemodinamical criteria of equalty of the diameters; making a complementary temporary A-V shunt.In 1982 we began to - use distal A-V shunt.In 1983,isolated popliteal venous valv transplant,becouse of the same phisiopatological criteria that Psatha - use to made his discontinuated external popliteal valv.In 1984 we sistematized the use of Venous transplant.So,if we make one by pass even at femoral or popliteal level,we ever use a 5-to-8,end-to-end cm superficial vein transplant,but when we make more than one,given the difficulties to made a 5-to-8 cm,end-to-end,popliteal anastomosis,we can make,at popliteal level a 4 cm,end-to-end by pass , or a longer one in end-to-side or side-to-side.Surgical findings - are the bassament of them.In 1985 we bigan to work with all principals venous va cular Services in our country.Fron that merge: The use of Valv-less Protocol and the introduction of group IV of the-classification of cronical venous inssufficiency in the above mentionated protocol.In the same year,we sistematized the use of distal A-V shunt in venous transplantation in cases of:

-More than one by pass,...or

-Forced valv

ACTUALLY,we totalized 39 Venous transplantation

Double transplant	single	06
	double	02
Single transplant	femoral	06
	politeo	25

Post operative evolution,must to be controlled by clinical ,Non invasive and invasive methods.

In Clinical Criteria,we must to consider:A drastic reduction of the oedema and asociated symptoms

A close of the venous-Ulcer

A recovery of working-capacity possibility

In Non Invasive Criteria:Doppler:recovering of Valsalva Manouver cantention and proximal augmentation negative

Reflux IPG:Recovering of valvular time

SPG in MVO or VO/VC,must be normal

Invasive Criteria are absolutly indicated for the other ones.If we are planing to make a phlebgram(ascending)it's better to make - first a phlebodynamomanometry,looking for the during excercise ve - nous presures.Also,if we made a descending phlebogram to a double - transplant(femoral and popliteo)we are going to see only the upper valv,if it is working perfectly.

Also there are no the best option,in comparison with Venous Valv Transposition,are there the most frecuent surgery recourse.

We report 90% of permeability in more than 5 years.

One of our patients death becouse a Ulcerated Colitis in an e-mergency-abdominal episode

One of our patients,the number seven expierence,present a venous transplant thrombosis becouse of a forced valv and we never have seen any more after we made a distal A-V shunt in dubds cases.

Six of all needs to use elastic vandaje or stokes,becouse of re cidual oedema.

Until now,we never have seen venous aneurism in a transplanted-segment(tahery)but,we must to enfatized that we ever use superficial veins in five to eight centimeter-segment

From 1984,we do not close the distal A-V shunt becouse it gives to the system anterograde venous hiperflux.

COMMENTS:When we take into account the fact that valveless-PTS, is the illnes that most affets the working-capacity in man,to obtain that a patient who formarlly was condemned to rest and inactivity , with the improductivity that this intrains,can now be rehabilited - does not call for any further comments.

BIBLIOGRAPHY

1-Bergan J,Yao ST:Venous Problems.Chicago,1978;Yearbook Medical Pub.

2-Dall'Aglio O:Sistema Venoso Profundo Avalvulado.Rev.Ana.Flebología diciembre 1981.Volumen III nº3 pag.174/176

3-Dall'Aglio O,Kenny J & Berro N:Síndrome Post Trombótico.Rev.Ana.de Flebología.Vol.I nº 2 pag.87/88.1977

4-Dall'Aglio O:Síndrome Post Trombótico.Ed.Celcius.Bs.As.Ana.1989

5-Simkin R:Várices Ulceras y Angiodisplasias.Libreros Lopez.B.A.1991

6-Taheri SA,Lazar L,et al:Vein Valve Transplant.Surgery Vol.91 nº 1 pp 28-33.1981

7-Tahery SA:Status of vein valve transplant after twelve months.Com. 060 of the programe and abstracts International Vascular Symposium London.UK.1981

Phlébologie 92. Eds P. Raymond-Martimbeau, R. Prescott, M. Zummo.
John Libbey Eurotext, Paris © 1992, pp. 1222-1223

Post-thrombotic syndrome venous valve transposition : surgical procedures

Osvaldo Dall' Aglio, *et al.*

Department of Vascular Surgery, Universidad Nacional de la Plata, Clínica Avenida, calle 11 n° 1018, La Plata, Provincia de Buenos Aires, CP 1900, Argentina.

Venous Transposition began in 1980 with Kistner and Queral & Whitehouse for the upper(femoral)forms.In 1981 we include distal (popliteal) and totals ones,and in 1991 the combinated (high plus distal).Actually,we intented to present a clasification that easily permit a total comprehension of the problem.

We classified the pathology according to the place to be transposed in: A (Altas or Hight:Femorals)

B (Bajas or Distal:Popliteals)

C (Combinated : Popliteo-Femorals)

T (totals)

<u>In A</u> (Femoral)cases,we've got the possibility to use Kistner or Queral technics(A,B,C).In all this,we prefer Queral procedures,becouse Kistner one are,for us,a litle bit troublesome and may be - thrombogenous.In Queral,we've got expierence with A and C modes.

<u>In B</u> (Popliteal)cases,we descrived Parvous Saphnous vein and - Gastrocnemius vein possibilities,or both in the same time.

<u>In C</u> (Femoro-popliteal or combinated)we use the sumatory of A plus B surgical possibilities

<u>In T</u> (total)We present the possibility to make a total femoro-femoral transposition between a valveless principal femoral vein , and a accesory or parasit valvulated femoral vein

With out dubs,venous trasposition is the better option in venous valv reconstruction,but it's only a radiological finding.When the reconstruction is a litle bit forced or when we make a combinated resolution,we use distal A-V shunt

Casuistic

Group A(Parcial femoral) Queral "A" :02
Queral "C" :01

We do not use Kistner nor Queral "B"

Group B(Parcial popliteal)

-with Gastrocnemious Vein :01

-with parvus saphenous Vein :02

-with G.V,plus P.S.Vein :01

Group C(Combinated popliteo-femoral)

using P.S.V plus L.S.Vein :02

Group T(Totals)

using Accesory Femoral Vein :05

Actually,we totalized 14 cases.

We use distal A-V shunt in 3 cases: 1 in group B with a double transposition of gastrocnemious and Parvus Saphenous Veins

2 cases of combinated popliteo-femoral,using Long Saphenous Vein for the upper,and Parvus Saphenous Vein for the distal

Until now,we never have seen complications.

100% of good results.

COMMENTS:In a Post Thrombotic Syndrome,it's very important to make a carely diagnosis,becouse cases like that,are only radiological findings,during the diagnosis process.

BIBLIOGRAPHY

1-Bergan J and Yao J:Venous Problems.Year book Medical publishers . Chicago.1978

2-Dall'Aglio O.:Valvuloplastía fisiológica por transplante mas transposición venosa.6ª Sesión Científica AMA.Sociedad de Flebología y Linfología.1981

3-Dall'Aglio O.:Síndrome Post Trombótico.Ed.Celcius.Bs.As.1989

4-Hernan EJ et al:Descending Venography:a method of evaluating lower extremity venous valvular function.Radiology 137:63.1972

5-Kistner R.and Ferris EG.:Technique of surgical reconstruction of femoral vein valves.Bergan and Yao(EDS)Operative technique in vascular surgery.New York Grune and Stratton p.291/300.1980

6-Pietravallo A.:Flebopatías superficiales y profundas,p 340/341.Publicación del Dto.Médico Ciba-Geigy Argentina

7-Queral L et al:Surgical correction of chronic venous insufficiency by valvular transposition.Surgery 87-688/95.1980

8-Simkin R:Várices,Ulceras y Angiodisplasias.Libreros Lopez.B.A.1991

Phlébologie 92. Eds P. Raymond-Martimbeau, R. Prescott, M. Zummo.
John Libbey Eurotext, Paris © 1992, pp. 1224-1226

Vein-vein bypass with valvuloplasty in the post-thrombotic syndrome

Roberto Simkin, Juan Carlos Esteban, Ruben Bulloj

Quintana Private Hospital, Malabia 3166, Buenos Aires, Argentina.

Deep thrombophlebitis leaves serious sequels in patients improperly treated.At present due to the fact that thromboflebitis is better understood and to the use of anticoagulants,it is less frequent.Nevertheless, after a number of years, many patients show a clinical picture of chronic venous insufficiency.This is brought about by chronic venous hypertension which is the result of a permanentocclusion of the deep venous system or vascular dilation and destruction.

In this paper we shall describe our experience with the final stage,using techniques which have advanced considerably in the last few years allow for a different prognosis for this type of patients

To better understand the different types of surgical management of the post thrombotic syndrome in the various stages,we have classifield it as follows.In the post thrombotic non recanalized the authors describe the,Palma's ,Warren's,Dale's,Izquierdo's and the personal thechnique (Simkin).In the Post thrombotic syndrome recanalized (valveless) the authors describe the, Taheri,Kistner"s Queral's ,Psataquis,and the associated techniques .All this techniques are associated to the arteriovenous temporary fistulae. There are anatomically thrombogenic zones,i.e. the crural arch withthe superior deep femoral veins; the illiac intercrosing, illiac veins and the left illiac artery;Hunter's canal:superficial femoral and popliteal veins.The illiac intercrossing described by Cocket appears as the cause of acute thromboflebitis in ours stadistics an must be taken into account because the pronosis of the treatment willdepend on the solution to the anatomical problem that is ,on the descompresion of the illiac vein compressed by the artery,followed by the clearing of the distal thrombosed venous trunk.

Materials and Method:

1-Non recanalized post thrombotic Syndrome:

Since we began our experience with surgery of the non recanalized syndrome,13 cases of direct femoro femoral by pass (Warren 's) operation,with homolateral internal saphenous vein were carried out,with temporaryarteriovenous fistulae in the last 8 cases.

In those cases where a temporary arteriovenous fistulae was used it was closed three weeeks later and a very important dilation of the grafted vein could be observed.Of the 8 cases ,in the period of two years,three shwoed oclussion,with the patiens returning to the pre operative condition.The remain cases are in in good condition until the present time.In one of them,no clear remission of the symptoms could be observed, and the oedema and venous claudication persist.In our series, we had 19 cases of crossed by pass with Palma's technique, 11 cases with temporary arteriovenous distal fistula,for which the saphenous vein was used.In one case, the phlebographic studies showed occlusion in the inmediate post operative period.In anauther case it was necessary to reoperate after a two hours due to obstruction of the by pass.A good flow and permeability were obtained and are maintained until the present time.In this case,we beleve the inmediatye obstruction was due to the fistula being to long and once it was modified,it remained permeable during the three remaining weeks.The others cases had a good evolution,with an evident remission of the syntomatology and oedema or ulcer.

2-Recanalized Post Thrombotic Syndrome(valveless).

We shall summarize the results obtained on a total 42 patients operated upon with the various techniques.Intraluminal (Simkin's) Valvuloplasty:4 cases with very good inmediste results,atthough the long term results are less than 50 per cent improvement. Femoral valvuloplasty (Tahery) venous venous by pass 8 cases,with good inmediate results ,although the long term imrpvment is in the order of 60 per cent.All the cases were characterized by relapsed of the malleal oedema.The transposition (Queral's) technique 11 cases with which the best inmediate and late post operative result were obtained,with 90 per cent improvements.Two cases of open ulcers healed completely,one of the cases had an oedema which decreased by nearly 80 per cent and the other patients showed a marked decrease in distal hypertensive symptomatology. Valvuloplasty (femoro-popliteal by pass) it was carried out simultaneously in two cases with very encouragin post operative results ,although the long term improvementhas yet to be evaluated

Discussion:

The results obtained with venous revascularization by means of by pass, since 1971 when this type of surgery was first applied, have been extremely encouraging.The evaluation of all cases is done by means of: Phlebomanometry,of great value in the post-operative period;Dynamic Isotopic Phlebography with a CRT screen. The surgery of venous reflux (valveless-recanalized) has had variations lately due to the implementation of new surgical techniques.Our patiens are evaluated on the basis of phlebomanometry and their clinical condition.A case is considered to have a good or excelent evolution when the ulcers close in the inmediate post operative period or if the claudicating pain or oedema disappear. Moderate when said synptoms decrease by 50 per cent and bad when the pain ,oedema and venous claudication persist, and even more so when there is a relapse of an ulcer. In our opinion, the ideal technique or treatment to solve the serious venous hipertension problems caused by the post thrombotic syndrome has not yet been found,but there currently exist techniqu witch, properly applied, can help omprove the patients life style.

References:

Bauer G:"A Roentegenologic and clinical study of the sequels of the Thrombosis",Acta Chirurg,Scand,86:174,1942.

Cocket F:"Abnormalities of the deep veins of the legs",Post Grad, medic.Journ 1964,30:512-18.

Felder D,Murphy T,and Ring: " A posterior facial approach to the comunicating veins of the legss" Surg Gyn.and Obst 1955:100,730.78

Palma E: "Surgical treatment of acute thrombophlebitis and post thrombotic syndrome".VI Latin American Congress of Angiology, 1962

Palma E,Esperon R,:"Surgical Treatment of the post thrombotic phlebitis syndrome by transplantation of the internal saphenous vein" Angiologia Ap.1959,vol XI ,No 2 .

Simkin R: "Venous Diseases" Lopez PUb.1979,Buenos Aires Argentina.

Simkin R : " Varicos Veins,Ulcers and Angiodisplasias",Lopez Edito 1991,Buenos Aires Argentina.

Vollmar J:"Vascular Endoscopy,Posibilities and limits of its clinicals aplication",Surg.Clin.Noth America 1974;54:111.

Kistner R.L.:"Surgical repair of the incompetent femoral vein valve"Arch Surg,100:1336-1342,1975.

Queral L:"Surgical correction of chronic deep venous insuficiency by valvular transposition",Surgery,87:688,1980.

Phlébologie 92. Eds P. Raymond-Martimbeau, R. Prescott, M. Zummo.
John Libbey Eurotext, Paris © 1992, pp. 1227-1229

An evaluation of femoral vein valvuloplasty, selection of patients by descending venography. Operative technique and results

C.A. Kruse, R.C. Webb Jr, C.J. Bos

Departments of Surgery and Radiology, Saint John's Hospital and Health Center, Santa Monica, California, USA.

This presentation is an evaluation of two techniques of femoral vein valvuloplasty on the deep venous system to control or improve those difficult cases of recurrent ulceration or skin changes. This procedure deals with those patients without a history of deep venous thrombosis but with recurrent skin changes after greater and lesser saphenous vein ligation and stripping with multiple counter ligations for incompetent perforator veins. Primary superficial vein varicosities on the basis of isolated sapheno-femoral or perforator valve incompetence seems unlikely. As suggested by others, there may be a congenital or developmental weakness in the valve system on a global basis. Our patient selection was by digital subtraction descending venogram -- ordered on the basis of a high index of suspicion based on 30+ years of clinical experience. No screening test is presented -- although others (Raju, S., 1983 & Christopoulos, D. & Nicolaides, A.N., et al, 1988) have published unique screening methods.

Femoral vein valve incompetence was first treated by Kistner of Honolulu, Hawaii, USA in 1968. He used a vertical incisional approach, reporting on 17 limbs in 14 patients (Kistner, R.L., 1975). An alternative approach by a transverse incision above the valve leaflets was developed by Raju of the University of Mississippi, USA. With the vertical incision of Kistner -- great care is necessary to make the venotomy through the junction of the two cusps on the anterior aspect of the vein. A fine Prolene suture is placed at the valve cusp juncture which can usually be seen through the vein wall just to one side of the anterior surface. Sometimes this is difficult to see, but absolutely necessary to avoid damage to the vein cusps themselves. Two to three minutes after 5000u of Heparin IV, the vein is opened. The redundant leaflets can be seen with magnification, although they are very thin and filmy in appearance. A 7-0 Prolene suture is passed through the vein wall, picking up the edges of the valve cusps and then passing the reefing suture out again and tying the same on the outside of the vein wall. It may take several such interrupted reefing sutures to take up the slack in the valve leaflet at each valve commissure. With this approach, the two valve leaflets must be carefully reapproximated anteriorly, and the venotomy closed with a continuous suture. The "strip test" is done to test valve competency.

The transverse incision (Raju, S., 1983) is placed well above the valve cusps to avoid injury to same. The transverse incision seemed to allow the operator to more adequately estimate the necessary size and number of the interrupted reefing sutures to take up the slack in the valve leaflet at each commissure. However, visualization of the thin valve leaflets was more difficult when the vein was initially opened -- even with magnification. The CFV, PFV and the SFV are exposed initially. <u>It is important</u> that the valve repaired be the first major valve just at or below the confluence of the profunda femoris and the superficial femor-al veins -- so as to avoid reflux from the profunda system through the incompetent superficial femoral vein valves --if valvuloplasty is done at the common femoral vein level.

In this short presentation, one patient is presented in detail. This 61-year old female initially had bilateral greater and lesser saphenous vein ligations and stripping with multiple counter ligations by the author in 1981. In spite of faithfully wearing gradient pressure elastic hose of 30-40 mm Hg strength daily while continuing to work as a secretary in the aerospace industry, she developed recurrent stasis dermatitis of both ankles. Ascending venograms in 1983 had revealed no evidence of deep venous thrombosis or obstruction. Impending ulceration of the left medial malleolar region with secondary infection was ultimately treated by resection of the area and a split thickness skin graft to the <u>left</u> lower extremity in <u>1986</u>. This healed well, but ultimately, in spite of continued use of compression to control any venous stasis, the skin graft area began to "weep." Stasis dermatitis persisted over the <u>right</u> lower extremity. Therefore, bilateral digital subtraction <u>descending</u> venograms (Kruse, C.A., et al, 1989) were carried out via a catheter placed in the common femoral veins which demonstrated "marked incompetency of the valves in the upper portion of the femoral veins bilaterally." This patient had a femoral vein valve repair on the <u>left</u> side by <u>transverse</u> <u>incision</u> above the valve leaflets in 1987 and on the right side by a <u>vertical</u> <u>incision</u> valvuloplasty in 1988. After the right femoral vein valvuloplasty, a fluid collection continued to recur in spite of <u>repeated</u> <u>aspirations</u> of the operative site. Because of swelling of the distal thigh area a repeat <u>ascending</u> venogram was carried out. This revealed wide patency of the iliac veins, femoral veins, and popliteal vein. The clear aspirate revealed an albumin content -- consistent with peripheral lymph fluid. The <u>edema</u> <u>subsided</u> <u>after</u> this <u>fluid</u> <u>sac</u> <u>was</u> <u>removed</u> -- relieving pressure on the femoral vein.

Postoperative descending venograms were obtained. In October, 1987, the valve at the upper end of the left superficial femoral vein appeared highly competent. In November, 1988, when the right side was studied, there was some mild to moderate incompetency of the valve in the upper portion of the <u>right</u> femoral vein during the Valsalva maneuver. The skin changes distally were improved or controlled in spite of the less than 100% competency of this valve repair. The <u>left</u> lower extremity, some 11 months following valvuloplasty, showed some tendency to stasis dermatitis above the skin graft -- prior to complete control by Compression Sclerotherapy of persisting incompetent perforating veins below the knee. In 1989, skin changes were controlled or improved over both lower extremities and there was no further edema of either extremity. The patient is now going without her gradient pressure hose on an intermittent trial basis at the present time.

Two complications in the five limbs operated were the formation of a cystic space due to a persistent lymph collection. This occurred in limbs operated via the vertical venotomy - and where chronic lymphadenitis was evident, secondary to prior or ongoing skin changes. This illustration shows the "mesothelial-lined sac" and the healed operative site in a 6 foot, 6 inch, 240 lb. male in whom a right valvuloplasty was performed one year previously. His distal right lower extremity remains improved.

IN CONCLUSION: Clinical improvement was obtained in all 5 limbs (4 patients) but persistent lymphorrhea occurred in 2 -- treated surgically at 6 and 12 months post-valvuloplasty. Vertical venotomies were used in these 2 limbs and transverse venotomies in the other 3 limbs. A long longitudinal incision over the femoral vein allowed better visualization of the valve cusps, but it was more difficult to estimate the number or size of the reefing sutures to produce a competent valve. The transverse incision seemed to allow the operator to more adequately estimate the necessary size and number of the interrupted reefing sutures to take up the slack in the valve leaflets at each valve commissure. However, visualization of the thin valve leaflets was more difficult when the vein was initially opened. Pre and postoperative digital subtraction descending venograms were obtained in all patients for this study.

REFERENCES:

Christopoulos, D. & Nicolaides, A.N., et al, (1988): Venous Reflux: Quantification And Correlation With The Clinical Severity Of Chronic Venous Disease.
Br J Surg 1988 Apr; 75(4): 352-6

Kistner, R.L. (1975): Surgical Repair Of The Incompetent Femoral Vein Valve. Arch Surg 110 (11): 1336-42, Nov 1975.

Kruse, C.A., Webb, Jr., R.C., Bos, C.J. (1989): An Evaluation Of Femoral Vein Valvuloplasty: Selection Of Patients By Descending Venography - Operative Technique And Results. 10eme Congres Mondial Union Internationale De Phlebologie. Poster Session.

Kruse, C.A., Webb, Jr., R.C., Bos, C.J. (1990): An Evaluation Of Femoral Vein Valvuloplasty: Selection Of Patients By Descending Venography - Operative Technique And Results. Scientific Exhibit At The Clinical Congress, San Francisco, CA., October 7-12, 1990, Of The American College Of Surgeons.

Raju, S. (1983): Venous Insufficiency Of The Lower Limb And Stasis Ulceration: Changing Concepts And Management.
Ann Surg 197: 688, 1983.

Phlébologie 92. Eds P. Raymond-Martimbeau, R. Prescott, M. Zummo.
John Libbey Eurotext, Paris © 1992, pp. 1230-1233

Reconstructive venous valvular surgery : preliminary experience and perspectives

Pietro Belardi, Germano Lucertini

Cattedra di Chirurgia Vascolare, Università degli Studi di Genova, Viale Benedetto XV, 10 16132 Genova, Italy.

Deep venous insufficiency is commonly the most severe type of the chronic venous disease. The management had great development during the last three decades. Role of conservative measures (hygienic rules, elastic stocking and pharmacotherapy) is defined. They have application always in each case. Surgery must be associated with these in symptomatic legs. Today surgery consists of several procedures, some of which are alternative. Conventional surgery, constituted by communicating veins interruption and stripping, is widely validated. These procedures must be performed in each case requiring surgical treatment. New trends of the last three decades are constituted by attempts for recovery of valvular function in the deep venous system. Such techniques, complementary to conventional surgery, are the most ambitious expression of the modern venous surgery. At the present time several surgical techniques for correction of deep venous valvular incompetence are known.

We have examined our experience to identify criteria and properties of some procedures for venous valvular reconstruction.

Material and methods

We have performed a retrospective study relating cases of deep venous insufficiency treated by venous valvular reconstruction. In all cases surgical procedure on deep veins was associated with subfascial interruption of communicating veins and stripping of greater and/or lesser saphenous veins, if it had indication.

Three limbs with deep venous insufficiency (grade II) (1) and grade 2 or 3 reflux (2) for valvular ring dilatation received venous cuff. Two females (one with bilateral lesion), aged 18 and 19, were operated upon. Assessment of results was found on clinical evaluation, Doppler C.W., photoplethysmography, strain-gauge plethysmography and ascending venography (descending venography too in one extremity). Surgical procedure is constituted by implantation of Dacron cuff, 4 cm long, around the proximal segment of the superficial femoral vein, immediately under the junction with the deep femoral vein (3). Follow-up ranged 6 through 12 months.

Venous valvular transposition was performed in 2 limbs (2 females, aged 55 and 41). Surgical indication was postthrombotic syndrome grades III and II (1) with recanalization of the infrapopliteal, popliteal and superficial femoral veins. The injured proximal segment of the great saphenous vein was utilised to correct venous valvular function (4). Results were

evaluated according clinical examination, Doppler C.W. and ascending venography. Follow-up was 10 and 11 years.
Venous valve transplant was performed in 8 lower extremities (7 patients, 4 males and 3 females, age ranging from 29 to 64 years, mean 48). Indication to surgery was postthrombotic syndrome grade III (6 cases) and II (2 cases) (1) with recanalization of infrapopliteal, popliteal and femoral veins. Transplant was performed at the above knee popliteal level through posterior (5 cases) or medial (3 cases) approach (5 6). A segment of ipsilateral great saphenous vein (4 cases) or brachioaxillary vein (4 cases) was utilised. A PTFE cuff was implanted around the transplanted venous valvular segment. Assessment of results was made according clinical evaluation, Doppler C.W., photoplethysmography and ascending venography. Follow-up was 6 to 26 months.

Results

With regard to venous cuff, all 3 lower extremities operated upon showed improvement. It is associated with correction of venous valvular incompetence, as Doppler C.W. and descending venography confirmed, and normalisation of photoplethysmographic venous refilling time.
Based on clinical criteria, Doppler C.W. and venography, one limb operated upon for venous valvular transposition showed satisfactory results, while in the other ulcer recurred.
Thrombosis was never observed in the venous valvular transplant group. Valvular incompetence developed in 2/8 (25%) cases, in which a segment of the ipsilateral great saphenous vein was utilised. Based on patency and valvular competence of the graft and clinical presentation, the results were positive in 4/8 (50%) cases. Beyond the 2 cases with valvular incompetence of the graft, venous valvular graft failed to yield satisfactory clinical results indeed in 1 limb for unrecovered ulcer and in 1 limb for recurrence of ulcer.

Discussion

At the present time several surgical procedures are available for correction of deep venous valvular incompetence. They have been proposed, modified and investigated relating their pathophysiological bases in the last thirty years. Today criteria of application for different surgical techniques can be defined.
On the basis of our experience, limited up today only to three surgical techniques and few cases, it is possible to define some important trends.
Dilatation of valvular ring, characterized by very large deep veins and secondary valvular incompetence, can be solved by venous cuff. This is a rational and effective surgical technique. Such device limits mechanically the venous dilatation, restoring valvular competence. The surgical technique can correct fully hemodynamic changes according our own observations, despite correction of valvular incompetence is performed at a single level (superficial femoral vein). It can be employed in cases with reflux grade 2, 3 and 4. Thereafter it is important to select the cases according to descending venography (or duplex scanning) and to investigate them by noninvasive and invasive examinations for the follow-up. Doppler C.W., photoplethysmography and strain-gauge plethysmography, beyond ambulatory venous pressure measurements, are looked adequate to the aforementioned aim in our series.
Applications of venous valve transposition are not numerous in the treatment of postthrombotic venous valvular incompetence. The procedure requires an uninjured great saphenous or deep femoral vein (7-12). Such condition is infrequent found indeed in limbs

with postthrombotic venous femoropopliteal lesion for concomitant change of those veins. This consideration justifies a very few cases in whom the procedure can be employed.
Venous valve transplantation can be stressed today as the most rational and functional procedure. It allows the correction of valvular incompetence at single level using an injured venous segment (5 11-14). More pathophysiological investigations showed critical importance of the lower extremity distal veins to determine venous hemodynamic conditions (15-18). Considered these aspects, the popliteal level seems to be preferred. These considerations induced us from the beginning to perform this surgical operation at the popliteal level. Our results, likely to the ones of other authors (5 6 10-14), are encouraging.
Surgery of deep venous valvular incompetence have overcome pioneer's phase. We are waiting still for validation by wide series of more centres for some surgical techniques. We believe that some procedures are to be considered in therapeutical armamentarium. Venous valve transplant are looked as the best therapeutical option for its properties. It can be performed quite in all cases of deep venous valvular incompetence and its results are very promising indeed.

REFERENCES

1. O' Donnell TF Jr. Clinical diagnosis and classification of chronic venous insufficiency. In: Rutherford RB, ed. Vascular surgery. Third ed. Volume II. Philadelphia: WB Saunders, 1989: 1504-12.
2. Herman RJ, Neiman HL, Yao JST, Egan TJ, Bergan JJ, Malave SR. Descending venography; a method of evaluating lower extremity venous valvular function. Radiology 1980; 137: 63-9.
3. Hallberg D. A method for repairing incompetent valves in deep veins. Acta Chir Scand 1972; 138: 143-5.
4. Kistner RL, Sparkhul MD. Surgery in acute and chronic venous disease. Surgery 1979; 85: 31-43.
5. Taheri SA, McHugh W, Pendergast D, Meenaghan M. Results of vein valve transplant after 6 years. In: Sakaguchi S, ed. Advances in phlebology. London-Paris: John Libbey Eurotext, 1987: 99-102.
6. Nash T. Long term results of vein valve transplants placed in the popliteal vein for intractable post-phlebitic venous ulcers and pre-ulcer skin changes. J Cardiovasc Surg 1988; 29: 712-6.
7. Johnson ND, Queral LA, Flinn WR, Yao JST, Bergan JJ. Late objective assessment of venous valve surgery. Arch Surg 1981; 116: 15461-6.
8. Ferris EB, Kistner RL. Femoral vein reconstruction in the management of chronic venous insufficiency: a 14-year experience. Arch Surg 1982; 117: 1571-9.
9. Huse JB, Nabseth DC, Bush HL Jr, Widrich WC, Johnson WC. Direct venous surgery for venous valvular insufficiency of the lower extremity. Arch Surg 1983; 118: 719-23.
10. Raju S. Venous insufficiency of the lower limb and stasis ulceration. Changing concepts in management. Ann Surg 1983; 197: 688-97.
11. Perrin M, Hiltbrand B, Bolot JE, Genevois A. Résultats de la chirurgie veineuse restauratrice dans les reflux de la voie veineuse profonde au niveau des membres inférieurs. In: Davy A, Stemmer R, eds. Phlébologie 89. London-Paris: John Libbey Eurotext; 1989: 1085-6.
12. Sottiurai VS. Surgical correction of recurrent venous ulcer. J Cardiovasc Surg 1991; 32:

104-9.
13. Eriksson I, Almgren B. Influence of the profunda femoris vein on venous hemodynamics of the limb. Experience from thirty-one deep vein valve reconstructions. J Vasc Surg 1986; 4: 390-5.
14. O'Donnell TF, Mackey WC, Shepard AD, Callow AD. Clinical, hemodynamic, and anatomic follow-up of direct venous reconstruction. Arch Surg 1987; 122: 474-82.
15. Shull KC, Nicolaides AN, Fernandes é Fernandes J, Miles C, Horner J, Needham T, Cooke ED, Eastcott FHG. Significance of popliteal reflux in relation to ambulatory venous pressure and ulceration. Arch Surg 1979; 114: 1304-6.
16. Strandness DE Jr, Langlois Y, Cramer M, Randlett A, Thiele BL. Long-term sequelae of acute venous thrombosis. JAMA 1983; 250: 1289-92.
17. Moore DJ, Himmel PD, Sumner DS. Distribution of venous valvular incompetence in patients with the post-phlebitic syndrome. J Vasc Surg 1986; 3: 49-57.
18. Belardi P, Lucertini G. Postthrombotic syndrome: correlations between clinical status, location of venous involvement and ambulatory venous pressure. In: Davy A, Stemmer R, eds. Phlébologie 89. London-Paris: John Libbey Eurotext, 1989: 248-52.

Phlébologie 92. Eds P. Raymond-Martimbeau, R. Prescott, M. Zummo.
John Libbey Eurotext, Paris © 1992, pp. 1234

Venous-venous by pass associated distal arteriovenous fistulae

Roberto Simkin, Ruben Bulloj, Juan Carlos Esteban

Quintana Private Hospital, Malabia 3166, 1425 Buenos-Aires, Argentina.

This video shows a Warren's operation with distal arteriovenous temporary fistulae inside into the calcaneus tunnel between the posterior tibial artery and vein.
In this case the patient has an obstruction on the popliteo femoral area but with a nice distal venous layer.
This was possible to see at the phlebography done before the surgery .The patient presents intermitent venous claudication and big oedema,which increaase during the day.
The non invasive studies show the related obstruction and the the phlebodinamometry shows the important increase of the venous pressure.
The surgical thechniques used were by disectioning the saphena venous from the superior area of the thight and anastomosing it to the distal layer.
That contributes to the descomposition of the hipertension systemdue to the obstruction.
After that it is necesary to disect the posterior tibial artery and the posterior tibial vein by sectioning it and anastomosing it to the artery.
In this way we can see a good flow closing it by points.
It is necesary to leave the arteriovenous fistulae for three weeks.
After that we clouse definitively with local anesthesia.

Phlébologie 92. Eds P. Raymond-Martimbeau, R. Prescott, M. Zummo.
John Libbey Eurotext, Paris © 1992, pp. 1235-1237

Surgical treatment of chronic venous ulceration

Ralph G. DePalma, M.D.

George Washington University Medical Center

Venous hypertension causes changes at the capillary level wich ultimately results in ulceration. Since Linton's teaching in 1938[1], it has been considered important to interrupt incompetent communicating and perforating veins to control skin changes of venous stasis. A variety of operations evolved. In 1975[2], a modified operation was developed using Linton's principles to interrupt perforating and communicating veins t minimize transmission of venous hypertension to the skin and subcutaneous tissues. This technique employed a series of bipedical flaps in the natural skin lines which provided access to offending veins in the lower part of the leg. In 1979[3], a follow-un report detailed experience in 68 extremities among 53 patients followed up to 12 years. Four failures were related to failure to use continued support or lateral occurrences related to later development of short saphenous or lateral perforator hypertension. Further techniques have been used to interrupt communicating and perforating veins employing a shearing phlebotome described by Edwards[4] and others[5] to devide the perforating veins of the postero medial arcade.

Indications and Pre-operative care

All patients are initially treated conservatively for at least three months using Unna paste boots, bedrest, elevation. If they fail this treatment, they are considered candidates for surgery. Forty-eight additional extremities in 39 patients were operated on between May, 1980 through January, 1992 using modifications of the initial technique and the sharing operation. All patients are evaluated for superficial venous incompetency by physical examination, continuous Doppler ultrasound probe and, since 1987, duplex scanning. To supplement these examinations, especially to plan ligations in the infracrural region where gastrocnemius or Boyd's perforators were present, intraoperative varicography is used. Operations were planned with information about major leak areas. In operations done after 1985, the operative technique was altered for the medial perforator approach using the shearing phlebotome and as described recently.

Results

In cases requiring skin grafts, patients remained at strict bedrest in a posterior splint for at least seven days. Broad spectrum antibiotics are used pre and postoperatively and anticoagulation with heparin is used beginning 36 hours postoperatively. All patients are fitted with pressure gradient support stockings with pressure of 30 mm of Hg at the ankle before leaving the hospital.

With the skin line incisions, there was primary healing in all except one patient in whom healing at the ankle was delayed for 21 days. The shearing operation reduced the need for but did not eliminate extra incisions for high pressure veins. In 12 extremities in which the skin grafts were applied, hospitalization postoperatively ranged from 7--18 days. However, hospitalization has generally been reduced to a period of about 3--4 days for severe stasis changes not requiring skin grafts.

Of 39 patients operated on since 1980, there were again 4 recurrences. The most troublesome occurred in a patient with a thrombosed venacave who refused caval reconstruction. His hospitalization required the longest interval. This recurrent episode was related to non-compliance. Another recurrence was related to cessation of wearing support stockings with ulceration in the upper third of the leg where a residual problematic perforator reappeared in the infracrural area. This reinforces our intraoperative use of varicography. Two other recurrences were related to breakdown laterally after lesions had been healed medially.

Comment

These patients are relieved of time-consuming and expensive clinic care following surgery. The individual must recognize a requirement for the idefinite use of graded support hose; however, these can be prescribed at a lighter weight and are, therefore, better tolerated.

We recommend triamcinolope cream (.025%) to areas of hyperpigmentation for the long term. This possibly reduces the inflammatory changes related to release of irritating enzymes and cytokines from stagnant white cells escaping from capillaries.

Summary

This risks of operation are minimal and satisfactory healing of ulceration can be maintained in most cases. The author recently used valvuloplasty in conjunction with skin grafting and removal of communicating veins where indicated by descending venography. Ultimately, these operations will need to be compared with classic procedures for venous ulceration.

References

1. Linton RR: The communicating veins of the lower leg and the operative technique for their ligation. Ann Surg 1938; 107:582.

2. DePalma RG: Surgical therapy for venous stasis. Surgery 1975; 76:910.

3. DePalma RG: Surgical therapy for venous stasis: Results of a modified Linton operation. Am J Surg 1979; 137:810.

4. Edwards JM: Shearing operation for incompetent perforating veins. Br J Surg 1976; 63:885.

5. Simpson CJ, Smellie GD: The phlebotome in the management of incompetent perforating veins and venous ulceration. J Cardiovasc Surg 1987; 28:279.

Phlébologie 92. Eds P. Raymond-Martimbeau, R. Prescott, M. Zummo.
John Libbey Eurotext, Paris © 1992, pp. 1238-1239

Modification of the PALMA operation : a new operative technique

Gy. Acsády

*Cardiovascular Surgical Clinic of Semmelweis Medical University,
1122 Budapest, Városmajor u. 68, Hungary.*

The two critical points of the cross-over vein grafting (op.sec. PALMA) are:
1) not to be any torsion of the saphenous vein,
2) the end-to-side anastomosis not to be stenotic.

The first problem can be eliminated with a careful operative technique.
The second point is a very difficult question and it depends not only on the surgical technique, but it depends on anatomical factors, too. If these anatomical conditions are not adequate (obesity, cicatrization etc.) in these cases an angulation develops in the area of the end-to-side anastomosis and it causes a relative stenosis (Fig. 1.).
Avoiding this problem I introduced a new operative solution.
It consists of two parts: (Fig. 2.)
1) resection and ligation of the occluded common femoral vein under the inquinal ligament,
2) end-to-end anastomosis between the saphenous and the common femoral vein.

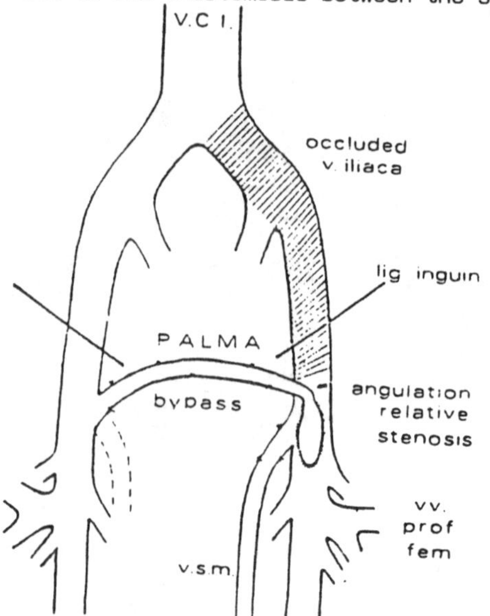

Fig. 1.

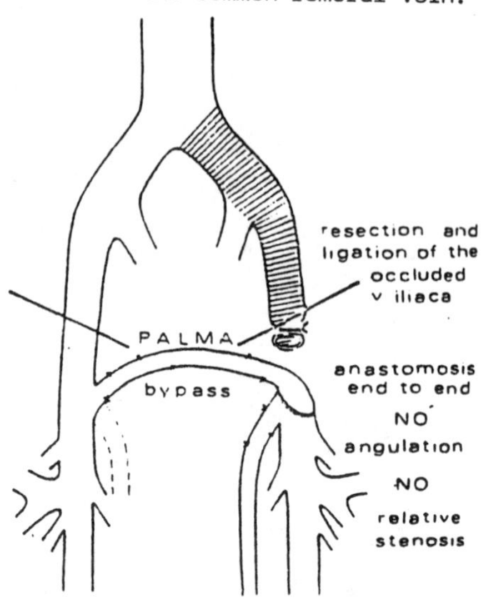

Fig. 2.

Advantages of the new method are: (Fig. 3.)

1) the resection of the occluded vein interrupts the pathological reflexes
2) in the case of the end-to-end anastomosis there is no angulation, there is no relative stenosis, therefore, the venous run-off and the hemodynamic effect will become better
3) there is no need for preparing temporary arteriovenous fistula.

18 female 22 male age: 23-68 ys	ORIGINAL OPERATION (end to side anastomosis)			MODIFICATED OPERATION (end to end anastomosis)		
NUMBER of OPERATIONS	20			20		
NUMBER of REOCCLUSIONS	8 (40%)			3 (15%)		
POSTOP. MORPHOLOGY	PATENT	REOCCLUDED		PATENT	REOCCLUDED	
		DEVELOPMENT of COLLATERAL SYSTEM	RECANALI-ZATION		DEVELOPMENT of COLLATERAL SYSTEM	RECANALI-ZATION
	12	2	6	17	3	-
POSTOP. FUNCTION	FREE of COMPLAINTS	IMPROVED	UNCHANGED	FREE of COMPLAINTS	IMPROVED	UNCHANGED
	12	2	6	17	3	-

Fig.3. Correlations between morphology and function after the original and modificated Palma operations

RESULTS

1) patients are getting on speedily and long-lastingly without complaints (the pain and the constant oedema disappears and the leg ulcer heals-up within a short time)
2) the occurence of the reocclusion is rarer than at the traditional PALMA operation.

On the basis of the above mentioned facts I suggest wide-ranging application of this new modification of the PALMA operation.

REFERENCE

Acsády Gy., Lengyel I. Modification between histomorphological and pathobiochemical changes leading to primary varicosis. Proceedings of the 10th World Congress Union Internationale de Phlebologie, Strasbourg 25-29 September 1989 John Libbey, Paris 1989

Théorie et pratique de la cure hémodynamique de l'insuffisance veineuse profonde par dévalvulation

Dr J.Rinieri-D.Mellière et collaborateurs

Hopital Henri Mondor Créteil France

La CHIVP est une thérapeutique chirurgicale qui, réalisant un ensemble de ligatures sélectives est destinée à traiter une insuffisance veineuse profonde par dévalvulation. Deux principes sont fondamentaux :

- une veine incontinente n'assure aucun retour veineux en orthostatisme et présente une circulation inversée
- cette veine inefficace développe une circulation collatérale du fait de l'augmentation de pression qu'elle engendre. Mais cette circulation parallèle est en fait neutralisée par la veine malade qui réalise un shunt rétrograde.

Des ligatures section sont proposées en tenant compte des axes veineux uniques à faible collatéralité (veine poplitée, fémorale commune et veine iliaque externe) dont la perméabilité est indispensable.
Cette théorie originale repose sur des arguments physiques, cliniques anatomiques et fonctionnels.
La stratégie est discutée sur la cartographie hémodynamique des veines profondes produite par l'examen doppler duplex orthostatique. Les premiers cas traités semblent confirmer le bien fondé de cette théorie.

Venous valve substitution: A new technique

Timothy J. Sloan, M.D. F.A.C.A.

UCMS, Yuba City California

A new technique of venous valve substitution has been devised for postphlebitic syndrome. Utilizing a cryopreserved pulmonic valve allograft, placed into the common femoral vein, a patient with postphlebitic syndrome, had complete recovery of postphlebitic syndrome, with total loss of pain, dissolution of chronic venous stasis ulcers, and return to daily work of at least 12 hours per day with no debility. Follow up at 30 months with duplex scanning clearly demonstrates patency and competency. Presented is the rationale as to the use of the cryopreserved allograft and the surgical technique employed. Based on a 2 1/2 year follow up, the prognosis is excellent for these patients. The supply for cryopreserved allograft (Cryolife, Mariette, GA) is almost limitless of any size, the surgical procedure is facile. Judging from these results, the cost of the cryopreserved valve is justified especially when considering the savings saved in medical bills, and return of the patient to the work-force.

Phlébologie 92. Eds P. Raymond-Martimbeau, R. Prescott, M. Zummo.
John Libbey Eurotext, Paris © 1992, pp. 1241-1243

Surgical treatment for lower limb chronic venous thrombosis

B. Augusto Diaz, Karolina Diaz, Miguel Bermeo

Instituto de Angiología, cirugía vascular e impotencia sexual, Av. de la República 770 y Eloy Alfaro, Quito, Ecuador.

In phlebological practice is frequent to discover, accidentally, some compensated or not compensated venous damages.

Just after executing a complete clinical study, including doppler, ecography, gammagraphy and plebography procedures, we are able to determine the appearance of venous post-thrombotic pathology, compensated or not compensated, by multiple natural pathological collateral ways. Observing those natural venous reconstruction changes, we accept to perform, with certain success, venous and venovenous grafts and by-pass.

Since about eleven years ago, we began to execute these procedures well understood that in past decades reconstructive and functional vein surgery had been an exceptional procedure, and was limited for its great number of failures.

During last years, this kind of procedures arises due:

1. An adequate sellection of the type of venous pathology upon which we can work with good possibilities of success: thrombosis and extraluminal compression.

2. Good knowledgement of appropriate material to use for this kind of procedure.

3. A great advance in management and knowledgement of coagulation, anti-coagulation, plate aggregation and reological circulatory features.

4. An improvement in surgical technique at different areas of human body, where pathological frequence is greater.

5. Knowledgement of the different kind of procedures to be used as: anathomical and extra-anathomical by-passes and transpositions.

Diagnosis is difficult, clinical anamnesis and physical examination give us about 70%. There are multiple auxilliary procedures to improve diagnosis and those are divided in: routine and special tests which give us the last 30% diagnosis, those are: doppler, ecography gammagraphy and specially phlebography, which permits us, in a best way, to have the conviction of a clear and precise diagnosis, and also it help us as a comparative basis for an adequate treatment and a definitive prediction.

According anathomical topography location, we divide deep venous thrombosis of lower limb in: foot, leg, thigh and ilio-cave areas, and in conformity with this, we execute our treatment as follows:

a) On foot area, we only use clinical treatment and we divide it in two parts: basic and anti-coagulant. Basic means elastic contention, physiotherapy, anti-static position plus medicamentous drugs as anti-inflamatory and anti-aggregate. For anti-coagulant treatment we use Heparine and Natrium Warfarine.

b) On leg venous thrombosis we just recommend the same clinical treatment.

c) At thigh level and due to the shrotness of the deep venous system we beleive in the importance of compensation and dis-compensation -our own concept-.

   The compensation statemen may be both: radiological or physiological. The radiological and physiological compensation statement may co-exist together, but, in some cases, radiological compensation statement may co-exist with physiological dis-compensation statement.

   There is a physiological compensation statement when venous insufficiency symptomatology is not present and when distal venous pressure is within normal limits. Dis-compensation statement will be the one in which there appear a venous insufficiency symptomatology as edema, cianosis, venous turgescence, pain, venous dilatation and distal venous hipertension.

   Those concepts are very important for the treatment of ilio-femoral or femoro-popliteo venous thrombosis by grafts or by-pass or venous transposition.

   Physiological compensated statement do not need any kind of surgical treatment.

d) Ilio-cava venous thrombosis have been divided in four groups:

   1. Iliac bilateral venous thrombosis in which we advise to perform a surgical treatment with one or bilateral axilo-femoral grafts (we have not any case performed)

   2. Iliac one lateral venous thrombosis in which we perform femoro-femoral or sapheno-femoral derivations, according Palma's technique, plus our modifications.

   3. One lateral ilio-femoral thrombosis in which we execute sapheno-femoral, contra-lateral derivations associated with sapheno-poplitea venous by-pass and sometimes varicotomies

and ligatures.

4. One or bilateral iliac-venous thrombosis plus spontaneous dis compensated recanalization in which the elective treatment is valvular transplantation. (we have not get any case).

In this moment, I must tell you that we call dis-connective surgery to all procedures of dis-connection of superficial axis from deep axis, such as: partial ligatures, scaled ligatures, perforant ligatures and veno-extraction. On the other hand, we call connective surgery to all procedures for establishment of venous circulation such as: by-pass, and transpositions.

SURGICAL TECHNIQUE

In one lateral iliac or ilio-femoral thrombosis we perform sapheno femoral or sapheno-venous by-pass with Palma's technique, modified in some way by us.

In femoro-popliteal obliterations we perform venous transposition technique which means to cross saphenous vein behind sartorious muscle.

In femoral or femor-popliteal thrombosis we had performed 7 sapheno femoral derivations by transposition of saphenous vein to the popliteal or femoral vein and only 3 cases of femoro-femoral free grafts.

In one lateral iliac or ilio-femoral thrombosis, we had performed 33 connective surgery procedures. 20 of them were sapheno-femoral and 13 were sapheno-saphenous by-pass.

27 procedures were made in males and 6, in females. We have 15 samples of connective surgery, 12 simple connective surgery plus dis-connective and 6 connective surgery plus dis-connective plus elastic contention.

We have had 24 iliac venous thrombosis and 9 ilio-femoral venous thrombosis

Phlebography control showed us at the post-operatory phase: 27 permeable cases, 4 obliterated cases and 2, without control. After 24 months, 20 were permeable, 4 obliterated and 9 without control.

CONCLUSIONS

1. Anathomical ethiological classification is necessary.

2. Phlebographic tests are extremely important.

3. Knowledge of surgical technique is recommeded.

4. Experience in handling anti-coagulation, anti-aggregation and reological features is required.

5. Arterio-venous fistulae is not indispensable.

Phlébologie 92. Eds P. Raymond-Martimbeau, R. Prescott, M. Zummo.
John Libbey Eurotext, Paris © 1992, pp. 1244-1246

Diagnosis and management of venous trauma

Svatopluk Kaspar, Vobotil Zbynek

Department of Surgery, Faculty of Medecine, Charles University, Hradec Králové, Czechoslovakia.

INTRODUCTION

Although a great deal of attention has been paid to vascular trauma, most of the emphasis has been on arterial rather than on venous injuries. Major venous trauma, however, occurs often in combination with or isolated from arterial injury.
The optimal management of major venous injuries continues to be a controversial topic. It may not initially appear to be as challenging and dramatic as managing injured arteries, but bleeding from injured veins can be even more difficult to control appropriately end even more frustrating to work with. The interruption of a major vein, particularly in the lower extremities, can be associated with acute venous hypertension, and there is the potential for long-term sequelae associated with chronic venous insufficiency.
Stimulated by the American military experiences during the Vienam War, there has been an increased interest in a more aggressive approach to the repair of injuries of large caliber veins. Most clinical reports to date are of high-velocity military injuries and may not be entirely applicable to civilian trauma.
The purpose of this report is to present our updated experience with different approaches in the treatment of major venous injuries in our civilian practice.

PATIENTS AND METHODS

The records of 99 patients (77 men, 22 women) with serious civilian vascular injuries treated in our institution in 18 year period were analysed. More then one third of the whole series sustained venous trauma - there were 21 venous injuries associated with arterial injuries, and 14 isolated venous injuries with intact arterial tree. These combined venous injuries had been sustained to the internal jugular (1), brachial (10), iliac (1), femoral (4), and popliteal veins (5). Distribution of the isolated venous injuries were as follows: the external jugular (1), internal jugular (1), brachial (1), portal (1), caval (1), external iliac (4), common femoral (2), and popliteal (3). The etiology of these injuries was blunt trauma in most cases, iatrogenic injuries to the venous system were noted six times. Management of injured veins consisted of end-to-end repair (10), lateral repair (12), vein graft (6), prosthetic graft (1), and vein ligation (6).

RESULTS

There were no perioperative deaths in these 35 patients and no postoperative symptomatic pulmonary embolus was diagnosed. The limb salvage rate was 100 per

cent.
In the group of isolated venous injuries, eight patients were personally assessed and long-term results were evaluated by clinical examination and ultrasound or phlebography in the period ranged from 1 to 10 years after the operation.
In eight cases of reconstructed veins, only one saphenous vein interposition graft was occluded, the reconstruction was patent in seven remaining patients.

DISCUSSION

The surgeon has two goals when approaching venous injuries. The first one is to ensure that the limb survives the acute trauma and the second one is to restore the long-term venous function.
Ligation was standart therapy for venous injuries during World Wars I. a II. Data collecting during Korean and particularly the Vietnam conflicts, however, raised questions regarding this practice.
Hughes (1954) drew attention to the fact that in cases with concomitant arterial and venous injuries, where the veins were ligated, some limbs required amputation despite apparently successful repair of the artery. Limb loss has been reported mainly following popliteal vein ligation (Rich et al., 1974; Pasch et al., 1986). Examination of the amputated extremities showed patent arteries and venous congestion due to venous thrombosis distal to ligation.
Rich (1982) and others have emphasized the importance of venous repair, rather than simple ligation, to prevent the sequelae of chronic venous hypertension.
The suspicion that repair might be associated with an increased incidence of thrombophlebitis and/or pulmonary embolism has been shown to be very improbable on the basis of experience from Vietnam Vascular Registry (Rich et al., 1974).
At least four different methods of venous repair are described. These are:
1) lateral suture repair; 2) end-to-end anastomosis; 3) venous patch graft;
4) venous replacement graft. The use of prosthetic material in these injuries is generally no standart practice. While some suggest that lateral repairs produce optimal patency rates, more complex repairs can produce satisfactory long-term results, too.
The critics of repair of major peripheral veins trauma often compare the effect of a major venous ligation on the peripheral circulation to the manner in which a deep vein thrombosis affects the venous drainage of the limb. But it must be emphasized that the occlusive effect of a deep vein thrombosis is often gradual, allowing time for neigbouring callaterals to develop. No such time is availabele following venous ligation (O'Reilly et al., 1980).
The critics of venous repair conclude also that a substantial percentage of such veins will thrombose in postoperative period (Meyer et al., 1987), yet Phifer et al. (1985) reported on a small series of patients in which venous patency was proved by venography 6 to 20 years after femoral vein repair.
We suggest with others (Buice et al., 1990; Rich, 1988) that the benefits of repairing major venous injuries include:

1. enhancement of venous outflow, resulting in better success in repair of a concomitant arterial injury;
2. decreased likelihood of postoperative swelling, venous stasis, and postphlebitic syndrome;
3. even short term patency (1 to 3 days) of venous repair may allow for increased venous outflow from the extermity before the development of collateral venous channels that are stimulated at the time that primary repair undergoes thrombosis (Rich, 1974). Also later recanalization of a short venous segment at the repair site which is thrombosed is possible (Rich, 1988). Better patency rates can also be achieved by performing A-V fistula distal to the venous reconstruction (Richardson et al., 1986).

The only disadvantage of venous repair is the time required to execute it and possibly the only indication for venous ligation are complex lacerations or associated injuries that require priority (Aitken et al., 1989).

CONCLUSION

In major vein trauma, an attempt should be made to repair the vein unless other life-saving procedures require priority. Whenever possible, lateral suture or vein patch seem to be the ideal types of repair. However, excellent results can be obtained with end-to-end anastomosis or venous interposition graft, too.

REFERENCES

Aitken, R. J., Matley, P. J., Immelman, E. J.: Lower limb vein trauma: a long-term clinical and physiological assessment. Brit. J. Surg. 76, 585-508 (1989)

Buice, W. S., Hollenbeck J. I., McElwee, T. (1990): Isolated iliac vein injury from blunt trauma. Surgery 107, 350-352

Hughes, C. W. (1954): Acute vascular trauma in Korean War casualties: An analysis of 180 cases. Surg. Gynecol. Obstet. 99, 91-100

Meyer, J., Walsh, J., Schuler, J. et al. (1987): The early fate of venous repair after civilian vascular trauma. Ann Surg. 206, 458-464

O'Reilly, M. J. G., Hood, J. M., Livingston, R. H. et al. (1980): Penetrating injuries of the popliteal vein: a report on 34 cases. Brit. J. Surg. 67, 337-340

Pasch, A. R., Bishara, R. A., Schaler, J. J. et al. (1986): Results of venous reconstruction after civilian vascular trauma. Arch Surg. 121, 607-611

Phifer, T. J., Gerlock, A. L., Rich, N. M. et al. (1985): Long term patency of venous repairs demonstrated by venography. J. Trauma 25, 342-346

Richardson, J. B. Jr., Jurkovich, G. J., Walker, G. T. et al. (1986): A temporary arteriovenous shunt (Scribner) in the management of traumatic venous injuries of the lower extermity. J. Trauma 26, 503-508

Rich, N. M., Hobson, R. W., Wright, C. B. et al. (1974): Repair of lower extremity venous trauma: a more aggressive approach required. J. Trauma 14, 639-652

Rich, N. M. (1982): Principles and indications for primary venous repair. Surgery 91, 492-496

Rich, N. M. (1988): Management of venous trauma. Surg. Clin. N. Amer. 68, 809-821

B.
VEINES SUPERFICIELLES
SUPERFICIAL VEINES

Phlébologie 92. Eds P. Raymond-Martimbeau, R. Prescott, M. Zummo.
John Libbey Eurotext, Paris © 1992, pp. 1249-1251

Conservative surgery for primary varicose veins of the lower limbs : clinical, instrumental, histopathological follow-up in 4 years

L. Corcos, G.P. Peruzzi, V. Romeo, T. Procacci, S. Dini*

*General Surgery Inst., Ferrara University, Italy. *Morbid Anatomy and Histology Inst., Florence University, Italy.*

INTRODUCTION

Limited surgery for varicose veins of the lower limbs (VVLL) is currently preferred over extensive procedure (1,2,3). A better knowledge of saphenous system's pathophisiology (4) and a more frequent demand for autologous vein graft led many Authors to experiment new conservative and reparative surgical techniques in the treatment of VVLL (5,6,7,8,9,10,11,12,13,14).
Since Sept. 1988 we have performed n.78 of these operations (11,13) using different, variously combined methods as follows: (Fig. 1)

- External valvuloplasty (Vpl) of sapheno-femoral junction (SFJ)
- Crossectomy (Cross)
- Hemodynamic correction (HC) of the saphenous system, according to others Authors' proposal (8,9,11,13)
- Subfascial ligation (Lig) of communicating veins of the leg (CV)
- Varicectomy (Var)
- Sapheno-popliteal ligation

During our preliminary experience we did not take patient age, duration of the disease or its degree and extension into consideration (4,6,10,11,12,13,14).
We only excluded cases with unsatisfactory echographic imaging of sapheno-femoral valve (15), recent or previous thrombophlebitis and sclerotherapy, deep venous pathology.
Our propose is now to analyze our results, related to clinical, instrumental and histopathological finding, and try to deduce more precise indications.

MATERIALS AND METHODS

All 78 patients were selected and 70 controlled by means of clinical-instrumental investigations (doppler CW, HR echography).
In 63 patients an intraoperative venous biopsy (mainly a LSV fragment) was performed, over 69 operations (6 bilateral).
N.54 Vpl out of 58 were controlled with an intraoperative doppler or duplex examination.

N. 47 cases underwent preoperative and postoperative non invasive venous pressure (VP) measurements. N.7 with symptoms of chronic insufficiency were subjected phlebography of the deep veins.
Table I shows the combination of methods employed in six groups of cases. Complementary sclerotherapy for reticular varicose veins and/or telangectases (in a few cases for residual truncular varicose veins) was performed postoperatively in N.17 patients. N.76 patients were treated with anticoagulats for 7-15 days.
Follow up of N.70 cases,out of a total of 78, has been completed from a minimum of 6 months to a maximum of 3 years and 6 months.

RESULTS AND DISCUSSION

Results have been divided into three groups (Tab. I):

Excellent: disappearance of varicose veins and symptoms, disappearance or consistent reduction of reflux, no complications.
Good: reduction of varicose veins, disappearance or reduction of symptoms, disappearance or reduction of reflux, reversible complications.
Poor or none: persistence or recurrence of varicose veins, symptoms and reflux.

The best results were obtained in groups 1,5,6 (patients with limited and early VVLL) and in group 3 (patients with extensive VVLL, submitted to Vpl+HC+Var).
Thrombosis occurred in N.13 cases (LSV): in 5 of them it was localized below the Vpl and in 8 in the distal segments of LSV.
Failures of Vpl appeared to be related to the age of disease (50% of cases with more than 20 years history). Thrombosis was due to a surgical error in 2 cases (exclusion of a LSV segment) and in the others, developed spontaneously.
In N.63 LSV biopsies a high degree of intimal damage was observed in 62.2% of cases with postoperative LSV thrombosis. No thrombotic event occurred in N.7 cases with normal intimal layer. No relation has been established between patient age and disease. Sclerosis of the middle coat appeared related to the history of varicose disease: a high degree of sclerosis was observed in 50% of cases with VV LL lasting more than 20 years and a normal media was present in 20% of patients with excellent and good postoperative results (4,6,10,12,13).
N.8 reoperations have been performed (N.5 Vpl explant and saphenectomy, N.3 second HC). N.17 patients have been subjected to complementary sclerotherapy, mainly for treatment of reticular VV and telangectases.
In 38 LSV of limbs with excellent or good results, postoperative VP became normal. Maintenance of SFJ obtained with Vpl gives better VP normalization compared with others Authors results obtained with Cross+HC (4,9,12,13).

CONCLUSIONS

Encouraging results have been obtained in our 4 years of experience and observations:
- techniques are easy performable and well tolerated (outpatient surgery);
- they have to be limited to early, not complicated VVLL;
- varicectomy has to be associated in order to obtain immediate clinical and

cosmetic results;

- Thrombotic risk has to be prevented with correct technique and anticoagulants.

TABLE I

PRIMARY VVLL:N.70 CONSERVATIVE AND REPARATIVE OPER. .RESULTS AFTER 4 YEARS									
GR	OPERATION	N	EXCELLENT	GOOD	POOR	LSV T	REOP.	SCLEROTH.	NOT CONTR.
1	Vpl Vpl+Var Vpl+CV Lig	11 2 6	14	1	2	2	3	7	2
2	Vpl+HC	23	8	5	6	4	1	3	4
3	Vpl+HC+Var	16	13	1	2	4	3	5	0
4	Cross+HC	10	6	2	0	1	0	1	2
5	HC	6	5	0	1	1	1	1	0
6	HC+Var	5	4	1	0	1	0	0	0
	TOTAL	78	50	9	11	13	8	17	8
	CONTROLLED	70	71.4%	12.8%	15.7%	18.5%	11.4%	24.2%	1.26%

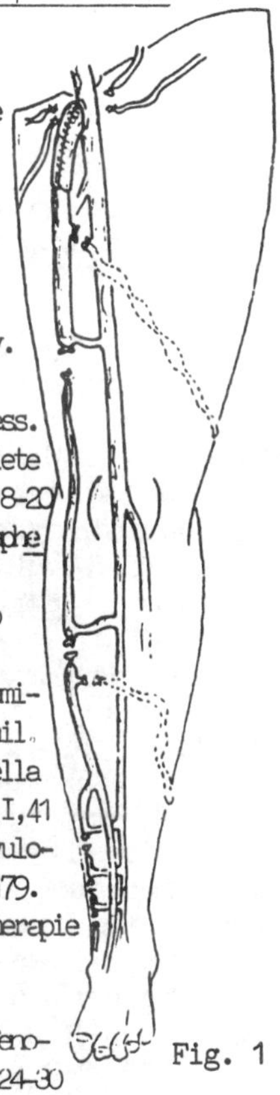

Fig. 1

REFERENCES

1-Negus D. (1986): Should the incopetent saphenous vein be stripped to the ankle Phlebology, 1, 33-36.

2-Darke S.G. (1991): Chronic venous insufficiency should the long saphenous vein be stripped? In Vascular Surgery. Current Question. Aires A.B.Barros D'Sac Eds. Oxford, 207-218.

3-Helsted M.,Hessefeldt-Nielsen J. et al.(1991):Partial versus total strippingof the great saphenous vein evaluated by strain-gauge plethysmogarphy. Phlebology 6,227-232.

4-Corcos L. (1992): Il ruolo delle safene nel ritorno venoso. Min Angiol. in press.

5-Bihari I. (1989): Saving the greater saphenous vein for prostesis with incomplete ligation in varicose cases. Phlebologie '89. Davy-Stemmer Eds.J.Libbey Ltd.1018-20

6-Corcos L.,Peruzzi G.P. et al. (1991): Valvuloplastie externe de la jonction sapheno-femorale. Phlebologie, 2, 497-508.

7-Belcaro G. (1989): Plication of the sapheno-femoral junction:an alternative to ligation. Phlebologie'89. Davy-Stemmer Eds. J.Libbey Ltd. 990-991.

8-Franceschi C. (1988): Theorie et pratique de la cure conservatrice et hemodynamique de l'insuffisance veineuse en ambulatoire. De l'Armancon Ed. Precy sous Thil.

9-Consiglio L.,Giorgi G. (1990):Risultati della CEC delle varici. valutazione della pressione venosa dell'arto operato con flebodinamometro di Varady. Flebologia,I,41

10-Donini I,Corcos L.(1991):Preliminary results of external sapheno-femoral valvuloplasty: a trial by the Italian Society of Phlebolimphology. Phlebolgy,6,167-179.

11-Corcos L.,Donini I. (1991): Konservierende und rekonstruktive chirurgische therapie bei ausgewahltel fallen von varikosis der uteren extremitaten,teil 1. Vasomed aktuell,8/91,16-19.

12-Corcos L.,Peruzzi G.P. (1991): La valvuloplastica esterna della giunzione safeno-femorale. III Intern.Congress Phlebolimphology Ferrara 1991. Abst.Book. pp.6.24-30

13-Corcos L.,Peruzzi G.P. et al (1992): Risultati e considerazioni sulla Valvuloplastica associata alla correzione emodinamica venosa. Flebolinfologia,II-2,in press.

14-Corcos L.,Peruzzi G.P. et al. (1992):Indication and exclusion criteria for external valvuloplasty of sapheno-femoral junction. XI Congress U.I.P. Montreal 1992. In press.

15-Peruzzi G.P,Romeo V. (1991): L'ecodoppler in flebolinfologia. Flebolinfologia, 1,5.

Phlébologie 92. Eds P. Raymond-Martimbeau, R. Prescott, M. Zummo.
John Libbey Eurotext, Paris © 1992, pp. 1252-1254

External valvuloplasty of the sapheno-femoral junction and tributaries preservation

Paolo Zamboni, Vincenzo Gasbarro, Enzo Pozza, Dino De Anna, Anna Paola Murgia, Annibale Donini, Vittorio Bresadola, Alberto Liboni

Department of Surgery, the University of Ferrara, 44100 Ferrara, Italy.

INTRODUCTION

Histological observations and a review of literature has led us to the convinction that sapheno-femoral reflux in early varicose vein syndrome is due to a separation of valve cusps in a dilated phlebosclerotic vein wall. External valvuloplasty of the sapheno-femoral junction restores valve function by reducing vein wall dilatation; for this purpose an external prosthetic perforated support of PTFE or Dacron has been used surrounding the dilated proximal long saphenous vein.

PATIENTS AND METHODS

A total of 30 patients underwent operation under local anaesthesia for the following indications: primary and early varicose veins, symptoms of venous insufficiency, sapheno-femoral reflux, ecographic evidence of normal valve cusps (pre-and/or intraoperative). Exclusion criteria were : previous or recent thrombophlebitis (endothelial damage and increased thrombotic risk); previous or recent sclerotherapy (endothelial damage and increased thrombotic risk) and local and/or general contraindications. Through an inferior transverse inguinal approach, careful dissection of the sapheno-femoral junction was performed, as for conventional saphenous ligation. Collateral veins of the terminal saphenous vein were ligated and divided, or, when possible, preserved, expecially those of important size. The terminal and subterminal valves were located by vein wall dilatations, in order to decide the lenght of prosthesis (5-7 cm). When pre-operative ultrasonography failed to show any valve leaflets, intraoperative echography was employed, and if the images were still not satisfactory, conventional saphenous ligation was performed. In total, 12 cases were operated on using a Dacron monovelour patch and 18 with PTFE patch (0.4-0.6 mm thick, 6-7 mm wide and 5-7 cm long.) The graft was placed round the proximal saphenous vein, removing any excess. The patch was secured by a continous or interrupted anterior suture of 6/0 PTFE suture for the PTFE grafts and 6/0 polypropylene suture for Dacron monovelour. The patch was perforated using a punch instrument or Pott' scissors whether at the sites of the tributary veins or of the stumps. The collateral veins or their stumps were inserted through the "windows" in the graft. After securing the graft, intra-operative Doppler examination of the long saphenous vein, just below the lower edge of graft, was performed, using the Valsalva and/or compressive manouvres. This instrumental control was useful in detecting residual reflux and saphenous vein patency and gave the opportunity of performing correction by valvuloplasty or conventional surgery. All patients were treated with antiplatelet drugs.

RESULTS

Follow-up was undertaken from 6 to 41 months postoperatively by monthly clinical examination, continuous wave Doppler, high resolution (HR) echography and Doppler venous pressure measurements. In twelve cases descending venography was used postoperatively (18-24 months) in order to demonstrate restored valvular function. This examination was performed with a controlateral femoral approach, in orthostatism under Valsalva manoeuvre: images always showed disapperance of reflux. Ascending phlebography , performed in four cases, showed a reduction in size of the internal Saphena vein. Complications were less than 12% and disappearance of sympthoms were recorded in 72%, as well as reduction in varicose veins (96%), disappearance of reflux (96%) and L.S.V. patency (96%). Saphena thrombosis occured in one case and was treated with emergency operation (short stripping). All cases were operated on in day surgery.

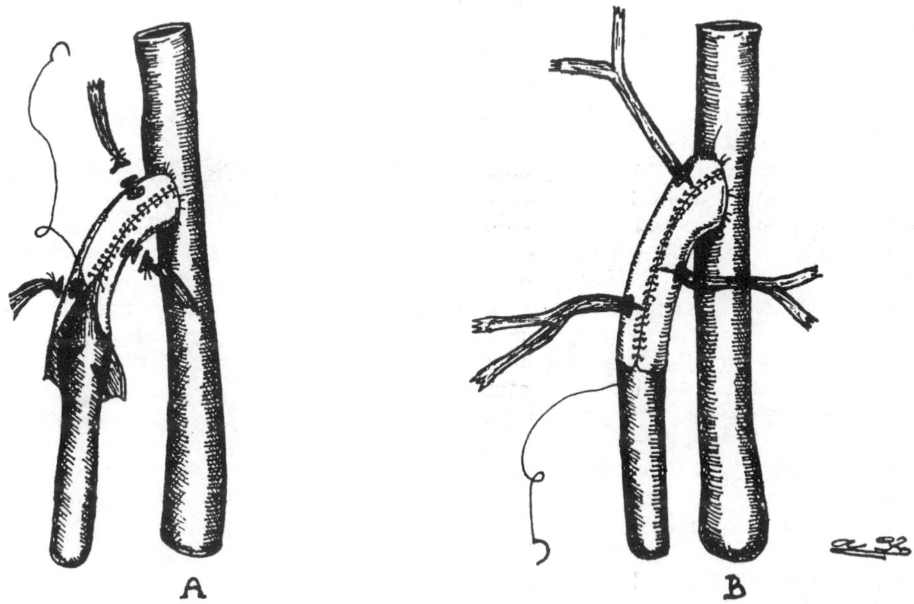

FIG. 1: External valvuloplasty of the S-F junction using perforated prosthesis without (A) and with (B) tributaries preservation.

DISCUSSION

Pre-operative and/or intra-operative H.R. echography is the main diagnostic step for successful surgery:evidence of valve leaflets in a dilated vein wall is necessary in order to plane reparative and conservative surgery. The perforated prosthesis is a surgical expedient that avoids compression between the graft and the walls of the tributary vein stumps, and in case of preserved collateral vein, allow us to performe the venoplasty around the saphena. Not compressed stumps, that were inserted through the holes of the graft, reduce the risk of thrombosis because there aren't deformation of the Saphena lumen with consequent turbolences and reduction of flow. Tributary preservation, thanks to perforated prosthesis, emphasize the conservative and hemodynamic aim of the operation. Flush ligation is advisable only in case of little collateral veins.

In conclusion, the results of EV-SFJ are encouraging, but longer evaluation is required. The method must be based on adequate preoperative assessment and careful selection of cases. Intra-operative diagnostic instrumental examination is also necessary for successful surgery. Further follow-up and advances in techniques and technology should lead to improve results. It will be interesting to find out whether the operation, which maintains the haemodynamic importance of saphenous drainage while controlling reflux, can modify the natural history of varicose disease. Another advantage is preservaton of the saphenous vein as a possible arterial graft.

REFERENCES

Corcos L., Zamboni P., Liboni A. (1989): External valvuloplasty of the s-f junction in early varicose veins of the lower limbs. Phlebologie 89, eds. A. Davy, R. Stemmer, pp. 1025-27, Libbey ed. Paris.

Cotton L.T., (1961): Varicose veins: gross anatomy and development. Br. J. Surg. 48: 489-499.

Edwards J.E., Edwards E.A. (1940): The saphenous valves in varicose veins. Am. Heart J. 19: 338-51.

Hallberg D.A., (1972): A method for reparing incompetent valves in deep veins. Acta Chir. Scand., 138: 143-5.

Rose S., Ahmed A., (1986): Some thoughts on the ethiology of varicose veins. J. Cardiovasc. Surg. 27: 534-43.

Zamboni P., Liboni A. (1991): External valvuloplasty of the s-f junction using perforated prosthesis. Phlebology 6: 141-47.

Phlébologie 92. Eds P. Raymond-Martimbeau, R. Prescott, M. Zummo.
John Libbey Eurotext, Paris © 1992, pp. 1255-1257

External valvuloplasty of the long saphenous vein by heterologous material : clinical survey and operated patients follow-up

Sergio Mancini, Giuseppe Botta, Simonetta Massi, Carla Ruggieri

Institute of General Surgery, University of Siena, Bracci Avenue, 53100 Siena, Italy.

ABSTRACT

Exsternal valvuloplasty of the long saphenous vein is a surgical technique whose aims is the abolition of the ostiale reflux in selected patients carachterized by saphenous-femoral cross insufficience at an early stage. The operation involves bringing the edges of the preostial valve closer together, using an external bandage made from heterologous material (P.T.F.E or Dacron). The preostial valve is found in the section of the long saphenous vein which, in conjuction with the preostial valve, is the centre of olivary dilation. The Authors clinically and instrumentally evaluated 24 patiens who had received the operation, with follow-up of up 30 months after the operation. The results obteined confirmed the experiments carried out with a physical model on removed section of long safphenous vein: the external valvuloplasty of the long saphenous vein can prevent ostial reflux.

KEY WORDS: Long saphenous, Varicose vein, Valvuloplasty.

INTRODUCTION

The anatomical studies carried out by Edward (1937-1940) and Cotton (1961) on 200 veins removed, mainly from the lower limbs, of patients suffering with varicose veins revealed the following:

1) structural alterations in the valves were never found, whereas, on the contrary, alteration in the nearly parietal tissue were costantly found.
2) the only valve which is costantly present is the preterminal valve (98.1% compared with 93.4% for the ostial valve).

Psaila and Melhuish (1989) compared normal and varicose veins, finding in the latter an higher elastic fibre content and a smaller amount of collagen, wich explains the lower resistance of the vein walls to stretching forces.

In the normal veins both the perivalvular and non valvular walls were analysed.

It was established that the perivalvular wall had a distinatly lower resistance than the non-valvular wall, calculated to be 50% lower. From what had been observed, it was concluded that the varicose distress depends not so much on an original alteration of the valves but more so of the walls, particularly perivalvular walls.

If this is true, for those patients in the initial stages of the distress it may be concluded that by correcting the ectasia of the parietal-valve complex, drawing the valve edges together, we can stop the pathological reflux.

MATERIALS AND METHOD

The use of the external plastic for the preostial valve is a surgical technique aimed to terminating the reflux which is caused by an insufficient femoral-saphenous junction leaving in situ the long saphenous vein.

The operation, performed under local anaesthetic, consists of wrapping an autologous (ring or peduncle) or prosthetical material around the preterminal valvular complex. This is than tightened around the vein until the edges of the valve come closer together, regaining doppler control. Finally it is firmly attached to the perivein by stitcnes.

The operation is proposing in all cases which the long reflux does not exceed the lower third of the thigh.

Our technique was undoubledly developed in such a way that the anatomical composition of the junction remains unaltered, but in the cases wich involved breaking the collaterals we had to be more prudent for two reasons:

1) in the eventuality that, after a period of time, a new reflux was revealed, we had to be sure that this was not due to an alteration in the contemption of the valve, or a perforant lower down which did not allow the collateral circles to be fed from above.

2) in case conditions were created which did not allow the plastic to remain in situ (eg. thrombosis), the stripping of the long saphenous vein would be much quicker and simpler.

RESULTS AND DISCUSSION

Twenty-four operations involving the external valvuloplasty were carried out.

In the first 3 cases cribrose ring bandages were used and the reflux reappared after two months. An ecograph of the last section of saphenous vein revealed that the diameter of the vein had returned to it's previous dimention. This signified that the external plastic had subsided, probably due to a vascular sufference, which with time brought necrosis.

This first partial success urged us to experiment with a vascular peduncle taken from a cribrose strip, which was used as the plastic. This new idea was tried on four patients, however it did not resolve the problem, but did make a significant improvement. In fact, these four patients after approximately 2 months of having received the operation showed a reflux which slowly reduced until it was eventually present only at the start of the test of Valsalva.

This ultrasonographic aspect, present in all cases, was explained by a partial suffering of the more distal part of the peduncle (this intending the part fixed to the perivein).

In effect, total coliquification of the plastic was not produced, as in the previous operations, only a relaxing of the binding around the valvular complex. Occurred in actuality, the part of the cribrose bandage which was not affected by suffering, remained attached to the walls creating, with time, a perivenous sclerosis capable of returning partial control to the valvolar apparatus.

Out of the 4 patients, clinical case n^ 4 recovered control of the long saphenous vein.

The others obviously remain under strict observation and only in future will we be able tell exactly whether the perivenous sclerosis will be capable of correcting the residual reflux.

Having great faith in the concept which composed the first part of our clinical experience, we wanted to experiment with the use of a heterological material, obviously without the innerent problems of vascolarization.

We chose P.T.F.E., 6 mm in diameter, and applied it adapting the same method as before.

The 17 cases operated on have so far shown no signs of reflux. All patients were dismissed on the same day as the operation and have not shown any post-operative complications.

REFERENCES

BASMAJAN J.V.: "The distribution of valves on the femoral external iliac and common iliac vein and their relationship to varicose veins". Surg.Gyn.Obst.1952,95:537-541.

BIHARI I.: "Saving the greater saphenous vein for prothesis, with incomplete ligation, in varicose cases". Phlebologie 1989. A.Davy,R.Stemmer eds.1989,John Libbey Eurotext Ltda. pp.1018-1020.

CAMILLI S. e COLL.: "La venoplastica esterna nella terapia dell'insufficienza valvolare venosa profonda primitiva. Risultati a distanza in 21 casi operati".Monduzzi ed. Bologna 1988 XXVI World Congr. I.C.S. Milano 1988.Cardiovasc.Surg.II:IX 83.

MANCINI S.,MARIANI F.: "La plastica esterna della valvola preterminale della vena grande safena con materiale eterologo (PTFE)" Atti Chir.Ivrea, maggio 1991.

MANCINI S.,MARIANI F."La valvola esterna della valvola preterminale della vena grande safena.Follow-up dei pazienti operati". Atti I^ Congr.Naz. di Cortona, sett.1990.

Phlébologie 92. Eds P. Raymond-Martimbeau, R. Prescott, M. Zummo.
John Libbey Eurotext, Paris © 1992, pp. 1258-1260

Indications and exclusion criteria for external valvuloplasty of sapheno-femoral junction

L. Corcos, G.P. Peruzzi, V. Romeo, T. Procacci, S. Dini*

*General Surgery Inst., Ferrara University, Italy. * Morbid Anatomy and Histology Inst., Florence University, Italy.*

INTRODUCTION

On the basis of international reports, wich demonstrated that primary venous valve incompetence is secondary to vein wall dilatation, we concluded that sapheno-femoral junction (SFJ) incompetence may be repaired by means of external support, as already proposed and experimented in deep venous surgery. For references see our previous papers(1,2,3,4).
Our proposal has been named External Valvuloplasty (Vpl) of SFJ.
Initially it was only performed in patients with limited and early varicose veins of the lower limbs (VVLL) (1). Later, our preliminary encouraging results led us to employ the Vpl in the treatment of extensive VVLL combining it with other methods (5,6,7). This new technique,performed without taking into account patient age or the stage of the varicose disease, gave us the opportunity to verify the behaviour of valve repair in different situations and using different materials (4,7). Our latest results and histopathological observations have been examined in order to make the point of patients selection and indications for operations.

MATERIALS AND METHODS

Over three years we have performed N.54 Vpl of SFJ in patients selected by means of clinical and instrumental investigations (doppler CW, HR echography, non invasive venous pressure measurements). At our hospital Dacron and PTFE tubular prosthesis were used and compared with other methods and materials in a multicenter trial (4). The conclusions of this study led us to choose PTFE prosthesis definitively and to perforate it in cases with huge collateral stumps, in order to avoid vein wall deformation (8).
N.54 cases were subjected to ultrasound postoperative examinations and intraoperative venous biopsy of LSV or peripheral vein.
N.47 cases were controlled with intraoperative doppler examination.
N.49 patients were treated with anticoagulants for 7-15 days.
In 47 cases deep and superficial venous pressure (DVP and SVP) measurements were performed before and after the operation. N.36 postoperative controls were normal

(competent Vpl-disappearance of reflux) and were comparable with results of demolitive surgery (sapheno-femoral ligation or disconnection).
Follow up = min. 6 months - Max. 3 years and 6 months.
The results were related with venous biopsies performed in the same patients.
In the meantime an histopathological examination of saphenic valves, taken during traditional demolitive operations for VVLL, was performed.
Relationships between surgical results, histopathological observations and stages of disease have beeen established.

RESULTS AND DISCUSSION

Table I summarizes the clinical and instrumental results in 54 surgically treated patients.

TABLE I

RESULTS IN N.54 EXT. VPL OF SFJ.FOLLOW UP FROM 6 TO 42 MONTHS.		
STABLE DISAPPEARANCE OF SYMPTOMS	N.42	% 77.7
STABLE DISAPPEARANCE OF REFLUX	N.37	% 68.5
PARTIAL RECURRENT OR RESIDUAL REFLUX	N. 6	% 11
COMPLETE RECURRENT OR RESIDUAL REFLUX	N.11	% 20.3
LSV THROMBOSIS	N. 5	% 9.2
PROSTHESIS INFECTION	N. 1	% 1.8
(Total recurrent reflux = 31.4%		

In all cases submitted to intraoperative doppler examination reflux disappeared at the time of the operation. In N.5 patients residual reflux was observed during the first ultrasound control, performed a few days after the operation. In N.7 cases intraoperative doppler ex. was performed and in 5 of them recurrent or residual reflux has been found. In 5 patients an early LSV thrombosis occurred, wich recanalize spontaneously in 4 patients. In N.2 cases terminal valves were involved and reflux recurred in two months time.
Three venous aneurysm of SFJ were subjected to external Vpl. One of them was related to postoperative LSV thrombosis and in the other two intraoperative doppler ex. demonstrated persistent reflux. In these last two cases a traditional SFJ ligation was performed immediately. A severe deformation of valvular structure and parietal wall was observed when we opened the LSV surrounded by prosthesis.
With the exception of these cases, all recurrences appeared from a minimum of 12 months to a maximum of 2 years. This indicates that parietal repair did not prevent valvular atrophy. In N.36 cases SVP normalized after Vpl and their mean decrease appeared more significant than in cases submitted to traditional ligation, as reported by other Authors (9). Further VP controls are still being performed in our patients with omogeneous methods. A few cases with pathologic DVP were also normalized.
Our histopathological observations demonstrated the following:
- N.5 incompetent Vpl have been explanted and valves were found to be atrophic or totally lacking; vasa vasorum were normal and a low degree fibrosis was observed.
- LSV thrombosis appears to be related to high degree of intimal damage in the parietal vein wall. In N.2 cases with mild intimal damage anticoagulants were administrated and LSV thrombosis occurred (7).
- N.40 vein valves, mainly taken from LSV segments, were studied with optical micro-

scopy. No alterations were observed in the specimens from patients suffering from VVLL for less than 20 years. Mild alterations in the insertion of the cusps were present in patients with more than 20 years history of venous disease. Severe alterations of the whole valve structure were observed in some patients with VVLL for more than 30 years. Stable results after Vpl have been obtained in 86.6% of the patients with early VVLL (less than 10 years), in 40% with VVLL for more than 10 years and in 42.8% with VVLL for more than 20 years. In this last group complete recurrent reflux reached 50%.

ERRATA **Page 2, line 24:**

"... In N.7 cases intraoperative doppler ex. was not performed ..."

CONCLUSIONS

A very careful diagnostic approach is necessary before performing external Vpl of SFJ. Intraoperative doppler examination is fundamental.
Venous aneurysm must not be treated with Vpl. The degree of intimal damage is not predictable and all patients must be given postoperative anticoagulant treatment.
Cases with high risk of thrombosis must be excluded: previous or recent thrombophlebitis or sclerotherapy and preparation for major surgery.
Valvular atrophy develops more frequently in patients with long standing disease and only early VVLL can be submitted to Vpl. Maintainance of SFJ outflow has an haemodynamic significance, as shown by VP measurements wich are being subjected to further verifications.

ERRATA **Page 2, line 44:**

"...In N.2 cases with mild intimal damage anticoagulants were not administrated ..."

REFERENCES

1-Corcos L.,Peruzzi G.P. etal.: Preliminary results of external valvuloplasty in sapheno-femoral junction insufficiency. Phlebology, 3:197-202,1989.

2-Corcos L.,Peruzzi G.P. et al.(1991): Valvuloplastie externe de la jonction sapheno femorale. Phlebologie,2,497-508.

3-Corcos L.,Peruzzi G.P. et al.(1989):External valvuloplasty of the sapheno-femoral junction in early varicose veins of the lower limbs. Phlebologie '89. A.Davy, R.Stemmer Eds.,pp1025-1027. J.Libbey Eurotext Ltd.

4-Donini I.,Corcos L. et al. (1991):Preliminary results of external sapheno-femoral valvuloplasty: a trial by the Italian Society of Phlebolymphology. Phlebology,6,167-179.

5-Corcos L.,Donini I. (1991):Konservierende und rekonstruktive chirurgische therapie bei ausgewahlten fallen von varikosis der unteren extremitaten,teil 1. Vasomed aktuell,8/91,16-19.

6-Corcos L.,Donini I. (1990): Reparative and conservative surgery in selected cases with varicose veins of the lower limbs. In European-American Symposium on Venous disease. Wien 1990. Abstr.Book I,4,A-7.

7-Corcos L.,Peruzzi G.P. (1992): Conservative surgery for primary varicose veins of the lower limbs: clinical,instrumental,histopathological follow-up in 4 years. XI World Congr. U.I.P. Montreal 1992. In press.

8-Zamboni P.,Boatto R. et al. (1990): La protesi fenestrata nella riparazione del giunto safeno-femorale dilatato ed insufficiente. Flebolinfologia,I-2,59-63.

9-Consiglio L.,Giorgi G. (1990): Risultati della chirurgia emodinamica conservativa delle varici (CEC). Valutazione della pressione venosa dell'arto operato con il flebodinamometro di Varady. Flebologia,I-1,41-44

We would like to tank W.Pabisch S.p.a. for his contribution.

Phlébologie 92. Eds P. Raymond-Martimbeau, R. Prescott, M. Zummo.
John Libbey Eurotext, Paris © 1992, pp. 1261-1262

External bounding of the saphenofemoral junction with a dacron ring

Andras Hetenyi

Department of Vascular Surgery, Magyar Imre Hospital H-8400 Ajka, Hungary.

Large number of patients with varicose veins have incompetent, mildly dilated but neither elongated, nor tortuous long saphenous vein /LSV/ in the thigh.The origin of the varicosity is the insufficiency of the saphenofemoral valve. These veins may be used theoretically in the future as an arterial graft in peripheral or coronary bypass surgery.

Our aim was to decrease the pressure and the regurgitated volume affecting the LSV in erect position with external bounding the upper insufficiency point - the saphenofemoral junction - and in this way to decrease or to stop the main hemodynamic factors of the progression of the varicosity.

Before surgery we have made clinical and Doppler examinations in supine and erect position, but no phlebography.

Operative technique: groin dissection - careful approach of the saphenofemoral junction /only 1-2 tributary veins are divided/ - narrowing of the inflow tract of LSV by means of a Dacron ring, external diameter 5 mm /Fig.1/ - removing the varicose tributary veins in the thigh and in the calf with meticulous regard of the trunk of LSV.

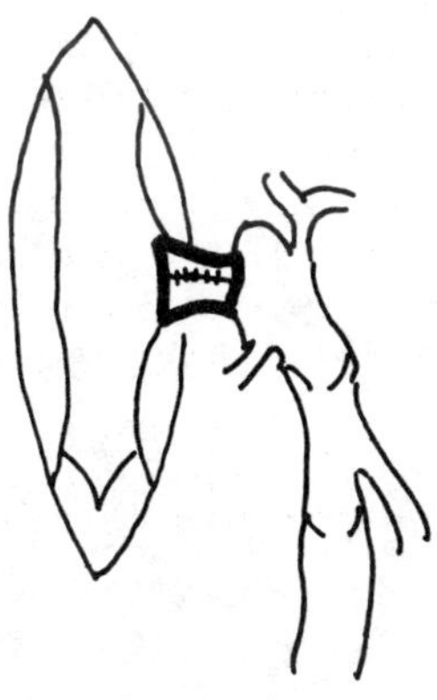

Fig.1.

We followed 81 patients during 5 years. The early results were very promising. One year after the surgery the dilatation of the LSV in the thigh regressed in all cases, ulcers are healed. The reflux left of the 90 % of the cases, and flow was always centripetal to the effect of the muscle pump.
Five years after the surgery 37 patients were without recurrency and in these cases there was no retrograde flow in the LSV at Valsalva maneuvere. At 20 of these patients the varicosity was originaly Hach II. type.
At 39 patients developed a recurrency. At Valsalva there was always a retrograde flow. Varicography was made in 12 cases. At the saphenofemoral junction the lumen of the LSV was only 1-2 mm. During Valsalva there was a visible regurgitation. We didn't find valves in the iliac and communis femoral veins, the superficial femoral vein was intact in all cases. Another possibility of the recurrency was the insufficiency of the Dodd perforating vein.
By varicography we observed in many cases a fluctuation of calibre of LSV trunk remaining secretly for the clinical examination.It made retrospectively uncertain that the vein really could have been useful as a long arterial bypass.
Altogether in 11 cases occured redo surgery /flush ligation and stripping of the LSV/.
However at five patients with known femoropopliteal arterial occlusion and mild LSV varicosity we performed first the external bounding of LSV junction, and after 4-8 months we made a regular bypass operation using the LSV trunk. The LSV diameter decreased in all cases compared to the first operation.

Our conclusions are:

1. The external bounding of the saphenofemoral junction with a Dacron ring didn't provide durably shelter from the recurrency of LSV varicosity despite favourable early results.

2. This operation is acceptable only in selected cases: at young patients in the Hach II. stadium of the varicosity /sufficient LSV valves in the mid-thigh/ and at femoropopliteal arteriosclerosis with mild LSV varicosity as a preparative operation.

3. It is probable, that with the more efficient examination /Duplex scan visualisation of the incompetence, but not copletly destructed subterminal valve of the LSV/ the surgical results can be considerably curable, but it is undoubted, that after interventions preserving the insufficient LSV trunk we have to reckon with a greater recurrency rate.

C.
MEMBRE INFÉRIEURE
LOWER EXTREMITY

Aesthetic reconstruction of the lower extremity

Gabriela Guzman-Stein, James C. Grotting, R. Jobe Fix and Luis O. Vasconez

University of Alabama at Birmingham

The initial phase of amazement with reconstruction by means of transposition or transplantation of a variety of tissue flaps has progressed to its present phase of refinement. With inflation of medical cost, seemingly the reconstructive surgeon is challenged to shorten the reconstructive process while providing the optimal result.

The current period of refinement in lower extremity reconstruction may «jump» steps in the reconstructive ladder and selectively choose that alternative which will offer not only the best coverage and resolution of the initial but the most aesthetically pleasing result with the advantage of a single operation. We review the systematic approach to flap selection relating the role of specific flaps to other methods in the reconstructive ladder for specific defects in the region. Specific information regarding the sign techniques and possible complications are presented.

Reconstruction of the lower extremity with vascular disease

Gabriela Guzman-Stein, James C. Grotting, R. Jobe Fix and Luis O. Vasconez

University of Alabama at Birmingham

With the introduction of muscle flaps and with the liberalized use of micro surgery for reconstruction of difficult problems in the lower extremity, surgeons are able to salvage limbs in patients who formerly might have had amputations. However, many patients with severe peripheral vascular insufficiency non-amenable to conventional arterial procedures eventually will require amputation. The use of microvascular tissue transfer as an adjunct toward arterial reconstruction has expanded the horizons on limb salvage inpatients with advanced arterial scleroses or non healing ischemic or irradiated ulcers. We review our experience.

Phlébologie 92. Eds P. Raymond-Martimbeau, R. Prescott, M. Zummo.
John Libbey Eurotext, Paris © 1992, pp. 1266-1269

Prevention of complications and correction of post operative problems in lower extremity reconstruction

Gabriela Guzman-Stein, Luis O. Vasconez, James C. Grotting

The most common complication seen in lower extremity reconstruction with transposed or microsurgically transplanted flaps are vascular thrombosis and recurrence of infection. These complications frequently represent errors in judgment or technical misadventures. Seemingly, failure of the operation to solve the initial problem adequately may result from what the surgeon though was an "insignificant" oversight or "calculated risks". For example the mistaken belief that a healthy flap will take care of an established infection. This may eventually result in chronic draining sinuses around an otherwise technically well executed flap.

Vigorous surgical debridement is the most relevant principle in reconstruction of the wounded extremity. The first step is to debride necrotic tissue to get rid of the infection. The next step is to obtain coverage. Adequate surgical debridement goes hand and hand with any reconstructive alternative. Both are associated with technically well executed operation which will lead to a healed. uninfected wound.

Avoiding Complications by Proper Patient Selection

According to Khouri and Shaw (Ref. 1) the failure rate for free flap reconstruction in the lower extremity (8%) as compared to other body areas (3%) is due to the degree in injury. Those patients which are severely comminuted or who have displaced fractures, long bone gaps, extensive soft tissue losses, and devascularization have the highest flap failure rates in their studies and others.

Adequate selection of who should and who should not be reconstructed instead of being primarily amputated should not be overcome by the surgeon's desire of performing a sophisticated reconstructive procedure. Some of these individuals, for example, with Type IIIC injuries can be spared from prolonged hospitalization, huge hospital costs and obtain an early recovery and return to work by a well performed amputation and prosthesis.

Vascular Disorders

There are a variety of factors that should alert a reconstructive surgeon to potential complications. Patients over the age of 50, smokers, or with diminished distal pulses or diabetics may have elements of arteriosclerotic vascular occlusive disease. This patient should be carefully evaluated preoperatively by arteriography. Patients with history of ischemic vascular disease or diabetic ulceration may require stage or simultaneous distal revascularization and microsurgical flap construction.

Likewise, superficial varicosities, skin discoloration, ulceration, unexplained edema, new or chronic of the lower extremity should alert the surgeon of the presence of venous insufficiency and possible difficulties with the outflow selection. Suitable vein grafts in these patients can also be a problem and should be addressed before surgery.

With identification of patients with vascular spastic disorders such as renal disease or patients with hemolytic disorders, and sickle cell disease, it is important to take preventive measurements, special pharmacological manipulation in some cases that will improve the odds.

Hypercoagulability should be specifically looked for especially in smokers and in those patients who have a major trauma like a crushing injury requiring transfusion. If hypercoagulability is anticipated, it is advisable to consider early use of anticoagulation to diminish intraoperative thrombosis.

Arteriography

The primary reason to perform preoperative angiography is to identify the main contributing vascular supply to the injured lower extremity. In order to minimize the irritant effects of the contrast agent, arteriography should be performed more than 48 hours prior to free flap transfer.

Wound Factors

Predictable, high rates of success for lower extremity reconstruction are best achieved when the patient, the wound, and the surgeon are all adequately prepared. The earlier stable coverage can be obtained the greater the liklihood of avoiding infection. But the single most important factor in preventing subsequent complications is debridement. Management of dead space, whether created surgically or traumatically, is the central issue in successful treatment of leg wounds, as well.

Refinement in the Choice of Donor Tissue

The surgeon should be familiar with a member of donor areas and avoid the urge to make a field work-horse flap the answer to every problem. In choosing a donor site the surgeon should critically check the particular site in that particular patient rather than assume that the patient will conform to the standard. Hobbies, sports, and work related areas should be taken into consideration before the decision is made.

General Consideration in Anesthetic Care

Careful attention to the patient's core temperature and circulation, fluid volume are important for success. Care in regard to each of the above should begin preoperatively, maintain transoperatively and continue postoperatively. Elderly and debilitated patients or those with associated medical problems should be monitored with an arterial line and CVP monitoring. Vasopressors should be avoided or used only as a last result in those patients who are undergoing microvascular reconstruction.

Post Traumatic Vessel Disease

After trauma to the lower extremity a widespread change occurs in the vessel wall and perivascular tissue at the injured extremity. The zone of trauma extends beyond the original site of injury and should strongly be avoided. Acland[2] Sites three hallmarks of the established conditions: 1) loss of normal easy plains of dissection between the vascular sheet and artery and between arteries and veins; 2) loss of vasavasorum, and 3) market tendency to vasospasm.

Tunnels

All tunnels made to accommodate flaps or flap vessels are potentially hazardous.

Thrombosis

The most likely time for thrombosis to occur is within the first several hours following anastomosis in the case of microvascular surgery of flap transfer. It is far better to reexplore the anastomosis. If there are periods when the flap becomes pale or venous congested. Pharmacological manipulation or application of leeches play no role in the treatment of vascular thrombosis. Careful determination of the cause of thrombosis should be done to be able to correct adequately and salvage the flap. "Most flaps die on the table".

Monitoring

The purpose of flap monitoring is to give an easy warning sign of circulatory compromise. At the present time no perfect monitoring system has been developed. There is no substitute for periodic observation of the flap by the surgeon and skilled personnel.

References

1. Khouri, RK, Shaw, WW: Reconstruction of the Lower Extremity with Microvascular Free Flaps: A 10 Year Experience with 304 Consecutive Cases. Journal of Trauma: 29:1086-1094, 1989.

2. Acland, RO: Refinements in Lower Extremity Free Flap. Clin. Plast. Surg. 17:733-744, 1980.

3. Shestak, KC, et al: Expanding The Horizons in Treatment of Severe Peripheral Vascular Disease Using Microsurgical Techniques, Plast. Reconstr. Surg. 85, (3): 406-411, 1990.

Phlébologie 92. Eds P. Raymond-Martimbeau, R. Prescott, M. Zummo.
John Libbey Eurotext, Paris © 1992, pp. 1270-1272

Liposuction of the calves and ankles

Richard A. Mladick, M.D., F.A.C.S.

Center for Cosmetic Plastic Surgery, Inc., 1037 First Colonial Road, Virginia Beach, Virginia 23454 U.S.A.

The Illouz technique of lipoplasty is a safe and successful technique for reducing fat bulges and contouring the body. While the early applications were primarily for bulges of the saddlebags, hips, and abdomen, the author began to suction calves and ankles starting in 1983. During the past ten years, he has built up an extensive series presently numbering almost one hundred patients who have had lipoplasty contouring of the calves and ankles. In all cases, the patients have been very positive and pleased about the correction.

Patient selection

The ideal patients for this procedure are those who desire a correction of fat (heavy) calves and ankles. The age range has been from the early twenties to the mid fifties. Patient must have realistic goals. A history of thrombophlebitis and deep vein thrombosis would be considered a contraindication for this procedure

Diagnosis and classification

Legs may be classified as circumferential heavy or localized heavy legs. The circumferential heavy legs are thick and fat from the knee all the way to the ankle. In the localized type, the calf is acceptable but there is a noticeable heaviness and bulges in the lower half of the leg. The ankles often have definite bulges over the lower lateral fibular and medial tibial regions. When examining the patient, it is helpful for the patient to stand flat footed and then stand on the toes. Standing on the toes tightens the underlying muscles and allows the surgeon to check the pinch test without pinching any underlying tissue. The pinch test must measure at least 2 cm. If there is any question of deep vein competency, the patient is referred for a vascular workup.

Plan of treatment

Preparation for surgery includes instructions to stop aspirin, alcohol, and tobacco ten days prior to surgery and the daily use of a surgical soap starting three days before surgery. The expected degree of improvement is thoroughly discussed with the patient and all possible complications are outlined. The proposed incisions are demonstrated.

On the day of surgery, the patient is marked in the standing position. The legs are marked with a topographical marking. Four or more incisions are used for each leg; two in the knee region, medial and lateral, and two in the ankle region, medial and lateral. Because these incisions are so small, usually less than 1 cm., they do not leave significant scarring. Often times, an additional incision is made in the mid line anterior lower leg for a small 2 or 3 mm. cannula that requires only a 1/2 cm. incision. In localized cases, only the lower half of the leg is suctioned. In the circumferentially heavy leg, the entire leg is suctioned from the knee to the ankle, except for a small area over the achilles tendon.

Technique

General anesthesia is used with the patient in the supine "frog" position for the medial legs and ankles. For the lateral legs and ankles, the patient is turned at the waist to the supine-lateral-decubitus position. Most of the legs are suctioned using a long 3 or 4 mm. cannula. Before beginning suction, the cannula is passed at the most superficial level possible just below the dermis. This pretunneling loosens up the separation of the skin from the underlying fat and allows for very accurate fat removal. The technique requires considerably more skill than suctioning the saddlebags or the abdomen. The surgeon should have extensive experience with liposuction before trying the calves and ankles. There is no tolerance for irregularities and the technique must be done with careful feathering in the localized cases so as not to leave a sharp edge of a depression but rather a blending in from the suctioned area to the nonsuctioned area. In the circumferential areas, it is important for the surgeon to completely suction the whole leg without leaving any gaps.

After the first leg is completed, it is immediately wrapped firmly from toes to knee with a sterile six inch ace bandage. When the second leg is completed, it is also wrapped with a six inch ace bandage. Then the first leg is unwrapped and the incisions closed. After closing the incisions on both legs, firm support hose is applied. The legs are then wrapped with six inch ace bandages over the support hose. The patient is started on the intermittent compression device while in the recovery room.

The average amount removed from circumferential cases is approximately 650 cc. The average amount removed from a localized case is approximately 220 cc. each leg.

Results

The results have improved as the experience has increased. It is common to decrease the calf circumference by 2 to 4 cm. and the ankle circumferency by at least 1 to 2 cm. Approximately one hundred patients have now been treated with this technique and six have required touch-up procedures. Fig. 1.

Complications

The complications with this technique have been extremely few and minor. There have been no hematomas, infections, or skin sloughs, but the incisions have remained noticeable in some patients for a number of months. In the beginning, before we used the intermittent compression device, it was common for the legs to remain edematous for many months. For the past three years, we have used an intermittent compression device beginning almost immediately after surgery and it is not unusual for the patient to be over most of their edema in six to eight weeks.

While it is not unusual to see some slight subcutaneous irregularities during the first three or four weeks, they disappear and smooth out nicely without any further treatment. There have been no significant permanent dents, divots, or irregularities in any of these patients. The bruising is surprisingly minimal. There has been no permanent staining of the lower leg skin from bruising. Since all of the patients had been done with a computerized suction machine, we have been able to monitor the exact blood loss and we have not had any significant blood loss over 500 cc. No patients have required transfusion. All patients had the subcutaneous fat preinjected with a dilute solution of xylocaine with epinephrine.

Summary
In summary, lipoplasty of the calves and ankles is an extremely rewarding procedure for those patients with very heavy, fat legs. The procedure is more difficult than the usual lipoplasty procedure because, in the lower legs, there is only one layer of fat as compared to the abdomen or saddlebags where there are two layers.

REFERENCES

Mladick, R.A. (1990): Lipoplasty of the calves and ankles. Plast. & Reconstr. Surg.86, 84-93.

XVI.
ANESTHÉSIE
ANESTHESIA

Phlébologie 92. Eds P. Raymond-Martimbeau, R. Prescott, M. Zummo.
John Libbey Eurotext, Paris © 1992, pp. 1275

Propositions techniques dans l'anesthésie de la chirurgie ambulatoire des varices

William Taieb, Olivier Musard

9, rue de Turin, 75008 Paris, France.

L'anesthésie peut être un obstacle à la chirurgie ambulatoire des varices.Pour nous,en pratique libèrale,la solution est univoque,après plusieurs tentatives techniques.

PROTOCOLE OPERATOIRE :
L'anesthésie pèri-durale est la solution idéale pour la chirurgie ambulatoire des éveinages saphènes. Les phlébectomies limitées peuvent être pratiquées sous anesthésie locale.

ARGUMENTS EN FAVEUR DE NOTRE ATTITUDE :
1/ medico-légale :
durée minima d'hospitalisation : 6 heures.
2/ anatomique :
Un bloc crural ou sciatique est insuffisant pour la plupart des éveinages.
3/ pratique :
Confort du patient et du chirurgien.
4/ Inocuité :
aucune gène post-opératoire.
CONCLUSION :
Nous proposons une solution univoque dans le cadre de l'anesthésie de la Chirurgie ambulatoire des varices :
" la pèridurale ".

Phlébologie 92. Eds P. Raymond-Martimbeau, R. Prescott, M. Zummo.
John Libbey Eurotext, Paris © 1992, pp. 1276-1279

Surgical-anaesthesiological approach in the treatment of lower extremities varices under D.H. regime

Mauro Casagrande, Albino Visintin, Vittorio Antonaglia, Darno Cosulich

Private medical-surgical nursing home Sanatorio Triestino S.p.a. Trieste, Italy.

INTRODUCTION

In our phlebologic activity of the last four years 356 patients have received surgical treatment. Suppression of long and/or short refluxes was the technique used, under general anaesthesia with controlled ventilation. Our cases showed a negligible number of surgical complications, so that patients were readly discharged. The number of minor complications related to general anaesthesia instead advises against short-term discharge. Therafore an alternative anaesthesiological method was called for, in order to ensure the patient's ready recovery and his early discharge. The advantages of outpatient surgery an anaesthesia are known:

1) patients can go back to their families within a few hours, they are free to walk about and no nursing is required;
2) removal of some postoperative complications such as hospital infections and thrombo-embollic events;
3) reduction of costs related to the stay in hospital.

Taking into account the most recent literature and our clinical experience, the anaesthesiological technique that ensures the fastest functional recovery associated with analgesia, amnesia and immobility during surgery is the one that couples local anaesthesia with "cross" by means of intravenous sedation and hypnosis during stripping. The purpose of this work is the perioperative assessment of a group 86 patients in relation to complications and comfort in order to check the new anaesthesiological method.

MATERIALS AN METHODS

86 patients have been threated for 18 months - 45 under General Anaesthesia (group A) and 41 under Local Anaesthesia and intravenous sedation (group B). The average age of the two groups was the following:

A) - 47.5 - B) - 49.3. Most patients belonged to ASA 1 and 2. In group A) there are 9 ASA 3 and in group B) - 7 ASA 3.

Group A) redceived the following treatment: 7 long Stripping, 2 short S., 30 short S. + phlebectomies, 2 small saphenas, 1 small saphena + short S. + phlebectomies, 3 Cross revisions.

Group B) 1 long S., 4 short S., 26 short S. + phlebectomies, 6 small saphenas, 3 small saphenas + short S. + phlebectomies, 1 cross revision.

The anaesthesiological treatment includes:
Group A) intubation,machanical ventilation, inhalation anaesthesia and curarization.
Group B) - perioperative sedation by means of Midazolan 5 mg. bolus plus 0.2 mg./Kg./hr.;
- subcutaneous infiltration in the Cross area with a linear multi-injector and in the phlebectomy area with Mepivacaina 0.5-1% (from 80 to 120 mg of Mepivacaina as a whole), 150 mg being the maximum dosage; in three cases the periadventitial infiltration of the saphena femoral junction was performed;
- hypnosis at the time of stripping by means of Propofol (1.5-2 mg/Kg) and possibily maintenance in infusion at 4 mg/Kg/hr.
The sedation`level during surgery was evaluated by means of Wiilson's and David's Sedation Scores. Vital parameters were monitored by non-invasive BP, ECG monitor. During the hypnotic stage ventilatio was provided by mask and administration of O_2 and the depth of hypnosis was assessed by means of the pupillary diameter, BP and breathing.
Duration of surgery ranged between 20 minutes and 1 hour and 30 minutes. The hypnotic stage never exceded 10 minutes. The postoperative assessment was carried out according to the recovery of the state of consciousness and comfort status. Immediatly after surgery response to simple orders, presence of pain and nausea were considered and evaluated with a score index. Three hours later the the same evaluation was repeated considering pain with analogical-visual scale and functional recovery by means of the performance status. Moreover postoperative complications were investigated (urinary retention, cephalea, pharyngodynia, myalgia, tooth avulsions, hyperthermia).

STATISTICAL EVALUATION

Methods of multivariate analysis were applied. The Cluster Analysis of 86 patients characterized by 14 variables (Table 1) was carried out, identified by the presence-absence criterion, and using the Jaccard similarity index. The Cluster Analyses of variables were carried out using the correlation coefficient as similarity index and the trend of patients and variables according to the correlation coefficient.

List of variables:
1) Long stripping + phlebectomy
2) Short stripping
3) Short stripping + phlebectomy
4) Small saphena
5) Small saphena + short stripping + phlebectomy
6) Cross revision
7) Immediate nausea
8) Immediatle pain
9) Response to simple orders
10) Nausea three hours after surgery
11) Pain three hours after surgery
12) Gait
13) Postoperative complications
14) ASA

RESULTS
The Dendogram of the 86 patients detects Clusters (Fig.1). Cluster A includes 19 patients showing postoperative complications: 2 of them

had been treated with our method (nausea and pain immediately after surgery).
Cluster B includes 2 patients showing complications characterized by nausea immediately after and three huors upon surgery, and one patient complaining of pain immediately after surgery: all three of them had been treated under general anaesthesia. The Dendogram of (Fig. 2) points out the competition of complication-indicating variables. The order of the variables parameters (Fig. 3) on the first axis detects a gradient among variables that is characterized by the Performance Status (V-12) and variables corresponding to the complications arising after surgery. The distribution of patients referring to the x axis is conditioned by the presence of such variables and the group of patients that is close to the right-hand variables (V-13-10-7-8-11) is the one treated under general anaesthesia. The evaluation of the sedation level during surgery according to Wilson's and David's scale scored between 3 and 4. During the stripping stage the administration of Propofol was followed by a 15% decrease in the systolic and diastolic pressure. The study concerning secondary complications of anaesthesia pointed out only the presence of nausea and vomit.
In group A) (general anaesthesia) 9 patients suffered from nausea immediately after surgery and 7 patients three ours later with six episodes of vomit.
In group B) omly one patient complained of nausea immediately afeter surgery. Pain was evaluated according to the presence-absence criterion immediately after surgery and by means of an analogical-visual scale three hours later.
In group A) immediate and delayed pain was complained of by 10 patients with an average VAS value equal to 5, three hours after surgery.
In group B) pain immediately after surgery was complained of by 3 patients and three hours upon surgery-by 1 patient whose VAS value was equal to 4.
All patients of group B) immediately after surgery showed ready recovery of the state of consciousness with performance of simple orders and suitable verbal answers. Three hours after surgery they were able to walk about freely and to perform skilled movements, so that they were discharged.

DISCUSSION

The clinical outcome and the interpretation of the multivariate analysis results are extremly favourable to the applications of our method. On the other hand the limited number of patients treated so far does not enable us to express a definite judgement, yet it induces as to carry on our study. Our method was shown a very low incidence of minor complications. The comfort that we have registered was confirmed by patients who appreciated sedation and anaesthesia status without recalling any unpleasantness as to the anaesthesiological and surgical procedure. The patients showed full functional recovery so that, provided with the necessary instructions for the following 24 hours, they were discharged without esitation.

Fig. 1: Dendogram of patients
Fig. 2: Dendogram of variables
Fig. 3: Order of variables and patients

REFERENCES

1) BISHOP-JARRET: "Out patient varicose vein surgery and local

anaesthesia". Br.J.Surg 73:821-822 1986

2) EICHELTER P. : "Stripping in regional femoral conduction block - V European American Symposium of Venous Diseases" Vienna 1990

3) NEGUS J.N., WHITE P.F.: "Use of sedative infusion during local and regional ànaesthesia". Anaesthesiology 1988,69

4) LAGONEGRO M., FEOLI E.: "Analisi multivariata di dati". Manuale d'uso di programmi BASIC per PC. Libreria Goliardica Trieste.

5) WILDI O., ORLOCI L.: 1980 "Menagement and multivariate analysis of vegetations data". Berichte Nr 215. Idtituto Federali di Ricerche Forestali. CH 8903 Birmensdorf.

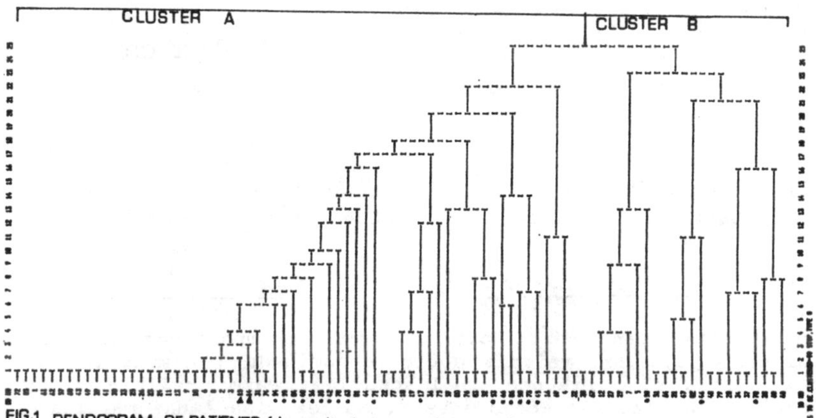

FIG.1 DENDOGRAM OF PATIENTS (Jaccard's index, medium joint)
• minor complications - general anaestesia
▲ - " - " - our methodic

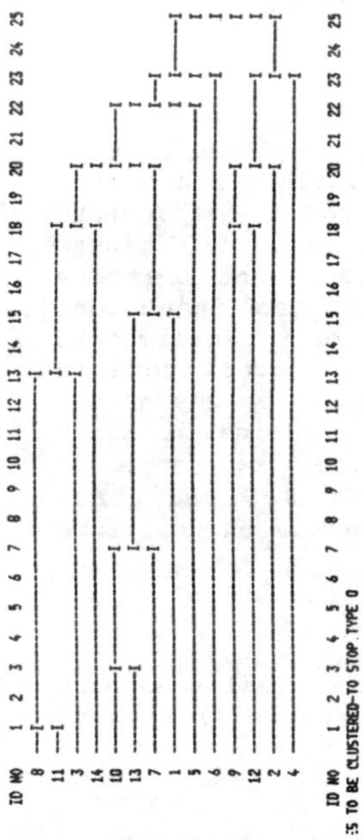

FIG.2 DENDOGRAM OF VARIABLES (coeff.correlations, medium joint)

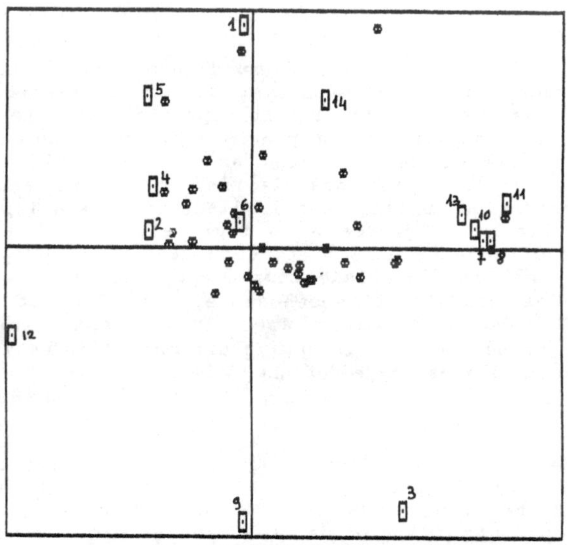

FIG.3 ORDER OF VARIABLES AND PATIENTS
▯ variables
⊗ patients

Phlébologie 92. Eds P. Raymond-Martimbeau, R. Prescott, M. Zummo.
John Libbey Eurotext, Paris © 1992, pp. 1280-1282

L'anesthésie locale au cours de la phlébectomie ambulatoire selon la méthode de R. Muller. Appréciation du risque par dosage de la lidocaïnémie

J.P. Vidal-Michel*, J.M. Trauchessec, R. Vergereau, J. Arditti**, J.H. Bourbon**, J.J. Bonerandi

** Service de dermatologie, Hôpital Ste-Marguerite, Marseille, Pr. J.J. Bonerandi, 270, Bd de Sainte-Marguerite, B.P. 29, 13277 Marseille Cedex 9. ** Laboratoire du Centre Anti-Poisons, Pr. J. Jouglard, Marseille, France.*

Les méthodes ambulatoires prennent de plus en plus d'importance dans le traitement des varices, pour des raisons socio-économiques : diminution de l'hospitalisation, reprise plus précoce de l'activité. Parmi celles-ci, la phlebectomie en ambulatoire selon la méthode de R. Muller vise à une meilleure qualité esthétique. Le plus souvent réalisée au cabinet du médecin, outre ses problèmes techniques propres, elle nécessite d'évaluer le risque général posé par l'injection de fortes doses d'anesthésiques locaux (par rapport aux doses utilisées en chirurgie dermatologique courante).

METHODE

L'anesthésie se fait par une succession d'injections de 0,5 à 1 ml étagées d'environ un à deux centimètres depart et d'autre du trajet variqueux avec une aiguille de 24 G 3/4. Les injections sont superficielles. Le produit est injecté rapidement. Le test d'aspiration est pratiqué systématiquement. Afin de diminuer le nombre de piqûres et de pousser l'anesthésique plus lentement certains utilisent des aiguilles intra-musculaires, réalisant ainsi des injections traçantes. L'anesthésique utilisé est la lidocaïne (1) à 1 p. cent conservée au réfrigérateur. Elle est injectée à la température de 2 à 5 degrés, pure ou parfois diluée à 25 p. cent ou à 50 p. cent dans du sérum physiologique glacé, réalisant ainsi une cryoanesthésie complémentaire. Pour les besoins de notre étude, nous avons utilisé l'anesthésique pur. Pendant tout le temps de l'injection le médecin converse avec le patient, surveille son état; obnubilation, logorrhée, pâleur feront interrompre l'injection. La surveillance de la tension artérielle est systématique.

ETUDE

Notre étude porte sur une série chronologique de 50 interventions réalisées dans le service du Pr J.J. Bonerandi, Hôpital Sainte Marguerite (Marseille); sept hommes et quarante trois femmes de 18 à 71 ans, allant de 48 à 103 kilogrammes.
Aucun des sujets n'a reçu dans les jours précédents ou juste avant l'intervention de prémédication.
Chez tous les patients l'interrogatoire à la recherche de réactions allergiques, incidents ou accidents à la lidocaïne (2,3,4,5) a été négatif; le bilan paraclinique (examen cardio-vasculaire, bilan hépatique et de la coagulation, écho-Doppler veineux) s'est avéré sans anomalie particulière pouvant contre-indiquer l'intervention.
Les dosages de lidocaïne dans le sang veineux périphérique ont été effectués par la méthode F.P.I.A. (Fluorescence Polarisation Immuno Assay) au temps T.O., à 30 mn, à 60 mn, à 90 mn, à 24 et 48 heures lorsque cela a été possible.

Le prélèvement pratiqué au temps T.O. avant toute injection permet de juger de la fiabilité de la méthode de dosage. Les résultats sont exprimés en mg/ml.
Le dosage de l'adrénalinémie n'a pu être réalisé. Cependant, aucune variation notable de la tension artérielle n'a été notée durant no interventions.

INTERPRETATION DES RESULTATS

D'après les Laboratoires R.B. (dictionnaire Vidal) une dose de 200 mg de lidocaïne injectée par voie sous-cutanée au niveau de l'avant-bras donne, une demi-heure après l'injection, des concentrations de 0,3 à 0,5 mg/ml. La dose maximale pour une anesthésie locale ne doit dépasser 200 mg pour un adulte de 70 kg (2,9 mg/kg) pour la forme sans adrénaline (1 flacon de 20 ml à 1 %) et 500 mg (7,1mg/kg) pour les formes avec adrénaline (2,5 flacon de 20 ml à 1 %).
Rappelons que la dose thérapeutique en cardiologie se situe aux concentrations plasmatiques comprises entre 1 et 5 mg/ml.
Au cours de notre étude, tous les taux plasmatiques de lidocaïne sont très inférieurs aux taux toxiques. Nous nous sommes fixé comme limite de sécurité le taux de 2 mg/ml, qui représente la moitié de la limite inférieure des taux considérés comme toxiques sur le plan neurologique (dont les premiers signes, rappelons-le, sont : paresthésies, angoisse, logorrhée, facilement curables par oxygénothérapie et diazepam) et le douzième des taux toxiques sur le plan cardio-vasculaire (24 mg/ml). Pour des doses allant de moins de 5 mg/kg à plus de 15 mg/kg, malgré une grande variabilité d'un sujet à un autre (parfois de 1 à 10), les concentrations sanguines se situent toutes au-dessous de 2 mg/ml.
Le taux maximum obtenu avec la lidocaïne adrénalinée, pour une dose de 700 mg pour un sujet de 65 kg (10,9 mg/kg), ne dépasse pas 1,8 mg/ml
Dans un cas, chez une femme de 32 ans, nous avons atteint la dose de 16,1 mg/kg soit 890 mg pour 55 kg, sans dépasser un taux de 1,3 mg/ml.
Dans un autre cas, chez une femme de 58 ans pesant 65 kg, nous avons dû utiliser de la lidocaïne à 1 p.cent non adrénalinée ; pour une dose de 400 mg (soit 6,2 mg/kg) le pic plasmatique a été de 0,7 mg/ml.
Les faibles taux plasmatiques retrouvés nous conduisent à quelques réflexions :
- la tolérance de l'anesthésie locale est-elle due :
• au métabolisme propre de la lidocaïne dans les tissus graisseux sous-cutanés,
• à la méthode elle-même qui consiste à faire des injections de 0,5 à 1 ml d'anesthésique étagées le long du trajet variqueux, diminuant ainsi le rapport quantité d'anesthésique/surface cutanée et par là même son passage plasmatique.
En raison de la multiplicité des points d'injection, on aurait pu se demander si une certaine quantité d'anesthésique ne s'éliminait pas au point d'injection ou d'incision pour l'éveinage, mais cela n'est pas le cas en pratique.
• à la vaso-constriction induite par le froid (anesthésique injecté entre 2 et 5 degrés) venant s'additionner à la vaso-constriction créée par l'adrénaline.

CONCLUSION

La pratique de l'anesthésie locale au cabinet du médecin est dénuée de risques majeurs, bien que les doses utilisées au cours de la phlébectomie ambulatoire soient très supérieures aux doses habituelles pratiquées en chirurgie dermatologique courante.

Table 1 : Tous les résultats sont rapportés dans le tableau suivant :

cas	sexe	age	poids	Vol	Qt inj. mg	mg/kg	t= 0	30 mn	1 h	90 mn	24 h	48 h
1	F	42	58	50	500	8,6	0	0,4	0,4			
2	F	39	55	40	400	7,3	0	0,3	0,3			
3	F	45	53	35	350	6,6	0	< 0,1	0,2	0,25		
4	F	51	52	35	350	6,7	0	0,3	0,4			
5	F	32	50	35	350	7,0	0	< 0,1	< 0,1			
6	F	18	75	17	170	2,3	0	< 0,1	< 0,1			
7	F	46	55	42	420	7,6	0	0,1	0,2			
8	F	66	55	40	400	7,3	0	0,2	0,2			
9	F	42	58	53	530	9,1	0	0,1	0,2		0,1	
10	F	58	65	40	400	6,2	0	0,7	0,6			
11	F	46	57	70	700	12,3	0	0,2		0,2	0,2	

12	F	56	52	46	460	8,8	0	0,5	0,6			
13	H	68	67	45	450	6,7	0	0,9	0,8			< 0,1
14	F	31	57	40	400	7,0	0	0,15			0,1	
15	F	43	54	70	700	13,0	0		0,5			
16	F	49	60	65	650	10,8	0	0,15				
17	F	48	55	50	500	9,1	0	0,3				
18	F	71	57	50	500	8,8	0	0,2	0,2			
19	F	71	57	45	450	7,9	0	0,2	0,2			< 0,1
20	F	41	50	55	550	11,0	0	0,9	0,9			
21	H	64	74	50	500	6,8	0	0,6	0,5			< 0,1
22	F	62	53	25	250	4,7	0	0,4	0,4			< 0,1
23	F	52	79	30	300	3,8	0	0,1	0,2			
24	F	48	47	30	300	6,4	0	0,8	0,6	0,4		
25	F	81	48	42	420	8,8	0	0,8	0,6	0,6		
26	H	68	67	31	310	4,6	0	0,5	0,6			< 0,1
27	F	45	52	45	450	8,7	0	0,2			0,4	
28	F	34	48	40	400	8,3	0	0,5	0,6			< 0,1
29	F	49	55	43	430	7,8	0	0,4	0,6	0,8		< 0,1
30	F	46	58	21	210	3,6	0	0,2	0,1	< 0,1		< 0,1
31	F	64	64	60	600	9,4	0	0,3	0,4	0,3		< 0,1
32	F	49	59	60	600	10,2	0	1	1	1,1		0,4
33	F	43	58	54	540	9,3	0	1,1	1,2	1		0,3
34	H	48	65	70	700	10,8	0	1,6	1,8	1,5		
35	F	65	66	60	600	9,1	0	0,6	0,8	0,7		< 0,1
36	F	41	56	80	800	14,3	0		1,2			
37	F	37	63	50	500	7,9	0	0,3	0,2	0,2		
38	F	65	67	46	460	6,9	0	0,4	0,4	0,3		
39	F	68	57	55	550	9,6	0	0,2	0,4			< 0,1
40	F	32	55	89	890	16,2	0	1,3	1,3	1		< 0,1
41	H	48	100	60	600	6,0	0	0,1	0,2	0,2		
42	F	53	65	60	600	9,2	0	0,4	0,3	0,3		
43	F	38	55	55	550	10,0	0	0,4	0,5	0,4		
44	F	46	87	60	600	6,9	0	0,1	0,5			
45	F	54	53	60	600	11,3	0	0,2				
46	H	63	103	80	800	7,8	0	0,8	0,9			
47	F	29	55	50	500	9,1	0	0,8	0,9			
48	H	48	100	95	950	9,5	0	0,2	0,5			< 0,1
49	F	50	50	80	800	16,0	0		0,6			
50	F	23	55	75	750	13,6	0	0,6	0,6			

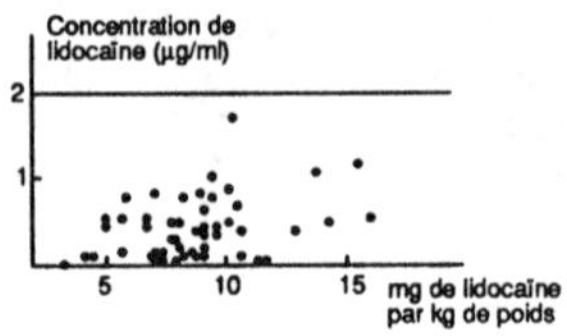

Fig. 1 En abscisses : doses administrées en mg/kg.
En ordonnées : concentrations plasmatiques en µg/ml.
On s'est fixé le seuil de 2 µg/ml comme limite de sécurité.

REFERENCES

1. Roujas F., Perney C. - Pharmacologie des anesthésiques locaux. Encycl. Méd.-chir. Anesthésie Réanimation, A 10, 1975.

2. Abijaoude F., Fischler M. - L'anesthésie locale au cabinet du praticien. Dermatol. prat., 1988, 30, n°19, 27-29.

3. Incaudo G., Schat Z., Patterson R., Rosenberg M., Yamamoto F., Hamburger R.N. - Administration of local anesthetics to patients with a history of prior adverse reactions. J. Allergy. Clin. Immunol., 1978, 61, 339-345.

4. Moneret-Vautrin. - Les réactions adverses aux anesthésiques locaux. Conceptions actuelles. Stratégies diagnostiques. Aspects préventifs. All. Immunol., 1985, 17, n° 7, 369-377.

5. Monneret-Vautrin. - Accidents immédiats aux anesthésiques locaux pluralité des mécanismes éthiopathogéniques et incidents pratiques. Médecine et Hygiène, 1981, 39, 112-117.

XVII.
TRAITEMENT DES ULCÈRES DE JAMBE
LEG ULCER TREATMENT

Phlébologie 92. Eds P. Raymond-Martimbeau, R. Prescott, M. Zummo.
John Libbey Eurotext, Paris © 1992, pp. 1285-1287

Venous ulcerations of the lower limbs : our medical cases contribution

Giovanni Perdonò

Via Borreani Dagna n° 9, 17014 Cairo Montenotte (SV), Italia.

INTRODUCTION

"Venous ulcerations" are defined as the trophic lesions, which usually cause complications in both, in the varicous disease and in the post-thrombotic syndrome at the third stadium, characterizing the differences and the possible connections. Undoubtedly, such diseases are very important, especially considering the social and individual costs. Therefore, a right clirical program imposes a careful differential diagnosis, a proper therapy as well as the complication and relapse prevention.

PHYSIOPATHOLOGY: OUTLINES

The reflux and the venous stasis represent the common beginning of all the venous lesions. In the varicous disease the reflux is caused by the incontinence of the saphenic crosses, added oro not to the incontinence of the deep circulation, following the valvular apparatus destruction, after the recanalization of the thrombus, and the centrifugal reflux, subsequent the valve's damage of the communicating circulation, have a great weight. The reflux and the venous stasis cause some typical systemic alterations (hemoviscosity rise, reduced clearance of potentially thrombogenicus elements, deficit of the fibrinolytic system) and district alterations (pericapillary fibrin abnormal deposition with reduced metabolic excange og the tissues and with local ischemia, as shown by Browse and Burnard).

Traumatic events, new disease attacks or intercourrent pathologies, break the precarius homeostatic equilibrium, producing the appearance of the trophic lesions, distinguished by the site (in the post-thrombotic syndrome, the leg third lower, along the Achilles tendon and near the site of the failing communicating veins, in the varicous disease, along the collaterals veins and the saphena sections).

Dimensions and appearance:small,but deep in the post-thrombotic syndrome; very large, but superficial in the varicous disease. Quickest and propitious development in the varicous disease, more "troubled" course in the post- thrombotic syndrome.

PATIENTS, MATERIALS AND METHODS

Our clinical cases comprehend two hundred patients, treated during four years, of both sex, aged between 35 and 85; 40 per cent of them were suffering from isolated thrombotic disease and the remaining 60 per cent having some typical disease (diabetes, arterial disease, heart disease, arterial hypertentient suffering from rheumatoid arthritis and from a multiple ulceration in the course of the paraneoplastic phlebothrombosis.Each patient was undergone a general clinical and vascular check-up, inclucommon therapeutic program was formulated. It included:

- causal therapy of the systemic pathology (diabetes, heart disease, etc.);
- medical phlebological therapy, using some specific venous tropism drugs,

Dypiridamol, heparinsodium, GAGS, according to particular necessities;
- local therapy, including the lesion cleaning and the edema reduction.

The cleaning comprised surgical or chemoproteolytic courretage, associated with local treatment by the following cures:

- tratment by imbricated sticking-plaster, according to Beyton (50 cases): it was the first method that we applied, but subsequently we left it, notwithstanding the excellent results, due to its poor praticalness and to the easy allergy it causes; its low price is very favourable;
- washings and compresses using iodic polyvinylpyrolidone (Betadine), (30 cases): good results, no collateral effects, reasonable cost;
- elastic stocking (Douderm), (20 cases): it gives excellent results in patients having some severeskin allergic reactions and some characteristic ulcerationsfrom a plentiful exudation; conta-indicated in collagenous disases, in allergic vasculitis and in lesions of the bones and the tendons; the high costs and the difficulty to find it are unfavourable;
- bovine collagene (Proteita), (10 cases): excellent resuts, especially in presence of very wide lesions, easily handy, but very higt price and many difficulties to find it;
- treatment by ichthyol + zinc oxide (Icthioplast), (60 cases) or by zinc oxide alone (20 cases):that's our favourite method of therapy, sometimes giving very good resulta in a short time, reasonable cost, that can be further on reduced if prepared at the moment. We lay stress on the bigpraticalness, but, at the same time,the frequent appearance of the sensitization and the skin intolerance;
- complementary sclerotherapy of the varicous collaterals veins by Polidecanolo or hypertonc glucose (20 cases): quik venous lesions recovery, but we need a great experience, in order not to cause additional iatrogenic eschars, making the sclerosing fluid gone out in the perivenous tissue,already chronically sick.

It's better to avoid the systemic and local antibiotic therapy (but in course of chemoproteolysis, frequently being on sale such substances associated to topic antibiotics such as Neomycin and Bacytracin); it's also better to avoid the steroyds for topical use, except in case of very aching ulcerations, as sometimes we find in case of necrotizing vasculitis, collagenous diseases and diabetes with neurovascular complications. We have to use very cautiously vaseline gauzes and other emollients, anyway, only if the skin appears very dehydrated.

The supportive treatments, as Dakey-Carrel's solutions, ammonium derivatives, hydrogen peroxide, chrome Mercury, Castellani solution and potassium permanganate, are considered by us very useful, in order to stimulate the tissue-granulation and to prevent the bacterial and mycotic overlaps.

It's better to make the edema's cleaning exclusively by physical means, avoiding the diuretic treatment and limiting at the most the use of anti-exudation substances, as Benzidamina and Escina.

At te beginning, we applied the rest in bed for some days, the limbs being raised; later, faithful to principle of the early mobilization, we prefered a pre-care by presso-therapy or by inextensible bandage plus foam rubber bandages, in order to cause a considerable increase in work-pressure.

Afterwards, the reduction was progressively kept by the elastic stocking and then by first or second class stocking, according to the venous basic disease and under the management of the venous pressure measuring by Doppler. Such cure is very useful for the "mixed" ulcerations, in addiction to an arterial disease, vherein the work-pressure must always be lower the perfusion pressure, in order to avoid the ischemic suffering of the nether limbs.

<u>The relapses prevention</u> is related to three elements:

- the correction of the systemic disease, that are able to induce to a tissutal lack of balance, favouring new development poussèes of the primary venous disease;
- the correction of the venous failure by medical therapy, modfyng the hemostatic and fibrinolyric lacks of balance and by elasto-compressive therapy, considered "the first and last drug". Suchtreatment is very important in the varicous disease, because the elastic compression, even thoug restricted to the first class, helps in the preservation of the peripheral orthodromic flux, invigorating the communicating circulation, even if such elastic compression can't be opposed to the "venous escape" through the incontinent crosses. the elasto-compressive therapy is also very

important in the post-thrombotic syndrome, wherein a more efficacious compressure is able to limit the reflux through the venous deep circulation with no valves, and is also able to oppose to the centrifugal reflux, caused by the muscolar pump, in case of irreversible lesions of the valvular piercing apparatus irreversibly damaged;
- surgical tratment of the superficial and deep venous failure (respectively saphenectomy in 40 cases and 10 operations for ligation of failing communicating vessels, according to Linton): the patients, who accepted our suggestions and have been sent to the surgeon, don't show relapses so far.

RESULTS

The right application of our method allowed the complete recovery in 196 cases, in a period from two weeks (a young man suffering from post-traumatic ulceration on idiopathic varices) to one year (old woman, motionless on the Bath-chair, suffering from iatrogenic ulceration and from rheumatoid arthritis). We point out two failures for two patients, absolutely intolerant to the medical and physical prescriptions, and also two immediate relapses, due to the impossibility to rapidly and radically correct the venous basic disease. We report thirty relapses during a period from six months to two years, for the patients to whom a surgical procedure has been proposed; twenty patients, persuaded of its necessity, didn't suffer from further relapses.

DISCUSSION

The real unitary etiology of the venous lesions allows the substantially unique therapy, even though using the proper nuances, both in the case of the trophic complications of the varicous disease and of the post-thrombotic syndrome.
An effective general therapy, directed to the basic venous disease and to the accompanying pathologies, a correct local methodology, hinging on essential bases, such as the cleaning and the reduction, and a rational and timely surgical suggestion, let to solve every kind of trophic lesion, eliminating or putting off the relapse risk. It's advisable to remember that the largest lesions, typical in the primary varocous disease, are the most rapidly curable, as remarked in the case of aour patient suffering from paraneoplastic phlebotrombosis. On the contrary, in the post-thrombotic syndrome, also the small lesions may take a muddy-looking, as if they express the district and systemic deep lack of balance, characterizing such disease, that, moreover, often is no efficacously treatable surgically.
In conclusion, we point out that, although a large number of local methods have been presented, we ourselves don't support the superiority of one therapeutic treatment in comparison with the others: each therapy must be made to measure, according to the kind of venous disease, to its clinical staging and to special requirements of the single patient.

BIBLIOGRAPHY

Abbondati A. e al and Perdonò G: Ulcere flebostatiche degli arti inferiori: revisione della casistica e nuove proposte terapeutiche. Rivista Generale Italiana di Chirurgia, 1985.

Barnes R.W. and Collicot P.E. and Sumner D.S. and tradness D.E.: Non invasive quantitation of venous hemodynamic in the post-phlebitic sundrome. Arch. Surg. 107:108, 1973.

Bassi G. and Stemmer R.: Traitments mécaniques et fonctionnels en flébologie. Ed. Piccin, 1984.

Bergan J.J. and Yao J.: Venous problems. Year book medical published inc. Chicago, 1981.

Browse N.L. and Gray L. and Morland M. and Jarret P.E.M.: Blood and vein wall fibrinolytic activity in health and vascular disease. Br. Med. J. 1:478, 1977.

Cancelli O. and Mallamaci G.: Le ulcere degli arti inferiori: diagnosi e trattamenti. Raffaello Cortina editore, Milano 1985.

Linton R.B.: the post-thrombotic ulceration of the lower extremity: its etiology and surgical treatment. Ann. Surg. 138:415, 1953.

Phlébologie 92. Eds P. Raymond-Martimbeau, R. Prescott, M. Zummo.
John Libbey Eurotext, Paris © 1992, pp. 1288-1290

Dissolution of wound coagulum and promotion of granulation tissue under DuoDERM™

George W. Cherry*, Michael J. Lydon, Jerry J. Hutchinson, Mark Rippon, Terence J. Ryan*

** Department of Dermatology, The Slade Hospital, Oxford, UK. Wound Healing Research Institute, Newtech Square, Deeside, Clwyd CH5 2NU, UK.*

The use of occlusive dressings with adequate support therapy has become part of the regimen in managing patients with chronic venous ulcers. These dressings have been shown to alter the microenvironment of wounds and enhance re-epithelialization. (Alvarez et al, 1983) In clinical studies with the hydrocolloid dressing DuoDERM™ we have observed liquefaction of eschar and increased granulation tissue in patients with venous leg ulcers. (Cherry et al 1984)

The pathophysiology of venous ulcers has been shown by Burnand (1982) and others to include impaired tissue fibrinolysis with concomitant fibrin deposition. Fibrin has been shown to be present around capillaries appearing as a fibrin cuff in histological sections of lipodermosclerotic skin or biopsies from leg ulcers.

The present studies were designed to explain our own clinical observations and to formulate a working hypothesis for healing of chronic wounds under occlusive hydrocolloid dressings.

MATERIALS AND METHODS

Clot lysis *in vitro*

The fibrinolytic capacity of wound dressings was assessed by overlaying a fibrin clot with 1 ml of phosphate-buffered saline (PBS) containing a known weight of test dressing material. Fibrinolysis was quantified by measuring the change in height of fibrin gels at 24-hour intervals. (Control experiments have validated this technique by demonstrating that change in gel height is linearly related to release of ^{125}I-fibrin degradation products from radiolabelled clot).(Lydon et al, 1989)

Porcine full thickness wound model

For fibrin clot dissolution studies, full-thickness dermal wounds 1.3 cm in diameter were made in six Landrace pigs. Fibrin clots were prepared from human fibrinogen 1.0 mg/ml (Kabi Vitrum, Stockholm, Sweden) containing a trace of ^{125}I-labelled fibrinogen. Fibrinogen (0.2 ml) clotted with thrombin was immediately introduced into the wounds and fibrin polymerization was visible within a few minutes.

After clotting, the wounds were dressed with either a nonocclusive dressing (NA Johnson & Johnson, Slough, England) or DuoDERM™. A hand-held scintillation probe was used on days 0, 1, 3 and 5 to monitor the radioactivity of the clots.

Laser Doppler Flowmetry

Post-operative perfusion readings were taken at various times from porcine full thickness wounds using a PF2 Laser Doppler Flowmeter (Perimed) with a Large Integrating Area Probe.

Immunolabelling for fibrin in venous ulcers

Punch biopsies (3 mm) were taken from the granulation tissue in the centre of venous ulcers. A monoclonal antibody specific for human cross-linked fibrin was used to label deposits of fibrin and visualized with fluorescein isothiocyanate (FITC) labelled second antibodies.

RESULTS

Clinical observations

In our clinical studies we have consistently observed liquefaction of fibrinous eschar at the wound surface under DuoDERM™ followed by development of a well-vascularized granulation tissue. Biopsies taken from the bed of venous ulcers and stained with a monoclonal antibody specific for cross linked fibrin clearly show pericapillary fibrin deposition.

Fibrinolysis

In the presence of DuoDERM™ complete *in vitro* clot lysis was observed after 24 hours incubation, compared with only 25% clot lysis by the other dressing.

In a series of experiments designed to assess fibrinolysis in a porcine full-thickness wound model ^{125}I-labelled fibrin clots were formed in the wound cavity and clot dissolution estimated by dissipation of radioactivity. Typical results showed a significantly increased fibrinolysis under DuoDERM™ compared with non-occlusive treatment.

Angiogenesis

Development of a well vascularized granulation tissue is a consistent observation in patients treated with DuoDERM™. Laser Doppler flowmetry showed an increased blood flow in DuoDERM™ treated wounds compared to control treatments ($p<0.025$) confirming blood vessel counts.

DISCUSSION

These studies have shown that DuoDERM™ dressing has fibrinolytic activity and can promote fibrinolysis at wound sites. In addition we have presented quantitative evidence demonstrating differential angiogenesis under occluded versus air-exposed wounds and under different occlusive dressings. Taking these observations in concert with the mass of clinical evidence we have further developed the thesis that chronic ulceration associated with venous insufficiency is a consequence of impaired fibrinolysis. Chronic refractory wounds might respond to occlusive treatments which serve to enhance the natural fibrinolytic system.

Cellular events might also be promoted via eschar breakdown under DuoDERM™ which may yield polypeptide fibrin-degradation products with cell stimulatory activity.

REFERENCES

Alvarez, O., Mertz, P. and Eaglestein, W.H.(1983): The effect of occlusive dressings on collagen synthesis and re-epithelialization in superficial wounds. J. Surg. Res.35:142-8

Cherry, G.W., Ryan, T.J. and McGibbon D. (1984):Trial of a new dressing in venous leg ulcers. The Practitioner 228: 1175-8

Burnand, K.G., Whimster, I.,Naidoo, A. and Browse N.L. (1982) Pericapillary fibrin in the ulcer-bearing skin of the leg. The cause of lipodermatosclerosis and venous ulceration. Br. Med. 285: 1071-2

Lydon, M.J., Hutchinson, J.J., Rippon, M., Johnson E.,de Sousa, N., Scudder, C., Ryan, T.J. and Cherry G.W. (1989): Dissolution of wound coagulum and promotion of granulation tissue under DuoDERM™ In Wounds: A compendium of Clinical Research and Practice 1: Number 2: 95-105

Phlébologie 92. Eds P. Raymond-Martimbeau, R. Prescott, M. Zummo.
John Libbey Eurotext, Paris © 1992, pp. 1291-1293

The distal long saphenous vein in recurrent venous ulceration : a preliminary report

David Negus

Lewisham Hospital, London, UK.

Venous ulcer recurrence can usually be prevented by ligation of incompetent perforating and saphenous veins, with the addition of knee length elastic compression stockings in patients with deep venous incompetence (2). Recurrent ulceration in patients with deep vein incompetence, following perforating and saphenous vein ligation, is an extremely difficult treatment problem, particularly as the cause of such recurrent ulceration is by no means clear. It has been suggested that it is the result of high ambulatory venous pressures in the deep veins being transmitted to the subcutaneous tissues by multiple small, clinically undetectable, perforating veins (1). This hypothesis becomes unnecessary when careful consideration is given to the venous anatomy of the foot and ankle. The long saphenous vein does not communicate directly with the calf and ankle perforating veins and these communicate with the posterior arch vein. There are, however, one or two previously unrecognised tributaries of the long saphenous vein which communicate with the corona phlebectatica just below the medial malleolus.

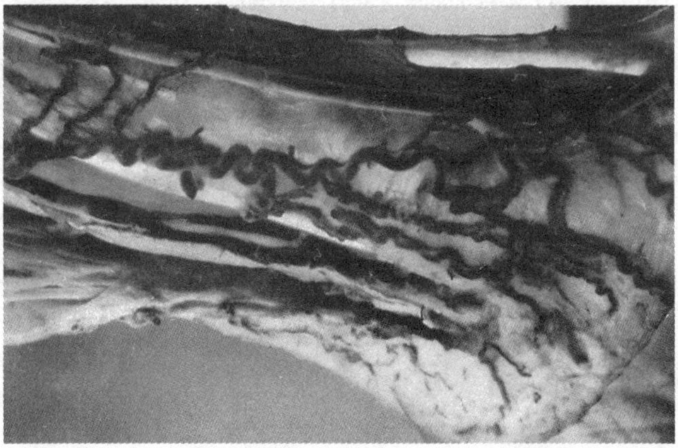

Fig. 1. Dissection of corona phlebectatica and communications with long saphenous vein.

This communication is physiologically important, when it is remembered that the long saphenous vein starts at the medial end of the dorsal venous arch of the foot, which itself communicates with the plantar venous network through the metatarsal perforating veins.

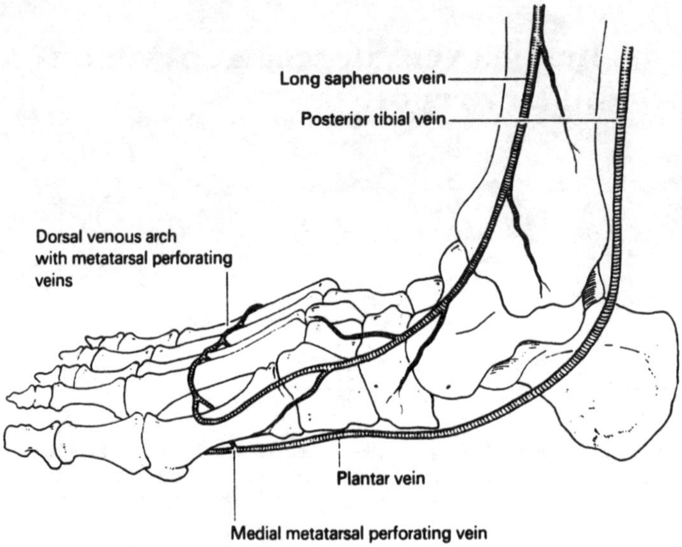

Fig. 2. Communications between dorsal venous arch and plantar veins.

In patients with deep venous incompetence, therefore, high pressures in the deep veins of the leg will be transmitted to the corona phlebectatica through the plantar veins, the metatarsal perforating veins, the dorsal venous arch and the distal long saphenous vein.

Pressures have been measured in the distal long saphenous vein in four patients with deep vein incompetence and with recurrent ulceration following previous calf perforating vein and saphenous vein ligation. Pressures were measured at rest and on passive exercise in the anaesthetised patient with the affected leg dependent. Venous pressures were measured before and after occlusion of the distal saphenous vein, and this significantly reduced exercising systolic pressures (85-140 mm Hg) to 38-68 mm Hg.

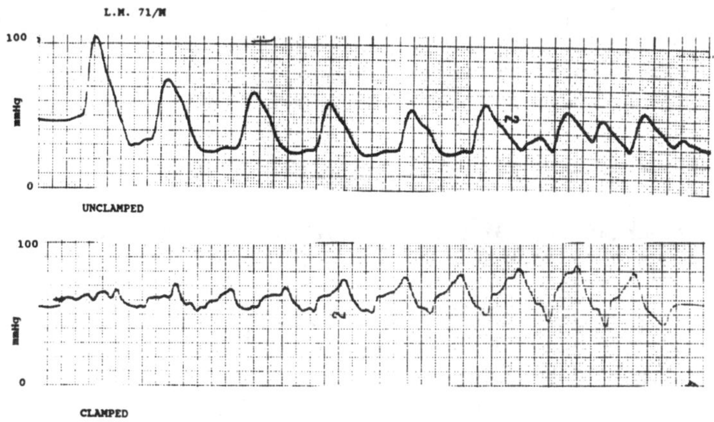

Fig. 3. Exercising pressures in long saphenous vein in foot before and after distal occlusion

Following pressure measurement, the distal long saphenous vein was divided and ligated and the incision closed.

RESULTS

Three out of the four recurrent medial ulcers have healed following distal saphenous ligation; all patients continue to wear knee length compression hosiery. In one patient, the medial ulcer healed satisfactorily but he subsequently developed a lateral venous ulcer. This was treated by ligation and division of lateral perforating veins and also ligation of the lateral limb of the dorsal venous arch. This ulcer has also remained healed.

CONCLUSIONS

The numbers of patients investigated and treated are too small to allow any firm conclusions, but it is tentatively suggested that the distal long saphenous vein acts as the "additional perforator" in patients with deep venous incompetence and that its ligation will prevent high pressures in the deep veins of the leg from being transmitted to the corona phlebectatica with beneficial effects on ulcer healing.

REFERENCES

1. Bjordal R I (1989): Pressure of flow measurement in venous insufficiency of the legs. In Controversies in the Management of Venous Disorders, eds Eklof B, Gjores J E, Thulesius O, Berqvist D, p 34. London: Butterworths

2. Holme T C, Negus D: The treatment of venous ulceration by surgery and elastic compression hosiery; a long-term review. Phlebology 1990; 5: 125-128.

Phlébologie 92. Eds P. Raymond-Martimbeau, R. Prescott, M. Zummo.
John Libbey Eurotext, Paris © 1992, pp. 1294-1296

Topic and general antibiotic therapy of lower limbs' venous ulcers

C. Bonifati, M. Campagnoli, G. Piovera, C. Strarosti

Casa di cura « S. Maria Delle Grazie » Voghera (PV), Italy.

SUMMARY

The authors have taken into consideration a very controversial subject in angiology: the use of antibiotics in the treatment of lower limbs' venous ulcers.

In this regard we selected three homogeneous groups of 15 patients who were being tested for the first time and suffered from infected venous ulcers supported by coltural examination and antibiogramma.

The first group was treated with topic antiseptics, the second group with antibiotics for local use finally the third group had a topic and general antibiotic therapy using two different antibiotics.

The results have confirmed the effectivenes of the antibiotic therapy in the treatment of infected venous ulcers provided it is aimeded and limited in time.

Even more brilliant results have followed the combined topic and general therapy, therefore the authors' present trend is to associate when possible two antibiotics of different classes.

INTRODUCTION

Angiologists are daily required to solve a very thorny problem: infections of lower limbs' vonous ulcers. The difficulties they come up against when treating this disease, which, of course, doesn't tend to a spontaneous recovery, are considerably increased in case of a bacterial contamination.

Besides angiologists meet with another difficulty: that of codifying a standardized therapy, especially because of the different individual reaction.

The use of antibiotics in the treatment of lower limbs' infected venous ulcers provoked a great deal of controversy.

Our dissartation aims at weighing up the real effectiveness of such therapy.

MATERIALS AND METHODS

We selected 3 homogenous groups. Each group consited of 15 patients who were examined by us for the first time and who were suffering from infected venous ulcers on their lower limbs as it was proved by a coltural examination and antibiogramma.

The first group was treated with topic antiseptics, the second group with antibiotics for local use; the third group, at last, was treated with two specific antibiotics of two different classes: suitable for a local use, the other for a general one.

The dressing was daily replaced and checks were carried out after 7 and 14 days'therapy.

After this period a new coltural examination was carried out. During the first visit we collected the following data: age, concomitant pathologies, the time in which the ulcer appared, and subjective and objective symptopatologies.

Among the 45 patients we had initially analysed, we finally treated 58 venous ulcers classified in two classes.

The patients'age variee between 22 and 85. The eziopathogenesis of the ulcer was proved by doppler velocimetria, of course by a precise clinica examination and by eventual hemato-chemical checks. During the period of our study each patient was treated with eparina 12500 U.I:die given with only one subcutaneous provision.

The patients soffering from concomitant pathologies continued their specific pharmacological treatment; these diseases had already seemed to be well controlled when our analysis started.

Absolute criteria of exclusion were: a recent(within 6 months before) mycardiac infarct,pathologies of different nature which had not been conterbalanced,neoplasie and/or cachexies,and other concomitant infective processes.

Our analysis lasted 7 months; we didn't remark any meaningful seasonal influence modifying the infective process positively or negatively. Having one patient belonging to one group often depends on a criterion of causalness: however by the end of the treatment we and managed to obtain a good homogeneity including many different elements (eziologia, age, concomitant pathologies, and so on).

RESULTS

The coltural examinations were carried out on all the vascular ulceres (58) at the beginning of the treatment and after a 14 day-therapy.

From the bacteriological results we could draw some deductions. The infections of venous ulcers are often difficult to write out in a short time, consequently they delay the cicatrization of some months.

From or study we could remark that at the end of the treatment 46,5% of the ulcers were still infected. Yet this percentage is widely modsified in connection with the therapy adopted: as a matter of fact while the first group, which was treated with antiseptics, still presented 75% of the ulcers infected, in the second group the percentage was clearly lower (42,1%), and it was even lower in the third group (21,1%).

Consequently what would seem advantageous is the use of antibiotics, and most of all the association, when the antibiogramma makes it possible, of 2 antibiotics of 2 different classes, one for a local use and the other for a general one.

Considering the data we had got, we couldn't show a statistically meaningful stronger resistance of some particular bacterial stocks, even if the presence of a mixed bacterial flora can undoubtedly influence the final result in a negative way.

The results were finally analysed by taking into account the type of vascular ulcer.

DISCUSSION

The sterilization of an ulcer is the first fundamental remedy warranting its future recovery; sometimes the infection, provoked by a mixed flora in particular, represents a serious problem for the doctor ant it often makes the patient suffer a lot.

In the light of these presuppositions, we compared the 3 different types of therapeutic approach looking for the best solution.

Altough the individual reaction depends on many elements, some of whiwh are not controllable or foreseeable,we can affirm that the antibiotic therapy represents an efficacious remedy. In particular what proved to be really efficient is the combination of 2 antibiotics of 2 different classes,one for local use and the other for a general one, provided it is aimed at and limited in time.

If you don't obtain any valuable results after two weeks' treatment you'd rather try with another therapy, in order to avoid causing any resistance or sensitization.

Every type of venous ulcer can benefit by the antibiotic therapy; yet compromising the microcircle seriously would prevent the absorbtion of the medecine.

The therapy we suggest keeps its present effectiveness, by shortening the times of cicatrization and considerably reducing any eventual aggravations of relapses.

REFERENCES

- Borri P., Seghezzi R., Campagnoli M., Bonifati C., Di Cello G., Invernizzi R., Strarosti C.: USO DELLE FITOSTIMOLINE VEGETALI NEL TRATTAMENTO DELLE ULCERE VASCOLARI DEGLI ARTI INFERIORI. Rass.Int.Cl.e Ter.vol. LXII n.24 pagg.1473-1485, 1987.
- Campagnoli M., Seghezzi R., Bonifati C., Di Cello G., Gallarini A., Invernizzi R., Piovera G., Strarosti C.: CADEXOMERO IODICO: UN NUOVO PRESIDIO TERAPEUTICO NEL TRATTAMENTO DELLE ULCERE VASCOLARI DEGLI ARTI INFERIORI. Atti del VI Congresso Nazionale di Flebologia. Roma 8-11 nov. 1989. pagg.401-404.
- Curri S.B.: LE MICROANGIOPATIE, Milano, Inverni della Beffa. 1986.
- Mollo P.,De Palo F.,Centra L.R.:IL COLLAGENE ETEROLOGO NEL TRATTAMENTO DELLE ULCERE FLEBOSTATICHE. Giornate Nazionali di Angiologia 1991. Minerva Angiologica, Suppl.2 vol.16 aprile-giugno 1991. pagg.321-322. Milano 23-29 giu.91.

Phlébologie 92. Eds P. Raymond-Martimbeau, R. Prescott, M. Zummo.
John Libbey Eurotext, Paris © 1992, pp. 1297-1300

Technique CHIVA dans le traitement de l'insuffisance veineuse superficielle

A. Bahnini, C. Franceschi, X. Mouren, E. Kieffer

Service de Chirurgie Vasculaire, Groupe Hospitalier Pitié-Salpêtrière, 83, Boulevard de l'hôpital, 75013 Paris, France.

La cure CHIVA ou Cure Conservatrice Hémodynamique de l'Insuffisance Veineuse en Ambulatoire propose une approche hémodynamique de l'insuffisance veineuse des membres inférieurs. Bien que l'insuffisance veineuse ait des étiologies et des déterminants très variés, la cure CHIVA permet de corriger le désordre le plus facilement accessible à la thérapeutique c'est-à-dire le désordre hémodynamique.

Le but de l'opération est de diminuer l'hyperpression veineuse proximale en réduisant l'importance du reflux veineux superficiel et en drainant le reflux résiduel dans les veines compétentes du système veineux profond au travers de veines perforantes continentes. En effet, la pression hydrostatique étant nécessaire mais non suffisante à l'apparition des varices, il faut essayer d'en atténuer l'effet en fractionnant la colonne de pression que constitue l'axe incontinent variqueux ou non. La veine est donc interrompue à différents endroits sélectionnés par l'exploration écho doppler et permettant d'éliminer les principaux points de fuite et de drainer la veine sous jacente vers le système profond qui fonctionne à la façon d'une pompe aspirante lors de l'effort musculaire.

BILAN ECHO-DOPPLER ET MARQUAGE PRE-OPERATOIRE

En pré-opératoire, cette technique nécessite une évaluation extrêmement précise du système veineux profond, du système veineux superficiel, des veines perforantes, des veines iliaques et de la veine cave inférieure. Ce bilan est réalisé grâce à un appareil d'échographie doppler pulsé en position couchée et debout et après activation de la pompe musculaire du mollet. L'exploration permet de réaliser une cartographie extrêmement précise des systèmes veineux des membres inférieurs. Les points où le système veineux superficiel doit être interrompu sont identifiés et marqués sur la peau sous contrôle écho doppler de façon à ce que chaque segment veineux superficiel obtenu puisse se drainer dans une veine compétente lors de l'activation de la pompe musculaire.

Les shunts veino-veineux sont également identifiés et interrompus. Les veines variqueuses du réseau quaternaire qu'il est impossible de drainer sont exclues par la ligature de leur segment proximal et la vidange de leur segment distal.

TECHNIQUE CHIRURGICALE DE LA CURE CHIVA

- Hospitalisation :

En pratique, les patients sont admis à jeun en milieu chirurgical en début de matinée et autorisés à regagner leur domicile quelques heures après la réalisation de la procédure. Le bilan pré-opératoire, en dehors du bilan échographique est inutile sauf chez les patients à risque pour lesquels un bilan minimum est demandé. Les patients sont invités à raser le membre inférieur opéré de l'aine jusqu'aux orteils avant la réalisation du marquage.

- Anesthésie :

Dans l'immense majorité des cas, on réalise une anesthésie locale à la xylocaïne à 1 %. Celle-ci est complétée à la demande par une diazanalgésie dont la nécessité dépend de l'état d'anxiété variable d'un patient à l'autre. La présence d'un anesthésiste est néanmoins souhaitable devant le risque possible bien qu'exceptionnel d'un choc lors de l'anesthésie locale ou plus banalement d'un malaise vagal ou d'un état d'agitation anxieuse.
L'injection se fait en sous-cutanée à l'aide d'une aiguille intra-dermique au niveau des sites de marquage. Au niveau de la crosse saphène interne, il est nécessaire d'effectuer outre l'anesthésie sous-cutanée, une injection de xylocaïne sous le fascia.

- Technique chirurgicale :

Après désinfection de la peau du membre en évitant d'effacer le marquage, et installation de champs stériles, l'anesthésie locale est effectuée chez un malade conscient et coopérant. La technique consiste à déconnecter chirurgicalement les circuits veineux superficiels en fonction des indications présices portées sur la feuille de marquage établie en pré-opératoire. Les ligatures sont effectuées au fil de nylon inerte (polypropilène) et non pas au fil résorbable de façon à éviter l'apparition de granulome inflammatoire dû à la résorbtion. Lorsqu'une crossectomie saphène interne est indiquée, l'abord de la veine est effectuée par une incision dans le pli inguinal. L'interruption de la crosse se fait au ras de la veine fémorale commune en respectant la perméabilité des branches de façon à conserver un flux rétrograde à faible pression.

L'interruption veineuse se fait habituellement par une section-ligature, la simple ligature n'étant pas suffisante à l'obtention d'un résultat durable. L'incision est refermée par un surjet intra-dermique.
La crossectomie saphène externe s'effectue de la même façon, si possible au ras de la veine poplité. En cas de crosse haute, on peut exclure le moignon résiduel en le tordant sur lui-même à plusieurs reprises de façon à supprimer le cul-de-sac puis à le nouer en le fixant de façon à éviter la détorsion. En cas de crossectomie saphène externe, une anti-coagulation efficace est prescrite pendant 8 jours et un contrôle écho-doppler au 4ème et 8ème jour évite de méconnaître l'éventuelle thrombose du cul-de-sac saphène externe et l'extension possible du thrombus à la veine poplitée ou aux veines jumelles.
L'abord des autres sites de marquage au membre inférieur se fait le plus souvent par des incisions de 2 mm. La veine est extraite à l'aide d'un crochet puis sectionnée entre 2 ligatures. Il est d'usage de réséquer un segment veineux d'au moins 1 cm entre les ligatures afin de limiter le risque de recanalisation.
L'exclusion d'un segment veineux est réalisé par la ligature des veines d'alimentation en laissant ouverte l'extrémité veineuse du segment concerné. Il est possible d'en exciser une partie en enroulant l'extrémité non ligaturée sur une pince. Une fois le segment veineux exclus, vidé de son contenu, les incisions ne saignent plus.
La reprise de la déambulation est quasiment immédiate. La contention élastique est assurée pendant une dizaine de jours par des collants ou des mi-bas à contention légère. Les patients sont invités à marcher le plus possible de façon à faire fonctionner la pompe musculaire mais à éviter la station debout prolongée. La reprise d'une activité normale peut être très rapide et varie de quelques heures à quelques jours après l'intervention selon les individus et le type de travail qu'ils effectuent.

En conclusion, le film vidéo qui est présenté montre précisément la réalisation de la cartographie veineuse et de la cure chirurgicale par la technique CHIVA chez une patiente ayant une importante insuffisance veineuse superficielle du membre inférieur. Les résultats à moyen terme de la cure CHIVA sont excellents à la condition d'une technique impeccable appuyée sur une analyse hémodynamique précise. Ces deux aspects de la méthode sont indissociables et soulignent la nécessité d'une collaboration étroite entre échodopplériste et chirurgien.

REFERENCE

FRANCESCHI C. - Théorie et pratique de la cure conservatrice et hémodynamique de l'insuffisance veineuse en ambulatoire. Précy-sous-Thyl. Editions de l'Armançon 1988.

USE OF SUCREAM IN THE TOPICAL TREATMENT OF VENOUS LEG ULCERS

Lopez, Lazaro, MD; Artaza, Heriberto, MD

Hospital Nacional, Havana, Cuba

Eighty patients with venous ulcers (varicose and postphlebitic) of the lower extremities, with an evolution ranging from less than one year to more than 20, were treated with a sugar-derived, cream-like ointment, Sucream (50 patients), and placebo (30 patients).

The clinical essay was carried out under ambulatory regime, patients having no changes in their living habits, but receiving per os Vitamin A (25000 U), and Vitamin C (500 mg) daily.

Treatment ranged from 10 to 90 days. Results show a significative response towards healing in patients treated with Sucream (84%, $p<0.001$), compared to those treated with placebo. Aspects related to material, method and results are shown in graphs and tables.

Phlébologie 92. Eds P. Raymond-Martimbeau, R. Prescott, M. Zummo.
John Libbey Eurotext, Paris © 1992, pp. 1302

Endoscopic subfascial discision of perforators (ESDP) of lower leg in the therapy of venous leg ulcer

Janusz S. Targonski

Department of General Surgery, Municipal Hospital, Gartenstrasse, 5802 Wetter, Germany.

ESDP and eventuel cure of saphenous junction were carried out on 13 limbs in 12 patients of mean age of 60 years with so called"therapy resistent",opened lower leg's ulcer of many years duration.

On 5 limbs varices operation were done in the past.All patients had praeoperatively Doppler venpus examination,ascending venography and ambulatory venous pressure measurement.

In the postoperative period were once ulcer necrosis,twice wound infection,twice paresthesia of saphenous nerv and six times tension and swellimg of lower leg observed.

Follow up period 6-21 months(mean 1 year)showed 4 paresthesia of branch of saphenous nerv.The leg's tension and swelling were recovered,anyway by two patient after 4 and 6 months after operation. All ulcer were healed and 7 0f 12 patients were wearing supporting stockings.

ESDP allow radical,exactly cure of medial and posterior group of lower leg perforators.This is especially by patients with bad skin, subcutaneus tissue induration and varices combined with lymphstasis advantaged against other procedures.27 ESDP carried out on patients without ulcer showed postoperative 4 calv tension and 2 paresthesia of saphenous nerv of short duration.

The operation's technic is on video presented.

#Dedicated to Chief of Dep.of Surgery D.Sipreck for 100 years anniversary of Municipal Hospital

The mucopolysaccharide content of venous ulcers, its distribution and function related to dressing type.

Kevin F M Patrick, *Stephen I White, Douglas Queen
Elaine Johnson, Michael J Lydon

ConvaTec Wound Healing Research Institute, Clwyd, U.K.
*Department of Dermatology, Clatterbridge Hospital, Merseyside, U.K.

Hyaluronic acid (HA), is a linear polymer of repeating N-acetylglucosamine-glucuronic acid disaccharides, and belongs to the class of polysaccharides known as Glycosaminoglycans. HA is known to occur in the early stages of wound healing and to be involved in the formation of granulation tissue. Other mucopolysaccharides are also known to occupy the wound matrix in the later stages of healing wound. Our current work, using biopsy material from patients with venous ulcers, has demonstrated the presence of HA together with other mucopolysaccharides in the wound matrix of venous ulcers. The current study has examined the mucopolysaccharide content of venous ulcers under a variety of treatment regimes, including dry dressing control, polyurethane film and hydrocolloid dressing. The findings to date suggest that dressing type may influence the deposition and relative proportions of mucopolysaccharides present within the wound matrix of venous ulcers.

Phlébologie 92. Eds P. Raymond-Martimbeau, R. Prescott, M. Zummo.
John Libbey Eurotext, Paris © 1992, pp. 1304-1306

Treatment of microcirculatory skin disorders in venous stasis or insufficiency of the lower limbs

Sergio B. Curri, Giancarlo Aldini, Ezio Bombardelli*

*Center of Molecular Biology, via G. Cagliero 10, 20125 Milan, Italy. * Indena SpA Res. Lab., via Ripamonti 99, Milan, Italy.*

1) The arterio-arteriolar component of microcirculatory disorders.

In chronic venous diseases of the lower limbs there are more or less severe changes of the skin microcirculation, detectables with capillaroscopic methods (Fagrell,1992). Alterations of the smallest blood vessels have been described also in the subcutaneous tissue and in the muscles of thighs, knees, legs, foot plant and finger tips (Curri,1987-1988). The morphofunctional patterns of capillaries and venules are well known and characterized by dilation, endothelial injury, microaneurisms, wall changes, sludge, halo formation, microhaemorrhages, rarely thrombosis (Fagrell,1979;Andreozzi,1989;Curri, 1991). On the contrary, only little attention has been given to the functional and morphological patterns of the smallest arteries during the progressive development of the microcirculatory skin, adipose tissue and muscle pathological changes provoked by CVI. The changes are precocious, initially focal and after much or less diffuse: the wall alterations of the small arteries are indistinguishable from an arteriosclerotic microangiopathy (Curri,1987,1988,1991). Endothelial swelling, increased deposition of P.A.S-positive glycoproteins, dissociation and degenerative changes of the smooth muscle cells and finally newforming of collagen fibers with wall sclerosis are common findings also in relative young subjects.Worsening of these patterns has been described after pregnancy. Very few instrumental findings on the so called "arteriolar component" of venous diseases are disposable. Laser-Doppler measurements (Belcaro,1986; Del Guercio et al.,1988; Binaghi et al.,1989) and video-photometric dynamic capillaroscopy of the big toe nailfold or foot back (Conti al.,1989) or the combination of these two methods (Fagrell, 1979, 1992) don't offer, in our opinion, clear and clinically useful elements for a better understanding of the problem concerning the involvement of the smallest arteries in chronic venous insufficiency of the lower limbs.

2) New proposals for the treatment of skin microcirculatory disorders in chronic venous stasis or insufficiency.

Up to date, a pharmacological treatment of the microcirculatory skin disorders in chronic venous stasis or insufficiency of the lower limbs, with a specific activity on the smallest arteries and precapillary arterioles and increasing their vasomotility and "pumping functions" (Curri, 1992) to remove the stasis at capillary-venular le- have been not proposed for topical administration. The drugs given percutaneously in ointmens or gels are the so called "phlebotonics" or antioedema active principles. Recently, we have found that Phospholipids give rise with such molecules to stable complexes, endowed different polarity and biological activity (Bombardelli and Curri, 1989). These complexes have been characterized by 1H-NMR, 13C-NMR, 31P-NMR and FT-IR. Phosholipid molecules are physiological carriers for the complexed drugs and favours their crossing through the epidermal barrier (Curri, 1989-1992). Among the complexes obtained, those with specific vasoactivity on the smallest arteries have been selected. Aim of the research was a longer lasting specific activity unfolds in the target sites, skin and hypoderma, and the lowering of the active dosis to reduce undesired side effects in long term treatments. Natural derivatives and synthetic or semisynthetic vasoactive molecules complexed with Phosphatidylcholine have been examined:
A): Natural Derivatives: Troxerutine ***(7.3'.4'-trihydroxyethyl-rutine, Quercetine, Gingkolides from Gingko biloba, Catechins, Silimarine;***
B): Synthetic or semisynthetic drugs: Buflomedil HCl, Iloprost.
The *evaluation* of the activity for all the drugs was clinical and instrumental (Computerized High Performance Contact Thermography, infrared Photo-Pulse Plethismography and Laser-Doppler Flowmetry computer-assisted; Optic Probe Video-Capillaroscopy acc. to Curri). Short term evaluation: (basis vs. 15, 30, 45, 60 min after treatment: Quercetine, Silimarine, Catechins, Iloprost; Long term (30-60 days): Troxerutine, Buflomedil HCl, Gingkolides from Ginko biloba.
Modalities of application: liposomal-like water microdispersion in vials directly applied on the skin of the lower limbs from foot to thigh, gently massed up to penetration trough the epidermis.
Dosis: PC-complexes of Troxerutine, Quercetine, Gingkolides from Ginko biloba, Catechins and Silimarine 30-50 mg/ml, daily 10 ml; Buflomedil HCl 50 mg/ml, 5 ml x 2; Iloprost 0.5-10 ng/ml, 1-5 ml.
Patients: PC/Troxerutine: short term 30 healthy controls (18 f., m.a. 24+/-4.78 y.); long term 112 cases (82f., 30 m., m.a. 43+/-18.6 y.) suffering from CVI; PC/Quercetine, PC/Silimarine, PC/Catechins: short term, 15 healthy controls of both sexes (m.a. 22+/-2.64 y.); PC/Iloprost: short term 20 healthy volunteers of both sexes (m.a. 24+-3.6 y.); long term (10-15 days) 20 f. patients with CVI (m.a. 40+/-9.2 y.); PC/Gingkolides: short term 30 helthy controls of both sexes (m.a. 24+/-2,8 y.); long term 45 f. cases with CVI (m.a. 48+/-22.9 y); PC/Buflomedil HCl: more than 400 patients with peripheral vascular diseases (Curri, 1991): with CVI 46 patients (m.a. 38+/-77.2 y.). Comprehensively 642 observations have been up to date submitted to the "Trans-Epidermal Barrier" (T.E.B.) treatment acc. to Curri (1989, 1990, 1992).

3) Results and concluding remarks.

All the examined vasoactive drugs carried by Phosphatidylcholine molecules show a microvasculokinetic effect on the smallest skin artees, improving the capillary volaemia by means of an more or less remarkable increase of the vasomotility or sphygmicity (Curri, 1992).

The most interesting have been PC/Troxerutine,PC/Buflomedil and PC/Iloprost.After the T.E.B. application the increase of the skin temperature, of the Laser-Doppler signals, of the i.r.Ph.P.P. waves hahave been sometimes surprising, and so far the recrutement of capillaries.Significant improvements of the symptoms have been observed with PC/Troxerutine and PC/Buflomedil. Therefore,it is possible using simple procedures to obtain entirely new species of compounds, which may find useful applications in Phlebology for the long term treatment of skin microcirculatory disorders. The advantages against the oral administration or topical treatments with ointments are the reduction of the active dosis, as compared with the "free" (uncomplexed) drug, the gradual onset of action, the longer activity on the target size and the practical absence of undesired side effects,because the slow passage (Berra et al.,1989) from the tissue-to the blood department.

REFERENCES

Andreozzi.G. (1989): Il microcircolo nell'insufficienza venosa cronica. In *Microcircolazione 1989*,ed.M.Tesi,pp.69-80.Bologna:Monduzzi Editore SpA.

Belcaro,G.V.: (1985): Evaluation of the veni-vasomotor response by-a Laser-Doppler fluxmeter in patients with varicose ulcers due chronic venous hypertension.In *Phlebology'85*,pp.549-550.London: John Libbey & Company.

Berra,B.,Rapelli,S. et al. (1989): Aspetti della farmacocinetica Trans-Epidermal Barrier (TEB) del Buflomedil cloridrato complesso so fosfolipidico in forma liposomal-like. In *Microcircolazione 1989*, ed.M.Tesi,pp.439-446.Bologna:Monduzzi Editore SpA.

Binaghi,F.,Cannas,F. et al. (1989): Studio del microcircolo cutaneo mediante Laser-Doppler in pazienti con insufficienza venosa cronica.Implicazioni clinico-terapeutiche. In *Microcircolazione 1989*,ed.M.Tesi,pp.273-277. Bologna: Monduzzi Editore SpA.

Bombardelli,e.,Curri S.B. et al. (1989): Complexes between Phospholipids and Vegetal Derivatives of Biological Interest.*Fitoterapia*,suppl.nr.1,60,1-9.

Conti,E.,Emiliani,I. et al. (1989): Prospettive di ricerca con l'ul'utilizzo della capillaroscopia dinamica computerizzata (Capiflow). In *Microcircolazione 1989*,ed.M.Tesi,pp.265-272. Bologna: Monduzzi SpA.

Curri,S.B. (1987): Correlazioni microvascolo-tessutali e stasi venosa:alterazioni dei microvasi e dei tessuti cutaneo,adiposo e muscolare. In *Atti IV Congr.it.Flebologia*,pp.265-284. Bologna: Monduzzi SpA.

Curri,S.B. (1988): L'interessamento del microcircolo cutaneo,adiposo e muscolare nella stasi venosa cronica degli arti inferiori. In *Flebolinfologia* vol.I,pp.31-41. Roma: Salus Ed.int.

Curri,S.B. (1989) : Liposomes of vasoactive drugs:new approaches for the treatment of peripheral vascular diseases (PVD).In *15th World Congr.int.Union of Angiology*,Rome 17-22 Sept.,Abstr.p.122.

Curri,S.B.: (1991) Caracteres morpho-fonctionnels de l'ulcere variqueux. *Arteres et Veines* 10,297-305.

Fagrell,B. (1979): Local microcirculation in chronic venous incompetence and leg ulcers.*Vasc.Surg*.13,217-225.

Fagrell.B. (1992): Consequences des modifications microcirculatoires sur le development des ulceres veineux. *XIIeme Congr.int.Acquisitions Nouvelles en Angio-Phlebologie*,La Baule 3-4 Avril 1992.

Phlébologie 92. Eds P. Raymond-Martimbeau, R. Prescott, M. Zummo.
John Libbey Eurotext, Paris © 1992, pp. 1307

The accelerated treatment program for venous leg ulcers

D. Brian McDonagh

Vein Clinics of America, 1101 Perimeter Drive, Suite 615, Schaumburg, Illinois 60173, USA.

Almost all leg ulcers are due to underlying venous pump failure, with or without varicose veins. The Accelerated Treatment Program (A.T.P.) treatment protocol was developed from a 10 year experience on hundreds of leg ulcer patients. It is a non-surgical ambulatory program. Clinical nursing staff who are very well trained in ulcer care and isometric compression wrapping are key factors in a successful program.

The Accelerated Treatment Program removes the edema and helps the ulcer to heal by augmenting the failing venous pump. This is achieved with isometric compression bandaging. It improves the venous pump action at the calf muscle by increasing the venous outflow during ambulation. Initially, patients are seen daily, but subsequently the treatment intervals are increased as the ulcer heals. This program produces the fastest response curve. The advantages include i) immediate ambulation ii) short healing time iii) rapid elimination of pain and drainage iv) high patient acceptance.

The A.T.P. is a necessary ingredient to healing leg ulcers especially the more complex cases. The A.T.P. makes definite demands on the provider with regard to frequency of treatment and well-trained/expert staff.

Phlébologie 92. Eds P. Raymond-Martimbeau, R. Prescott, M. Zummo.
John Libbey Eurotext, Paris © 1992, pp. 1308

Effects of paratibial fasciotomy on the macro-and microcirculation of venous leg ulcer patients

W. Vanscheidt, P. Bräutigam, J. Kreitinger, E. Schöpf

Department of Dermatology, University Hospital, D-78 Freiburg, Germany.

Paratibial fasciotomy was shown to be effective in the treatment of conservatively therapy-resistant venous leg ulcers(1).
Since this surgical procedure consists of a combination of fascia splitting and perforator dissection, the hemodynamical effects were hitherto not clear.
TcPO2 (44 0C), d-PPG, LRR were performed on the proximal leg ulcer edge before and 2, 6 and 10 days after paratibial fasciotomy.
D-PPG failed after paratibial fasciotomy, the venous refilling time could not be prolonged by this operation. Therefore this operation does not seem improve the macrocirculation of venous leg ulcer patients.
Significant immediate increases of tcPO2 after fasciotomy could be demonstrated.
Measurement of tcP02 in six patients 8 weeks after paratibial fasciotomy confirmed the findings of an increase of transcutaneous oxygen tensions either.

This is an evidence that the effect of the fasciotomy splitting is presumably a rather acute improval of the impaired microcirculation in chronic venous insufficiency. Paratibial fasciotomy does not improve the impaired hemodynamic of venous leg ulcer patients.

References

Hach, W., Vanderpuye R: Operationstechnik der paratibialen Fasziotomie. Med. Welt 36:1616-1618, 1985.

Linton RR: The Postthrombotic Ulceration of the Lower Extremity: its etiology and surgical treatment. Ann. Surg. 38: 415-433, 1953.

Vanscheidt W, Wokalek H, Glatz E, Wenz W, Schöpf E: Paratibiale Fasziotomie bei Atrophie blanche. Phlebol. Proktol. 18:40-42, 1988.

La chirurgie globale des ulcères d'origine veineuse

J.M. Junod

La relative fréquence des ulcères d'origine veineuse, leur caractère torpide, rebelle et douloureux, ainsi que leur importance socio-économique justifient une véritable panoplie de traitements plus ou moins énergiques et plus ou moins efficaces. Il importe donc de connaître et de choisir nos moyens d'action, qui doivent viser autant les causes que les conséquences. Traiter un ulcère par des moyens purement dermatologiques, c'est méconnaître la complexité du problème, c'est négliger les causes pour ne s'attacher qu'aux effets. Il importe de préciser les localisations et l'ampleur de la pathologie veineuse afin de traiter celle-ci d'une manière adéquate.

Nous décrivons ici une technique chirurgicale qui, sur plus de quatre cents cas, nous a donné une très forte proportion de bons résultats. L'essentiel, c'est le choix des malades et de leurs ulcères. Il est évident qu'un état général très déficient interdit les traitements agressifs, encore que les indications soient très larges: il n'y a,par exemple, pas de limite d'âge, et nous avons opéré avec succès plusieurs nonagénaires. Quant aux ulcères eux-mêmes, il faut surtout reconnaître ceux qui n'ont pas besoin d'être greffés. S'ils sont très superficiels, propres et entourés d'une peau assez saine, ils guériront par la simple compression et les autres moyens conservateurs. À l'opposé de ces «bons cas», nous avons ceux qui font le désespoir du malade et du médecin, les ulcères torpides, géants ou multiples, en guêtres, à sol scléreux, entourés d'une peau atrophique.

Exciser l'ulcère et pratiquer une greffe de peau implique un double choix: quel genre de greffe et quel traitement veineux? Pour les greffes, il faut connaître celles qui ont le plus de chances de succès. Ce ne sont pas les greffes pédiculées, dangereuses en cas de «cross leg», ni les greffes minces parce qu'elles restent minces et fragiles, ni les greffes de peau totale parce qu'elles ne prennent pas.

Phlébologie 92. Eds P. Raymond-Martimbeau, R. Prescott, M. Zummo.
John Libbey Eurotext, Paris © 1992, pp. 1310

The surgeons part in the treatment of venous ulcerations

Werner Weissenhofer

Rudolfinerhaus, A-1190 Vienna, Austria.

Pathophysiologic and rheologic considerations lead to vascular surgical treatment of venous ulcers of the lower limb. The elimination of incompetent perforating veins is possibly the most important part of the procedure. Direct approaches are often impossible due to skin alterations. Surgical approaches along LINTON´ line (DODD´ operation) enable the surgeon to ligate incompetent perforating veins of the COCKETT´ groups, as the classic venous ulcer is situated in this region. Further procedures, like stripping, local excision and skin grafting can be done in the same session as well as step by step. Our favourable experience of eight years with 133 patients demonstrates well the possibilities of surgical treatment. Healing of ulcers in a mean observation period of 3,6 years took place within 7 months. The permanent healing rate amongst patients remaining in our interdisciplinary treatment system is over 80 per cent. In our opinion an interdisciplinary approach including vascular surgical means markedly increases the chances for success.

References

Cockett, F.B. (1955): The pathology and treatment of venous ulcers of the legs. Br.J.Surg. 43, 260-278.

Dodd, H. (1964): The diagnosis and ligation of incompetent perforating veins. Ann.R.Coll.Surg. Engl. 34, 186-196.

May, R. (1974): Chirurgie der Bein- und Beckenvenen. Stuttgart: Georg Thieme Verlag.

Negus, D. and Friedgood, A. (1983): The effective management of venous ulceration. Br.J.Surg. 70, 623-627.

Recek, E. (1971): A critical appraisal of the role of ankle perforators of the genesis of venous ulcers in the lower leg. J.Cardiovasc.Surg. 12, 45.

Weissenhofer, W. und Ittner, G. (1985): Die Dodd´sche Operation. Indikation, Methode und Resultate. Angio Archiv 11, 89-90.

Weissenhofer, W. and Politzer, P. (1989): Surgical management of venous ulcerations. Phlébologie ´89, 1205. London: John Libbey Ltd.

LE TRAITEMENT DES ULCERES VEINEUSES "DIFFICILES"

PAOLICELLI D.,CROCETTI N.,CAVALLOTTI A.,DI PINTO R.

Hôpitale S.Camillo De Lellis de Rome

La maladie variqueuse a une remarquable importance sociale. Dans les Etats Units à cause de cette pathologie on perd 6 millions de jours ouvrables par an.En Italie 2 millions.La complication la plus gênante du phlébopatique est l'ulcère. Durant les dernières années nos éfforts ont été addressées vers la recherche d'un traitement qui fusse:I)le plus possible ambulatoire 2)le plus possible durable 3)qui permettisse de continuer le travail.Dans cet étude nous presentons notre experience sur les lesions trophiques"difficiles",c'est a dire les ulcères qui n'aboutissent à la guérison que très lentement.Le traitement proposé consiste en une crossectomie en ambulatoire des crosses safeniennes incontinentes,suivi,à partir d'une semaine après l'intervention,par la sclérose des varices et des perforantes incontinentes,en commencant de celles qui se trouvent au-dessous de la lesion.Une efficace contention et un traitement topique sont toujour utilisées.Aussitot que l'état de la lésion le permet on execute une greffe cutanée en îlots.Les controles à 5 ans sont très satisfaisants.

Phlébologie 92. Eds P. Raymond-Martimbeau, R. Prescott, M. Zummo.
John Libbey Eurotext, Paris © 1992, pp. 1312-1314

Venous ulcers at lower limbs : treatment with mesoglicano for topical and systematic use

F. Rück, D. Valenghi, M. Agostini, L. Morotti

Lovere Hospital, General Surgery Department (Chief : Dr. L. Beluffi), Italy.

Venous ulcers at lower limbs: treatment with mesoglicano for topical and systematic use.

Dr. F.Rück, Dr. D.Valenghi; Dr. M.Agostini; Dr. L.Morotti.
Lovere Hospital - General Surgery Department - Chief: Dr. L. Beluffi.

Venous ulcers recognize, as main etiologic agent, the alterations of the vein parietal permeability, being veins subjected to a hypertension regimen caused by the communicans valvular failure.
Permeability alteration is liable for aedema as to the escape of liquids, for fibrinogen which changes into fibrin and causes cuffing around capillaries. The passage of oxygen and feeding substances from blood to tissues is thus obstructed causing the tissue necrosis processes to start.
The correct phlebostatic ulcer treatment aims to remove fibrin cuffing, to restore vascular permeability and to reduce venous stasis.
So we have studied the efficacy of the treatment with mesoglicano both for topical and systematic use. Mesoglicano is a product extract from mammals aorta and consists for 83% of "heparan sulphate" and 17% of "dermatan sulphate", molecules belonging to the "glycosamino glycans" family. They fulfil an antithrombotic and profibrinolitique action, an improvement of the endothelial selective permeability at endothelial level.

MATERIALS AND METHODS

16 patients underwent the medical treatment: 10 women and 6 men with an average of 65 years suffering from venous ulcers with postphlebitic syndrome.
As for the control group 10 patients have been selected: 6 women and 4 men suffering from venous ulcers at lower limbs.
All patients underwent a topical ulcer detersion by means of Glucose at 5% with Rifocin and a compressive bendage.
Furthermore the group underwent the treatment with mesoglicano (Prisma Mediolanum Farmaceutical-Milan) according to the following therapeutic scheme:

- Mesoglicano phials, two im/per day for 15 days;
- 50 mg mesoglicano tablets, two per day for 45 days
- Mesoglicano phials for topical use.

The treatment required 60 days. The ulcers were measured every week and "mapped" once a month.

All patients were hospitalized, even for short time, and underwent the routine hematochemical examinations.

RESULTS

All patients underwent a clinical control after 60 days treatment. The following parameters were considered: the general symptomatology i.e. aedema, flush, pain, feeling of burn, heat, paresthesia, cramps, and the ulcer characteristics, such as extension, depth, base and edges conditions.

50% of the 16 patients undergone the treatment, completely recovered from ulcer, 30% improved their ulcer, 15% remained stationary and 5% got worse.

As for 90% of the cases a complete remission of the subjective symptomatology occured.

As far as 10 patients of the control group is concerned, 60% of the cases improved their ulcer condition, 35% of the cases remained stationary and 5% of the cases recovered their ulcer.

DISCUSSION

The results of this treatment confirm the efficacy of the mesoglicano given to patients suffering from venous ulcers, as it helps to re-activate the tissues and as a consequence it shorts the ulcer recovery times.

The system by which mesoglicano acts, consists in reducing the venous hypertension, in activating the fibrinolysis, in re-establishing and controlling the endothelium permeability.

In particular, I think that the topical use of mesoglicano phials has been useful in shortening the ulcers recovery times.

REFERENCES

1. Agrifoglio G. Di Perri T., Strano A.
   Studio multicentrico sull'efficacia e la tollerabilità del mesoglicano in pazienti affetti da malattia venosa.Farmaci,13,89.
2. Allegra C., Bonifacio M., Riccioni C., Tonelli V.
   Mesoglicani e flebopatie. Contributo clinico-sperimentale.
   Minerva Medica, 77, 1887-1892, 1986.
3. Anzivino F.
   Studio clinico sull'efficacia del mesoglicano nelle insufficienze venose croniche e arteriopatie obliterative croniche degli arti inferiori.
   IX Congresso Nazionale della Società Italiana di Patologia Vascolare, 53-58, 1987.
4. Bracale G. C. et al.
   "L'attività terapeutica del mesoglicano per os nelle flebopatie. Valutazione clinica ed emocoagulativa".
   Minerva Medica, 77, 1919, 1986.

5. Cancelli O., Mallamaci G.
"Le ulcere degli arti inferiori".
Raffaello Cortina Editore, 1985.
6. Castriotta G., Ambroso G.A.
Efficacia del mesoglicano nel trattamento della insufficienza venosa cronica degli arti inferiori e delle sue complicanze.
4° Congresso Italiano di Flebologia, 1003-1009, 1987.
7. Coppi G., Silingardi R., Vecchiati E., Giovannoni M.
Sull'utilizzo del mesoglicano nel trattamento delle flebopatie degli arti inferiori.
IX Congresso Nazionale della Società Italiana di Patalogia Vascolare, 71-75, 1987.
8. Croce E., Sanzone E., Barresi A., Iapichino G.
Trattamento delle ulcere postflebitiche con mesoglicano ad alte dosi. Primi risultati.
Gazzetta Medica Italiana, Archivio per le Scienze Mediche, 146, (6), 273-277, 1987.
9. Petruzzelis V., Velon A.
"Rilievi clinici e ossimetrici cutanei sull'attività del mesoglicano somministrato per os (100 mg/die) nelle dermatiti, flebopatiche".
Minerva Medica, 77, 1911, 1986.
10. Romagnoli G.
Il mesoglicano nel trattamento delle ulcere venose degli arti inferiori: studio clinico.
Minerva Medica, in press.
11. Spinella G.
Risultati clinici con l'impiego del mesoglicano nel trattamento dell'insufficienza venosa cronica (IVC) degli arti inferiori: studio di un campione di pazienti ambulatoriali.
IX Congresso Nazionale della Società Italiana di Patologia Vascolare, 77-81, 1987
12. Vercelloni M., Cogo R., Furcolo F., Monzani G., Casali W., Di Franco G.
Studio clinico sull'efficacia del mesoglicano nel trattamento delle flebopatie degli arti inferiori.
La Clinica Terapeutica, 115 (3), 173-176, 1985.

Phlébologie 92. Eds P. Raymond-Martimbeau, R. Prescott, M. Zummo.
John Libbey Eurotext, Paris © 1992, pp. 1315-1317

The reversed dermal graft for treating chronic varicose ulcers

Alina Fratila[1], E. Rabe[1], U. Schultz-Ehrenburg[2], H.W. Kreysel[1]

[1] *Dermotology Clinic, University of Bonn, Germany.* [2] *Dermatology Clinic, University of bochum, Germany.*

Introduction:

The reversed dermal graft has been used for almost eighty years for different plastic reconstructions. Since 1953 the reversed dermal graft has also been used for covering chronic stasis leg ulcers, decubital ulcers, diabetic leg ulcers, and defects on the plantar aspect of the foot or bare bones. In order to treat or only to improve the supra- and/or subfascial venous insufficiency which causes the chronic stasis leg ulcers, crossectomy with short stripping and then paratibial fasciotomy have to be performed. At the end of the operation the ulcer is then covered with a reversed dermal graft and a split-thickness skin graft simultaneously. This modification of the surgical technique has proved that covering defects in a one-stage procedure with both grafts is indeed a good solution, because immediate postoperative care will be two weeks shorter. This was the period surgeons used to wait until the split-thickness skin graft had been put on the reversed dermal graft, of course using a second anaesthesia. On the other hand, the general postoperative care of ulcers, which is used to heal secondarily within months after crossectomy with short stripping, will now be months shorter.

Operating technique:

The donor area has to be as wide as the surgical defect and twice as long. We start raising a thick split-thickness skin flap, half the length of the defect, and continue without interruption after having switched the dermatom to raise a very thin split-thickness skin flap. The first thick flap is then cut off. This flat is used to cover the dermal graft. The second thin flap remains attached to the skin, i. e., pedicled at one end. The underlying dermis is then taken like a dermal graft - without subcutaneous tissue - and the dermis donor site is immediately closed by suturing the pedicled flap. The first half of the donor area, i. e., of the thick split-thickness skin graft, will epithelize spontaneously. The dermal graft is then reversed and placed in the debrided ulcer's bed, i. e., the former superficial surface is placed face down in opposition to the recipient bed. In this manner the numerous small vessels of the papillary dermis will anastomise easily and quickly with the ulcers bed even if the areas are poorly vascularized. The dermal graft is then covered with the thick split-thickness skin graft and both are together sutured into place. A pressure dressing, as in case of a full thickness skin graft, is applied and left in place for five days.

Discussion:

The reversed dermal graft has several well recognized advantages:

1. The free dermal graft is uncomplicated and takes even on bare bone without periosteum. Due to turning over the dermal graft, the numerous very small vessels of the papiliary dermis make connections more easily with the bed of the ulcer, even if this is poorly vascularized.

2. Compared to a conventional split-thickness skin graft of equivalent thickness, the dermal graft shrinks much less, i. e.,

15 % or a bit more.

3. In areas that carry too much stress, the graft can be derm-abraded and covered with another split-thickness skin graft 16 days later (so called overgrafting).

4. The donor area of the dermal graft is immediately closed. It heals very quickly, painlessly and has no tendency to "trap-door" (pincushioning).

The modification we propose reveals further advantages. First, the ulcers heal within two to three weeks (not months as when they heal secondarily). Second, covering the ulcers bed simultaneously with reversed dermal graft and split-thickness skin graft shortens the postoperative care by two weeks and eliminates a second anaesthesia. Last but not least, the cosmetical and mechanical results are much better than in case of using a split-thickness skin graft alone, because the two grafts match better at skin level and can withstand more weight.

Initially, the operating technique was sceptically received. The possible survival of epidermis cells was a concern for getting epithelcysts. Thompson checked the literature and studied the developement of buried dermis grafts. He found that formation of epidermoid inclusion cysts usually resulted from the sebaceous glands and hair follicles of the dermis graft but then usually underwent dissolution within twelve weeks. The sweat glands and arrector muscles of hair persist indefinitely but do not cause any clinical complications.

If the defect to be covered is an ulcer and the patient also has deep venous insufficiency, the postoperative result has to be preserved by having the patient wear supportive stockings after the reverse dermis grafting.

Phlébologie 92. Eds P. Raymond-Martimbeau, R. Prescott, M. Zummo.
John Libbey Eurotext, Paris © 1992, pp. 1318-1320

The influence of dressing on venous ulcer healing

M.C. Stacey, A. Jopp-McKay, P. Rashid, S. Hoskin

University Department of Surgery, Fremantle Hospital, Alma Street, Fremantle, Western Australia.

INTRODUCTION

The effectiveness of different dressings on the healing of chronic venous ulcers remains questionable. Frequently, claims are made that particular dressings produce faster time to healing of an ulcerated limb. However, there is no good evidence for these claims. Deficiencies in studies comparing different dressings include treating ulcerated limbs with more than one aetiology (Robinson 1988), using different bandaging regimens in the different dressing groups that are compared (Kikta & Schuler et al 1988) and in using inadequate measures of healing such as reduction in size at a given time interval (Ormiston, Seymour et al 1985). The only effective measure of outpatient dressings is total healing of the ulcerated limb (Stacey, Burnand et al 1991).

This study was a prospective randomised trial in which three different dressings were compared to assess whether they had a direct influence on the time to total healing of chronic venous ulcers.

METHODS

The dressings employed were a zinc oxide impregnated stockingette (Acoband, Auspharm), a zinc oxide impregnated paste bandage (Viscopaste, Smith & Nephew) and a calcium alginate fibre dressing (Kaltostat, Phaulding Pharmaceuticals).

The following investigations were performed to determine the aetiology of ulceration: venous refilling on photoplethysmography, resting ankle/brachial Doppler arterial pressure index, full blood picture and ESR, Urea and electrolytes, liver function tests, blood sugar, rheumatoid factors. A full history and examination were also performed. For the purposes of this study only ulcers with a minimum diameter of 0.5cm and a maximum diameter of 10cm in the longest diameter were included.

The ulcerated limbs were dressed in a standard manner at an out-patient Leg Ulcer Clinic. Viscopaste was applied in a spiral fashion from the base of the toes to just below the knee, Acoband was also applied from the base of the toes to just below the knee, and Kaltostat was applied only over the ulcer itself. Over each of these dressings two elastocrepe bandages were applied from the base of the toes to just below the knee and a tubigrip stockingette (Seton) was placed over the bandages to keep them in place. The dressings were changed once weekly.

Dressings were continued for 9 months or until the limbs had healed. Treatment was considered to have failed if the limb remained unhealed at nine months, if there was marked deterioration of the ulcer with a rapid increase in size such that the outpatient treatment could no longer be justified, or if over any three month period there was a failure of the ulcer to reduce in size. Patients were considered withdrawals from the study if the dressings had to be discontinued for reasons other than failure of the ulcer to heal. These causes of withdrawal included allergy to the dressings, excessive pain with the application of the dressing, the development of cellulitis in the leg, or if the patient had some medical or personal reason for which they were unable to continue the dressings.

RESULTS

113 patients with 133 ulcerated limbs were entered into the study. The median age was 74 years with a range of 31 to 92. There was 67 females and 46 males entered into this study. 43 ulcerated limbs were randomised to Viscopaste, 46 to Kaltostat and 44 to Acoband. There was no significant difference in the age or male:female ratio of patients in these three treatment groups. There was no difference in median ulcer size for the 3 groups: Viscopaste 3.7cm^2 (1.5-57.5), Kaltostat 3.4cm^2 (2.6-61.3), Acoband 3.0cm^2 (2.4-75.4) The mean ulcer sizes were also similar to those in other studies but these are a misleading representation of ulcer size due to the distribution of the data - (Viscopaste 10.8cm^2, Acoband 9.9cm^2, Kaltostat 10.7cm^2. A total of 21 limbs were withdrawn from the study for reasons unrelated to healing in the ulcer (Table 1).

TABLE 1: TIME TO TOTAL HEALING OF EACH TREATMENT GROUP

WITHDRAWALS

	Viscopaste	Acoband	Kaltostat
Allergy	2	1	1
Pain	1	1	3
Cellulitis		1	3
Medical/Personal	2	3	3
Total Withdrawals	5	6	10
Completed Trial	38	38	36

There was no clear difference in pressures achieved under the dressings in the three treatment groups in either erect or supine position using a Medical Stocking Tester (Salzman). The median pressures in the erect position were 41mmHg at the ankle, 47 mid calf and 44 upper calf, and in the supine position - 31mmHg at the ankle, 34 mid calf and 32 upper calf.

The time to total healing in the three groups is shown in Fig 1. Healing after 3 months was 66% for Viscopaste, 50% for Acoband and 45% for Kaltostat. The healing of limbs dressed with Viscopaste was significantly better than the healing with Kaltostat ($p<0.05$) and that with Acoband ($p<0.05$) (Log rank analysis). There was no significant difference in the healing between Acoband and Kaltostat.

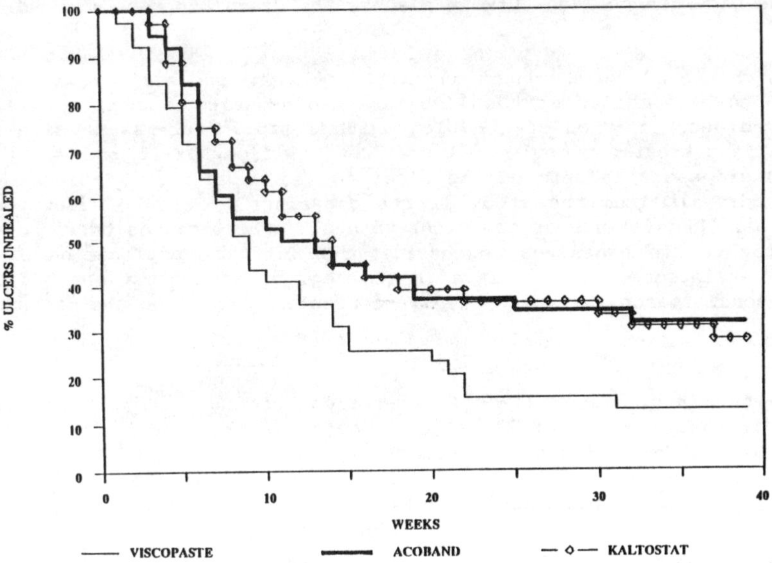

Figure 1. Time to Total Healing of each Treatment Group

DISCUSSION

This study clearly demonstrated improved healing when a zinc oxide impregnated paste bandage was used under compression bandaging compared to the use of zinc oxide impregnated stockingette or a local alginate fibre dressing.

The reasons for these differences need to be considered. Clearly the topical zinc oxide has no direct influence on ulcer healing when compared to an alginate dressing (Acoband and Kaltostat). The major difference, however, would seem to be in the extra bandaging that the paste bandage employs. The paste bandage consists of a zinc oxide impregnated non-stretch cotton bandage, which could have some added effect on the venous return during exercise.

There was, however, no difference in the pressures obtained at rest in patients with any of the three dressing regimens. Clearly the ability to assess the influence on venous return of different bandages and dressings is limited by the tools available. The implication of this study would be that on exercise the non-stretch bandage of Viscopaste implies some added improvement in venous return compared to the compression bandaging employed in the other two groups.

REFERENCES:

Kikta M J, Schuler J J, Meyer J P, et al. (1988): A prospective, randomized trial of Unna's Boots versus hydroactive dressing in the treatment of venous statis ulcers. *J Vasc Surg*. 7: 478-83.

Ormiston M C, Seymour M T J, Venn G E, Cohen R I, Fox J A. (1985): Controlled trial of Iodosorb in chronic venous ulcers. *Br Med J*. 291: 308-310.

Robinson B J. (1988) Randomized comparative trial of Duoderm vs Viscopaste PB7 bandage in the management of venous leg ulceration and cost to the community. In: *Beyond Occlusion: wound care proceedings*, ed. T J Ryan, Royal Society of Medicine, London. 101-4.

Stacey M C, Burnand K G, Layer G T, Pattison M, Browse N L. (1991) Measurement of the healing of venous ulcers. Aust NZ J Surg. 61: 844-848.

-POST- THROMBOTIC HIPODERMITIS: A PERSONAL THECNIQUE-

G. Scipioni - G. Perilli - A. Scipioni

Servizio di Flebologia Chirurgica Ospedale S.Eugenio Roma, Italia

We report our personal experience, with the surgical treatment of post-thrombotic hypodermitis.

This technique consists of the elimination of saphenous reflux by saphenectomy, ligation of all perforating veins of the leg, stripping the venous arch of the foot and creating a series of small fascialwindows below the area of inflammation.

Thus, with a minor surgical procedure, deep drainage accross the fascial aponeurosis is allowed.

In our series of 12 patients, with a follow-up of two years, 10 area disease free and 2 show significant improvement.

Resultats preliminaires de l'utilization de tendon artificial dans la correction du reflux veineux profond dans la sindrome post-phlebitique.

Paolo Detullio, Marco Lombardi, Michele Vitali, ^Attilio Manfredi.

Divisione di Chirurgia Generale. USL 6. Borgo Val di Taro (PR)

^Cattedra di Chirurgia Generale. Università degli Studi di Parma. Parma (ITALY).

La thérapie de la sindrome post phlebitique sévère et resistente a la contention elastique et a la medication veino-active est essentialment chirurgicale et les procedures utilisés sont rappresentées par valvuloplasties, transposition d'un axe avalvulè sur un axe dont les valvules sont restées compétentes ou l'interposition d'un segment veineux valvulè. Le caractere comune de ces méthodes est la necessitè de traumatiser les tissus veineuses avec une percentuelle trés haute de complications, que sovent donnes des resultats mediocres. Les auteurs présentent les resultats preliminaires de l'utilisation du tendon artificial dans la correction du reflux veineux profond sur l'expérience de 6 cas traitè, les principes de tecnique chirurgicale, le follow-up avant et post-operatoire des malades et les eventuales complications.

Phlébologie 92. Eds P. Raymond-Martimbeau, R. Prescott, M. Zummo.
John Libbey Eurotext, Paris © 1992, pp. 1322-1324

Factors associated with healing venous ulcers

P.J. Franks[1], C.J. Moffatt[1], N. Bosanquet[3], M. Oldroyd[1], R.M. Greenhalgh[1], C.N. McCollum[2]

Departments of Surgery, [1] Charing Cross and Westminster Medical School, London, [2] University Hospital of South Manchester, Manchester and [3] Department of Social Policy, Royal Holloway and Bedford New College, Egham, UK.

Community leg ulcer clinics have been shown to provide an effective means of ulcer treatment with a cumulative healing rate for venous ulcers of 67% at 12 weeks rising to 81% after 24 weeks of treatment (Moffat *et al* 1992). Despite this success, some ulcers heal more slowly than others, and there remains a small number of patients who fail to heal despite intensive assessment and therapy. As part of the investigation of the effectiveness of community ulcer clinics, patients were interviewed prior to the start of their treatment regime to observe which factors influenced healing rate.

PATIENTS AND METHODS

All patients who presented within two years of six community ulcer clinics being established in Riverside Health Authority with venous ulceration were included in this study. All patients were assessed to determine the cause of ulceration and only those with ankle brachial pressure indices (ABPI) >0.8 were included and treated with the four layer bandage high compression system (Blair *et al* 1988). Prior to the start of treatment patients were interviewed about their previous medical history, mobility and social history. The area of leg ulceration was traced onto clear actetate sheets which were later measured using computer planimetry.

Analysis was by life table for time to complete healing. Ulcer details eg. size and duration of ulceration, were analysed for each limb separately. Those factors associated with the patient, eg. general medical history, mobility were analysed for each patient. Patients with bilateral ulceration were analysed for the larger ulcer.

Statistical comparison was made using the logrank method, with a relative risk (RR) and 95% confidence intervals (95%CI) calculated from the hazard rates. A stepwise Cox proportional hazards model was used to identify independent risk factors for venous ulcer healing.

RESULTS

Of the 554 ulcerated limbs 477 were considered to be venous in origin. The overall healing rate was 67% at 12 weeks rising to 81% by 24 weeks. Ulcers present for 1-6 months did not heal more slowly than those present for less than one month (RR=1.05, 95%CI 0.81- 1.37, p=0.702), but those present for longer than 6 months healed significantly more slowly (RR=0.52, 95%CI 0.40-0.69, p<0.001), fig 1.

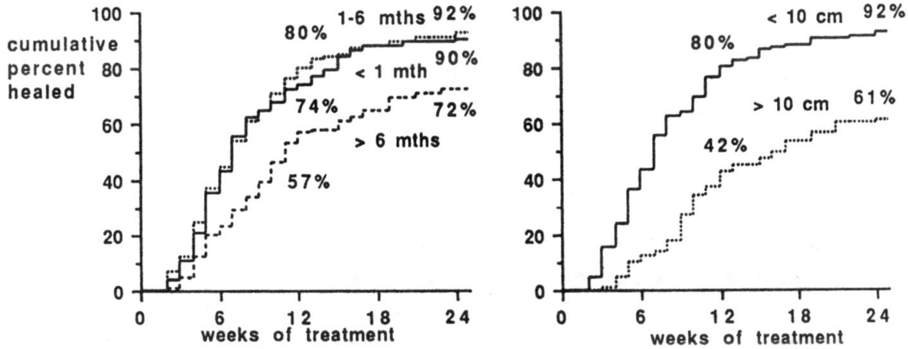

Fig. 1. Life tables of time to heal in ulcers of differing duration and size

Large ulcers (>10 cm^2) healed significantly more slowly than small ulcers (<10 cm^2), RR=0.40, 95%CI 0.32-0.51, p<0.001, fig 1.

Table I. Univariate analysis of risk factors healing for venous ulceration using the four layer bandage technique

Factor	n	risk	n	risk	RR	95%C.I.	p-value
Sex (M vs F)	137	3.1	270	4.0	0.78	0.63-0.98	0.027 *
Weight (<60kg vs 60-80kg)	106	3.3	168	4.2	0.88	0.67-1.14	0.317
Weight (<60kg vs >80kg)	106	3.3	128	3.1	1.12	0.84-1.49	0.437
Hypertensive (Y vs N)	79	4.3	326	3.5	1.19	0.91-1.54	0.198
Diabetic (Y vs N)	21	3.8	384	3.6	1.02	0.65-1.61	0.909
DVT (Y vs N)	47	2.6	351	3.8	0.83	0.60-1.16	0.262
Smoker (Y vs N)	85	3.9	320	3.6	0.99	0.77-1.29	0.980
Fixed limb (Y vs N)	78	1.8	329	4.6	0.51	0.38-0.69	0.001 *
Mobility (chair vs none)	27	2.0	232	3.9	0.53	0.33-0.85	0.004 *
Mobility (aid vs none)	148	3.7	232	3.9	0.96	0.77-1.19	0.703
Place of treatment (home vs clinic)	37	2.0	368	3.9	0.62	0.42-0.91	0.008 *

On univariate anlaysis male sex, limitations of mobility and fixed limb were risk factors for the ulcer failing to heal. Those treated at home also healed slower than the clinic patients.

Table II. Stepwise Cox model to determine independent risk factors for ulcer healing. Values are corrected for age and sex, given by order of fit into the model.

Factor	RR	95% C. I.	p-value
1. Ulcer size (>10cm^2 vs <10cm^2)	0.49	(0.37-0.64)	<0.001
2. Fixed joints (Y vs N)	0.52	(0.37-0.71)	<0.001
3. Ulcer duration (>1m vs <1m)	0.52	(0.39-0.70)	<0.001
4. Ulcer duration (<1m,>6m vs 1-6m)	0.60	(0.46-0.79)	<0.001
5. Mobility (aid vs none)	0.73	(0.57-0.93)	0.010

Stepwise Cox model results are given in table II. When corrected for age and sex ulcer healing was significantly associated with mobility, fixed joints, ulcer duration and ulcer size.

DISCUSSION

This study has identified a number of factors which are important in the healing of venous ulcers. Mobility is clearly a major factor in healing, both general and limb mobility. Walking, even with an aid improves venous function and increase the chance of healing quickly. Community clinics, where patients go to be treated rather than being treated at home may help this by getting patients out and exercising. Size and duration of ulceration are both independently associated with failure to heal. This demonstrates the need for early referral when the area of ulceration is still small and easily treated. With late referral small ulcers may develop into large chronic ulcers which will be more difficult to heal.

REFERENCES

Blair SD Wright DDI Backhouse CM Riddle E McCollum CN (1988): Sustained compression and healing of chronic venous ulcers. Br Med J 297, 1159-61

Moffatt CJ. Franks PJ Oldroyd M Bosanquet N Greenhalgh RM McCollum CN (1992). Evaluation of community leg ulcer clinics. In Phlebologie '92. Actes du XI Congres Mondiale Union de Phlebologie. Canada. John Libbey

Phlébologie 92. Eds P. Raymond-Martimbeau, R. Prescott, M. Zummo.
John Libbey Eurotext, Paris © 1992, pp. 1325-1327

Randomised trial of an occlusive dressing in the treatment of chronic non healing leg ulcer

C.J. Moffatt, P.J. Franks, M. Oldroyd, R.M. Greenhalgh

Department of Surgery, Charing Cross and Westminster Medical School, London, W6 8RF, UK.

INTRODUCTION

Venous ulcers are a common source of morbidity in the elderly population and place a heavy burden on Health Service resources. A wide variety of methods have been advocated to treat leg ulceration but few have been asseessed in randomised trials.

The four layer bandage sytem (Blair *et al*, 1988) has been used to treat venous ulcers in a hospital research clinic. Published results demonstrated a cumulative healing rate of 74% at 12 weeks. More recently, this technique has been taken into the community where similar results have been obtained by the community nurses under the direction of the Vascular Surgical Service at Charing Cross Hospital (Moffatt 1991).

The normal dressing applied in with the four layer bandage is a simple non-adherent (NA) dressing. Small trials of alternative dressings have not found significant improvements in healing from this simple approach (Backhouse *et al* 1987, Blair *et al* 1988). Despite the success of the bandage system, there remain a number of patients who fail to heal following compression. These patients either fail to respond completely, or reduce in size initially, leaving a residual ulcer which subsequently fails to heal. Occlusive dressings are used in chronic non healing ulcers because they are able to stimulate granulation and promote angiogenesis (Handfield-Jones *et al* 1988). The aim of this trial was to observe whether an occlusive dressing (Comfeel, Coloplast) could improve healing in patients with resistent ulcers when compared with the non-adherent dressing normally used.

PATIENTS AND METHODS

All patients were drawn from the Charing Cross Ulcer Clinic or the Riverside community ulcer clinics. The entry criteria were that the patient was suffering from a venous ulcer which (1) had failed to heal within 24 weeks of high compression therapy, or (2) which had failed to reduce in size by more than 20% of its original size within 12 weeks. Patients with arterial disease were excluded in the initial asessment if their ankle brachial pressure index (ABPI) was less than 0.8. Those with a known allergy or other contraindications to the products were not included. All patients gave written consent to take part in the trial, and the protocol was agreed by the local ethical committee.

A sample size of 30 patients in each group was calculated assuming a background healing rate of 10% over a further 12 weeks of treatment in the control group, and an improvement in healing by 30% up to 40% (power=80%, level of significance=5%).

Randomisation took place by assigning sequential numbers to each patient as they entered the trial, and relating this number to a randomisation group. The new treatment regime was started on the day of randomisation. At each follow up clinic the wound was cleaned and measured using computer planimetry and the ulcer was then dressed using the randomised dressing and rebandaged using the same four layer bandage technique in both groups.

The main end point for this trial was the time to complete healing. Comparison of life tables up to 12 weeks of treatment was made using the Logrank method. Presenting comparisons were made using Chi squared or Mann-Whitney U-test as appropriate.

RESULTS

Sixty patients were entered into the trial and randomised. Table I gives a comparison of the presenting features of the two groups. Patients were followed up to 12 weeks with the exception of four patients, two who refused to continue with the treatment and two patients who died within the 12 week period. The life table takes these withdrawals and deaths into consideration.

Table I. Comparison of presenting features of the two randomised groups. Continuous variables are presented as median (range)

	Dressing type		
	NA	**Occlusive**	**p-value**
Sex (female)	18 (60%)	15 (50%)	0.60
Age (years)	71 (26-87)	74 (50-89)	0.37
Diabetic	3 (10%)	0 (0%)	0.24
Hypertensive	4 (13%)	3 (10%)	0.99
Ulcer size (cm^2)	6.7 (2.6-14.9)	7.3 (1.3-66.3)	0.39

After 12 weeks of treatment, 7 (23%) in the NA group and 13 (43%) in the occlusive dressing group had healed completely . Cumulative healing rate was 17% in the NA group and 46% in the occlusive dressing group. The relative risk of healing in the occlusive dressing group was 2.25 (95%CI 0.88 to 5.75, p=0.077) that of the NA group (Fig 1).

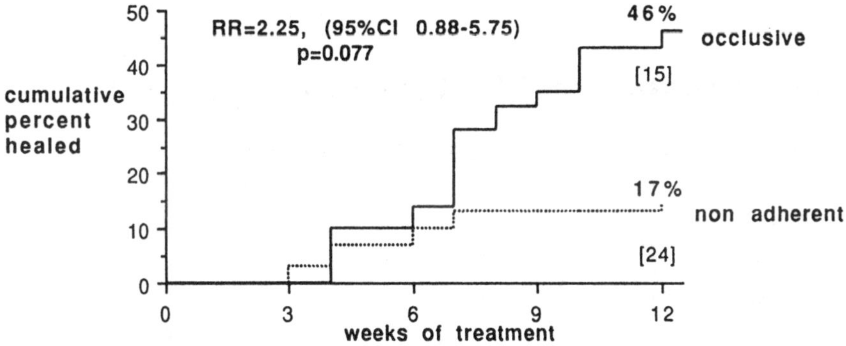

Fig 1. Cumulative healing rates for chronic non healing venous ulcers

DISCUSSION

Although previous research has shown that high compression bandaging will heal most venous ulcers rapidly (Blair *et al* 1988), there remain a group of patients who respond slowly to this method of treatment. The results from this small randomised trial of an occlusive dressing has indicated a need for further investigation of this dressing type in patients with venous ulcers which fail to respond to high compression therapy. Despite a relatively short follow up of 12 weeks, 43% of patients healed with occlusive dressings compared with only 23% in the non-adherent dressing group. Based on these healing rates it is calculated that a trial of 180 patients (90 in each group) would detect a significant difference over a similar follow up period (90% power, 5% significance).

REFERENCES

Backhouse CM Blair SD Walton J McCollum CN (1987): A controlled trial of occlusive dressings in the healing of chronic venous ulcers. Br J Surg 74, 626-7

Blair SD Wright DDI Backhouse CM Riddle E McCollum CN (1988): Sustained compression and healing of chronic venous ulcers. Br Med J 297, 1159-61

Blair SD Backhouse CM Wright DDI Riddle E McCollum CN (1988): Do dressings influence the healing of chronic venous ulcers? Phlebology 3, 129-134

Handfield-Jones SE *et al* (1988): Comparison of hydrocolloid dressing and paraffin gauze in the treatment of venous ulcers. Br J Dermatol 121, 425-427

Moffatt CJ. (1991): Community clinics for leg ulcer management. Wound Management 1(2), 6-9

Phlébologie 92. Eds P. Raymond-Martimbeau, R. Prescott, M. Zummo.
John Libbey Eurotext, Paris © 1992, pp. 1328-1330

Varicose ulcers : treatment with « bioprocess »

E. Liguori

Chief of vascular surgery service, Army Hospital of Rome, Italy.

Venous ulceration is a troublesome and disabling complication, which remains one of the most difficult problems to treat.

The principal physiological abnormality behind this ulceration is raised venous pressure in the lower limb caused by varicose veins; deep vein reflux produced by deep vein thrombosis or primary valve failure, or isolated incompetence of perforating veins (1).

The fundamental approach in treating of leg ulcers associated with chronic venous insufficiciency remains the permanent control of pathological pressure , which is primarily achieved by phlebosurgery, sclerotherapy and / or conservative coompression therapy.

The persistently raised pressure in both the deep and superficial veins of the leg and the congestion in the perivascular tissue lead to the deposition of hemosiderin, with pigmentation of the skin over an area which may be several centimeters in diameter and is characteristically situated on the medial aspect of the shin. The skin in this area is normally thin and easily traumatized.$ 2)

Consequently , venous congestion combined with ischemia, the cytotoxic effect of the oxygen metabolites , the damaging action of the proteolytic enzymes; and the irritation of the effused blood pigment cause it to be indurated. Even a minor injury may then precipitate the development of an ulcer, usually a few centimeters above the medial malleolus immediately superficial to the point of the emergence of a perforating vein. (3)

The present study was designed to examine the role of a new occlusive skin dressing , called "bioprocess by Farmitalia Carlo Erba", in healing of venous ulcerations.

MATERIAL and METHODS

This is a prospective randimized controlled trial conducted on consecutive patients with venous ulceration occurring for the first time and presenting to the Vascular Surgery Service of the Rome Army Hospital.

Randomization was done by drawing sealed anvelopes (alternating sequence).

Treatment started immediately after the diagnosis was made and was conducetdd on an out-patient basis.

Patients were initially recruited if they had noncircumferential ulceration located on the medial side of only one leg,less than 10 cm2 in area, occurring for the first time, not previously treated, and not infected or associated with abnorm leg edema.

The patient was judged suitable for this study only if there was no evidence of surgery or injection sclerotherapy for varicose veins or if the surgical therapy was schedulated after the healing of the ulceration.

Diabetes , hypertension, arterial occlusive diseases and any form of collagen diseases was investigated.

Venous ulceration was diagnosed from the history , clinical examination and Doppler C.W. , Duplex scanner assessment andDoppler assessment of the arterial pressure at the ankles to confirm that the ulcers were venous.

The presence of long or short saphenous incompetence and varicosity was noted by using the non invasive investigations , incluting the Color flow.

The treatment consists in use of "bioprocess 3 to dress the ulceration of fifteen patients , while five patients were dressed using the cotton gauze.

Any devitalized skin surrounding the ulceration was removed by warm olive oil.

The ulcer was then washed with physiological saline and any loose tissue removed.

After the dressing a below-knee graduated compression bandage was applied over the dressing.

This procedures was repeated every day for 7 days and then weekly until the ulceration had healed or the study reached its end point.

Patients were advised to sleep with the foot of the bed raised, to avoid long period of standing without exercising the calf pump , to walk whenever possible , and to drink f watere

The size of the ulcer was measured before the treatment and then at 2,3,4 and8 weeks afterwards. Healing was defined as complete granulation and epiyhelializatior of the ulcer. The end point for this study when the treatment code was broken was 2 mounths after therapy had started.

RESULTS

The patients studied had a mean age of 56 years with range 33-72.

The male/ female ratio was 1: 2.

The size of ulcers was:

group	pretreatment	2 weeks	3 weeks	4weeks	8weeks
bioprocess	4.4 ± 0.5	3.2± 0.4	2.0 ± 0.3	0.8 ± 0.2	0.2 ± 0.1
Cotton gauze	4.2 ± 0.4	3.3 ± 0.3	2.9 ± 0.4	1.9 ± 0.4	1.2 ± 0.3

The statistical significance ($p<0.05$) was evaluated in healing rates among the study grpup using the Wilcoxon's statistict.

DISCUSSION

Venous ulcers are common and cause considerable morbility in the adult populaion. Since healing may be slow or never achieved , ulcers create persistent and substantial demands on resources. A wide variety of treatments has been used but it is generally agreed that elevation of the leg and a good compression bandagong are the central importance to encourage small ulcers to heal. This study was conducted on patients presenting for the first time with untreated venoss ulcers.

The present investigation demonstrated a good results using "bioprocess" dressing of the ulcers , but we emphatize that long term healing of venous ulcers can be achieved by saphenous stripping and/or ligation of incompetence perforating veins in patients with normal deep veins. Similar results can be achieved in patients wiIth incompetence of both the deep and perforating veins by the addition pf permanent knee-length graduated elastic compression stockings.

REFERENCES

1) Corwall J.V. : Leg Ulcers: epidemiology and aetiology Br. J. Surg. 73, 693, 1986

2) Curri S.B., Liguori E. : relazione tra sintomi di stasi venosa cronica degli arti inferiori e sintomi di stasi venulare mammaria. Min. Ang. 14,165,1989

3)Browse N.L. ,Burnand K.G. The cause of venous ulceration Lancet 2,243,1982

Phlébologie 92. Eds P. Raymond-Martimbeau, R. Prescott, M. Zummo.
John Libbey Eurotext, Paris © 1992, pp. 1331-1333

Oxygénothérapie hyperbare et ulcères

J.P. Millien, J.M. Coget, R. Nevière, D. Mathieu, F. Wattel

Service d'Urgence Respiratoire, de Réanimation Médicale et de Médecine Hyperbare, Hôpital A. Calmette, CHRU de Lille, 59037 Lille Cedex, France.

L'OXYGENOTHERAPIE HYPERBARE (OHB) est une modalité d'administration de l'oxygène par voie respiratoire sous une pression supérieure à la pression atmosphérique. Les effets recherchés de l'OHB en pathologie vasculaire sont directement liés à l'apparition d'une pression partielle d'oxygène élevée, dont la principale conséquence est l'augmentation de l'oxygène dissous dans le plasma. L'OHB permet donc de suppléer éventuellement à un défaut de perfusion tissulaire. A côté de cet effet de suppléance, on constate un effet bactériostatique et bactéricide, une stimulation de la phagocytose des polynucléaires et un effet trés favorable sur la déformabilité du globule rouge. On conçoit donc aisément l'intérêt de l'OHB dans la pathologie ulcéreuse, où il existe toujours un défaut d'oxygénation tissulaire locale et une tendance à la surinfection.

Si l'hypoxie tissulaire est le denominateur commun de l'OHB, il nous apparaît important d'avoir des critères objectifs permettant d'une part de poser les indications de l'OHB et d'autre part de vérifier la bonne administration du traitement. Actuellement, notre attitude vis à vis des ulcères de jambe est dictée par la mesure des pressions transcutanées d'O2 (PtcO2) en hyperbarie, associée au flux laser doppler. Les mesures sont effectuées le long des trajets vasculaires ainsi qu'en périphérie des zones ulcérées. Dans le cas où il existe une hypoxie à l'état normal, les PtcO2 sont alors abaissées. On réalise ensuite la mesure sous oxygène en hyperbarie, et si l'on assiste à une élévation de ces valeurs, c'est à dire, à une correction des PtcO2, on peut en conclure que le traitement par OHB permettra la normalisation des pressions tissulaires d'oxygène et exercera donc un effet cicatrisant et anti-infectieux. Dans le cas où cette hypoxie ne se corrige pas suffisament sous oxygènothérapie hyperbare, la pathologie n'est pas alors justifiable de cette thérapeutique.

Nous avons pu ainsi montrer dans une série de patients présentant des ulcères d'origine artérielle ou mixte, l'importance de la mesure des PtcO2 péri-lésionnelles qui permettait de classer les patients en deux groupes : l'un qui tirerait bénéficice de l'OHB et dont l'évolution serait favorable et l'autre dont l'état local n'est absolument pas modifié par l'OHB et dont l'évolution conduit malheureusement à l'amputation. Il est capitale de noter que cette différence n'apparait pas dans les mesures réalisées en air ambiant ni en oxygène normobare. Seules, en fait, les mesures réalisées en oxygène hyperbare permettent cette classification. Nous avons donc décidé d'appliquer la règle suivante, en ce qui concerne les ulcères artériels ou mixtes : - une PtcO2 inférieure à 50 mmHg, lorsque le sujet respire de l'oxygène pur, à 2,5 ATA signe un échec constant, et donc nous amène à conseiller une amputation, - une ptcO2 supérieure à 200 mmHg, en OHB à 2,5 ATA correspond à un succés constant.

De même, dans une autre série comportant des patients diabètiques, présentant soit des lésions d'ulcère sur pied diabètique, soit des lésions de mal perforant plantaire, nous avons pu également vérifier que la mesure des PO2 transcutanée péri-lésionnelle permettait également d'établir cette classification. Mais à la différence des lésions d'ulcère sur artérite, le niveau critique des PtcO2 était nettement SUPERIEUR chez les patients diabètiques, que chez les patients artéritiques. On peut considérer que pour obtenir une réponse satisfaisante, il est nécessaire de porter l'indication d'OHB pour une valeur de la PtcO2 supérieure à 400 mmHg. Cela rend compte, vraisemblablement des troubles spécifiques de la microcirculation rencontrée au cours de la maladie diabètique. Parallèlement, aux mesures de PtcO2, nous réalisons systématiquement une étude du flux microcirculatoire cutané par flux doppler laser. Cette mesure, nous permet d'une part, d'enregistrer le flux basal, et surtout, d'autre part, de constater ou non la présence d'une vasomotricité spontanée. Cet examen est particulièrement utile pour les ulcères rencontrés chez les diabètiques. En effet, il est fréquent de rencontrer une absence de vasomotricité spontanée avant toute thérapeutique par OHB et de constater une réapparition de cette vasomotricité spontanée aprés plusieurs séances d'oxygénothérapie hyperbare.

On voit donc que l'oxygénothérapie hyperbare peut être bénéfique dans les ulcères de jambe, mais que son indication doit reposer sur des critères paracliniques bien définis. Cependant, il existe également des critères cliniques qu'il convient de ne pas oublier avant de proposer à un patient, porteur d'ulcères, une thérapeutique par OHB.

Dans les ulcères artériels, les indications de l'OHB sont dictées par trois impératifs : - échec d'un traitement médical ou chirurgical, bien conduits, - augmentation de douleurs avec aggravation des lésions, - développement d'une surinfection ne répondant pas à une antibiothérapie.

On peut rattacher dans les indications des ulcères artériels, les ulcères artério-veineux, les angiodermites nécrotiques, les angéites inflammatoires et les ulcères capillaritiques. Le protocole d'indication et de thérapeutique est similaire.

En ce qui concerne, les ulcères diabètiques, et plus particulièrement les pieds diabètiques, outre l'intérêt de l'apport en oxygène, l'OHB permet lorsqu'il existe un syndrôme d'hyperhémie du pied diabètique, de réduire le flux sanguin d'environ 20 % et ainsi de diminuer l'oedème présent par l'action vasoconstrictive de l'oxygène.

L'ulcère veineux ne relève en principe pas de l'OHB, en effet, l'hypoxie est secondaire à la stase, qu'il convient de corriger en premier lieu. Cependant, quand les techniques de soins, de contention et les greffes de peau ont échoué, ou qu'il existe une atteinte ostéo-articulaire sous jacente, il est parfois utile d'envisager une oxygénothérapie hyperbare, dont le résultat est dans ces cas en règle remarquable.

L'oxygénothérapie hyperbare constitue donc une thérapeutique complémentaire trés utile dans les ulcères des membres inférieurs, pour lesquels les thérapeutiques habituelles n'ont pas amené de cicatrisation satisfaisante. C'est essentiellement dans les ulcères artériels, artério-veineux et chez le diabètique que l'OHB tient une place prépondérante. En dehors des critères cliniques qui doivent toujours être recherchés au préalable, l'indication de l'OHB dans la pathologie ulcèreuse est essentiellement dictée par la mesure des PtcO2, couplée au flux doppler laser. Ces mesures permettent de plus de juger de l'efficacité du traitement et de l'évolution de la pathologie.

BIBLIOGRAPHIE

1. BARR P.O., PERRINS D.J.D. Hyperbaric oxygen in peripheral vascular disease in : McCarthy ST (ed.). Peripheral vascular disease in the elder. Churchill Linvingston, Edinburgh, 1983, 87-92

2. BASS B.H. The treatment of variose leg ulcers by hyperbaric oxygen. Postgrad, Med. J., 1970, 46 : 497

3. BIRD A.D., TELFER A.B.M. Effects of hyperbaric oxygen on limb circulation. Lancet, 1965, 13 : 355-356

4. DAVIDSON J.A., DAVIDSON J.D., ENDICOTT Q., MASSARO H. Clinical experience with transcutaneous tissue oxygen measurements in nonhealing ulcers and compromised wounds (Abstract). J. Hyperbaric Med., 1986, J (3) : 169.

5. EMHOFF T.A., MYERS R.A.M. Transcutaneous oxygen measurements and wound healing. Maryland Institute for Emergency Medical Services Systems, Baltimore, 1984.

6. FAGLIA E., BARONI G., FAVALES F., BALLERIO G. Traitement de la gangrène diabètique par l'oxygène hyperbare. Journées de diabètologie de l'hôtel Dieu, Paris 1987. Flammarion Medecine Sciences, Paris, 1987, 209-216.

7. ORIANI G., MEAZZA D., FAVALES F., PIZZI G.I., ALDEGHI A., FAGLIA E. Hyperbaric oxygen therapy in diabetic gangrene. Journal of Hyperbaric Medicine, 1990, 5, 3 : 171-

8. HART G.B., STRAUSS M.B. Responses of ischemic ulcerative conditions to OHB. Hyperbaric Medicine, 312-314. G. Smith, Aberdeen University Press, Aberdeen, 1979.

9. KIZER K.W., KRAM J., DOBOS I. Hyperbaric oxygen therapy of refractory skin ulcers. Proceedings of the seventh annual conference on clinical application of HBO. Anaheim (CA), June 1982, 9-11.

10. VISONA A., LUSIANI I., RUSCA F., BARBIERO D., PAGNAN A. Hyperbaric oxygenation in the treatment of peripheral vascular disease. J. Hyperbaric Med., 1987, 2, 4 : 223-227

11. F. WATTEL, J.M. COGET, D. MATHIEU. Oxygénothérapie hyperbare et cicatrisation. Phlébologie, 1990, 43, 1 : 13-24

12. WATTEL F., MATHIEU D., COGET J.M., BILLARD V. Hyperbaric oxygen therapy in chronic vascular wound management. International College of Angiology, Rome, Italy, June, 1989, 59-

13. YAGI H. On the hyperbaric oxygen therapy for severe infected granulation wounds (ulcers) of upper and lower extremities. Jnp Hyperbar Med., 1987, 22, 1 : 27-40

14. ZEGHAL K., GESLIN P., MAUREL A., LAGRUE G., LHOSTE F. La vélocimétrie laser-doppler : nouvelle technique d'évaluation de la microcirlulation. La Presse Médicale, 15/11/1986, 15, 40

Phlébologie 92. Eds P. Raymond-Martimbeau, R. Prescott, M. Zummo.
John Libbey Eurotext, Paris © 1992, pp. 1334-1335

Pulsatile magnetic field in phlebology

Louis Grondin

Circularoty disease Center, Calgary, Alberta, Canada.

Although pulsatile-magnetic therapy is a relatively recent phenomenon in North America, World wide in the past 30 years, scientists and physicians in Germany, Russia and Romania, have been using magnetic forces and electro-pulsating magnets to treat many chronic and acute conditions.

In North America in recent years many convincing scientific publications have demonstrated the beneficial effect of electromagnetic fields in speeding the recovery from fractures. This has led, in 1979, to the approval by the F.D.A. of this therapeutic modality for the treatment of non-unions, failed fusions, and congenital pseudoarthroses.

Low intensity magnetic energy has also been employed by European investigators for treating chronic pain secondary to tissue ischemia and slow healing or non-healing vascular ulcers with encouraging results. The therapeutic effects of electromagnetic energy has been attributed to increased vascularization, and improvement of tissue oxygenation.

The effects of low frequency electromagnetic energy on the circulating peripheral blood has also been studied. And although no appreciable change in blood velocity or flow was demonstrated at a frequency of 5 hz. or less, significant increases in flow was observed at frequencies of 12 to 20 hz, (at an intensity of 5 gauss). Concomitant monitoring of cardiac output apparently indicate that the improved flow has resulted from vasodilatation and decrease in peripheral resistance. A concomitant one to four-fold increase of the tissue PAO2 has also been demonstrated, persisting in some instances for a period of several hours.

This has led us to explore its possible applications in venous diseases and more specifically in the post phlebitic syndrome.

REFERENCES

Lau,. B.H.S. Effects of low frequency electromagnetic fields on blood circulation,
Biophysics & Medicine Report, 1983.

Pasynkov, Konstantinova, Vlasova,
The therapeutic use of Alternating Magnetic Field in Chronic diseases of the veins of the lower extremity
Vestnik chirurgii imeni 19, 16-19, 1976

Pasynkov, Konstantinova and others
Magnetic Field Therapy (Polus 1)in Venous Diseases of the legs
Novosti medicinskoj techniki 3, 61-61, 1977

Leg Ulcers

Dall'Aglio Osvaldo

UNIVERSIDAD NACIONAL DE LA PLATA

In the plenary session,we're going to discuss some of our personal concepts about:Ethiology,diagnosis and treatment of venous leg Ulcers.

In Ethiology,we differenciate different Clinical Forms:
Sclero-Ulcer,Edematous and Mixed Forms

In Diagnosis:Non Invasive Methods:Doppler(patern of obstruction;P.of insuficiency or both)PPG(patern of venous reflux)SPG (patern of obstruction)Combinated "Avalvulated Patron"

Invasive Methods:Phlebomanometry(Venous presures) and Phlebography(anterograde and retrograde)

IntTreatment:We'll going to discuss:Sclero-Ulcer forms(Ito V)
Edematous forms,becouse of
Persisten occlution of the deep venous system,... or
Avalvulation

Phlébologie 92. Eds P. Raymond-Martimbeau, R. Prescott, M. Zummo.
John Libbey Eurotext, Paris © 1992, pp. 1337-1338

Surgical hemodynamic treatment and plastic repair, using mesh graft, of the venous ulcers

Dino De Anna, Enzo Pozza, Vincenzo Gasbarro, Paolo Zamboni, Francesco Mascoli, Giuseppe Fiorentini, Carlo Feo, Gian Franco Vettorello, Alberto Liboni

Department of Surgery, the University of Ferrara, 44100 Ferrara, Italy.

INTRODUCTION

L'ulcère variqueux des membres infèrieurs est la complication plus fréquent et redoutable vers laquelle peuvent évouluer soit l'insuffisance veineuse chronique que le syndrome post-phlébitique.
Il represente l' expression d'une altération du trophisme cutane.
Le moment étiopathogénéntique fondamental pour la formation de l' ulcère phlébostatique est représenté par une altération hémodynamique, causée par l' augmentation de la perméablitée pariétale, qui se traduit donc par une extravasation du fibrinogène dans l'interstice.
Le fibrinogène en s' organisant en polymères de fibrine crée une barrière à la normale perfusion nutritionelle et à la diffusion de l' oxigène avec une conséquente soufrance tissulaire et formation de l'ulcère.
Le traitment de l'ulcère veineux prévoit, à part la détersin et la stimulation de la granulation, l'emploi en premiére istance d'un bandage élastocompressif qui, en diminuant l'afflux sanguin au territoire des comuniquantes et du cercle superficiel, contribue à la réduction de l'ulcère sans pourtant la guérir.
Se traitement en effect n'elimine pas le moment physiopathologique fondamental de la pathologie: l' iopoertension veineuse du cercle profond. Pour cette raison, notre protocole est de préférence chirurgical et prévoid la saphénectomie radicale avec ablation du cercle veineux ectasique et la ligature des communiquantes incontinentes, cette dernièr phase étant indispensable pou bloquer le procès physiopatologique dégat superficiel causé par l' inversion de la circulation.
Pour l' approche chirurgicale de l' ulcère, nous avons proposé une méthode originale, héritée des chirurgiens plastiques, en alternative aux graffes dermo-épidermiques d' aprés Tirsh fréquemment accompagnées par des complications: la graffe "en grille".

MATERIAUX ET METHODES

Auprés de la Clinique Chirurgicale Générale de l' Université de Ferrarara du mois de Janvier 1986 au mois d' Avril 1992, 58 intervention reconstructives d' ulcère phlébostatique (U.P.) ont étà effectuées avec graffe "en grille"; 11 patients présentaient un quadre clinbique d' insuffisaince veineuse chronique, tandis que ches 31 patients l' ulcère représentait la séquèle d' un syndrome post-phlébitique. Au début, cette intervention était réservée aux patient soigneusement sélectionnés, mais pour les excellentes résultas obtenus, nous avons consideréé pouvoir élargir son indication, dans la phase successive, à tous les patients porteurs d' U.P. qui n' avaient pas de complications locales et/ou générales.

1) phase démolitive: elle comprende la crossectomie de la grande saphéne, le stripping long, les phlébectomies multiples, la ligature des communiquantes incontinentes avec une vaste bonification de la lé sion ulcèreuse jusqu'à la bande musculaire.
2) phase reconstructive: durant laquelle on réalise des prélèvements d' un lambeau dermo-épidermique de la quis omolatérale et son modelage en guise de grille comme l' AMPLIGRAFFE, qui en consent l' augmentation des dimensions de 2 à 8 fois. on réalize donc sa fixation avec des points détachés directment de la bande musculaire où se trouvait l' ulcère. Enfin, on procède à une médication avec bandage compressif.
Le patient doit observer le repos absolu jusqu' au 6º-7º jour, au moment de la premiére médication; la démission se fera en 12ª journée lorsqu' il sera possible vérifier que la graffe a pris et que réépithélisation a commencé.

RESULTAS
Les résultas obtenus sont très réconfortants: nous avons réussi a avoir une réusite de la graffe, rapide et compléte chez l'84% des patients, tandis que ches 6 patients, nous avons enrégistré une réussite partiale parce qu' elle etait conditionnée par de graves troubles hemodynamiques et throphiques avec une guerison en 20 jour environ. Nous avons rencontré seulment dans le 14% des patientes une legér oedém, rapidement réabsorbé, aux bordes de la graffe.

CONCLUSIONS
La technique de la graffe "en grille", pour le traitment des ulcères phlébostatiques garantit d' excellents résultats aussi bien du point de vue clinique qu esthétique: la guérison peut en effet etre considérée compléte aprés environ tre semaines de la date de l' intervention.
Nous avon auci mis en évidence que la graffe réussi efficacement meme si est réalisée directement sur la bande musculaire; ceci ne correspond pas avec la pensée des chirurgiens plastiques qui ritiennent indispensable, pou une réussite totale, un support dermique.
Les avantages de cette technique sont reconduisibles à:
1) la possibilité de prèlévement de peau de 2 à 8 fois plus petits que la surface de l' ulcère à réparer, avec une epargne remarcable des tissus.
2) un réussite rapide et totale meme dans des zones pas trés vascularisées, gràce à l' action bénéfique de la graffe "à grille", qui consent l' élimination des aires nécrotiques; ceci ne se vérifiait pas avec les graffes totales d' aprés Tirsh, qui favorisaient, au contraire, la formation d' abcéss et séromes.

BIBLIOGRAPHIE
BASSI G. (1974): L' ulcère et les dermatoses pre-ulcèreuse dans l' insuffisance primitive de la saphéne externe.
Phlebologie, 27, 119.

BELARDI P., BRESADOLA F., CAVALIERE P., NOCE P. (1986): Aspetti emoidinamici e clinici nella sindrome post-flebitica.
La Riforma Medica, 52.

DAVY A. (1974): Les varices.
Exp. Scient. Paris.

D. DE ANNA, V. GASBARRO, E. POZZA, S. INTINI, G. ANANIA, A. DONINI, P. CARCOFORO, I. DONINI. (1989): Le traitment chirurgical des ulcères variqueux: l' emploi des mesh-graft.
10ème Congr. Mond. Un. Int. Phleb., Vol. IIº -1187-1189
Strasbourg, 25-29 Sept. Jhon Libbey Eurotext London-Paris

Phlébologie 92. Eds P. Raymond-Martimbeau, R. Prescott, M. Zummo.
John Libbey Eurotext, Paris © 1992, pp. 1339-1340

Therapy by penthoxifylline in post-phlebitic leg's ulcers : clinical and $TcPO_2$ changes

E. Marchitelli, R. Pepe, R. Gloria, P.L. Bartoletti

Angiology Dpt. S. Eugenio Hospital U.S.L. RM 7 Rome, P.zzale dell'Umanesimo, n.10, 00144, Rome, Italy.

The cause of trophic lesions in patients suffering from chronic venous incompetence is still under discussion.

According to Browse and Burnard theory, the increased fibrinogen permeability due to venous stasis, causes the formation of "fibrin cuff". More recently, Thomas and Dormandy stress the importance of intravasal leukocytic accumulation, due to abnormal vein contraction reflex, as the main cause for decreased capillary perfusion. It is possible to integrate the two theories if we accept that the leukocyties entrapment due to hypoxya and connected with O2 free radicals and proteolitic enzymes released can cause a endothelial damage and altered permeability. Ischaemia, therefore, seems ultimately responsible for flebostatic ulcers. This has been proved conclusively by a definite reduction of O2 values tested with percutaneous oximeter.

The application of this simple and practical method, makes it possible to measure the diffusion of this gas at various epidermic levels and in particular in periulcerative areas.

We think it appropriate to apply this method not only at diagnostic stage but also in the course of different therapeutic treatments.

Amongst these the rational behind the use of penthoxifylline appears to be based on the drug's emorheological properties (increased deformation of erythrocytes and leukocytes, decreased aggregation of plaques ,increased t-PA, decreased antiplasmin activity) and parietal properties (stimulus of synthesis / release of prostacyclins).

MATERIALS AND METHOD

28 patients have been selected, 19 female and 9 male, of average age 48+-3, who have been suffering for some time from post-phlebitic ulcers and had previously undergone various treatments, either topical or general.

Preliminary instrumental screening, in addition to locating the spot of the original phlebitic injury, led to the exclusion of arterial origin of the ulcer.

TcPO2 data have been measured with a De Mori TcM2 machine equipped with two probes for the measurement of O2 tension in the intercostal and peri-ulcerative areas, both at the first observation and also during fortnightly controls over a period of two months. Size and characteristics of the ulcer have been measured at the first observation and then at four weeks intervals, in order to draw up a map of the situation and follow its development. Patients have then been divided in two groups at random: the first group, 15 patients, have been treated with 1.200 mg./die of penthoxifylline per os over an average period of two months. The second group, 13 patients, have not been treated systematically with any drug. All patients have also taken the ususal topical and elastic stokes.

RESULTS

Peri-ulcerative TcPO2 data obtained at the pre-treatment stage showed average values of 13:6 mm.Hg in all patients.

Of the 15 patients treated with penthoxifylline two had to discontinue treatment because of gastric intolerance;2 patients in the control group dropped out. All 13 remaining patients in the first group have shown a progressive reduction in the diameter as well as gradual cleansing of the ulcerative fundus, especially evident after one month treatment. Also, during the final check-ups a significant increase of TcPO2 values was noted, averaging 25+- 8 mmHg. By contrast, in the 11 patients who had not been treated, TcPO2 values did not show any significant increase in any of the check-ups carried out (16 +-2 mmHg).

At the end of the second month of observation, 6 of the patients treated with drugs showed complete re-epitelization.

The remaining 7patients (whose ulcer had a diameter superior to 5 cm at the initial stage) showed a reduction of the damage of 1/3 and a fundus which was clearly healing.

Only 2 patients in the control group had recovered by the end of the firts month and only 1 at the end of the second month.

At the end of the observation period, 5 of the remaining 7 patients showed a reduction in ulcer diameter inferior to I/3 of the initial size, whereas the remaining 3 did not show any significant change at all.

CONCLUSIONS

Although we must bear in mind the limits set by the few patients case studies, nonetheless from our investigation we can the duce that penthoxifylline may be considered a useful therapeutic aid in the treatment of throphic phlebostatic ulcer.

Its effectiveness is proved by the changes induced in transcutaneous oximetry values as a consequence of an improvement in rheology and therefore in chronic hypoxic conditions.

REFERENCES

BROWSE N.L.,BURNAND K.G.: The cause of venous ulceration. Lancet 1982; 2: 243-6

COLGAN M., DORMANDY J. et al: L'efficacia del Trental nella cura delle ulcerazioni venose. Atti XV Congr. Mond. I.U.A., ROMA 1989

DORMANDY J., THOMAS P.: The role of leukocytes in chronic venous insufficiency and venous leg ulceration. Phlebologie '89. Atti X Congr. Mond. U.I.F. JL Ed 1989:113-5

WIDMER L.K.,ZEMP E.,WIDMER M.T.H.,VOLLIN R.:Thromboembolic recurrence and post-thrombotic syndrome after deep vein thrombosis. Phlebology '85 Londra, JL Ed, 1986:556-8.

Regeneration of mesenchyma, primary demaged tissue in ulcus cruris venosum, by a local use of Bezafibrate (hypolipemic)

Mario Gligora, Croatian Medical

Association-Dermatology division Rijeka, Croatia

On the basis of the histopathologic and ultramicroscopic findings in ulcus cruris venosum (UCV) before and after the therapy with ointment consisting of 2% Bezafibrate, and on the basis of pathogenetic notion about forming of UCV, we think as a older authors that the primary damage in UCV is one that originates in mesenchyma, that is in blood vessels and collagen fibers of the dermis, caused by defect of microcirculation. After healing of necrotic UCV tissue in histopathologic finding newly created blood capilaries which are streching like a finger towards the epidermis dominate. In the ultramicroscopic finding those are huge capillaries with three to four pericytes with the nucleus rich with the organellae. The newly created collagen fibers in histopathological finding mostly are located subepidermaly, that is on the location of generation of reticular fibers in embryogenesis.

Our experience about treatment of outpatients with venous leg ulcers

P. Bonadeo, M. Hafner, G. Capaldi, R. Viticllo, M. Domanin

Istituto di Chirurgia Vascolare dell'Università di Milano

One hundred and thirty outpatients suffering from venous leg ulcers have been treated from october '89 to october '91 at the Vascular Surgery Institute of Milan University.

Ambulatorial treatment allows to decrease the cost in managing with this highly disabling pathology.

Our therapeutic management is founded on an accurate diagnosis, which is carried out through non-invasive methods like Duplex scanner and Doppler through a possible biopsy and a bacterial text as well as through a rational local medical treatment.

A more lasting and short-time healing is enable by individuation of etiopathogenesis of ulcerous lesion and by elimination of its causes.

The aim of this work is to define a therapeutic protocol which makes use of the various medical, surgical and sclerotherapical possibilities in relation to the etiopathogenetic and clinical aspects of lesion.

Phlébologie 92. Eds P. Raymond-Martimbeau, R. Prescott, M. Zummo.
John Libbey Eurotext, Paris © 1992, pp. 1342-1344

Clinical experimentation of a new microfibrillar structure cellulose membrane called « bioprocess » on ulcers found on the lower limbs. 50 case reports

Stefano Mancini, Giuseppe Botta, Simonetta Massi, Carla Ruggieri, Sergio Mancini

Institute of General Surgery, University of Siena, Bracci Avenue, 53100 Siena, Italy.

ABSTRACT

Fifty patients suffering from ulcers of different etiology, were treated with a new dressing consisting of a microfibrillar cellulose membrane. The membrane is synthesized in vitro from bacteria of the Acetobacter species kept on a vegetable extract culture: it is this which provides the membrane with an elevated biocompatibility. The results obtained were excellent and therefore the product, wich is called "Bioprocess", can be immediately included in the treatment of lower limbs ulcers.

KEY-WORD: Bioprocess, ulcers of lower limbs.

INTRODUCTION

There are numerous therapeutic protections which favour the healing of ulcer on the lower limbs, These may be classified into two fondamental groups according to their composition and mode of action:

1) semiocclusive and adsorbent treatments
2) biological treatment.

The biosynthetic cellulose membrane (BIOPROCESS) belongs to the first group.

It consists of microfibrillar cellulose structure obteined with advanced biotechnological process. It is synthesized in vitro from Acetobacter species bacteria, kept on a vegetable extract culture, which makes the membrane highly biocompatible with very little allergenic properties. The membrane is very thin (0.005 mm) and semitrasparent, allowing visual evaluation of the lesion progress, during the recovery stage. The semipermeable layer allows sufficient cutaneous transpiration, reducing risks of contaminatio and hydroelectrolytic and protein loss.

The use of active medicines in the repair of venous ulcers on the lower limbs must consider the fundamentals moments of teraphy: inelastic and pneumatic intermittent compression.

Surgical treatment is aimed at the interruption of the long and short refluxes (stripping, binding ained at the perforans, Felder's operation) and the cleaning of the ulcer fundus.

The various methods of dermal-epidermal graftings, (Davis or Reverdin's pastille, the Mesh-Graft ship) are only used when there is a notable loss of substances and topically applied medication have little effect.

The most important stages of the healing process are:

a) elimination of the necrotic fundus
b) formation of granular tissue
c) reepithelization.

The most important action of the active products is based on the last two stages mentioned above.

Bioprocess is almost an ideal treatment since, althagh it does not demonstrate a marked deasing action, it is able of accelerating the granulation process, reepithelializing and protecting the from bacterial and mycotic contamination.

CASE REPORTS

Bioprocess used in the treatment of traumatic, venous, arterial, mixed ulcers, as covers for skip and pastille dermal-epidermal graftings, on surgical incisions in general and particulary on inguinal incisions, on Felder's incisions and mini-incisions.

Fifty patients, a high percentage of which were female (ratio 2:1), were treated with Bioprocess. The average age was 65 years, with a minimun age of 47 years and maximum of 86 years. All lesions, except those made surgically, were treated according to our therapeutic protocol: photographic examination of the lesions, measurement of length and depth of the ulcer, position recording, biopsy of the edges and fundus, tiepid ozonized washes, chlorohexidine hydromassage, surgical curettagė of the edges and fundus until bleeding occurs under local anaesthetic, periulcerous application cutaneous disinfectants (Fucsina basica) and Ag-sulfodiazina ointment (Sofargen), followed by application of strips of zinc bandages. Tubegauz made from German cotton and rigid serf-adhesive bandages was applied to the limb. The patient, treated as above, wos then recalled after and 3 and 7 days during which he receaved intermittent pneumatic compression and manual lymphodrenage.

Wider and deeper ulcers require more complex treatement, for example the use of other products such as carboxymethylcellulose, with the aim of accelerating the cleaning of the wound and stimulating granular tissue growth. In doing this a possible coupling of the product with other products of different actions was attempted. Only when the site of the lesion was compatible and suitable for the application of the Bioprocess was the product systematically used.

Both faces of Bioprocess, the area of the ulcer and surrounding skin were washed with physiological solution. The membrane was then placed in a central position over the area of the ulcer and spread out with the finger until it passes substancially the edges of the lesion (4-5 cm), this way protecting the surrounding cutaneous tissue. Applying finger pressure to the area of the ulcer the membrane was dried with a hairdryer, which assured that it stuck completely to the sore and surrounding skin. To complete the treatment, the wound is covered with a steril mull tahen from a linen tube, and then tue classical protection with German cotton and a self-adhesive non elastic bandage.

DISCUSSION

The product, which we used in this experiment, responded in an excellent way, to our great satisfation. It is a low cost product, easily applied and scotches the general pain and sense of annoyance generated from the sore. It is ideal treatement for abrasions and traumatic ulcers, as well as for injuries protection, such as inguinal cutaneous incisions and the mini-incisions performed in Muller phlebectomy.

Another main use in the protection of skip and Davis dermal-epidermal graftings, as well as healing of the area from where the skip was withdrawed. In secernent ulcers the membrane can provoke periulcerous hypodermodermatitis, that obliges to application suspending, and it is treated for one or two weeks. Then the treatment with Bioprocess can recommence, up until complete recovery. The large quantity of fluid, which collects between the ulcer and the membrane, slowly unstucks the membrane from the surrounding skin, seeping outside the membrane and soaking the bandages.

It is clear that in the case, much is due to the weekly of the treatment, the check up time being too long. For this reason, secretory ulcers in particular, must be inspected at least every 3 days. Once the external medication has been removed, leaving only the membrane, fluid can then be removed by lancing the membrane and covering the incision point with a patch of the same product. It is advisable, once the fluid has been removed, to wipe the membrane with a piece of cotton soaked in physiological solution. This dermitis on one hand to squeeze out any remaining fluid between the skip and Bioprocess and an the other to prepare for the adhesion of the new membrane to the old one.

In cases, where the Bioprocess is particularly damaged, we recommend complete removal of the membrane and through cleaning of the skin underneath and the fundus ulcer, followed by reapplication of a new membrane.

When a crust forms, soft at first becoming harder, the membrane must not be touched, as crusting is sign of healing. The crust can be removed with anatomical pincers about 40 days after it first formed, leaving beneath it a completely reepithelialized surface.

In the initial stage of vasculitic lesions, the product assures a decrease and eventual disappearance of the pain, and rapid crust formation.

In lesions which appear following an injury to the feet, the product adjusts to the shape of the feet, assuring a quick recovery.

In post-sclerosis iatrogenic ulcers the product, applied after a quick exeresis of necrotic tissue, assure crust formation in two weeks on average.

REFERENCES

Alexander J. W., Wheller L. M.; Rooney R. C.: Clinical evaluation ou epigard, a new synthetic for homograft and hetero grafts shin. Trauma, 1973; 13 (4): 374-383.

Brown A. S.: Biologic dressing and skin substitutes clinics in plastic surgery. Vol. 13, N. 1, Januari 1986.

Katz S., McGinley K.: Semi permeable occlusive dressing. Arch. dermatol., 1986; 140: 58-62.

Neal D. E., Whalley P. C., Flours M. W.: The effects of an adherent polyurethane film and conventional absorbend dressung in patients with small partial thickness burns. Br. J. Clin. Prat., 1981; 254-257.

Pitanguy I., Salgado F.: Utilization of the cellulose pellicle as a biological dressing. Rev. Bras. Cir., 1988; 78 (5): 371-326.

Tavis M. J.: Current status of skin substitutes. Surg. Clin. NorthAm., 1978; 58 (6): 1233-1249.

Phlébologie 92. Eds P. Raymond-Martimbeau, R. Prescott, M. Zummo.
John Libbey Eurotext, Paris © 1992, pp. 1345-1347

Use of restore wound care dressing by incare in the treatment of venous stasis ulcers

Filippo La Torre, Attilio Nicastro, Francesco Stio, Paolo Pontone

III Department of Surgery, University « La Sapienza », Rome, Italy.

INTRODUCTION

Skin ulcers are among the most frequent symptoms of lower limb venous stasis, compounding the clinical picture of patients affected by varix, incontinence of perforing veins or deep vein disorders. The evolutionary symptom of phlebostasis are edema, pain and nocturnal cramps, along with other objective signs such as grave limb induration, skin's brownish hue, dermatitis and ulcerations. The latter can appear either spontaneously or as a result of micro trauma and are typically localized in the malleolar region, where pressure at the level of superficial veins is stronger. The signs and symptoms of phlebostasis, associated with ulceration bring about limitations to the limb's functional capacity and often impair the surgical treatment of the basic disease. Hyppocrates (460-377 b.C.) had already found a correlation between varicose veins and lower limb ulcers, against which he suggested the application of compressive dressings. The use of these dressings helps reducing pressure on the superficial vein level and increasing the venous flux of communicating and deep veins. For this purpose, one can use elasticized cotton stockings, gradual compression elastic stockings (Jobst), Una paste, Elastoplast, ankle boots and cloth-ankle boots with inflatable rubber cushion (Aeropulse). However effective they may as regards slight controlled phlebostasis, these remedies should supplement intensive treatment in the case of severe venous insufficience with ulcers. The treatment of phlebostatical ulcers is now a much disputed one; some authors suggest the topical use of cicatrizing dressings, the cleaning of lesions, the application of compressive cushions, skin grafts, etc. together with elastic dressings. The purpose of our experimental study was that of treating patient suffering from phlebostatic ulcers with an occlusive dressing (Restore In care) in order to evaluate the time for the wound to recover as compared to the time needed when elastic dressing is used.

MATERIALS AND METHODS

We selected 30 study patients (22F, 8M) with an average age of 48,4 (ranging from to 36 to 72). The patients, affected by phlebostatical ulcers of 2 to 4 centimeters in diameter, were divided into 3 homogeneous groups (A,B,C) of 10 patients each. Each group underwent a different kind of treatment: elastic dressing

was used for group A, elastic dressing plus Restore In care was used for group B; group C was only treated with Restore In care occlusive dressing.
Restore In care dressing consists of a flexible, sterile surface, impervious to micro organisms and biological fluids (faeces, urine). The dressings inner part is self sticking to the skin, has a wet layer and absorbs exudates in order to protect the ulcer from waste liquids.
Previous to the application of occlusive dressing, the ulcer must be cleaned and washed with Dakin solution. After wiping the skin and the ulcer thoroughly, the flexible surface was applied on the wound so as to cover the surrounding skin for 2,5 centimeters. As regards group A and B, the dressing consisted of elasticized cloth ankle boots, whose gradual compression was determined after Doppler fluximetric test. Patients were medicated and controlled every 3 days over a period of 60 days.

R E S U L T S

Results have been evaluated with reference to the average recovery time for each group. The average recovery time for group A patients was of 30 days (rangin from 22 TO 46). Group B patients recovered in an average time of 23 days (range 14-30); in group C the cicatrization took 25 days (range 14-35).

D I S C U S S I O N

The onset of ulcers in lower limb venous stasis is a frequent occurrence which compounds the basic symptomatologic picture and causes limitations to the limbs' functional capacity in the worst cases. Such project demands the impementation of preventive rules aimed at improving the haematic flow from superficial to deep circulation. The surgical treatment of venous insufficience caused by incontinence of communicant veins or by varix in lower limbs is the best therapeutical choice to be taken in an early stage before other signs and symptoms of serious venous insufficience arise. With phlebostatical ulcers caused by serious venous insufficience, in order to obtain better results of surgical treatment and post-operative lapse, a conservatory treatment is useful if we aim at the decompression of the superficial circulation and at a better dystrophic skin condition. For this reason elastic dressings are a unique and resolutive method even with larger ulcers. Controversies about the usefulness of direct intervention on the skin ulcers lead us to experiment the use of an occlusive dressing like the Restore Incareso as to evaluate the time of a complete skin recovery.
The results of our study demonstrate how the combined treatment (elastic dressing + Restore), helps healing ulcers in Group B patients in respect with the other two groups: 7 days less. If we take into consideration the recovery range, we will notice a difference of 16 days between group A and B. The treatment with Restore Incare (Group C) gave medium results in respect with the other two groups, but still good (average recovery time 23 days, maximum range 35). We will therefore affirm that Restore Incare proved to be effective in the treatment of phlebostatical ulcers and its action enhances the therapeutical benefits of compressive elastic dressings. Restore occlusive dressing is easy to use and, even without elastic dressing, patients can use it at home, by themselves, provided that ordinary hygiene rules are respected, alon with the right position a pressure increase of superficial circulation in lower limbs (use of elastic stockings, relaxed position with legs at a higher level in respect with that of vena cava, avoidance of long orthostatisms, etc.)

Our study was carried out on a limited number of cases and obtained very good results. We believe that it should be encouraged and carried out on a larger scale with more patients and a more heterogeneous picture of ulcers and venous insufficience.

R E F E R E N C E S

1) Jamieson V.G. et al: Management of venous stasis ulcer: long-term follow-up. Can. J. Surg., 33(3):222-3; 1990

2) Wattel F. et al: Hyperbaric oxygen therapy in chronic vascular wound management. Angiology, 41(1): 59-65; 1990

3) Stacey M.C. et al.: Calf pump function in patients with healed venous ulcers is not improved by surgery to the communicating veins or by elastic stockings Br. J. Surg., 75(5)/436-9; 1988

4) Kikta M. J. et al.: A prospective randomized trial of Unna's boots versus hydradactive dressing in the treatment of venous stasis ulcers. J. Vasc. Surg. 7(3): 478 83;1988

5) Laudanska H. et al.: In patient treatment of chronic varicose venous ulcers. A randomized trial of cadexomer iopine versus standard dressings. I. Int. Med. Res. 16(6): 428-35; 1988

6) Moglia R.M.: A prospective randomized trial of Unna's boots versus hydroactive dressing in the treatment of venous stasis ulcer.J. Vasc. Surg. 9(3):508; 1989

7) Sottiurai V.S.: Comparison of surgical modalities in the treatment of recurrent venous ulcer. Int. Angiol. 9(4):231-5; 1990

INTRAVENOUS AND ORAL PENTOXIFYLLINE TREATMENT FOR VENOUS ULCERS OF THE LEG

C. Barbarino

Service of Angiology Surgical Department
Hospital of Chioggia (Venice) ITALY

Twelve patients suffering by venous leg ulcers were randomized in 2 groups of 6 patients. The first group received a 7 day in-patient treatment comprising Pentoxifylline infusion 200 mg. i.v. twice a day together with Pentoxifylline 400 mg. by mouth 3 times a day, followed by a 60 day out-patient treatment with Pentoxifylline 400 mg. 3 times a day by mouth and compression bandaging of the affected leg. The second group received placebo treatment in place of Pentoxifylline, and subsequent out-patient compression bandaging for the same lenght of time. The results after 2 months of treatment were as follows : In the first group (treated with Pentoxifylline) the venous leg ulcer had healed in 4 cases and reduced in size in 2 cases ; In the second group (treated with placebo) the leg ulcer healed in only 1 case, and the ulcers reduced in size in the remaining 5 cases . These differences are statistically significant. Since Pentoxifylline is known to have fibrinolytic effects possibly mediated via leukocytes it is possible that it may be effective in healing venous leg ulcers in combination with compression bandaging .

Recurrent venous ulcers. An aggressive surgical approach.

Pereira Alves, J. Neves, A. Formiga, M. Neves

Hospital Dos Capuchos, Serviço 6, Unidade Vascular, Lisboa

Aim: Assess surgery in management of recurrent venous ulcers.

Methodology: 20 patients with recurrent venous ulcers study with complete medical history, doppler and plethismography (Phlebotest) at entry and 6 months after treatment. Phlebography and arteriography at demand. Surgery when presents: varicose veins / incompetent leg perforators / arterial disease.

Results: Operated on: 4 cases with primary long-term varicose veins / 3 cases with well developed leg perforators / 3 cases with arterial disease. The other 10 cases just trated with elastic stocks. After 1 year 15 maintain ulcers healed. 5 recurrence, 1 operated. All with non compliance with elastic support.

Le traitement chirurgical des ulcères mixte

G. Tuscano, R. Lonardi, G. Veronesi, C. Pepe, G. Sava, C. Ragazzi

Istituto Policattedra Patologia Chir. Cattedra Chirurgia Vascolare Universita Modena

L'ulcère de la jambe représente généralement la complication la plus courante de l'I.V.C. Mais pour les nombreux problèmes diagnostiques et thérapeutiques, il faut rappeler les ulcères mixtes, c'est-à-dire ceux où il y a une participation aussi bien de la circulation veineuse que de celle artérielle. Pour ces ulcères, afin d'éviter un échec ou une récidive, il faut programmer et traiter l'insuffisance artérielle et veineuse avec un timing soigné qui est en fonction d'un bilan diagnostique complet. L'expérience des auteurs se réfère à 16 cas traités de 1972 à 1990 à l'"Istituto di Patologia Chirurgica" de Modène, avec de bons résultats dans 62% des cas, discrets dans 30% et nuls dans 8%. Conséquemment à ces résultats, les auteurs exposent leurs critères de choix dans la programmation thérapeutique.

Phlébologie 92. Eds P. Raymond-Martimbeau, R. Prescott, M. Zummo.
John Libbey Eurotext, Paris © 1992, pp. 1350-1352

Ambulatory treatment of venous ulcer

Enrique G. Bertranou

Sección Flebología, Hospital Privado de Comunidad, Calle Córdoba 4545, 7600 Mar del Plata, Argentina.

SUMMARY:
The results of the first 22 months of ambulatory treatment of venous ulcers are presented. The basic features of the setting are: patient education, anti-stasis postures, exercise (walking) and a daily local treatment by the patient or his family based upon neutral soap lavage, zinc-neomicine ointment, cotton dress and permanent elastic bandage. Once the patient and/or family are well trained in ulcer dressing, the outpatient visits are monthly up to complete healing. Results: patients treated 282, being 191 women (age 69.0±11) and 91 men (age 67.9±12). Ulcer area in cm² 7.1 (median) 3.1, 23.6 (interquartile range). Ulcer "age" in months 4 (median) 2-12 (interquartile range). Risk factors of slow healing: obesity 50%; age >70 years 48%; ulcer "age" before treatment >12 months 36%; ulcer area >10 cm² 35.1%; no patient participation in the treatment 18%; diabetes 14%. Actuarial analysis considering complete healing as the event, showed a 66% non healed ulcers at the 3th month treatment, 34% at the 6th month, and 27% at the 8th month. The most important risk factor for slow ulcer healing is the "age" of the ulcer followed by the no patient participation. In conclusion: 1) The ambulatory treatment is well accepted and tolerated by the patient and family; 2) The number of outpatient visits and the cost of treatment are low; 3) The non healed ulcer rate is low; 4) The actuarial analysis is efficient to evaluate and compare treatments; 5) Risk factors of slow ulcer healing are stressed.

INTRODUCTION:
Venous ulcer is the end point of an unsatisfactory management of a long standing deep venous incompetence syndrome. The prevalence in general population varies from 0.4% following Anderson et al (1984) to 1% following Callam et al (1985). The treatment of the venous ulcer is expensive and time consuming. Added to this the social cost for patient, family, and community must be considered. Pathophysiology of venous ulcer showed by Partsch (1988) is as follows: valvular incompetence, venous reflux, chronic venous ambulatory hypertension, capillary dilatation, protein-rich edema, failure of fibrine clearence from pericapillary space due to inadequate fibrinolysis and lymph drainage, proliferation of fibres, pericapillary fibrin cuffs, diffusion block, local hypoxia, tissue

death. The purpose of this work is to present the results of an institutional approach of the treatment of venous ulcer, in an ambulatory setting.

PATIENTS AND METHODS:
During a period of 22 months in a 230 bed community hospital, 282 patients with venous ulcers were treated, being 191 women (mean age 69.0±11 years) and 91 men (mean age 67.9±12 years). The ulcer area in cm^2 was 7.1 (median) 3.1-23.6 (interquartile range). Five risk factors for slow ulcer healing were considered, being its prevalence in the study group as follows: 1) obesity 50%, 2) ulcer area >10 cm^2 40.8%, 3) "age" of the ulcer >1 year 36%, 4) no patient participation 18%, 5) diabetes 14%. The ambulatory treatment is based in a number of features such as: 1) implementation of a special unit for treatment of venous ulcers, 2) patient and family education about the pathology, 3) anti stasis postures, 4) excercise (walking), 5) permanent wear of elastic bandages, 6) perforating veins esclerotherapy in rebel ulcers, 7) a daily local treatment based upon neutral soap lavage, zinc-neomicine ointment and cotton dressing, and elastic bandage. Once the patient and/or the family are well trained in ulcer dressing, the outpatient visits are monthly up to complete healing. In cases of patient or family disability to perform daily dressing, institutional trained nurses do domicilliary treatment. In order to evaluate results of ambulatory treatment and influence of different risk factors in healing process, actuarial techniques were used following Kaplan et al (1958) considering complete healing as the event and patients in treatment by the end of the study period and patients lost in the follow up as censored patients. The results are expressed as a percentage of non healed ulcer with 70% confidence limits.

RESULTS:
The results of the ambulatory treatment are shown in figure I. By the 3th month of treatment 66% of the ulcers were non healed (70%-61% confidence limits); by the 6th month 34% (42%-26% confidence limits); and by the 8th month 27% (37%-19% confidence limits).
The study of risk factors influencing ulcer healing are shown in figure II. The most important risk factor for slow ulcer healing is the "age" of ulcer followed by ulcer area >10 cm^2 and no patient participation in the treatment. The other two risk factors are not relevant.

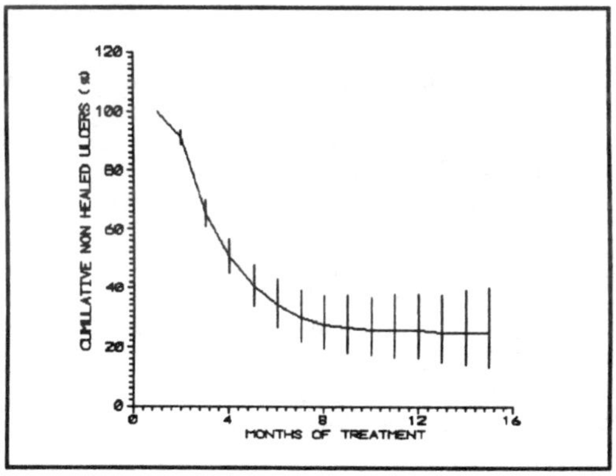

n=282
Percentage and 70% confidence limits.

FIG.I: Actuarial analysis of percetage of non healed ulcers.

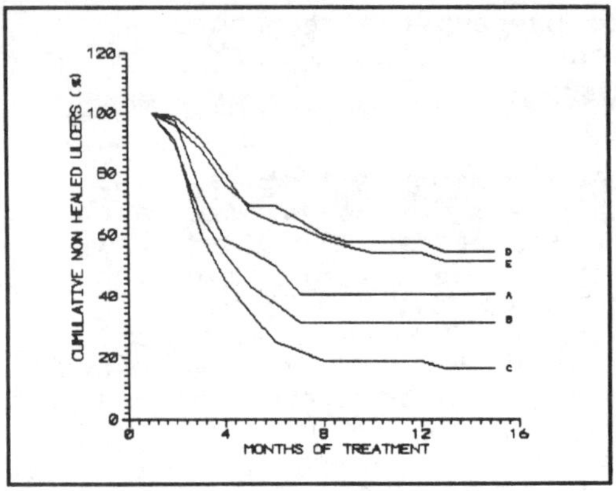

Risk Factors

A: No patient participation (n=52)
B: Diabetes (n=40)
C: Obesity (n=141)
D: Ulcer "age" > 12 months (n=82)
E: Ulcer area > 10 cm² (n=99)

FIG.II: Actuarial analysis following non healing risk factors.

DISCUSSION:
In a bibliographic search shortly after initiation of the ambulatory treatment during May 1990 the work of Hördegen (1989) was found, showing excellent results with similar treatment. A recent paper by Colgan et al (1990) reported a better result in ambulatory treatment of venous ulcer using oxpentifylline per mouth, compared with a placebo group. Considering the oxpentifylline group of 38 patients and using actuarial techniques Colgan showed 64% complete healing of venous ulcers by the 6th month of treatment. The present study on 282 venous ulcers, with alike mean age but bigger ulcer area and using similar actuarial techniques, shows a similar result expressed in a 66% complete healing by the 6th month treatment, considering the opposite of the figure I (complete healing = 1/non healed ulcers). The actuarial study of risk factors showed that obesity and diabetes are statistically less important than "age" of the ulcer and non participation of patient in treatment. No other data was found in the literature to be compared with the present study.

CONCLUSIONS:
1) The ambulatory treatment is well accepted and tolerated by the patient and family; 2) the number of outpatient visits and the cost of treatment are low; 3) the non healed ulcers rate is low; 4) the actuarial analysis is efficient to evaluate and compare treatments; 5) risk factors of slow ulcer healing are stressed.

REFERENCES:

Anderson E., Hansson C., et al (1984): Leg and foot ulcers. An epidemiological survey. Acta Derm. Venereol. (Stockh.) 64: 227-232.

Callam M.J., Ruckley C.V., et al (1985): Chronic ulceration of the leg: extent of the problem and provision of care. Br. Med.J. 290, 1855-1856.

Colgan M.P., Dormandy J.A., et al (1990): Oxpentifylline treatment of venous ulcers of the leg. Br.Med.J. 300, 972-975.

Hördegen K.M. (1989): Ulcus cruris - ambulante Behandlung und Ergebnisse. Schweiz.med.Wschr. 119, 1264-1269.

Kaplan E.L., Meier P. (1958): Nonparametric estimation for incomplete observations. Journal of Statistical Association 53, 457.

Partsch H. (1988): Investigations on the pathogenesis of venous leg ulcers. Acta Chir. Scand. Suppl. 544: 25-29.

Phlébologie 92. Eds P. Raymond-Martimbeau, R. Prescott, M. Zummo.
John Libbey Eurotext, Paris © 1992, pp. 1353-1354

Treatment of phlebopathic ulcers : our experience

G. Amisano, P. Milone

Casa di Cura Privata Eporediese S.p.A., Via Castiglia, 27, Ivrea, Italy.

Ulcers of lower limbs represent a common condition caused by many ethiological e-vents, but more frequently they are a conseguence of a pathological situation of venous system.

According to recent literature phlebopathic ulcers are present in 85% of the cases vs a 10% of arterious origin and a 5% of ulcers are due to a different cause.
Females are mostly affected. The venous insufficence causes a hypertension status which is responsable of an increased capillary permeability : thus fibrin and other factors in the perivasal space create an obstacle to oxygen perfusion lead - ing to tissutal sufference.

Phlebopathic ulcers are usually localized to medial lower third of the leg but sometimes they could extend over the whole circumference of the leg. Without a correct therapy the lesions can be very long and difficult and not rarely these patients can present recurrences.

Material and methods The study we present, concerns 970 patients, evalueted in period 1980-1990, aged between 38 and 88 years: in 124 patients (13%) the ulcers were bilateral. All patients underwent Doppler cw and/or DUplex Scanner studies.
The treatment was based on daily medications during which the ulcers were accura-tely cleaned and disinfected with topic application of antibiotic solutions. In the last three years the treatment has been improved with the application of a solution composed by "Propolis" associated with "Centella Asiatica" extract, with the aim of favouring and the cicatrisation of the ulcer.

When it was necessary we administered systemic drugs (anti-inflammatory) to the patients and corrected methabolic diseases.

In all patients a compressive bending was applied during the whole period of the treatment in association with a long term magnetotherapy and ozonotherapy.

Results A complete resolution of the lesions was achieved in a period of 4-10 weeks, according to the original dimentions of the ulcers.

In order to prevent possible recurrences, patients underwent a periodic follow-up.
At last a small part of the patients were treated surgically with saphenectomy as phlebectomy and/or sclerotherapy.

Conclusions It's Authors opinion that topic treatments are the most important means for reaching satisfactory results without forgetting however those complemen tary therapies such as magneto- or ozono-therapy and elasticcompression.

When necessary surgical approach could be undertaken in great consideration, not only as for as traditional saphenectomy goes, but also phlebectomy or sclerotherapy.

DISSOLUTION OF WOUND COAGULUM AND PROMOTION OF GRANULATION TISSUE UNDER DUODERM™

George W. Cherry, Michael J. Lydon, Jerry J. Hutchinson, Mark Rippon
Department of Dermatology, Slade Hospital, Oxford, UK
and Wound Healing Research Institute, Deeside, UK

Occlusive dressings have been used for many years to treat chronic wounds such as venous leg ulcers. The pathophysiology of venous ulcers is thought to involve impaired tissue fibrinolysis with the deposition of extravascular fibrin cuffs. The latter is associated with an impaired microcirculation as well as tissue breakdown and ulceration. Clinical observations have shown eschar liquefaction and increased granulation tissue growth in leg ulcers treated with the occlusive hydrocolloid dressing DuoDERM™.

The present study examines DuoDERM™ mediated fibrinolysis, demonstrating promotion of clot dissolution in a lysis assay *in vitro* and resolution of ^{125}I–labelled clots in experimental wounds. Furthermore, we have examined angiogenesis *in vivo* using immunofluorescent staining and Laser Doppler Flowmetry and shown significantly enhanced blood vessel counts and perfusion under DuoDERM™ compared with other dressings

An experimentally and clinically–founded hypothesis is proposed for the success of DuoDERM™ in the treatment of chronic wounds.

Phlébologie 92. Eds P. Raymond-Martimbeau, R. Prescott, M. Zummo.
John Libbey Eurotext, Paris © 1992, pp. 1356-1358

La pelote rétromalléolaire anatomique

Robert Stemmer, Christian Furderer

8, rue Auguste-Lamey, 67000 Strasbourg, France.

La gouttière rétromalléolaire interne est une région anatomique à haut risque pour les complications de l'insuffisance veineuse chronique.

La gouttière rétromalléolaire interne est comprise entre la saillie du tendon d'Achille et le bord postérieur, saillant, de la malléole, puis elle s'incurve autour de la partie inférieure de la malléole.

La profondeur de cette gouttière n'est pas uniforme. La proéminence de la malléole façonne cette gouttière, elle est la plus profonde à la hauteur de sa pointe.

Dans cette région se situe le point de départ des veines perforantes dont l'insuffisance a une grande importance hémodynamique. Dans son schéma exhaustif de toutes les veines perforantes du membre inférieur, VAN LIMBORGH les dénomme veines communicantes jambières médiales postérieures. En 1953 COCKETT les a qualifié du point de vue anatomique "medial ankle perforators" et de par leur rôle pathogénique dans les ulcères de jambe de "feeder veins".

D'après les dissections pratiquées par STAUBESAND et STEMMER, ces veines perforantes partent aussi bien de la veine jambière postérieure, que du tronc saphénien, mais le plus souvent des communicantes entre ces deux veines. Cette constatation contredit la division des veines perforantes de Cockett en trois groupes, telle qu'elle a été indiquée par HAEGER.

Dans une statistique de 408 ulcères de jambe d'origine veineuse, STEMMER note 71 % situés à la face interne, 14 % de la face externe et 15 % de la face antérieure des jambes. Cette grande fréquence de la face interne de la jambe s'explique par la présence de veines perforantes de Cockett insuffisantes. Il est licite d'admettre que le développement des hypodermites aiguës dans la même région est en rapport avec la même pathogénie.

La compression apporte une contribution décisive au traitement et à la prévention de ces complications. Or d'après la loi de Laplace une pression concentrique est peu efficace sur une surface plane et inopérante dans une gouttière.

Seule une compression excentrique positive sera à même de transmettre la compression dans la gouttière rétromalléolaire. Il s'agit alors non seulement de combler la gouttière pour la transformer en une surface plane, ce qui serait inefficace, mais de créer un rayon de courbure artificiel au-dessus de cette gouttière. A cet effet il est préférable que la pelote soit adaptée aux contours anatomiques de la gouttière rétromalléolaire.

Une étude anatomique par moulage d'une trentaine de gouttières rétromalléolaires libres de tout oedème a été effectuée. Elle a permis de déterminer leur profondeur moyenne. Le creusement débute progressivement au-dessus de la malléole et atteint son maximum dans la partie rétromalléolaire.

Un modèle adapté à la forme de la gouttière rétromalléolaire interne a été élaboré, avec une branche jambière couvrant les veines perforantes de Cockett et une branche tarsienne plus courte. Ces deux branches forment un angle droit centré autour de la malléole. Les deux faces de cette pelote étant symétriques, le même modèle peut être mis en place à droite ou à gauche.

Toutes les complications situées dans les gouttières rétromalléolaires, avant tout les ulcères, bénéficient de cette compression posée non pas directement sur la lésion, mais sur l'application locale protégée par une compresse.

Après guérison des ulcères de jambe de l'insuffisance veineuse chronique de la gouttière rétromalléolaire interne, la seule compression concentrique d'un bas médical ne suffit pas pour éviter des récidives. La pression doit être amenée dans cette gouttière par une pelote. La fixation de la pelote dans le bas complique son enfilage et ne s'est pas imposée.

Il suffit de mettre le bas de compression en place, puis de le récliner jusqu'à la cheville, de placer la pelote dans la gouttière, avec comme point de repère la malléole dans l'angle des deux branches, puis de remettre le bas en place. Le faible poids de le pelote et son élasticité s'adaptent à toutes les classes de compression. Le renforcement local de la pression dans cette région à haut risque de complications autorise même à porter des bas d'une classe inférieure.

La pelote rétromalléolaire anatomique répond à la conformation de la région à traiter et devrait faire partie intégrante du traitement compressif par bas destiné à éviter les récidives locales de complications de l'insuffisance veineuse chronique.

Bibliographie:

COCKETT, F.B., JONES, D.E. (1953): The ankle blow-out syndrome; a new approach to the varicose ulcer problem. Lancet, 1, 17 - 23.

HAEGER, K. (1966): Venous and lymphatic disorders of the leg. Bokförlaget Universitet Och Skola, Lund.

STAUBESAND, J., STEMMER, R. (1987): Etudes anatomiques sur la constance des perforantes de Cockett. Phlébologie, 40, 599 - 604.

STEMMER, R. (1971): La cicatrisation des ulcères de jambe d'origine veineuse. Phlébologie, 26, 151 - 164.

VAN LIMBORGH, J., BANCA, D.A., MIJERINK, J.H., LUIGIES, H.H. (1961): Démonstration d'un modèle anatomique des veines de l'extrémité inférieure. Phlébologie, 14, 175 - 182.

Phlébologie 92. Eds P. Raymond-Martimbeau, R. Prescott, M. Zummo.
John Libbey Eurotext, Paris © 1992, pp. 1359-1361

Surgical management of severe venous ulcer of the leg : follow-up studies of 100 patients

Hisashi Gotoh, Akihiko Matsumoto, Hiroto Matsumura, Makoto Mou

Department of Surgery, Yokohama City University School of Medicine, Yokohama, Japan.

Severe venous ulcer of the leg remains one of the most difficult to treat diseases. We already presented surgical management of venous ulcer of the leg indicated by our two-directional phlebography (Gotoh, H. et al., 1975). Because of chronicity of this disease, time is the most important factor in evaluating any kind of management of this disease.

The purpose of our paper is to show surgical management incoporating our two methods of phlebography, the first is already presented, and the second is phlebography to reveal circumferential veins beneath venous ulcer of the leg. In these 25 years, we performed operation to 100 patients of severe venous ulcer of the legs. Follow-up studies from 22 years to 1 year (average: 4 years) of all patients were presented in this paper.

Methods and Materials

There are many methods of phlebography presented by many authors (Massell, T.B.et al., 1957, DeWeese, J.A. et al., 1959).

The first method of our two-directional phlebography was already presented at 1975. The second method is also very simple as follows: patient was laid in supine position and rubber band tourniguet was tightend just below the knee. Before X-ray exposure, it is important to mark ulcer by some marker like fuse. Thirty ml of contrast medium was injected into dorsal vein in 30 seconds. After injection, postero-anterior and lateral exposure was made by comparing all the films obtained by two methods of phlebography, it became possible to evaluate the location of many abnormal veins beneath or around the ulcer with reasonable accuracy. We call the second method, as ulcer circumferential phlebography. The reason why we tried this method of phlebography was that the area of ulcer is always infected, indurated, edematous, so it is very difficult to observe varicose veins. By this method of phlebography, it became easy to observe occult, pathological veins beneath the areas of the ulcer. The finding of phlebograms became good guides for us to perform precice operation. As a result, long incision to leg according to Linton's (1977) or Lim's (1970) operation became unnecessary.

One hundred patients of venous ulcer of the legs were operated by the indidication of our phlebographies. Sixty seven patients were male and 33 patients were femal, age ranged from 20 to 69 years old.

Age distribution shows about 75% of the patients belongs to the age from thirty to fifty. Nineteen of these patients(19%) had had the ulcer for more than 10 year and 38 patients(38%) for more than 3 years. Usually duration of ulceration is very long in many patients.

Their phlebographical findings were classfied into 2 groups: primary varicose vein group(82 patients) and postphlebitic syndrome group (18 patients). It is the most impotant preparation that before operation, sufficient brushing out of ulcer exudate together with bacteria, tissue degradation products should be given to the anethetifized patients to avoid wound infection.

Fifty-three patients had undergone stripping of long saphenous main trunk and ligation and dividion of circumferential veins of the ulcer. Twenty-seven patients had undergone stripping of not only long but also short saphenous main trunk. To patients of postphlebitcf syndrome, stripping of long saphenous main tunk below the knee and short saphenous main trunk was mainly done. The reason why we perform only stripping of long saphenous main trunk below the knee in the cases of postphlebitc syndrome is that if rethrombosis occurs, residual long saphenous vein from the groin to the knee would be able to serve as collateral pathway and stripping below the knee would reduce local venous hypertention around ulcer. Postoperative intermittent drip infusion of low molecular weight dextran is very effective for early healing of the ulcer. Low molecular weight dextran is said to increase blood flow and improve microcirculation and lower peripheral resistance. Another effect of LMWD is antisludging effect. Practically, 500 ml of dextran, molecular weight 40,000 average was given as intravenous infusion on 3 or 4 consecutive days. One or 2 days rest, the protocol will be continued unitl the ulcer become healed.

Delayed small skin grafting was added to only 6 patients.

Results

As the results of our follow-up studies (average 4 years) 82 patients showed excellent results and 3 patients showed unchanged. Recurrent ulcers were noticed in 14 patients. Two cases of leg amputaion were included here. The main causes of recurrece were considered incomplete stripping of long and short saphenous main trunk. Additional operatin was effective to these patients. Linton' s operation was added to 2 patients at the time of reoperation.

Discussion

There are many hypothesis about the cause of venous ulcer. Usually venous hypertension and arteriovenous shunting are considered as the main causes. Browse (1982) and Burnand (1990) hypothesized a new theory. They sujested that a high ambulatory venous pressure within the calf-muscle pump is tranmitted through communicating veins to the superficial veins within the skin and subcutaneous tissues of the calf. As a result, fibrinogen, the most important molecule that accumulates within the tissues and the fibrin deposited around the capillary forms a barrier to the passage of oxgen and nutrients. This lead to cell ceath and ulceration.

We consider a high ambulatory venous pressure not only within calf-muscle pump but also within long and short saphenous veins will be the cause of ulceration. Apart from disputes, it is practically very essential to recognize pathological veins beneath ulcer bearing area.

As many authors stress on, time is one of the most important factors in determinating the effeicacy of the method of treatments.

It is also said that real effecacy of the methods must be judged in the light of a follow-up of 3 to 4 years at least.
The periods of follow-up studies for about 4 years will be precisely reasonable to evaluate the efficacy of our method of surgical management.

Summary

Surgical management of venous ulcer of the legs should be planned to individual patients and should be performed adequately. Our methods including phlebographies were very simple and effective and could be evaluated in long follow-up studies.

Reference

Burnand, K.G.(1990): Aetiology of venous ulceration. Brit.J.Surg. 77, 483. Browse, N.L. & Burnand, K.G.(1982): The cause of venous ulceration. 31, 243. DeWeese, J.A. et al. (1959): Functional asending phlebography of the lower extremity by serial long film technique. Ame. J. Roentg. 81, 841.
Goto, H. et al. (1975): Surgical management of severe venous ulcer of the leg indicated by two directional phlebography. Atti di Angiologia 1, 365. Centro Minerva Medica.
Linton, R.R.(1977): John Homan's impact on diseases of veins of the lower extremity, with special reference to deep thrompophlebitis and the post thrombotic syndrome with ulceration. Surgery. 81, 1.
Lim, R.C. et al. (1970):Subfacial ligation of perforating veins in recurrent stasis ulceration. Am. J. Surg. 119, 246.
Massell, T.B. et al. (1957): The problem of perforator localization in varicose veins. Arch. Surg. 75, 112.

Phlébologie 92. Eds P. Raymond-Martimbeau, R. Prescott, M. Zummo.
John Libbey Eurotext, Paris © 1992, pp. 1362-1364

The evolution of the surgical treatment of venous ulceration : a 35 year experience

C.A. Kruse

Departments of Surgery and Radiology, Saint John's Hospital and Health Center, Santa Monica, California, USA.

Treatment of venous ulceration is the control of venous stasis, whether by continuous compression and/or elevation. Subsequent obliteration of all varices is necessary to prevent recurrent ulceration.

Continuous compression is best supplied by an "ELASTOPLAST BOOT" which is placed on the lower leg from the ball of the foot to the knee after the leg is elevated and drained of venous blood. Prior to the application of the boot, the ulcer site is cleansed with Hydrogen Peroxide, after a smear of any exudate present is taken for culture and sensitivity for any pathogenic organism, particularly if there is surrounding cellulitis. Gentamicin cream is placed on the "infected" ulcer. An inner sterile dressing of 3 x 3 gauze squares and Kling is placed. The boot is allowed to remain in place for five to seven days or longer - then removed and replaced. Occasionally, with an unusual amount of edema or exudation, the dressing and boot was replaced in 24-72 hours. Gentamicin is a topical antibiotic that the pseudomonas aeruginosa organism is sensitive to. Only two cases of patient sensitivity to this topical antibiotic have been noted in many years' use of it.

With marked edema and cellulitis with ulceration, secondary to prior deep venous thrombosis - continuous elevation with wet to dry dressings and intravenous Gentamicin may be necessary. A hospital setting for this treatment may be necessary to obtain a clean granulating ulcer bed, prior to skin grafting. After a successful graft is obtained, then continued external compression with gradient pressure elastic hose is necessary to maintain normal leg size and a healed ulcer site.

The judicious use of the "Elastoplast boot" treatment method can be used in spite of diminished arterial flow - as illustrated by such healing in a 90 year old patient with absent femoral pulses, but with good capillary filling and warm feet on clinical examination.

Original surgical treatment of varicose veins was multiple local ligations of all palpable or visible varicose veins. Many persistent or subsequent varices were soon evident, even after a long tedious operation. The next advance in the surgical treatment was high and low (long and short) saphenous vein ligation (Ochsner & Mahorner, 1937). A positive Trendelenburg test correlated with an incompetent greater saphenous vein valve at the saphenofemoral junction. Varices over the distal posterior leg suggested similar valve incompetence at the lesser saphenous/popliteal vein junction. The stripping of the long saphenous vein from the groin to the ankle obliterated incompetent communicating veins as well. The same rationale and treatment was applied for the short saphenous varices. Other "counter" ligations are necessary for complete removal of all varices where larger collections of incompetent perforator veins are noted clinically and marked preoperatively. Transverse skin incisions (in the lines of the skin) give a good cosmetic result - in contrast to long vertical type incisions. Thus, a carefully carried out procedure gave good results but took a long period of operating time and a dedicated surgeon.

When there is a history of prior deep venous thrombosis and <u>recurrent</u> ulceration after adequate surgical treatment of the long and short saphenous systems and the incompetent perforating veins, subfascial ligation of the incompetent (persistent or recurring) perforating veins may be necessary (Blumenberg & Gelfand, 1978). This is illustrated by a 50 year old patient with recurring medial malleolar ulcerations over a several year period. He had prior bilateral deep femoral vein thrombosis (at age 18, subsequent to operation for acute appendicitis). This was proven on ascending venograms. Subsequent subfascial ligation of incompetent perforators via a long stocking seam posterior approach was successful in healing his stasis dermatitis and recurring ulceration. Continued external compression is necessary in such situations - to force the venous blood back "uphill" via the numerous small collateral veins. In the author's experience, obvious untreated superficial varicosities should be surgically removed as described above - in spite of proven prior deep venous thrombosis. This is the first step in the surgical management of same with usual healing of stasis dermatitis or recurrent ulceration. <u>No</u> untoward effect has resulted from this procedure in the author's hands. However, recurrent ulceration after surgical obliteration of the superficial system does warrant subfascial ligation of persistent incompetent perforating veins which may only be evident at the time of operation.

Both physician and patient have sought a shorter procedure with less anesthesia required and with acceptable post-treatment results. Selection of patients with incompetent long saphenous veins with a Doppler probe treated by high saphenous (flush) ligation and its branches, with perforating veins being treated by compression sclerotherapy, is a more recent advance (Sladen, J. G., 1986). This is followed by gradient pressure elastic hose for several weeks, or perhaps permanently in some cases. Careful follow-up and subsequent treatment of persisting or recurring varices should follow. A large localized mass of varices may require surgical treatment or removal under local anesthesia for a "complete" or good result. Again, a "transverse" incision (in the lines of the skin) makes for an excellent cosmetic result.

Without a history of deep venous thrombosis and recurrent ulceration after adequate greater and lesser saphenous vein surgery as described above, the patient should be studied for femoral vein valve incompetence by descending venography (Kruse, et al, 1989). If femoral vein valve incompetence is found, then valvuloplasty can be carried out on the first major valve just at or below the confluence of the profunda femoris and the superficial femoral veins - so as to avoid reflux from the profundus system through the incompetent superficial femoral vein valves (if valvuloplasty is done at the common femoral vein level). A transverse incision for the venotomy is preferred by the author, placed well above the valve cusp to avoid injury to same (Raju, S., 1983). In all these procedures, compression sclerotherapy can be used to treat persisting or recurring incompetent perforating veins.

Other variations of surgical treatment now being advocated are minute multiple incisions, using a button-hook type instrument to extract varices and obliterate their connections. This may be combined with selective stripping of incompetent truncal veins under femoral nerve block on an out-patient basis (Goren, G., 1992). Careful mapping of the superficial and deep venous systems by a properly executed Doppler Ultrasound examination, complimented by Duplex imaging, is an advance in patient selection for surgery and/or sclerotherapy (Raymond-Martimbeau, P., 1989). Venoscopy has also been suggested as an adjunct to surgical correction of reflux and for guided sclerotherapy (Biegeleisen and Nielsen, 1989). Preservation of the uninvolved greater saphenous vein is hopefully a dividend from the use of these newer techniques.

REFERENCES:

Biegeleisen, K. & Nielsen, R.D. (1989): Use of the Venoscope for the Treatment of Varicose Veins. 10eme Congres Mondial Union Internationale De Phlebologie, Vol 1: 419-22 (1989).

Blumenberg, R.M. & Gelfand, M.I. (1978): The Posterior Stocking-Seam Approach to Radical Subfascial Clipping of Perforator Veins. Am J Surg 1978; 136-2: 202-5.

Goren, Gabriel (1992): Personal Communication.

Kruse, C.A., Webb, Jr., R.D., Bos, C.J. (1989): An Evaluation of Femoral Vein Valvuloplasty: Selection of Patients by Descending Venography - Operative Technique and Results. 10eme Congres Mondial Union Internationale De Phlebologie. Poster Session.

Ochsner, R. & Mahorner, H. (1937): The Modern Treatment of Varicose Veins. Surgery, 2: 889, 1937.

Raju, S. (1983): Venous Insufficiency of the Lower Limb and Stasis Ulceration: Changing Concepts and Management.

Raymond-Martimbeau, P. (1989): Duplex Ultrasound, Colour Flow Doppler and Magnetic Imaging in Phlebology. 10eme Congres Mondial Union Internationale De Phlebologie. Vol 1, 351-53 (1989).

Sladen, J.G. (1986): Flush Ligation and Compression Sclerotherapy for the Control of Venous Disease. Am J Surg 1986; 152:535-38.

XVIII.
TRAITEMENT DES MALADIES THROMBO-EMBOLIQUE
THROMBO-EMBOLIC DISORDER TREATMENT

Thermograthic study of legs with post-phlebitic syndrome after different lines of management

Molokia F., Naga R.

Fac. of Med. Alexandria Univ.

Different types of management to improve skin pathology in post-phlebitic legs were compared. Thermometric changes at 20 points before and after management were recorded 1st: after walking without stocking, 2nd: after walking with stocking, 3rd: after leg elevation, 45h: after surgical correction of the main venous outflow (vein or porsthetic by-pass and valves segment implantation). Each group consisted of 20 legs. A similar number of normal legs was used as control. The data were analyses by computer study marked reversal to near normal valves at the medial aspect of the leg was after elevation followed by walking in elastic stockings. No significant changes were noticed after walking without stockings or surgical reconstruction.

The Surgical Management of the Varicose Disease in the Post-Thrombotic Syndrome

Galea Romeo Florin
University of Medicine Cluj-Napoca, the Second Surgical Clinic, str.E.Grigorescu 12o,34oo Cluj-Napoca, Romania

The anatomic disturbances from the deep venous system are responsible for the venous hemodynamic changes from the post-thrombotic syndrome. Venous hypertension is the main cause of the valve incompetence of the perforating and superficial veins which need surgical correction. The author presents his experience of 6 years in this field, aided by the clinical, phlebographic and Doppler tests. Through this information the patients could be fitted in one of the following syndromes: the obstructive, the substitution, the repermeation, and the restrictive syndrome. It also helps in the selection of patients for operation and in finding the best moment in the post-thrombotic syndrome evolution for the intervention upon the incompetent perforating and superficial veins or upon the deep venous system. Through this information we can understand better the significance of venous distension, venous insufficiency, venous hypertension, varicose veins with venous ulcer and the role of the muscular venous pump which is efficient or not. Those data are important for the therapeutic decision, either conservative or surgical.

Phlébologie 92. Eds P. Raymond-Martimbeau, R. Prescott, M. Zummo.
John Libbey Eurotext, Paris © 1992, pp. 1368

Therapeutic comparative trial of superficial vein thrombosis of the lower limbs : Fraxiparine® versus anti-inflammatory drug, a multicenter trial

J.P. Titon, J.J. Vaissie

Trousseau Hospital, Tours, France.

Objective

To assess the efficacy and tolerance of Fraxiparine® in the treatment of superficial vein thrombosis.

Patients and methods

Six centers participated in this controlled randomized trial ; 120 out-patients (40 patients per group) were included. Inclusion was decided on the duplex-scanning showing presence of a superficial vein thrombosis of the lower limbs, without any extension to deep veins.

Primary end-point criteria were represented by variations of length of the thrombi and vein repermeability as assessed by duplex-scanning perfomed on day 7.

Secondary end-point criteria were represented by changes of clinical symptoms and signs between day 0 and day 7.

Treatment

Treatment was allocated in a randomized way and given for a period of 7 days :

Group I :	patients received anti-inflammatory drug : 1 tablet of Naproxen® 550 mg once a day
Group II :	patients received fixed dose of Fraxiparine® : 6150 I U AXa, 1 subcutaneous injection of 0,6 ml per day.
Group III :	patients received adapted dose of Fraxiparine® : 61 I U AXa/kg bw, 1 subcutaneous injection per day.

Results

The three groups of patients were well matched for age, sexe, weight and height, as well as for incidence of risk factors which could predispose to the development of the thromboembolic disease.

There was no statistically significant difference between the three groups with regard to the regression of the thrombi's length and repermeability of the superficial veins.

Comparison of the evolution of clinical symptoms and signs, by the Lancaster and Irwin method, showed a statistically significant difference between the anti-inflammatory group and both Fraxiparine® groups ($p<0,05$).

Tolerance and acceptability were indentical in each group.

Conclusion

Fraxiparine®, subcutaneously injected, not only induces a similar regression of the thrombi than anti-inflammatory drug, but also is significantly more efficient than anti-inflammatory drug if we consider the regression of disability, local flusch, rubor, oedemia, and spontaneous pain.

Our experience about the treatment of axillo-subclavian venous trombosis

S. Manfrini, G. Azzena, A. Fugagnoli, G.P. Garutti

Istituto patologia chirurgica - University of Ferrara - Italy

As a patogenetic point of view, we essentially consider, with Donayre three forms of axillo-subclavian venous thrombosis: intrinsic, extrinsic and mixed. Intrinsic form is due to original alterations, caused by a physical-chemical nature of vascular endothelium or to a blood ipercoagulation. The extrinsic form, is identified in the so called"effort thrombosis" which corresponds to nosologic entity described by Paget in 1875, by Von Schroetter in 1884 and today recognized as "Paget-Schroetter syndrome". A typical mixed form example appears in operated breast tumours, irradiated or treated with chemiotherapy, where chemio-radiotherapy and mechanic venous aggressions and the lymphatic stasis are united. Authors report their experience about the diagnosis and the treatment of twenty cases. Discussion and results are reported.

THERAPY OF PRIMARY SUBCLAVIAN AXILLARY VENOUS THROMBOSIS

*E. Giraldi, *G. Spreafico, *A. Gongolo, P. Pavei, F. Schwan, R. Tasinato e U. Baccaglini

Clinica Chirurgica I, Universita' di Padova

*Presidio Ospedaliero Dolo - Venezia, Italy

The Authors report their experience in (PSAT) primary subclavian axillary thrombosis therapy. 8 patients were treated between September '87 to January '90. Because of the age of the patients (32 on average) and the early diagnosis (1-3 days) a fibrinolytique therapy with strepto or urokinase was carried out in most of the cases (5 out of 8) in order to recanalize the vein totally and to point out a possible compression in the upper thoracic outlet (CUTO). Three patients were treated only with anticoagulant therapy; the clinical result was inferior than that obtained with fibrinolytique therapy. Total recanalization was found on venography only in 3 patients (2 treated with fibrinolytique therapy and 1 with anticoagulant therapy): 2 of them had a venous comnpression in the upper thoracic outlet. Therefore a resection of the first rib was carried out. It is convenient to conclude that a PSAT should always be recanalized in order to point out and, in case, to treat a compression of the upper thoracic outlet surgically. The clinic-symptomatological improvement using fibrinolitique therapy seams to be far better than that obtainable only with an anticoagulant therapy.

BED-REST IS NOT NECESSARY IN WALKING PATIENTS WITH DEEP VEIN THROMBOSIS

Hugo Partsch, MD, Karin Oburger, MD, Adolf Mostbeck, MD, Beatrix König, MD, Horst Köhn, MD

H. Partsch, K. Oburger: Dept. of Dermatology,
A. Mostbeck: Ludwig Boltzmann Institute for Nuclear Medicine,
H. Köhn, B. König: Dept. of Nuclear Medicine, Wilhelminenspital,
A 1171 Vienna/Austria

The conventional therapeutic approach to treat a patient with deep vein thrombosis (DVT) is to administer intravenous heparin for 5 to 10 days and then to continue with oral anticoagulants starting with a crossover period of about 5 days. Most centers put the patient into bed, thereby hoping to avoid pulmonary embolism (PE) although this behavior is based more on tradition than on firm data.

It has been our policy for years not to immobilize ambulant patients with deep vein thrombosis but to encourage them to walk around with a firm compression bandage and to administer heparin subcutaneously(1). The aim of this prospective study was to detect the frequency of PE in mobile patients with acute proximal DVT extending into the pelvis who are kept walking with a firm bandage under heparin.

Patients

139 consecutive patients (53 male, 86 female, age 18-94 years, mean 70.1 y) with DVT extending into the pelvis proved by radionuclide venography were included in this prospective study. They were able to walk and did not keep strict bed rest for at least 36 hours prior to admission.

Methods

Radionuclide venography

After screening the patient by means of venous occlusion plethysmography, Doppler and Duplex-scanning, thrombotic involvement of the external and common pelvic vein was confirmed or excluded in every suspicious case by radionuclide venography using 99m Tc-labelled microspheres with a diameter of 10 - 20 micron (37 MBq in about 0.3 ml).

Lung imaging

The microspheres are trapped in the terminal pulmonary arterioles resulting in a perfusion scintigram of the lungs.

If perfusion defects are present, an additional inhalation scan using 99mTc DTPA-aerosol is performed. Perfusion defects mismatched to a normal inhalation scan and a normal X-ray are diagnostic for PE. In every patient a conventional perfusion lung scan was repeated after 11 days on the average by injecting the tracer into an arm vein.

Therapeutic regimen

Heparin was administered as a bolus intravenous dose of 5000 U, followed by subcutaneous injections of approximately 30,000 to 40,000 U per 24 hours. The heparin dose was adjusted to maintain the APTT at 1.5 to 2 times the control value. Subcutaneous heparin injections every eight to twelve hours were continued for 10-14 days. Oral anticoagulants were introduced after the second lung-scan, overlapping the last 4 days of heparin.Very firm compression bandages were applied to the diseased leg using non-elastic zinc plaster and short stretch material. The patients were encouraged to walk around.

Results

39 patients (28%) had a malignoma.

Pulmonary embolism before therapy

PE was detected by perfusion/ventilation imaging in 80 patients (58%). Only 11 patients (7.9%) presented with symptoms such as dyspnoea or chest pain. In 69 cases (49.6%) PE was clinically silent. 59 patients (42.4%) had no scintigraphic signs of embolism.

Pulmonary embolism 11 days after heparin, compression and walking

Lung scans were unchanged in 95 patients (68.3%), and improved in 33 cases (23.7%). New pulmonary emboli occurred in 10 patients (7.1%). No change of the pulmonary scan was observed in 55 patients without and in 40 patients with primary PE. A 80 years old patient with prostatic carcinoma died from massive pulmonary embolism verified by autopsy.

Discussion

Comparing data from the literature with our frequency of newly detected PE in pelvic vein thrombosis (7.9%), it is evident that our regimen of anticoagulation, compression- bandaging and walking-exercise in mobile patients is by no means more dangerous than bed-rest (Tab.1).

Table 1.: Frequency of PE before and after therapy. (Bed-rest in the first three reports, compression therapy and ambulation in our study.)

				Incidence of PE(%) before/after therapy	
Authors	DVT	Therapy	n	initial PE	new PE
Plate et	iliofemoral	heparin	29	45%	+11
	iliofemoral	surgery	20	45%	+20
Huisman et al.(3)	whole leg	heparin iv	95	51%	+8%
Albada et al.(4)	whole leg	heparin iv	98	47%	+13 %
		Fragmin iv	96	35%	+11 %
This study	iliofemoral	heparin sc, ambulant	139	58%	+8%

We feel that manipulations with a bed-pan, sudden mobilization after several days of bed-rest and all other well-known hemodynamic and respiratory risk-factors together with long lasting recumbency may even be more hazardous, especially in old patients.

Our data suggest that in ambulant patients seen at the clinic with the main symptom of an acute leg problem, the life-threatening danger of fatal pulmonary embolism has been already surpassed at the time when DVT is diagnosed. Provided adequate anticoagulation is instituted, the risk remains low even if patients are kept mobile with bandages.

The surprisingly high amount (28%) of malignant diseases is one argument to admit patients with a proximal DVT to the hospital even if they are kept ambulant. Another argument in favor of hospitalization is the need to monitor heparin therapy by frequent laboratory testing.

Provided these two problems can be solved also for outpatients, an ambulant care of mobile DVT patients would become possible.

Summary

In 139 consecutive patients (average age 70.1 y) seen at the clinic, walking with a swollen leg, diagnosis of acute DVT extending to the pelvis was confirmed by radionuclide venography using 99m Tc-labelled microspheres . 39 (28%) of these patients suffered from malignant disease.

Perfusion lung scans performed immediately after radionuclide venography were supplemented by inhalation scans (99m Tc-DTPA aerosol) in case of perfusion defects. Pulmonary embolism (PE) was found in 80 patients (58%), but only 11 (7.9%) had minor clinical symptoms. All patients were admitted to the ward, received heparin s.c.(35,000-40,000 U /24h), got firm bandages and were encouraged to walk.

After 11 days pulmonary scintigraphy was repeated and revealed no change in 55/59 without and in 40/80 with PE. 33 patients (41%) showed regression of their perfusion-defects.

11 patients (7.9%, 4 without and 7 with previous PE) developed PE. One 80 year old patient with prostatic carcinoma died from massive PE proved by autopsy.

When comparing this frequency of newly developed PE during ambulation with the occurrence of PE after bed-rest, according to the literature, it is not more dangerous for a mobile patient with proximal DVT to walk around with a firm bandage than to be put into bed. Therefore we recommend to treat mobile patients with DVT by anticoagulation, firm compression-bandages and by ambulation.

References

1 Partsch H, Oburger O, Mostbeck A. (1991): Häufigkeit von Lungenembolien bei Bein-/Beckenvenenthrombosen unter Antikoagulation, Kompressionsverband und Gehen. Phlebol 20,205-9.

2. Huisman MV, Büller HR, ten Cate, JW, van Royen EA, Vreeken J, Kersten M-J, Bakx R. (1989): Unexpected high prevalence of silent pulmonary embolism in patients with deep venous thrombosis. Chest 95,498-502

3. Plate G, Ohlin,P, Eklöf B. (1985): Pulmonary embolism in acute iliofemoral venous thrombosis. Br J Surg. 72,912-5

4. Albada J, Nieuwenhuis HK, Sixma JJ. (1989): Treatment of acute venous thromboembolism with low molecular weight heparin (Fragmin). Results of a double-blind randomized study. Circulation 80,935-409.

Phlébologie 92. Eds P. Raymond-Martimbeau, R. Prescott, M. Zummo.
John Libbey Eurotext, Paris © 1992, pp. 1373-1375

The post-phlebitic syndrome : thermal treatment with « calcium-sulfate » water

F. Rück, A. Giovanelli, A. Pecunia.

Angiology Service, Medical Centre Terme di Boario (BS), Italy.

The post-phlebitic syndrome: thermal treatment with "calcium-sulphate" water.

Dr. F.Rück; Dr. A.Giovanelli; Dr. A.Pecunia.
Angiology Service - Medical Centre Terme di Boario (BS) - Italy.

The post-phlebitic syndrome is a frequent intercurrent desease of phlebitis; for instance, in the U.S.A it has been estimated that 300/400.000 persons were suffering from this syndrome.
It has as main etiologic agent venous congestion, and is characterized by hypodermitis of the skin, aedema, cutaneous dyschromia and dystrophia.
Chrenotherapeutic treatment of phlebitis combined with techniques of physical therapy, is large developed in thermal centers beyond the Alps, above all in France and in Germany; in fact, there are some thermal centers which deal only with vein deseases. One of the most well-known is Bagnoles de l'Orne, in Normandy.
At Boario Terme Center, with the same weather as that in Bagnoles, it has been used a crenotherapeutic treatment with calcium sulphate water to improve venous congestion, to reduce aedema and trophic disorders. The purpose of the following text is the evaluation of the usefulness of thermal treatment, in patients suffering from phlebitic syndrome.

MATERIALS AND METHODS

The Angiology Service of Medical Center Terme di Boario has treated 300 patients suffering from post-phlebitic syndrome with calcium sulphate water from 1986 to 1991.
Patients, at admission, presented parestesias at lower limbs (in 80% of the cases), phlebodinia (in 95% of the cases), sensation of heaviness at lower limb, expecially in the evening (in 95% of the cases).
Sulphate-bicarbonate-alkaline-soily water or "Antica Fonte" calcium sulphate water of the thermal baths in Boario was used for the treatment.

The chemical composition of the same is shown in Table 1.

Tab.1 - "ANTICA FONTE" CALCIUM SULPHATE WATER. CHEMICAL COMPOSITION.
Components dissolved per litre.
- CALCIUM ION (Ca^{++}) 0,66000 g/l
- SULPHATE ION (SO_4^{--}) 1,56050 g/l
- MAGNESIUM ION (Mg^{++}) 0,04620 g/l
- CARBONATE HYDROGEN ION (HCO_3^-) 0,28265 g/l
- POTASSIUM ION (K^+) 0,00244 g/l
- SILICA (SiO_2) 0,02300 g/l
- FIXED RESIDUAL
  F. R. 180° 2,6600 g/l

The calcium sulphate waters constantly show some main properties:
- anti - aedema action, with particular reference to perimalleolar swellings;
- improved capillary circle distribution and regular defluction through the arteriovenous junctions;
- regression of the algic component at lower limb;
- reduction of the peripheral vascular resistances, which affects the hemic flow;
- central and peripherical sedative action.

The ion Ca and more generally the sulphate Ca, seems to assume specific therapeutic properties with typical antiphlogistic action.
The crenotheraupetic treatment (Fig. 1) consisted in cycles of hydrokinesy therapy (15-16 sessions) in the bath with "Antica Fonte" calcium sulphate water at a temperature of about 23°-26°, for the lenght of about 20 minutes each, with underwater ozoned massage at low pressure, repeated passages combined with hydrospouts for intensified massages. The phlebopathic patient undergoing this treatment was attentively checked on a general clinic and angiologic specialistic level and underwent a thermographic, plethysmographic, Doppler control.

Tab. 2 THERMAL METHODOLOGY BATHS WITH "ANTICA FONTE" WATER

- Temperature: not higher than 36° preferably around 23°-26° (heat causes further vein damage)
- Sessions: No. 15-18 (repeatable every 6 months)
- Session time: about 20 minutes
- Slow movements of lower limbs
- Underwater ozoned massage at low pressure
- Douche (hydromassage) in the clear varices
- Repeated passages combined with hydrospouts for intensified massages.

The crenotherapeutic treatment was associated with a

complementary treatment characterized by detoxifying and personalized diets, including the therapy per os with SILIA WATER, the use of elastic stockings connected with the gait on the different ways of a phlebitic walk.

RESULTS AND DISCUSSIONS

After each treatment cycle, patient underwent a check-up.

It was thus evidenced the almost total loss of sensation of heaviness at lower limbs (in 98% of the cases treated), of phlebodynia (in 95% of the cases treated), of parestesias (95% of the cases treated), of a notable reduction of the aedema (90% of the cases treated). The a.m. results confirm the usefulness and the efficacy of Boario "Antica Fonte" calcium sulphate water in the therapy of post-phlebitic syndrome.

The crenotherapeutic treatment determines an increase in the volume and in the speed of the vein circulation return which is of thermal and mechanic origin, followed by an increase in the cardiac output and span associated with a loss in the pressor values. The calcium sulphate treatments contribute in the phlebitic patient to the rechanalisation of the thrombosed vein trunks and to the regression of the periulcerous thrombosing capillaritis, achieving thus the regularisation of the microcycle. The aedemas of the limbs concerned, are favourably influenced by the thermal qualities of the waters. The consequent drop of the tissue pressure sollecitates the re-establishment of elastic structures and the reduction of fibrous connective.

In conclusion we can affirm that Boario "Antica Fonte" calcium sulphate Waters are useful in the treatment of many aspects of phlebopaties, especially in the treatment of the post-phlebitic syndrome.

REFERENCES

- Agus G.B., Costantini A. et al. (1986): Morphoystological study of microcirculation in patients with chronic venous insufficiency of surgical interest. In Phlebology 85, Negus et al.
- Caillé J.P. (1982): Phlebologie en pratique quotidienne. In expansion Scientifique Francaise. Paris.
- Chatard H. (1982): Hypodermite seléreuse. Phlébologie
- Deschamps P.N. (1958): Inections sous cutanes de gaz carbonique termal en angeologie. Angeologia, 10, n.3
- Gualtierotti R. (1981): Medicina Termale. Ed. Libreria del lo Studente. Milano
- Mercier R., Valette J., Vaneuville C. : Affections vasculaires des membres et Kinésithérapie. Maloine ED., Parigi 1970.
- Messina B., Grossi F. (1984): Elementi di Idrologia Medica. Ed. Seu. Roma.
- Tamburino G., Andreozzi G.M. (1984): The initial stage of venous diseases of lower limbs. M. Tesi, J.A. Dormandy. Ed. Pan Minerva Medica. Torino.

Phlébologie 92. Eds P. Raymond-Martimbeau, R. Prescott, M. Zummo.
John Libbey Eurotext, Paris © 1992, pp. 1376-1377

Follow-up studies of iliofemoral venous thrombectomy

Hisashi Gotoh, Akihiko Matsumoto, Hiroto Matsumura

Department of Surgery, Yokohama City University School of Medicine, Yokohama, Japan.

Comparing with conservative treatments, iliofemoral venous thrombectomy using Fogarty balloon catheter is considered to provide a better results in rapidly relieving the symptoms of acute thrombotic events and further reducing the risk of pulmonary embolism and Phlegmasia Cerulea Dolens. Evaluation of averating 8 years and 4 months follow-up studies of venous thrombectomy by means of pre-and post opertive phlebograms, questionnaire and personal contacts is reviewed in this operation.
The most important key point of this opertion is that catheterization and milking should be alternately repeated to remove thrombi as much as possible. By this method of operation, excellent or good results can be obtained not only in early stage but also in long follow-up studies. Seventy patients were followed-up by questionnaire and personal contacts.
A review of 136 thrombectomized patients and follow-up studies of 70 patients led us to the conclusion that venous thrombectomy is useful for relief of severe pain, swelling, and incapacity to walk and plays an important role in the prevention of postphlebitic syndrome.

Materials

In these 26 years, we experienced 408 patients of venous thrombosis of the extremities. On ehundred thirty-six patients, about one-third of all cases had accepted iliofemoral venous thrombectomy. There were ten pulmonary embolism and ten Phlegmasia Celurea Dolens. Two of each diseases were fatal. These patients included 54 males and 82 females, their ages ranged from 15 to 79 years old. The diagnosis of venous thrombosis is usually confirmed not only with clinical findings but also Phlebograms.

Operative Procedure

After identificatin of the thrombus within the femoral vein, 50 mg of heparin are given intravenouly to prevent propagation of the thrombus during extraction and to avoid further thrombus formation after thrombus is removed. Fogarty balloon venous catheter is inserted at first to distal part through transverse incision of femoral vein. After extraction of thrombus by catheter, the foot is forcibly milked, dorsiflexed and stretched, thus the thrombi are pumped proximally. Catheter has proved to be very effective in removing thrombi from the deep vein, while maneuver of milking have been effective in removing thrombi from branches to the deep vein. Then it is very important that catheterization and milking should be repeated alternately. We usually perform each manipulation 4 or 5 times.

When we insert catheter to the proximal part., meticulous, careful removal of thrombi is necessary not to push them out to the lung. Rough manupuration of catheter should be avoided. After removal of thrombi, femoral vein is irrigated with dilute heparin solution and closed with 5-0 arterial silk or polypropylene by running suture. We do not employ any other methods such as ligation, plicatin, clipping or temporary obstruction of the vena cava for prevention of pulmonary embolism. We have not experience of precise fatal pulmonary embolism except one doubtful case in these 136 series. After operation, supplemental treatments with heparin, low molecular weight dextran and urokinase are used for the period of about one week.

Result and discussion

In the immediate results of our thrombectomy, excellent results were seen in 28 patients. These patients demonstrated no abnormality with regard to patent deep vein and funcitonal valve on post-operative phlebograms. Good results were obtained in 104 patients. These patients showed clinical improvement despite near complete or partial deep venous obstruction were noted. 2 patients showed no clinical improvement. One out of the two aggravated patients developed Phlegmasia Cerulea Dolens reguiring amputation of the leg. Another exacerbated patients died 5 hours after operation but precise cause of the death was not determined because autosy was not available. Fatal pulmonary embolism had not occured during operation and post-operative course.

The results of the long term follow-up (avarage 8 years and 4 months) by means of personal contact and questionaire, excellent results were obtained in 46 patients, good results in 17 patients and almost no change in 7 patients. The fact that long follow-up results were better than the immeidate results probably means that good operation and precise supplimental treatments by drugs decide good long follow-up results.

There is controversy about destruction of valves by Fogarty balloon catheter (Edwards et al., 1970; fogarty et al., 1966; Goto et al., 1980; lansing & Davis, 1969; Willman V.L., 1974).

In our experiences, Fogarty catheter did not laead to any late venous insufficiency in those cases whose post-operative phlebograms showed patency of deep veins and normal valves.

In conclusion, iliofemoral venous thrombectomy is safe and useful for relief of complaints and plays an important role in the prevention of postphlebitic syndrome.

Refferences

Edwards W.M., Sauyers J.L., Foste J.H. (1970): Iliofemoral Venous Thrombectomy: reappraisal of thrombectomy. Ann. Surg., 171, 1961.

Fogarty T.J., Dennis D., Krppaehne W.W. (1966): Surgical management of Iliofemoral Venous Thrombosis. Amer J. Surg., 112, 211.

Goto H., Wada T., Matsumoto A. Matsumura H., Soma T. (1980): Iliofemoral Venous Thrombectomy: Follow-up studies of 88 patients. J. Cardiovasc. Surg. 21.341. Lansing A.M., Davis W.M. (1969): Five year follow-up study of Iliofemoral Venous Thrombectomy. Ann. Surg., 168, 620.

Willman V.L. (1974): Thrombectomy for Iliofemoral Venous Thrombosis: A position Against. In Varco R.L. and Delaney. J.P.: Controversy in Surgery. Philadelphia, W.B.S aunders Co.

Phlébologie 92. Eds P. Raymond-Martimbeau, R. Prescott, M. Zummo.
John Libbey Eurotext, Paris © 1992, pp. 1378-1380

Venous thromboembolism as a complication of bariatric surgery

G. Bajardi, G. Ricevuto, G. Mastrandrea, G. Pischedda, G. Rubino

Department of Surgery, University of Palermo, Palermo, Italy.

Obesity is a well known risk factor for venous thromboembolism (Juan-Vague Alessi 1990). Factors like lower limbs venous insufficiency, modifications of hemoreologic parameters, ipomobility, may cause in obese people higher incidence of post-operative thromboembolic complications, in particular after orthopedic, gynecologic and oncologic surgery (Pasulka et al. 1986). In this study we have considered thromboembolic complications in bariatric surgery.

Between March 1989 and December 1991, seventyfive (75) obese patients underwent, at our Institute, BilioPancreatic Diversion (BPD) for surgical treatment of morbid obesity. They were 28 men (37%) and 47 women (63%) with a mean age of 38 (18-61), mean weight of 130 Kg. (90-187), mean overweight of 72.5 Kg. (38.5-129.5) or 128% (64-225), and a mean BMI of 49 (37-73).

41 patients demonstrated by the time of intervention lower limbs venous insufficiency (54%), 26 lumbar arthritis (34%), 26 effort dispnea (34%), 17 sleep apnea syndrome (22%), 16 hypertension (21%), 8 diabetes (10%), 3 depression (4%), 1 atopic asthma (1%).

In every patient subcutaneous heparin (5.000 Units twice/day), preoperative hemodiluition, intraoperative lower limbs elastic bandaging and early postoperative ambulation were used as prevention of thromboembolic complications. The intervention (BPD) consists of a gastric resection, leaving a gastric pouch of 250-400 ml., and a small bowel bypass creating two separate pathways for food (2 meters) and bilio-pancreatic secretions (all the remaining small bowel), rejoning 50 cm. before ileo-caecal valve. Cholecistectomy was always performed if not done before.

Post-operative thromboembolic complications consisted in 1 case of clinically evident deep venous thrombosis (DVT) (1,3%), and 2 cases of pulmonary embolism (PE) (2,6%) of which 1 lethal . Other complications like gastric bleedings , wound disruption, asymptomatic gastric leak, and gastric outlet obstructions occourred in 8% of cases, for a total morbidity of 10% and a mortality of 1,3%.

The only clinically evident DVT, extended to common femoral vein, occourred on the 8th post-operative day and was successfully treated with intravenous heparin anticoagulation. Both the PEs occourred in patients without signs and sym ptoms of DVT; the first appeared on the 4th postoperative day and was successfully treated with heparin, the second appeared on the 15th post-operative day, after the patient had quitte the hospital, and resulted in patient's death despite heparin therapy.

Venous thromboembolism is a common complication following bariatric surgery. Many authors report these complications being responsible of morbidity and mortality too. We have considered, from the literature, 2979 cases submitted to different types of bariatric surgery interventions like Horizontal Gastroplasty (B. Doldi et al. 90), Vertical Banded Gastroplasty (Owen et al. 89), Roux-en-Y Gastric By pass (Lopez et al. 89), Jejuno-ileal Bypass (B. Doldi et al. 90), BPD (Scopinaro et al. 90) and Re-Do Bariatric Surgery (Schwartz et al. 88), analyzing death causes. PE caused 33% of deaths.

DEATH CAUSES AMONG 2979 BARIATRIC SURGERY INTERVENTIONS

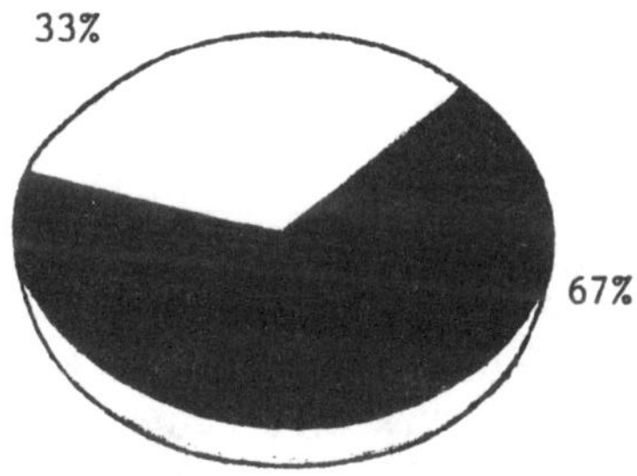

☐ PULMONARY EMBOLISM (33%)

■ Peritonitis (13%), Hypertemia (4%), CVA (4%) , Unknown (8%), Gastric Bleeding (8%), Septic Shock (8%), Pancreatitis (4%), Subdiaphragmatic Abscess (4%), Cardiac Shock (14%).

Data obtained from the following series:
Lopez 89, B. Doldi 90, Rucker 82, Owen 89, Scopinaro 90, Buckwalter 80, Schwartz 88

Many studies have been addressed to find out correlations between obesity and thromboembolism. Factors like hemoreologic parameters modifications have been demonstrated (Le Devehat et al. 90) in obese people, but their real implication in thrombogenesis is still debated.

In consideration of the difficulties still existing to assess which must be considered risk factors for venous thromboembolism in obese people, we believe that a particular effort must be made toward prevention of these complications, also because obesity often lowers the chance of an early clinical suspect of DVT. This prevention must be particularly careful when approaching bariatric surgery that, among its many aims, is intended to lower thromboembolic risk too.

The prophylactic methods we applied led us to a percentage of 1,3% for DVT and 2,6% for PE, similar to other bariatric surgery reports (Hall et al. 90), (Morino et al. 89) (Owen et al. 89).

Despite preventive measures venous thromboembolism is a persistent complication of bariatric surgery. Even if these complications are sometimes lethal the drastic improvement of the several risk factors connected with obesity, after achievement of a proper weight, still sustains the opportunity of this type of surgery.

REFERENCES

1) Juan-Vague I, Alessi MC: Le risque trombotique veineux chez l'obese.- In Jambon C "Obésité et pathologie de la circulation de retour". Solal Ed., Marseille 1990

2) Pasulka PS, Bistrian BR, Benotti PN, Blackburn GL: The risk of surgery in obese patients.- Ann. Int. Med. 1986, 104, 540-46.

3) B. Doldi S, Vita PM, Lattuada E, Restelli A, Micheketto G, Longoni F, Montorsi W : Gastroplastie horizontale dans la chirurgie de l'obésité morbide: une condamnation injustifiée?- Ann. Chir. 1990,5,356-61.

4) Owen ERTC, Abraham R, Kark AE: Gastroplasty for morbid obesity: technique, complications and results in 60 cases.- Br. J. Surg. 1989,76,131-35.

5) Lopez JF, Smart CR, Miller DK, Goodman GN, Ford CR, Filloux F: Traitement de la obésité morbide par dérivation gastrique. A propos de 1158 cas opérés.- J. Chir 1989, 126,5-12.

6) B. Doldi S, Vita PM, Restelli A, Micheletto G, Longoni F, Caspani P, Montorsi W : Y à-t-il encore une place pour le court-circuit jéjuno-iléal dans le traitement chirurgical de l'obésité morbide?- Ann. Chir. 1990,5,362-67.

7) Scopinaro N, Gianetta E, Friedman D, Traverso E, Adami GF, Vitale B, Marinari G , Cuneo S, Ballari F, Colombini M, Bachi V : La Diversione Biliopancreatica.- Atti XCII Congr. Naz. Soc. It. Chir., vol. 6°,39-64, Roma Ott. 1990.

8) Schwartz RW, Strodel WE, Simpson WS, Griffen WO : Gastric bypass revision: lesson learned from 920 cases.- Surgery 1988,104,806-12.

9) Rucker RD, Horstmann J, Schneider PD, Varco RL, Buchwald H: Comparison between jejuno-ileal and gastric by-pass operations for morbid obesity.- Surgery 1982, 92, 241-49.

10) Buckwalter JA, Herbst CA: Complications of gastric bypass for morbid obesity.- Am. J. Surg. 1980,139,55-60.

11) Le Devehat C, Khodabandehlou T, Boisseau M, Dougny M : Etude des paramètres hémorhéologiques dans l'obésité isolée.- In Jambon C "Obésité et phatologie de la circulation de retour". SOLAL Ed. Marseille 1990.

12) Hall JC, Mck Watts J, O'Brien PE, Dunstan RE, Walsh JF, Slavotinek AH, Elmslie RG: Gastric surgery for morbid obesity. The Adelaide study.- Ann. Surg. 1990, 211, 419-27.

13) Morino M, Robecchi A, Fronda GR, Toppino M, Scollo MA, Morino F : Chirurgie gastrique dans l'obésité morbide. A propos de 101 cas.- Ann. Chir. 1989,43,429-32

Phlébologie 92. Eds P. Raymond-Martimbeau, R. Prescott, M. Zummo.
John Libbey Eurotext, Paris © 1992, pp. 1381

Temporary caval filters and loco-regional thrombolysis in DVT

P. Mingazzini, P. Ventura, S. Zaccone, P. Bedoni*

*Department of General Surgery « S. Garberini », S. Carlo Hospital, Milan. * Department of General Surgery 8° fl., Carlo Hospital, Milan, Italy.*

DVT rappresents an unforeseeable pathology with high mortality and important morbility. Temporary caval filter rappresents now a real help for treatment of DVT and for prevention of pulmonary embolism.

Indications to use the temporary caval filter are:

- caval protection during locoregional thrombolysis;
- caval protection during thrombectomy.

Temporary caval filter is in teflon and has a central canal to make cavogram and infusion of thrombotyc agents and anticoagulants.

When DVT is diagnosed an ascendent phleoogram is necessary to value distal extention. Then the right basilic vein is pricked and before the guide then the filter are introduced.

THROugh the filter a cavogram is executed to value the thrombus proximal limit. Temporary filter is opened and thrombus is pricked with a catheter introduced through the filter central canal. Locoregional thrombolysis is started with 1/4 dosage to sistemic thrombolysis. If safena is using it is possible pricks it at the malleolus to execute a combined locoregional thrombolysis from high and low combined.

Good result of thrombolysis depends to the precocity of treatment, within 5 days from thrombotic event, and to a correct method.

We treated 4 patients with locoregional thrombolysis. Three patients had a femoro-iliaco-caval DVT while one had a femoro-iliac DVT.

The ricanalization of femoro-iliaco-caval tract has been complete in 3 patients while in the other one has remained iliac thrombosys.

In 3 cases we have used Urokinase with a 50.000 U.I./h dosage, in one RTPA wiht a 4 ml/h dosage.

There was anemia in 2 cases. One patient has showed hematoma in inguino-femoral place of prick, while the second has fall of Hb without hematoma.

This method has showed,if correctly used, a high efficacy. We have obteined complete ricanalizzation in 24-48 h, while sistemic thombolysis has had poor results even with high dosage of Urokinase (200.000 U.I./h).

Post-phlebitis syndrom may be avoided wiht a fast and precocious lysis, with low dosage because hemorragic complication and ictus are proportional to dosage used.

Fibrinolytic treatment in deep vein thrombosis

G.Gandarias, J.Ocana; E.Aracil, A.Utrilla, JM Egana, E.Puras, M.Lasso, I.Crespo, A.Chinchilla, F.Ortiz, J.Fontcuberta, L.A.Castrillo, C.Cuesta

Servicio de Angiologia y Cirugia Vascular, Hospital Ramon y Cajal, Apart. 34, 28034 Madrid, Espana

The socieconomical impact of deep vein thrombosis in based in his incidence in the general papulation and high cost.

A DVT episode will be present in 2.5 to 5% of the papulation, with 29% of them developing venous ulcers and 28% of them secondary varices with an estimated cost of 40.000$ (O'Donnel) in patients with postflebitic syndrome in a 10 years period.

Between 1984-1989 a total of 520 cases DVT had been treated in our hospital; 77 cases with fibrinolytic treatment, 12 cases with streptokinase and 65 cases with urokinase. We had 72 patients with inferior limb syndrome and 5 cases with superior extremity affectation.

Total lysis in 15 cases and no modification in 24 cases.

We had follow-up in 53 patients (72,6%) for a period between 1 and 4 years; 31 patients had no postflebitic syndrome, 15 had moderate affectation and 7 cases had severe postflebitic affectation.

Phlébologie 92. Eds P. Raymond-Martimbeau, R. Prescott, M. Zummo.
John Libbey Eurotext, Paris © 1992, pp. 1383-1384

A teleological approach to the treatment of superficial thrombophlebitis

George M. Robb

501-625 5th avenue, New Westminster, B.C. V3M 1X4, Canada.

Superficial thrombophlebitis occurs commonly following relatively minor trauma and often there is no history of trauma at all. However it nearly always occurs at the site of pre-existent varices. Keeping this in mind it is not unreasonable in many cases to regard the attack of superficial thrombophlebitis as an attempt on the part of the system to close off unwanted varices. Unfortunately this system of varicose vein eradication seldom works effectively in the long term and in most cases leads only to a temporary reduction in the varicose veins at the location. If this is accepted as a reasonable assumption, then it seems foolish indeed to treat the problem by trying to cut the process short with the use of drugs to limit the inflammatory response, and certainly the advocation of bed rest is hard to justify. Yet these two measures are the usual practice in most clinics today. Considering that in the average case bed rest is not as effective in controlling the pain as is exercise combined with the application of local pressure by means of an elastic bandage or stocking, there is even more reason to question the value of such a routine. In some areas patients with superficial thrombophlebitis are treated by anticoagulation but although this gives rapid relief of the symptoms one must remember that other methods are equally efficient in relieving symptoms and in addition afford a method of long term improvement in the basic problem.

After ruling out the possibility of deep vein thrombosis, which is usually very easy when the patient is first seen, the proposal is to deal with superficial thrombophlebitis by treating the underlying varicose veins by the simplest and most direct means available. Eradication of the veins involved in the phlebitis by surgical extirpation is not easy. However the same objective is achieved by sclerotherapy of the adjacent varices. This then gives the phlebitic process a better chance to achieve permanent obliteration of the involved varices.

CASE STUDY REVIEW

Number of cases reviewed	80	female	53
		male	27

Assessment of result:	satisfactory	improved	lost
Treatment modality			
Pressure bandage	31	4	7
Surgery	66		1
Sclerotherapy	29	1	0

When the trunk of the great saphenous vein is involved ligation and division at the saphenofemoral junction leads to rapid improvement in the phlebitis in most cases leading to early resumption of normal activities. Extirpation of varices involved in a phlebitic process is difficult to perform, and cannot usually be done very satisfactorily. However, in the large majority of cases this is not necessary and the same rapid relief of symptoms can be achieved by compression sclerotherapy of the patent varices around the area of phlebitis, application of local pressure, and initiation of a programme of active walking. Patients whenever possible are asked to walk for about one and a half hours per day - a much more acceptable request in most cases than enforced bed rest.

Phlébologie 92. Eds P. Raymond-Martimbeau, R. Prescott, M. Zummo.
John Libbey Eurotext, Paris © 1992, pp. 1385-1386

Lower limb thrombophlebitis : a new diagnostic and therapeutic approach

S. Michelini, A. Failla, A. Micci, A. Jantaffi, E. Cartoni, V. Podagrosi

Hospital « San Giovanni Battista » Acismom, Roma, Italy.

INTRODUCTION

Lower limb thrombophlebitis is one of the most common causes of temporary disability. Relapses are quite frequent and the involvement of the deep venous circulation can lead to an impairement of variable degree of the quality of the life.
Deep and superficial thrombophlebitis have different prognosis and require different medical and rehabilitative treatment. The clinical follow-up has a fundamental role but is not easily standardized.
Aim of the present work is a report on the usefulness of a safe, cheap, repetible and reliable method: **the venous treadmill stress test.**

MATERIALS AND METHODS

We studied 145 patients (56 males and 89 females aged 22 to 79 years) with lower limb thrombophlebitis (LLT). In 33 patients there was a deep involvement while in the other 112 the LLT was superficial.
All patients had periodic physical examinations and doppler studies. PT, PTT, fibrinogen, FDP, antithrombin III, coagulation factor VII, ESR, complement factors C3 and C4 were also periodically determined.
The patients with deep LLT were put on parenteral anticoagulative therapy (Calciparine 12,500 IU twice a day for 15 days) followed by an oral anticoagulative treatment. Phlebotonic, antiflogistic and steroid support was also given. Steroid drugs were expecially effective in younger patients because of the higher intensity of the flogistic reactive phenomenons.
Superficial LLT was treated with profibrinolitic drugs (heparansulphate 100 mg three times a day and glycosaminoglycan 50 mg three times a day).

All patients underwent a rehabilitative training consisting of 1) exercises of thoraco-diafragmatic respiration; 2) isotonic contraction exercises (under elasto-pressure) of all the muscolar groups of the lower limb; 3) lymphatic manual drainage according to Leduc; 4) presso-therapy and 5) elastic bandage.
The assessment of the effectiveness of the treatment is not easy because of the large amount of environmental and examinator-linked variables.
In order to get a more objective evaluation we used a venous treadmill test on 18 patients with deep LLT: blood pressure in tibial posterior vein was determined at rest both in orthostatism and in clinostatism by doppler test according to Bartolo. Then the patients were invited to walk on a treadmill (speed 3 Km/h, leaning 10 degrees). The exercise was carried out until pain raised. At this time superficial venous ectasies were often present. Blood pressure in tibial posterior vein was again determined.

RESULTS AND CONCLUSIONS

The values recorded by venous treadmill stress test on the normal side were always equal or slightly inferior to the basal ones while in the affected side they were up to 8 times higher than at rest.
After the treatment (mean duration 3 weeks) the mean increment of Antithrombin III was 18%. FDP and coagulation factor VII showed, an average decrease of 10%. Fibrinogen values showed a 15% decrease. Complement factors C3 and C4 normalized.
In all 18 cases of deep LLT treadmill test showed a progressive reduction of the tibial posterior vein pressure after stress, reflecting clinical and strumental improvement.
The treadmill stress test data accorded with the functional outcome and were useful in the choise of the long-term therapy.

REFERENCES

Antignani P.L., Di Fortunato T., Dragoni F., Arcresi P., Bartolo M. (1991) : Flebotrombosi e deficit di proteina C, proteina S e Antitrombina III. Atti 13^ Congr. Naz. Soc. Ital. Patol. Vasc. 24-26 giugno 1991.

Franco A., Richaud C., Bouchet J.Y., Piton J.L., Truche H., De Angelis M.P., Carpentier P. (1989) : Rehabilitation of patients with lower limb proximal deep venous thrombosis. 15th World Congress of Intern. Union of Angiology, Rome 17-22 sept. 1989.

Michelini S., Micci A., Iantaffi A., Cartoni E., Todini M.M. (1991) : Fattori di rischio emocoagulativi nella genesi delle tromboflebiti degli arti inferiori. Atti III Intern. Congr. of Phlebolymphology, Ferrara S. Marino 18-20 sept. 1991.

PENTOXIFYLLINE AND COMPRESSION BANDAGES IN THE TREATMENT OF SUPERFICIAL PHLEBITIS OF THE LOWER LIMBS

C. Barbarino

Service of Angiology Surgical Department
Hospital of Chioggia (Venice) ITALY

Ten patients were studied. All had superficial phlebitis of the lower limb. Five were treated with compression bandages and Pentoxifylline (5 days of 300 mg. Pentoxifylline i.v. plus 1,200 mg. Pentoxifylline orally). The other five patients were also treated with compression bandages but received 5 days of placebo therapy . At the beginning and the end of the study the following clinical variables were recorded : heaviness of the legs, pain, phlebodinia, orthostatic oedema and ankle circumference. The following non invasive tests were also performed: venous pressure by Doppler sonography and venous refilling time by plethysmography. After treatment with Pentoxifylline and compression bandages an improvement in clinical and non invasive measurements was observed as follows : Phlebitis resolved completely in 2 cases and showed a remarkable improvement in the other 3 cases. By comparison an improvement in clinical condition was seen in only 1 case receiving placebo and compression bandages . Our preliminary data show tha Pentoxifylline, in conjunction with compression bandaging, improves the venous return and the clinical symptomatology of patients suffering from superficial phlebitis of the lower limbs .

Regional lymphatic therapy in the treatment of acute thrombophlebitis

Dr. S.U. Jumabaev, V.A. Hakimov

The Republican Center of Clinical Lyphology

Complex regional lymphatic therapy is used in the treatment of 134 patients with acute thrombophlebitis of tower extremities.

Regional stimulation of lymphatic drainage and regional lymphatic antibioticotherapy was used in the complex of treatments. Manipulation was carried out once a day with the use of a single dosage of antibiotics of wide spectrum of effect. The course consisted of 5-7 treatments.

In the process of treatment one can achieve acceleration of regress of pathologic process on considerable reduction of concentration of used antibiotics and the decrease of injections in number.

XIX.
TRAITEMENT DE L'INSUFFISANCE VEINEUSE CHRONIQUE
CHRONIC VENOUS INSUFFICIENCY TREATMENT

Phlébologie 92. Eds P. Raymond-Martimbeau, R. Prescott, M. Zummo.
John Libbey Eurotext, Paris © 1992, pp. 1391-1393

Operative management of essential and post-phlebitic varicose syndrome : personal experience on 2000 extremities operated with a radical criteria

G. Pintos Díaz, E. Ramos Gato, M. Martínez Pérez, E. Senín Fernandez, J.A. Pintos Moreu, I. Lojo Rocamonde, R. García Casas

Department of Vascular Surgery, General Hospital of Galicia, Medicine School, Santiago of Compostela, Spain.

Introduction

The prevalence of varicose syndrome range between 4 and 50 per cent.Genetic factors, pregnacy and professional activity in bipedestation influence in a very significant way the development of the essential varicose syndrome.

Radical surgical treatment of varicose syndrome has shown better long term results than conservative treatment, but the recent appearance of new and less aggressive techniques has brought the reappearance of controversy about the suitability or not of persisting in the use of such radical criteria.

Material and methods

A total of 1,965 extremities were operated on in 1,146 patients (table I) in 88.7% of the cases the patient suffered essential varicose syndrome (table II) and in the 11.3% post-phlebitic syndrome(table III).

Table I.

Chronic Venous Insufficiency.

Patients: 1319*	Limbs operated:2000	
Etiology	NO. of patients	NO. of Limbs
Essential varicose veins	1146*	1774 (88.7%)
Post-phlebitic venous insuf.	189*	226 (11.3%)

*16 patients had primary varicose veins in one limb and post-phlebitic venous insufficiency in the other one.

Table II.

Essential Varicose Syndrome

NO. of patients		1146
Age: 12-84 years ($\bar{x}$=43)		
Sex: Male	363 (31.7%)	
Female	783 (68.3%)	
Clinical presentation		
Unilateral	327 (28.5%)	
Bilateral	819 (71.5%)	
NO. limbs explored		1965
Right	975 (49.6%)	
Left	990 (50.4%)	

Table III

Post-phlebitic Venous Insufficiency

NO. of patients		189
Age: 21 -78 years (x̄=49.7)		
Sex: Male	83 (43.9%)	
Female	106 (56.1%)	
Clinical presentation		
Unilateral	143 (75.7%)	
Bilateral	46 (24.3%)	
NO. of limbs explorated		235
Right	105 (44.7%)	
Left	130 (55.3%)	

Table IV

Physical Findings

	NO. of limbs	%
Long saphenous insufficiency.	1513	75.65
Short saphenous insufficiency.	247	12.35
Incompetence of perforating veins	429	21.45
Edema	887	44.35
Pigmentary changes	493	24.65
Eczematose dermatitis	48	2.4
Celulitis induration	375	18.75
Ulcer	483	24.15
Subjetive symptoms	1131	56.55
Phlebography	217	10.85

Long saphenous vein insufficiency (75.65%), communicating veins incompetency (21.45%) and induration celulitis with ulcer (24.5%)were the most frequent pathology (tablaIV).Ulcers were more frequent in the post-phlebitic syndrome(72.3%)than in the essential varicose syndrome(15.9%).

The surgical technique most commonly performed was the internal saphenectomy with complementary varicectomy and perforating vein ligature. Ulcer resection was performed on 30.3% of the extremities (table V).

Tabla V

Operative Management

	NO.	%
Internal Saphenectomy	1872	93.6
External Saphenectomy	680	34
Complementary varicectomy and perforans veins ligature	1948	97.4
Cockett´s technical	440	22
Ulcers/induration resection	539	26.9
Free skin graft(second time)	424	21.2

The results after ten years show a varicose veins recurrence of 10.7% in essential varicose syndrome and of 10.8% in post-phlebitic syndrome.Reappearance of ulcers show 5.7% in essential varicose syndrome and 30.3% in post-phlebitic syndrome.All cases were reoperated upon.(table VI and table VII).

The recurrence of ulcers was 4.4% in essential venose syndrome and 35.1% in post-phlebitic, needing reiterative grafts .(table VII).

Table VI

Late Development Post-operative

Recurrence of varicose veins

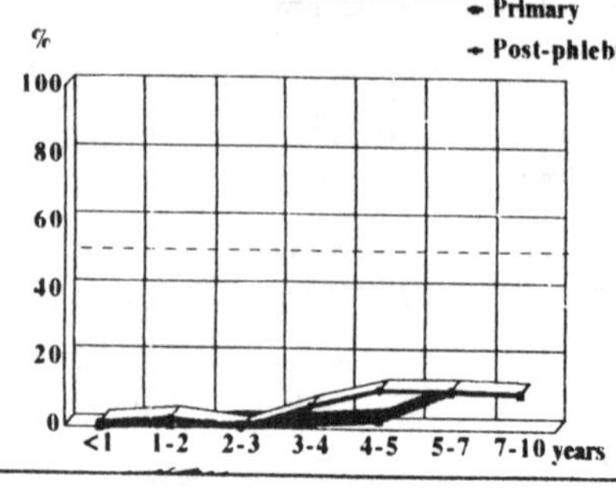

Table VII

Late Development post-operative

Recurrence of ulcers

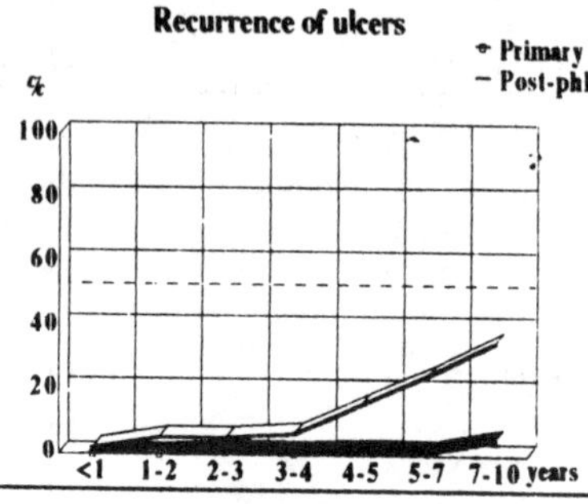

Discussion

Despite the fact that nowadays there is a trend towards the use of less aggressive techniques for surgical treatment of varicose syndrome(4,5) the results show that this generalized attitude causes a fall in its effectiveness, creating a greater varicose recurrence and a fall in the clinic improvement symptomatology(6).The excellent results obtained on our sample group,after 10 years,79.8% in cases of essential varicose syndrome and 67.6% in post-phlebitic syndrome, corroborates the advantage of our method of treatment.

The systematic surgery that we propose is the removal of the insufficient saphenous vein with ligature of communicating veins and extensive varicectomy by multiple incisions.

When an ulcer or indurated area is presented, a wide resection is performed including the surrounding tissue up to the dermic areas not affected by the venous stasis and penetrating up to the dermic areas not affected by the venous stasis and up to the muscular fascia ligating the insufficient perforated veins.

Plastic reconstruction is performed by free skin graft one to three months after initial surgery.At this point it must be remarked that a good aesthetic result can only be achieved by obtaining an adequate area for implantation of the skin graft, waiting for the tisular granulation to now to the surrounding skin level and ensuring complete freedom from infection.The sclerotherapy plays a complementary role on small superficial varicosities and on the recurrence of varicose veins.

The results obtained with this procedure has reassured for us that the approach of radicality in surgical treatment of varicose syndrome in the lower leg obtains the best long-term results.

References

1.-Beaglehole R.
Epidemiology of varicose veins
W.J.Surg.1986;10:898-902

2.-Burnham J.St.
Varicose veins: patient seletion and treatment.
In:Vascular Surgery.RutherfordR.B.Saunders Co.
Philadelphia.1989.pp 1512-1517.

3.-Vin.F. et Schadeck. M.
La maladie veineuse superficielle.
Ed. Masson.Paris 1991.pp.140-195.

4.-Francesci.Cl.
Teorie et practique de la cure C.H.I.V.A.
Ed. L´armmancon.Precy-souse-Thil.1988.

5.-Masson J.L.
Methode Carsena.Erradication ambulatoire des varices.
Ed Solal.Marseille.1991.

6.-Darke.G.S.
Recurrent varicose veins and shortsaphenous
insufficiency evaluation and treatment.
In:Venous Disorders.J.J Bergan and J.S.T.Yao.Saunders Co.
Philadelphia 1991.pp 217-232.

INDICATIONS ET MODIFICATIONS DE L´OPERATION DE COCKETT DANS LE TRAITEMENT DE L´INSUFFISANCE VEINEUSE CHRONIQUE. *Dr. Ermenegildo Alejo Enrici **.

Cete opération est absolument indiquée dans l´insuffisance du Circuit Veineux Amortisseur.

L´opération subfaciale préconisée par le celébre chirurgien anglais en 1956 a été réglée de cette maniére par l´auteur de cette communication.

I. Il est important de realiser la coloration des vaisseaux lymphatiques au moyen d´une injection sub-cutanée interdijitale et périplantaire interne de "bleu patente" á 5% pour éviter leur lésion intra opératoire.

II. L´incision prend naissance au-dessus de la "perforante" directe supérieure interne. Elle borde l´hypodermie indurée et elle se dirige ensuite vers la zone rétromalléolaire interne et, en arrivant á l´angle inférieur du malléolaire, elle le contourne vers l´avant, jusqu´a le naissance de la saphéne interieure.

III. Section de peau cellulaire subcutanée et aponeurose en bloc sans essayer de disséquer les noeuds variqueux pour éviter des défauts de cicatrisation.

IV. Identification des vaisseaux tibiaux postérieurs depuis la lére á la 3éme perforante directe en effectuant les ligatures au ras du paquet.

V. Résection de l´arc anastomatique inférieur et de la 4eme perforante".

VI. S´il existe simultanément un syndróme d´hyper-postomie, ligatire et section des branches artérielles affectées.

VII. En soulevant la masse musculaire, ligature des "perforantes" directes externes.

VIII. S´il y a insuffisances profondes segmentaires, ligature et résection.

IX. Dans tous les cas, la fermeture se réalise sur deux plans, l´un aponeurotique et l´autre de la peau.

Dans le Servicio de Flebolgía y Linfología del Hospital Militar Central se realixent 346 operations Cckett dans 2 étapes: la premiére, dans la que se effectue la operation classique (109 cas) et la 2º avec la technique que dans c´est communication se preconise (237 cas).

Dans le premier grupe Eut a niveau submalelar un 15,59 % de recidives (eczema et/out ulcere) contre 0 complicatins dans la 2º grupe dans le que se ajouté la resection de l´arc anatomique inferieur et la 4º perforant. En plus, dans c´est groupe, fisent mieux l´oedeme post-operatire (11,07 %) disparu (84,92 %) et reste le meme (4 %).

Dans le follow up de dix ans se apprecie l´apparition des varices residuares dans un (19,36 %) dans tous les cas furont traité avec solerotérapie.

C´est imprudent la complementation du crirugie subfaciale physiologique avec operations plastique que augmenterent l´oedeme post-operatoire dans l´estaditique d´une maniere signifacative. Il serait une agression directe contre le systeme lymphatique engendrant parfois une maladie plus mal que l´anterieur.

* Profesor Titular de Flebología y Linfología. Universidad Católica Argentina. Aramburu 352, Martinez, Provincia de Buenos Aires, Argentina. Te: 798-5613.-

CLASIFICATION CLINIQUE ÉVOLUTIVE DE L´INSUFFISANCE VEINEUSE CHRONIQUE ET LA RELATION AVEC LA THÉRAPEUTIQUE CHIRURGICALE. *Dr. Ermenegildo Alejo Enrici, Buenos Aires, Argentina *.-*

L´auteur de cette communication propose une classification dans lequelle se classent chonologiquement les divers etats cliniques que cette maladie peut présenter, lesquels marquent des regles thérapeutiques fondamentades.

I. *Sindrome post thrombonaire récent.*

Il commencence au moment méme oú s´installe la thrombose et finit avec la recanalisation du SVP. Le signe fondememtal est l´oedéme dont l´emplacement indique en géneral le lieu de l´obstruction. La thérapeutique s´adresse á la thrombose (anticoagulants - fibrinoli - tiques out thrombectomie plus une contension élastique externe suivant le stade de la maladie).

II. *Hyperthophie compensatrice de la bombe musculo - veineuse.*

Elle commence par la recanalization de la S.V.P. l´oedéme disparáint et on observe une augmentation de volume de la jámbe produit par l´effort que réalise le membre pour comperser l´hyperténsión veineuse profonde créée devant la lesion valvulo -pariétale que laisse la recanalisation post thrombonaire. Elle peut s´acompagner on non d´insuffisance perforante et superficielle produit du "blow out".

L´auteur considére que c´est le moment idéal pour propose unne chirurgie veineuse profonde quand l´organisme est capable de produire des baisses de tension compatibles avec une vie normale, surtout quand il s´agit de jeunes.

III. *Insuffisance veineuse chonique avancée.*

Cette étape se caractérise par l´apparition de deux grands indices symptomatiques -l´hypodermie indurée et l´oedéme. La chirugie sur le systéme perforant est absolument nécessaire pour couper les reflux trasversanx et, á partir de celle ci, il est nécessáire d´agir sur le systéme veineux profond.

IV. *Syndróme phlébo - arthrosique.*

Dans sa progression, la maladie a envahi les articulations produisant une rigidite da la regíon du tibia el de l´astragale qui annube le mécanisme de bombe soléaire -jumeau-. L´hypertension veineuse profonde devient permanente et il n´existe aucune solution clirugicale si, auparavent, on ne récupere pas ce mecanisme.

V. *Lymphoedeme posthrombonaire.*

Le plus grave de tous et d´une solution plus difficile. A partir de la lésion du S.V.P. il s´établit un oedéme permanent au flux important et bas en protéines. Les infections répétées qui trouvent dans ce cas un bouillon de culture propice,ajoutent á la lésion initiale l´obliteratión lymphatique chronique qui assombrit le pronostic vu qu´il n´y a actuellment aucune thépeutique adéquate pour sa récuperation.

Sur le total de les interventions realizes par le Servicio de Flebología y Linfología del Hospital Militar Central, Buenos Aires, Argentina, dans dix ans, l´insuffisance veineuse chronique les memes s´indiquent:

1º) Sindrome post thrombonaire récent, c´est exclusif de traitament médique.

2º) Sindrome d´hypertrophie compensatrice de la bombe VMA: 31 patients les indications chirurgicales furent,

a) 1 operation de Palma,

b) 1 operation de May Husni avec distel temporaire,fistula(FVA)

c) 1 Saphectomie interne, ligature de perforants FVA distel temporaire,

d) 27 cas, saphenectomie interne, ligature échelonnais et résection de trajet variqueux,

e) 1 operation de Cockett avec saphenectomie interne.

3º) Insuffisance veineuse chronique avancée, 439 operations de ligature subfaciale perforante (Cockett o Linton modifiqué) 12 complementé avec chirugie sur le SVP.

4º) Sindrome phlebo-arthrosique: 18 cas; 15 rétrograderent a l´étape anterieur kinesioterapie et aprés furent soumis a chirurgie sur le systeme perforant.

5º)Lymphoedeme posthrombonaire, 5 cas operé avec techniques Thompson. Dans c´est pathologie, les résultes ne furent pas satisfactoires.

L'effet hémodynamique au niveau poplitee de l'élastocompression exerce avec des bas élastiques dans les différents degrés de l'insuffisance veineuse chronique

Eugenio-O. Brizzio, Carmen Juan-Salvia

Laboratorio vascular periferico, Buenos Aires, Argentina

Les variations hémodynamiques dues à l'effet de la élastocompression ont été étudiées avec le Doppler dynamique et l'écho-Doppler couleur.

Les résultats obtenus pendant la marche ont été comparés entre les malades porteurs d'une élastocompression et chaussures adéquates, et malades avec une compression et chaussures inadéquates.

Cette étude a comme but d'évaluer l'effet négatif de la compression et chaussures inadéquates.

Phlébologie 92. Eds P. Raymond-Martimbeau, R. Prescott, M. Zummo.
John Libbey Eurotext, Paris © 1992, pp. 1399

Reduction of the dermal space in patients with dermato- and liposclerosis during the treatment of chronic venous insufficiency

H.A.M. Neumann

Department of Dermatology, University Hospital Maastricht, P.O. Box 5800, 6202 AZ Maastricht, The Netherlands.

Dermato- et liposclerosis is a serious sign of chronic venous insufficiency. It reflects disfunction of the microcirculation due to increased pressure at the venous side of the capillaries. Different plasma proteins leak out of the capillaries and induce a immunologic inflammatory process. Collagen I and III synthesis is increased. Skinbiopsies show a compact dermal collagen. The total dermal space is thicker than that of the surrounding normal looking skin.

In two studies we measured the mean dermal thickness before and after treatment.

Group I (12 patients) untreated patients with severe chronic venous insufficiency and dermato- et liposclerosis where treated for 2 months by compression bandage. Dermal thickness reduced from 2.8 to 1.4 mm.

Group II (10 patients) with dermato- et liposclerosis, who where well compensated for chronic venous insufficiency with compression hosiery are treated for 6 months with the anabolic steroid Stanozolol. Dermal space reduced from 1.6 to 1.3 mm.

Reduction of dermal space during treatment occurs partly by reduction of edema. On the other hand collagen synthesis can be influenced by steroids as Stanozolol for which the fibroblasts have a receptor. Longterm treatment of dermato- et liposclerosis leads to a normalization of the dermal collagen compartment.

Ultrasonographic Detection and the Role of the Perforating Veins in Primary Varicose Veins

Kenichi Koyano MD and Shukichi Sakaguchi MD
Hamamatsu University School of Medicine, JAPAN

In one hundred and nineteen limbs of eighty patients with primary varicose veins, ultrasonographic detection of the perforating veins was attempted to evaluate the diagnostic sensitivity and to elucidate the role of the perforating veins in primary varicose veins.
The positive predictive value of the ultrasonography for detecting the localization of the perforating veins was 89.8%. As previously reported we classified varicosities of the long saphenous vein into several types. Type I:reverse flow is revealed in the entire saphenous trunk from the saphenofemoral junction to the ankle. Type II:the reverse flow of the saphenous trunk is localized until the upper part of the lower leg. Type III,IV:the reverse flow is observed only in the thigh. The incidence of incompetent Cockett's perforators confirmed intraoperatively by Turner Warwick's test was significantly($P<0.05$) higher in Type I(52.6%) than in Type II(30.4%) and Type III,IV(18.2%). The results may suggest that the perforating veins act as drainage pathway at the bottom of the venous reflux and would become dilatated and incompetent with increase of the reverse flow.

Phlébologie 92. Eds P. Raymond-Martimbeau, R. Prescott, M. Zummo.
John Libbey Eurotext, Paris © 1992, pp. 1401-1403

Management of chronic venous insufficiency and its attendant complications in the aged

George M. Robb

501-625 5th avenue, New Westminster, B.C. V3M 1X4, Canada.

STUDY MATERIAL

For the purposes of this study the charts of 223 patients of eighty years of age and over, seen at this clinic over the past several years were reviewed. The average age in this group was 84.4 years. The reasons for attendance at the clinic are summarised as follows:

Arterial problems	69		
Venous problems	162	Most common complaint was of aching legs	
		Ankle swelling	42%
		Cellulitis	3%
		Ulceration	38%
		Bleeding	2%
		D.V.T.	1%
		Superf. thrombophlebitis	1%

Follow up was considered inadequate in 12%. Of the remainder the outcome of treatment was rated satisfactory in 73%.

COMPLICATIONS OF CHRONIC VENOUS INSUFFICIENCY

Oedema:

In these patients swelling of one or both ankles was the main complaint, and this interfered with the ability to walk or made management of the disabled patient more difficult. In all cases seen the swelling was thought to be venous in origin.When first seen the routine was to give small doses of furosemide by mouth - 20 mg. at 10 a.m. and at 2 p.m. daily. A tensor bandage with a medially placed sponge rubber pad was applied and the patient instructed to leave it undisturbed. After a week the situation was reviewed and the venous problems dealt with surgically in the early days with high ligation and multiple stripping with or without a fasciotomy type procedure, but later mainly by sclerotherapy. This was the most difficult group in which to achieve good results as the continuing cooperation of the patient in application of bandages or stockings was usually required, and for feeble patients this can be a major problem. Occasionally Lymphapress treatment also proved helpful in the management of the badly swollen leg.

Ulceration

Ulcers were treated initially by application of an occlusive pressure dressing. In some cases response was slow enough to warrant changing to a Viscopaste type bandage. Dressings were changed weekly or every two weeks. Coupled with this, sclerotherapy of the venous problem was undertaken, and every effort made to encourage the patient to increase walking as much as was reasonable. A few patients had to be hospitalised for skin grafting.

Cellulitis

A small number of patients presented with recurrent bouts of cellulitis. This was treated in the first instance by application of a medial pad and tensor bandage below the knee and institution of frequent short distance walks as soon as the pain allowed. This was then followed up by sclerotherapy of the offending varices.

Bleeding

This potentially serious problem has been seen more commonly in recent years than previously. The important point is that it requires immediate treatment, and this is most conveniently and probably best done by sclerotherapy. The veins that bleed are usually of the tiny "spider vein" variety and they yield better to sclerotherapy than to other forms of treatment. If one can find an underlying incompetent perforator or a large adjacent superficial varix, that can usually be treated in the same way. The application of local pressure is of course mandatory in the early phases of treatment. Bandaging is a dying art, it seems, and in this clinic bandages are applied by the staff rather than by outsiders.

Patient reviews

#A This spry old lady of 85 years of age attended complaining of the appearance of her legs and of some aching discomfort in the lateral leg region. These varices were treated by sclerotherapy and a satisfactory result achieved.

#BIRM This 80 year old lady was seen complaining of recurrent bouts of cellulitis in both legs. She was treated by bilateral high ligation and multiple stripping with right fasciotomy. Her recovery from this was uneventful and she had no further problems.

#B 82 year old male complaining of severe swelling of both legs. Very limited mobility led to inadequacy of the calf muscle pump action. This was managed mainly by elevation of both legs whenever possible and administration of furosemide. Attempts were also made to promote active movement but these did not meet with much success. These measures along with the use of elastic stockings led to a considerable improvement in the condition.

#NORG A 95 year old female presenting with ulceration in the lateral aspect of her right ankle. This was treated by occlusive pressure dressing and sclerotherapy of the offending varices. Healing of the ulcer was achieved.

SUMMARY

Age is not a barrier to effective treatment. With modern techniques it is possible to help most of the problems encountered in chronic venous insufficiency in old age with very satisfactory results. The thing to be avoided is a low expectation of improvement. Aged patients often need to have adequate help in the home situation to enable them to wear bandages or stockings as prescribed.

THE EFFICAY OF BUFLOMEDIL CHLORIDRATE IN PATIENTS AFFECTED BY CHRONIC VENOUS INSUFFICIENCY IN LOWER LIMBS: DOPPLER C.W. AND R.L.R. STUDY.

A.Grasso, C.Costanzo, O.F.Cormaci, C.Monachino, S.Romeo.

Cattedra e Scuola di Specializzazione in Chirurgia Vascolare
Direttore Prof. S.Romeo - Universita' degli Studi di Catania

Buflomedil chloridrate is a vasoactive drug. It is utilized in the treatment of A.O.C.P. because of its important effects on smooth muscular tunic of little vessels. This is essential to determine a microvascular circulation flow increase both in arterial and in venous district.

The authors evaluated these pharmacological effects in a group of 30 patients affected by chronic venous insufficiency of lower limbs. Drug somministration (Loftyl) was taken on during 60 days, with a dosage of 600 mg daily.

The authors evaluated also all subjective symptoms (heaviness, burn, nocturnal cramp, oedema) and some instrumental parameters: venous pressure by doppler velocimetry, venous repletion time (To) by R.L.R.. 65% of patients had a reduction of subjective sintomatology, especially about heaviness and nocturnal cramps.

Modifications of instrumental recording was significative in 58% of patients with doppler velocimetry and in 70% with R.L.R.

So the authors think that this drug may be utilized with great efficacy in the treatment of phlebopaties thanks to its strong therapeutic effect on microcirculation. An increased flow at this level takes to a reduction of stasis in venular district and, consequently, a reduction of stasis and venous pressure.

Phlébologie 92. Eds P. Raymond-Martimbeau, R. Prescott, M. Zummo.
John Libbey Eurotext, Paris © 1992, pp. 1405-1408

Adequate therapy of chronic venous insufficiency in patients with arterial occlusive disease

M. Emter, C. Shaper, K. Alexander

Medizinische Hochschule Hannover, Abteilung Angiologie, Karl-Weichert-Allee, D 3000 Hannover 61, Germany.

Incidence of venous insufficiency (cvi) in coincidence with arterial occlusive disease (paod) is discribed in literature from 10,0% to 15,8% in all angiological patients (4,5,6).
Therapy in venous insufficiency is to lower the venous hypertension in the extremity to have less edema-filtration (2). This mainly is reached by compression which reduces the venous cross-section, the venous volume in the leg and forces the blood-flow back to the heart (1,7). In contrary to that therapy of arterial occlusive disease is up to better the transmural pressure by a vasodilatation.
It is a great therapeutical problem if healing of a venous ulcer cannot take place because a compression-therapy would lower the arterial blood-flow so that a decompensation of the arterial occlusive disease would happen (3). This decompensation of the arterial component must be avoided.

In a study investigations were done on 42 healthy volunteers without arterial or venous defects (20 females, 22 males; 23 years to 53 years) and 22 patients with a arterial occlusive disease (IIb f. Fontaine; 8 females, 14 males; 53 years to 74 years). None of the patients had a diabetes mellitus or a endangiitis obliterans. In 16 patients a postthrombotic syndrome and in 6 patients severe varicose veins caused a venous insufficiency.
Each patient got a complete arterial and venous investigation; for testing what a compression therapy induces in a leg with arterial occlusive disease Ultrasound-Doppler for the arterial occlusive pressure (A. tib. post) was used as well as the maximal walking distance (ergometric : 3 km/h , 5% climax).
Transcutaneous measured oxygen pressure was got on the dorsum pedis. The test included measurement without compression, with compression-stockings class I, II, III and a compression - bandage, in each case in lying and standing position and during walking.

Results: It could be shown that during walking in healthy volunteers compression induced a decrease of arterial occlusive pressure related to the strength of compression and no decrease of tcPO2. All healthy volunteers still were in a "normal region" with a compression therapy.
In patients with paod it could be shown that arterial occlusive pressure was only reduced significantly by very strong compression (class III and bandages). TcPO2 is "tolerable" reduced by class I and II (significant), seriously by strong compression (class III and bandages)(significant).
But in none of the patients a reduction of his walking distance because of a compression (even with class III) took place.
The results showed that during lying compression should not be used in patients with paod. While standing and walking it should be tested wether an adequate compression would have a negative effect.
Compression therapy should not principally looked at contraindicated in patients with arterial occlusive disease especially because of the consequences of the venous insufficiency.

References

1) Bollinger, A.A. (1980) : Flußgeschwindigkeit in der Vena saphena und in der Vena femoralis mit und ohne Kompressionsverbände, SWISS med 2 , 61

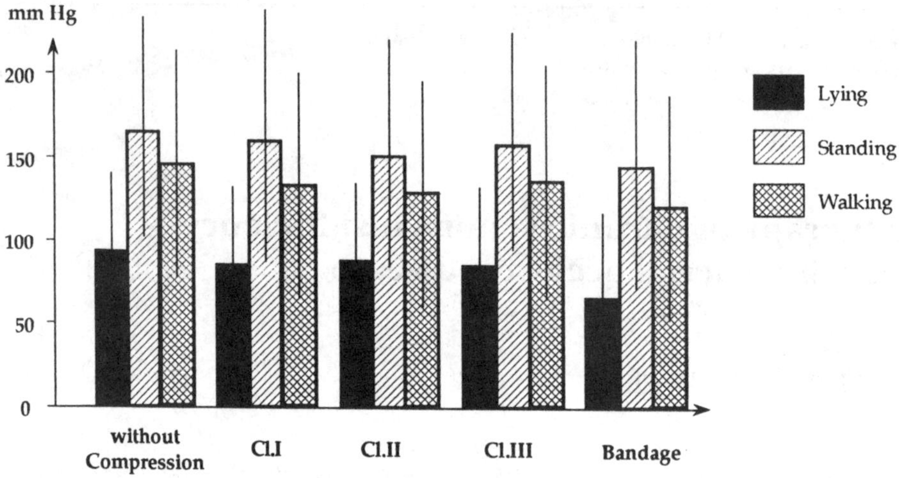

Arterial Occlusive Pressure of the A. tibialis post. during Lying, Standing and Walking in Patients with Arterial Occlusive Disease (n = 22) (IIb Fontaine) and Chronic Venous Insufficiency with Various Compréssion Therapies

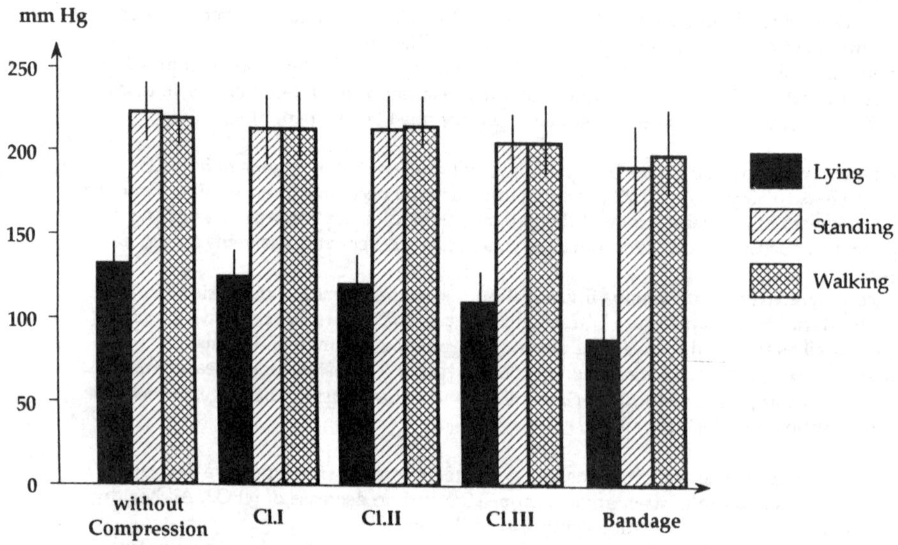

Arterial Occlusive Pressure of the A. tibialis post. during Lying, Standing and Walking in Healthy Volunteers (n = 42) with Various Compression Therapies

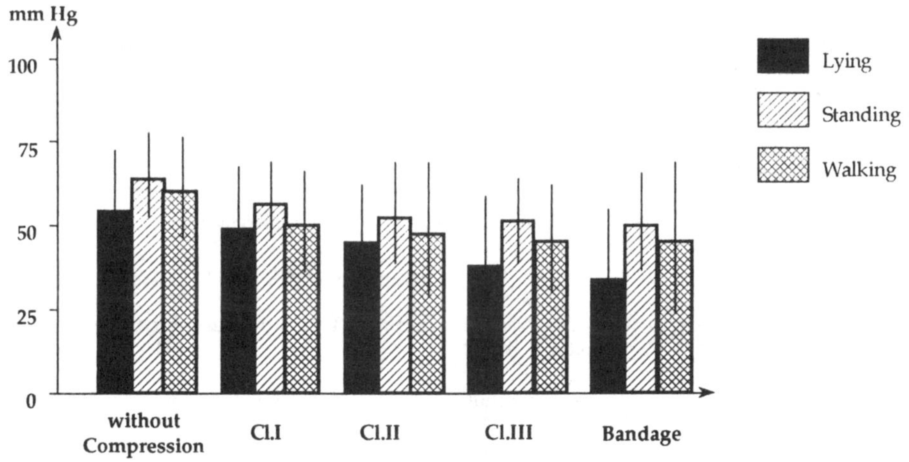

TcPO2 at the Forefoot During Lying, Standing and Walking in Patients with Arterial Occlusive Disease (n = 22) (IIb Fontaine) and Chronic Venous Insufficiency with Various Compression Therapies

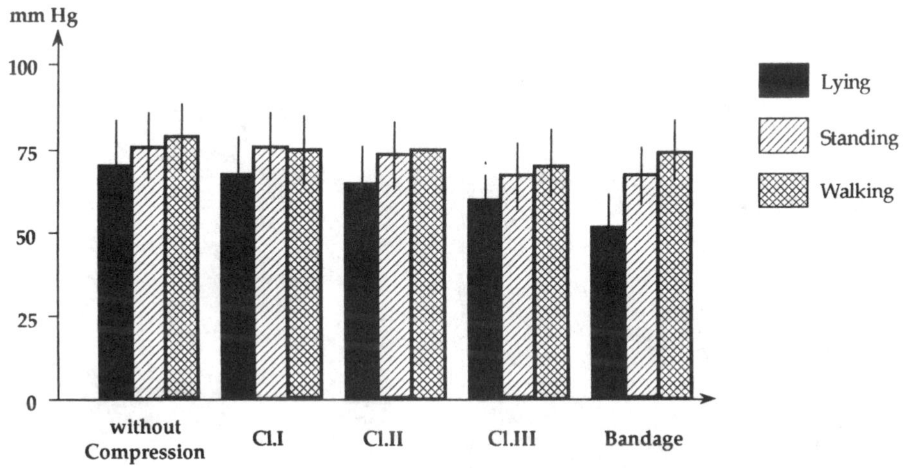

TcPO2 at the Forefoot during Lying, Standing and Walking in Healthy Volunteers (n = 42) with Various Compression Therapies

2) Emter, M., Pretschner, D.P., Hundeshagen, H., Alexander,K. (1987): Determination of Changes in the Intravascular and Extravascular Compartment in the Leg - The Engymetric Double Radionuclide Method-, Nuclear Medicine (New Trends and Possibilities in Nuclear Medicine), ed. H.A.E. Schmidt and L. Czernay, Schattauer Verlag ,265-269
3) Emter, M., Schaper, C., Alexander, (1990), Koinzidenz von arterieller Verschlußkrankheit und chronischer Veneninsuffizienz -ein therapeutisches Problem-, Phlebol. Proktol. 19, 215 -22
4) Fäs, J. (1973): Zur Frage der arteriosklerotischen Venopathie, Schweiz.Med.Wochenschr. 103 : 1189 - 1191
5) Großmann, K. Heerklotz, I., Basche, S. (1984) : Über die Kombination von arteriellen und venösen Gefäßkrankheiten, Z.ges.inn.Med. Jahrg. 39 Heft 4 : 59 - 63
6) Kappert, A. (1985) : Lehrbuch und Atlas der Angiologie, 11. Auflage Verlag Hans Huber, Bern, Stuttgart, Toronto
7) Partsch, H. (1978), Verbesserte Förderleistung der Wadenmuskelpumpe unter Kompressionsstrümpfen bei Varizen und venöser Insuffizienz, Phlebol.Proktol. 7 ,58 - 66

Authors address: Dr. Michael Emter, Medizinische Hochschule Hannover, Abteilung Angiologie, Karl-Wiechert-Allee, D 3000 Hannover 61, Germany

Phlébologie 92. Eds P. Raymond-Martimbeau, R. Prescott, M. Zummo.
John Libbey Eurotext, Paris © 1992, pp. 1409-1411

The Paratibial fasciotomy: a new method in the treatment of severe chronic venous congestion with recurring leg ulcers

R. Vanderpuye, R. Ritz-Schäfer, G. Salzmann, W. Hach

William Harvey-Klinik, Bad Nauheim, Germany

Since 1981 Hach's paratibial fasciotomy (PTF) is being increasingly used in the treatment of chronic-venous congestion with persisting ulcers, dermatolipofasciasclerosis and atrophie blanche. We now overlook more than 1550 successfull operations. In a retrospective study on 72 patients who underwent paratibial fasciotomy, we found a healing-quotient of 96% in respect to the leg ulcers.
The paratibial fasciotomy follows two principles :
The macrocirculation is improved by dissecting the perforating veins; the microcirculation, by severing the crural fascia. In our opinion this leads to improvement of tissue drainage in the compartment and to consecutive improvement of the oxygen diffusion.

PARATIBIAL FASCIOTOMY
- Indications -

- Persisting Ulcus cruris venosum
- Recurring Ulcus cruris venosum
- Atrophie Blanche
- Dermatoliposclerosis

Pic.1

Technically the operation is quite simple. Through a small skin incision on the inner side of the calf, proximal to the pathologically changed skin areas, the crural fascia is opened, the insufficient perforating veins are subfascialy, nonselectivly dissected and the crural fascia is split paratibialy over two thirds of the lower leg to the medial ankle. When leg-ulcers are present the paratibial fasciotomy is performed under perioperative antibiotic prophylaxis.

To avoid complications, such as damaging the posterior tibial artery, the saphenus nerve and the lymphatic system, a special set of instruments consisting of a blunt perforator-dissector and a protective fasciotom has been developed.

The improvement of the macro- and microcirculation is demonstrated in our prospective PaFas study, currently being conducted.
The haemodynamic parameters are measured by phlebodynamometry, photoplethysmography, venous occlusion plethysmography and transcutaneous oxygen-pressure measurements. After the operation these parameters react more noticably in cases of primary varicosis than in cases of postthrombotic syndrom. The drastic improvement of the microcirculation is demonstrated in the rise in transcutaneous oxygen-partial pressure (Pic 2)

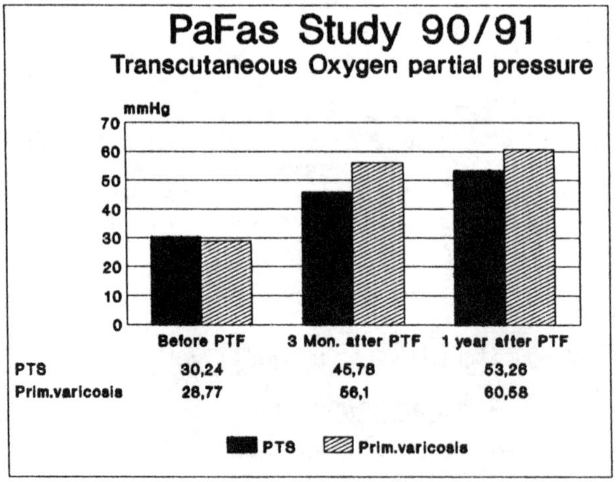

Pic.2

The healing rate of ulcers was found to be 96%, pain was eliminated in 85% and swelling of the lower-leg lessend in 65% of the patients who underwent Paratibial Fasciotomy.
In the treatment of chronic venous congestion the paratibial fasciotomy has brought a dramatic improvement of clinical symptoms through healing of the ulcers and reduction of pain.

The paratibial fasciotomy now offers for the first time the possibility for treating chronic venous congestive syndrome with an easy, low-risk, operation. It is still unclear whether the success can only be attributed to the dissection of the Cockett perforators alone or whether the incision of the fascia with the ensuing communication between the extrafascial and the intrafascial compartments has an additional effect on the microcirculation. Clinical results do speak in favour of this but final proof is still outstanding.

INDEX DES AUTEURS
Author index

Reproduction photomécanique
IMPRIMERIE QUAD PRINTING INC.
4555, Des Grandes Prairies (N° 65)
Montréal (Québec) Canada H1R 1A5

Août 1992
Imprimé au Canada